HAEMATOLOGICAL VALUES (CONTINUED

Analysis	Reference range SI units	Non-SI units
Differential white cell count		
Neutrophil granulocytes	2.0–7.5 x 10^9/l	2.0–7.5 x 10^3/mm^3
Lymphocytes	1.5–4.0 x 10^9/l	1.5–4.0 x 10^3/mm^3
Monocytes	0.2–0.8 x 10^9/l	0.2–0.8 x 10^3/mm^3
Eosinophil granulocytes	0.04–0.4 x 10^9/l	0.04–0.4 x 10^3/mm^3
Basophil granulocytes	0.01–0.1 x 10^9/l	0.01–0.1 x 10^3/mm^3
Mean cell haemoglobin (MCH)	27–32 pg	–
Mean cell volume (MCV)	78–98 fl	–
Packed cell volume (PCV) or haematocrit		
Male	0.40–0.54	–
Female	0.37–0.47	–
Platelets	150–350 x 10^9/l	150–350 x 10^3/mm^3
Red cell count		
Male	4.5–6.5 x 10^{12}/l	4.5–6.5 x 10^6/mm^3
Female	3.8–5.8 x 10^{12}/l	3.8–5.8 x 10^6/mm^3
Red cell lifespan		
Mean	120 days	–
Half-life (^{51}Cr)	25–35 days	–
Reticulocytes (adults)	25–85 x 10^9/l	25–85 x 10^3/mm^3
Transferrin	2.0–4.0 g/l	0.2–0.4 g/dl
Transferrin saturation		
Male	25–56%	–
Female	14–51%	–
Vitamin B$_{12}$	130–770 pg/ml	

Assistant Editors

Sunil Adwani BSc(Hons) M...
Specialty Registrar in General ...
Stirling, UK

J. Kenneth ...
Clinical Lect...
Pain M...

Jeh...
Specialist ...
Edinburgh, UK

Alan G. Japp ...
Specialty Registrar in Ca...
Edinburgh, UK

Nazir I. Lone MBChB M...
Specialist Registrar in Respiratory and ...
Northern Deanery, Newcastle-upon-Tyne, ...

Donald D. Noble MBChB MRCP
Specialist Registrar in Respiratory Medicine, Royal In...
Edinburgh, Edinburgh, UK

Sarah A. Walsh MB BCh BAO BMedSci MRCP
Specialist Registrar in Dermatology, Royal Infirmary of Edinburgh,
Edinburgh, UK

Consulting Editors

Nicki Colledge BSc FRCP(Ed)
Consultant Geriatrician, Liberton Hospital, Edinburgh and Royal
Infirmary of Edinburgh, Honorary Senior Lecturer in Geriatric
Medicine, University of Edinburgh, UK

Brian R. Walker BSc MD FRCP(Ed)
Professor of Endocrinology, University of Edinburgh, UK

A Davidson Title

Davidson's Essentials of Medicine

Edited by

J. Alastair Innes
PhD FRCP(Ed)
Consultant Physician
and Honorary Reader
in Respiratory Medicine
Western General Hospital,
Edinburgh, UK

CHURCHILL LIVINGSTONE
ELSEVIER

Edinburgh London New York Oxford Philadelphia St Louis Sydney Toronto 2009

CHURCHILL
LIVINGSTONE
ELSEVIER

First published 2009

ISBN: 9780702030017 Main edition
ISBN: 9780702030000 International edition

British Library Cataloguing in Publication Data
A catalogue record for this book is available from the British Library

Library of Congress Cataloging in Publication Data
A catalog record for this book is available from the Library of Congress

Notice
Knowledge and best practice in this field are constantly changing. As new research and experience broaden our knowledge, changes in practice, treatment and drug therapy may become necessary or appropriate. Readers are advised to check the most current information provided (i) on procedures featured or (ii) by the manufacturer of each product to be administered, to verify the recommended dose or formula, the method and duration of administration, and contraindications. It is the responsibility of the practitioner, relying on their own experience and knowledge of the patient, to make diagnoses, to determine dosages and the best treatment for each individual patient, and to take all appropriate safety precautions. To the fullest extent of the law, neither the Publisher nor the Editors assume any liability for any injury and/or damage to persons or property arising out or related to any use of the material contained in this book.

The Publisher

Printed in China

The publisher's policy is to use paper manufactured from sustainable forests

For Elsevier
Commissioning Editor: Laurence Hunter
Development Editor: Clive Hewat
Project Manager: Nancy Arnott
Designer: Stewart Larking
Illustrator: Robert Britton
Illustration Manager: Bruce Hogarth

Contents

Sir Stanley Davidson
(1894–1981)

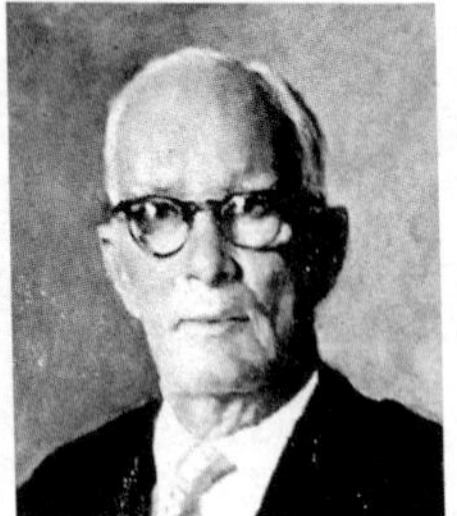

Davidson's Principles and Practice of Medicine was the brainchild of one of the great Professors of Medicine of the 20th century. Stanley Davidson was born in Sri Lanka and began his medical undergraduate training at Trinity College, Cambridge; this was interrupted by World War I and later resumed in Edinburgh. He was seriously wounded in battle, and the carnage and shocking waste of young life that he encountered had a profound effect on his subsequent attitudes and values.

In 1930 Stanley Davidson was appointed Professor of Medicine at the University of Aberdeen, one of the first full-time Chairs of Medicine anywhere and the first in Scotland. In 1938, he took up the Chair of Medicine at Edinburgh and was to remain in this post until retirement in 1959. He was a renowned educator and a particularly gifted teacher at the bedside, where he taught that everything had to be questioned and explained. He gave most of the systematic lectures in Medicine himself, which were made available as typewritten notes that emphasised the essentials and far surpassed any textbook available at the time.

Principles and Practice of Medicine was conceived in the late 1940s with its origins in those lecture notes. The First Edition was a masterpiece of clarity and uniformity of style. It was of modest size and price, but sufficiently comprehensive and up to date to provide students with the main elements of sound medical practice. More than half a century after its first publication, his book continues to inform and educate students, doctors and health professionals all over the world, and is the basis from which *Davidson's Essentials of Medicine* has been derived.

Portrait reproduced by courtesy of the Royal College of Physicians of Edinburgh.

Preface

In the 56 years since *Davidson's Principles and Practice of Medicine* was first published, the rapid growth in the understanding of pathophysiology, in the variety of available diagnostic tests and in the range of possible treatments has posed an increasing challenge to those seeking to summarise clinical medicine in a single textbook. An inevitable consequence has been a parallel growth in the physical size of all the major textbooks, including *Davidson*. This First Edition of *Davidson's Essentials of Medicine* seeks to complement the parent volume by helping those who also need portable information to study on the move—whether commuting, travelling between training sites and during remote attachments and electives.

For the first time, the core content from *Davidson* 20th Edition has been updated and condensed to a size which can easily accompany readers on their travels. Although the text is concise, every effort has been made to maximise the readability and to avoid dry and unmemorable lists; the intention has been to produce a genuine miniature textbook. The text draws directly on the enormous depth and breadth of experience of the parent *Davidson* writing team and presents the essential elements in a format to suit hand luggage. Key *Davidson* illustrations have been adapted and retained, and several new 'added value' sections have been included. A chapter on Interpreting Key Investigations introduces the reader to the key diagnostic tests; examples of typical OSCE scenarios are illustrated to prepare the reader for this ubiquitous examination format; and a chapter on Therapeutics describes the typical clinical use of the major drug groups.

In an age when on-line information is ever more accessible to doctors in training, most still agree that there is no substitute for the physical page when systematic study is needed. With this book, we hope that the proven value of the parent *Davidson* can be augmented by making the essential elements accessible while on the move.

First Editions are always written in a spirit of optimism, yet with the realisation that the enterprise is at best a judgement of the readers' needs. As such, your feedback and suggestions for improvement would be most welcome and valued.

J.A.I.
Edinburgh 2009

Acknowledgements

I am very grateful to Nicki Colledge and Brian Walker for their invaluable help and guidance in the early stages of the project, to my enthusiastic team of chapter editors, and to the original Davidson's chapter authors without whom the project would not have been possible. Thanks also to Laurence Hunter, Clive Hewat and Wendy Lee at Elsevier for their constant support and meticulous attention to detail. Finally I would like to thank my family for their encouragement during the gestation of this book.

J.A.I.
Edinburgh 2009

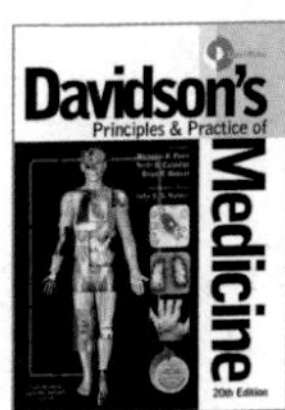

Contributors to *Davidson's Principles and Practice of Medicine*

The core of this book is based on the contents of *Davidson's Principles and Practice of Medicine*, with material extracted and re-edited to suit the format of this book. Although some chapters and topics have of necessity been cut or substantially edited, authors of all chapters drawn upon have been acknowledged here in recognition of their contribution to the parent textbook.

Chris Allen MA MD FRCP
Consultant Neurologist, Addenbrooke's Hospital, Cambridge, UK

Jeffrey K. Aronson MA MBChB DPhil FRCP FBPharmacolS FFPM(Hon)
Reader in Clinical Pharmacology, University of Oxford, UK; Honorary Consultant Physician, Oxford Radcliffe Hospitals Trust, Oxford, UK

Peter Bloomfield MD FRCP FACC
Consultant Cardiologist, Royal Infirmary of Edinburgh; Honorary Senior Lecturer, University of Edinburgh, UK

Nicholas A. Boon MD FRCP(Ed) FESC
Consultant Cardiologist, Royal Infirmary of Edinburgh; Honorary Reader, University of Edinburgh, UK

Andrew W. Bradbury BSc MBChB MD MBA FRCS(Ed)
Sampson Gamgee Professor of Vascular Surgery and Head of Educational Quality and Enhancement, College of Medical and Dental Sciences, University of Birmingham; Consultant Vascular and Endovascular Surgeon, Heart of England NHS Foundation Trust, UK

Leslie Burnett MB BS PhD FRCPA MAACB FHGSA
Director and Chief Executive, Pathology North, Royal North Shore Hospital, Sydney; Clinical Professor in Pathology, Northern Clinical School, University of Sydney; Adjunct Professor in Science and Technology, University of Technology, Sydney, Australia

Mark Byers MRCGP DA DipIMC
Lieutenant-Colonel, 3 Close Support Medical Regiment, Catterick Garrison, North Yorkshire, UK

Roger William Chapman BSc MD(Lond) FRCP(Lond)
Consultant Gastroenterologist/Hepatologist, John Radcliffe Hospital, Oxford; Honorary Senior Lecturer in Medicine, Oxford University Clinical Medical School, Oxford, UK

Nicki Colledge BSc FRCP(Ed)
Consultant Geriatrician, Liberton Hospital, Edinburgh and Royal Infirmary of Edinburgh; Honorary Senior Lecturer in Geriatric Medicine, University of Edinburgh, UK

Jane Collier MD FRCP
Consultant Hepatologist, John Radcliffe Hospital, Oxford, UK

Jenny I.O. Craig MD FRCP(Ed) FRCPath
Consultant Haematologist, Addenbrooke's Hospital, Cambridge, UK

Allan D. Cumming
MBChB MD FRCP(Ed) FRCP(Lond)
Director of Undergraduate Learning and Teaching and Professor of Medical Education, University of Edinburgh; Consultant Renal Physician, Royal Infirmary of Edinburgh, UK

Martin Dennis MD FRCP(Ed)
Professor of Stroke Medicine, University of Edinburgh, UK

Michael Doherty MA MD FRCP
Professor of Rheumatology, University of Nottingham; Consultant Rheumatologist, City Hospital, Nottingham, UK

Michael John Field MD BS BSc FRACP
Professor of Medicine, University of Sydney; Associate Dean and Head, Northern Clinical School, Royal North Shore Hospital of Sydney, Australia

Miles Fisher MD FRCP(Glas) FRCP(Ed)
Consultant Physician, Glasgow Royal Infirmary; Honorary Clinical Senior Lecturer, University of Glasgow, UK

Brian M. Frier
BSc(Hons) MD FRCP(Ed) FRCP(Glas)
Consultant Physician, Department of Diabetes, Royal Infirmary of Edinburgh; Honorary Professor of Diabetes, University of Edinburgh, UK

Jane Goddard PhD FRCP(Ed)
Consultant Nephrologist, Royal Infirmary of Edinburgh; Honorary Senior Lecturer, University of Edinburgh, UK

Ian S. Grant
FRCP(Ed) FRCP(Glas) FFARCSI
Consultant in Intensive Care Medicine and Anaesthesia, Western General Hospital, Edinburgh, UK

Neil Grubb MD MRCP
Consultant in Cardiac Electrophysiology, Royal Infirmary of Edinburgh; Honorary Senior Lecturer, University of Edinburgh, UK

Phil Hanlon MD FRCP FFPH MRCGP
Professor of Public Health, University of Glasgow, UK

Peter Clive Hayes MD PhD FRCP
Professor of Hepatology and Honorary Consultant Gastroenterologist, Scottish Liver Transplant Unit and Gastroenterology and Liver Unit, Royal Infirmary of Edinburgh, UK

J. Alastair Innes PhD FRCP(Ed)
Consultant Physician and Honorary Reader in Respiratory Medicine, Western General Hospital, Edinburgh, UK

George John MD FRACP FJFICM
Professor of Medicine, Christian Medical College, Vellore, Tamil Nadu, India

Alison L. Jones
BSc(Hons) MD FRCP(Ed) FRCP FiBiol
Professor of Medicine and Clinical Toxicology, School of Medicine and Public Health, University of Newcastle, Newcastle, Australia

Lakshman Karalliedde MBBS DA FRCA
Medical Toxicologist, Chemical Hazards and Poisons Division, Health Protection Agency; Visiting Senior Lecturer, King's College London, Department of Public Health Sciences, School of Medicine, London, UK

Peter C. Lanyon DM FRCP MRCGP
Consultant Rheumatologist, University Hospital, Queen's Medical Centre, Nottingham, UK

Diana N.J. Lockwood BSc MD FRCP
Professor of Tropical Medicine, London School of Hygiene and Tropical Medicine; Consultant Physician and Leprologist, Hospital for Tropical Diseases, London, UK

Christopher A. Ludlam
MBChB BSc PhD FRCP FRCPath
Professor of Haematology and Coagulation Medicine, University of Edinburgh; Director, Haemophilia and Thrombosis Centre, Royal Infirmary of Edinburgh, UK

Christian J. Lueck
PhD FRCP FRCP(Ed) FRACP
Head, Department of Neurology, Canberra Hospital; Associate Professor, Australian National University Medical School, Canberra, Australia

D.B.L. McClelland
PhD(Leiden) FRCP FRCPath
Consultant, Scottish National Blood Transfusion Service, Edinburgh, UK

Sara Marshall
MRCP(Eire) FRCPath(UK) PhD
Professor of Clinical Immunology, University of Dundee, UK

David E. Newby PhD DM FRCP
Professor of Cardiology, University of Edinburgh, UK

David Richard Oxenham
FRCP(Ed) FAChPM
Medical Director, Marie Curie Hospice, Edinburgh; Honorary Senior Lecturer, University of Edinburgh, UK

Kelvin R. Palmer MD FRCP(Ed)
FRCP(Lond) FRCS(Ed)
Consultant Gastroenterologist, Western General Hospital, Edinburgh, UK

Simon Paterson-Brown MS MPhil FRCS
Consultant General and Upper Gastrointestinal Surgeon, Royal Infirmary of Edinburgh; Honorary Senior Lecturer, University of Edinburgh, UK

Ian D. Penman MD FRCP(Ed)
Consultant Gastroenterologist, Western General Hospital, Edinburgh; Part-time Senior Lecturer, University of Edinburgh, UK

Stephen Potts MA FRCPsych
Consultant Liaison Psychiatrist, Royal Infirmary of Edinburgh; Honorary Senior Clinical Lecturer, University of Edinburgh, UK

Stuart H. Ralston MD FRCP FMedSci FRSE
ARC Professor of Rheumatology, University of Edinburgh; Honorary Consultant Rheumatologist, NHS Lothian, Edinburgh, UK

Jonathan L. Rees
BMedSci FRCP FRCP(Ed) FMedSci
Grant Chair of Dermatology, University of Edinburgh; Honorary Consultant, Lothian Health, University Hospitals Division, Edinburgh, UK

Peter T. Reid MD FRCP(Ed)
Consultant Physician and Honorary Senior Lecturer in Respiratory Medicine, Western General Hospital, Edinburgh, UK

Olivia M.V. Schofield FRCP(Ed)
Consultant Dermatologist, Royal Infirmary of Edinburgh, UK

Gordon R. Scott BSc FRCP
Consultant in Genitourinary Medicine and Honorary Senior Lecturer, University of Edinburgh, UK

Michael C. Sharpe
MA MD FRCP FRCP(Ed) FRCPsych
Professor of Psychological Medicine and Symptoms Research, University of Edinburgh, UK

Laurence H. Stewart
MD FRCS(Ed) FRCS(Urol)
Consultant Urological Surgeon, Western General Hospital, Edinburgh, UK

Peter Stewart FRACP FRCPA MBA
Clinical Director, Sydney South West Pathology Service; Associate Professor of Biochemistry, University of Sydney, Australia

Mark W.J. Strachan
BSc(Hons) MD FRCP(Ed)
Consultant Physician, Western General Hospital, Edinburgh; Part-time Senior Lecturer, University of Edinburgh, UK

David Richmond Sullivan FRACP FRCPA
Senior Staff Specialist, Royal Prince Alfred Hospital, Camperdown, New South Wales; Clinical Associate Professor, University of Sydney, Australia

Christopher B. Summerton
MA MD FRCP FRCP(Ed)
Consultant in Gastroenterology and General Medicine, Trafford Healthcare NHS Trust, Manchester, UK

Shyam Sundar
MD FRCP(Lond) FAMS FNA
Professor of Medicine, Institute of Medical Sciences, Banaras Hindu University, India

W.T. Andrew Todd
BSc FRCP FRCPS(Glas)
Consultant Physician, Lanarkshire Area Infectious Diseases Unit, Monklands Hospital, Airdrie; Honorary Senior Lecturer, University of Glasgow, UK

David F. Treacher MA FRCP
Consultant Physician in Intensive Care, Guy's and St Thomas' NHS Trust, London, UK

Neil Turner PhD FRCP
Professor of Nephrology, University of Edinburgh; Honorary Consultant Nephrologist, Royal Infirmary of Edinburgh, UK

Brian R. Walker BSc MD FRCP(Ed)
Professor of Endocrinology, University of Edinburgh, UK

Simon Walker MB BS(Lond) MA DM(Oxon)
Senior Lecturer and Honorary Consultant in Clinical Biochemistry, University of Edinburgh, UK

Ed Wilkins FRCP FRCPath
Consultant Physician in Infectious Diseases, North Manchester General Hospital, Manchester, UK

1

Good medical practice

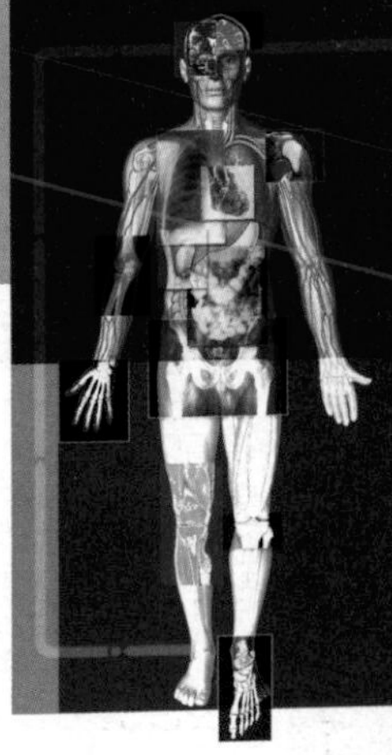

Patients (and doctors) differ in their beliefs, attitudes and expectations. Good medical practice requires the ability to recognise and respect these individual differences. This chapter describes how to:

• Provide patients and their families with complex information. • Discuss management options. • Reach appropriate ethical decisions within resource constraints.

THE DOCTOR–PATIENT RELATIONSHIP

While some medical knowledge is based on clear evidence, much reflects wisdom and understanding passed down generations of doctors over hundreds of years. This wisdom is central to how doctors and patients interact; it demands respect, and if combined with compassion, fosters the development of trust.

The doctor–patient relationship is itself therapeutic; a successful consultation with a trusted practitioner will have benefits irrespective of other therapies. It is also dynamic, bilateral, and influenced by differing attitudes and beliefs. Patients with chronic diseases increasingly interact with a multidisciplinary team of health professionals. The doctor usually leads in determining the overall direction of care but must also:

• Guide the patient through the unfamiliar language and customs of clinical care. • Interpret and convey complex information. • Help patient and family to participate in decision-making.

Regulatory bodies seek to define the duties of a doctor (e.g. Box 1.1), and many medical schools require students to sign an ethical code based on such statements.

1.1 THE DUTIES OF A DOCTOR REGISTERED WITH THE UK GMC

- Make the care of your patient your first concern
- Treat every patient politely and considerately
- Respect the patient's dignity and privacy
- Listen to patients and respect their views
- Give patients information in a way they can understand
- Respect the rights of patients to be fully involved in decisions about their care
- Keep your professional knowledge and skills up to date
- Recognise the limits of your professional competence
- Be honest and trustworthy
- Respect and protect confidential information
- Make sure that your personal beliefs do not prejudice your patient's care
- Act quickly to protect patients from risk if you have good reason to believe that you or a colleague may not be fit to practise
- Avoid abusing your position as a doctor
- Work with colleagues in the ways that best serve patients' interests

CLINICAL AND COMMUNICATION SKILLS

Good communication is the single most important component of good practice. Failures in communication are common, and lead to poor health outcomes, strained working relations, dissatisfaction, anger and litigation among patients, their families and their carers. Some common barriers to good communication are listed in Box 1.2.

At the beginning of a consultation, patients commonly feel ill and apprehensive. Their distress will be enhanced and communication impaired if the clinician appears indifferent, unsympathetic or short of time. First impressions are critical; the patient must be put at ease by a friendly and culturally appropriate greeting, with the clinician remembering to look at the patient, *not* the notes. The clinician must ensure that patients feel that they are the centre of interest, and should start by outlining the contents and agreeing the objectives of the consultation.

The main aim of a consultation is to establish a factual account of the patient's illness. In addition the clinician must explore the patient's feelings, their interpretation of their symptoms, and their concerns and fears, before agreeing a plan. These goals will not be met unless clinicians demonstrate understanding and empathy, not merely sympathy, which rarely helps. Many patients have multiple concerns and will not discuss these if they sense the clinician is uninterested, or likely to dismiss their complaints as irrational or trivial.

Careful questioning and listening will usually yield a provisional diagnosis, establish rapport, and determine which investigations are appropriate. The clinician must allow the patient to describe the problems with appropri-

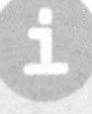

1.2 SOME BARRIERS TO GOOD COMMUNICATION IN HEALTH CARE	
The clinician	
• Authoritarian or dismissive attitude • Hurried approach • Use of jargon	• Inability to speak first language of patient • No experience of patient's cultural background
The patient	
• Anxiety • Reluctance to discuss sensitive or seemingly trivial issues • Misconceptions	• Conflicting sources of information • Cognitive impairment • Hearing/speech/visual impediment

ate, not leading or overbearing questions. Non-verbal communication is equally important. The patient's facial expressions and body language may betray hidden fears. The clinician can help the patient to talk more freely by smiling or nodding appropriately.

The doctor must always ensure that dignity is preserved and that the patient feels comfortable throughout the examination; this may entail the presence of a chaperone and always requires advance explanation of any examination.

INVESTIGATIONS

Modern medical practice is dominated by investigations. Judicious use of these is crucially dependent on good clinical skills. Indeed, a test should only be ordered if it is clear that the value of the result justifies the discomfort, risk and cost incurred. Clinicians should therefore draw up a provisional management plan before requesting any investigations.

THE 'NORMAL' RANGE

Although some tests provide qualitative results (present or absent), most provide a quantitative value. To classify quantitative resuts as normal or abnormal, it is necessary to define a 'normal range'. Many biological measurements exhibit a bell-shaped, 'normal distribution', described statistically by the mean value and the standard deviation (SD, which describes the spread of results). The 'normal range' is conventionally defined as the range which includes 95% of the population, i.e. two SDs above and below the mean. Results more than two SDs from the mean occur either because the person is one of the 2.5% of the normal population whose result is outside the normal range, or because their disease is affecting the test result.

In medicine, it is also important to define results which correlate with biological disadvantage. In some diseases, there is no overlap between results from the normal and abnormal population (e.g. creatinine in renal failure). In many diseases, however, there is overlap with the normal range (e.g. thyroxine in toxic multinodular goitre). The greater the difference between the test result and the normal range, the higher the chance that the person has a disease, but results within the normal range may be 'false negatives' and results outside the normal range may be 'false positives'. Similarly, when assessing quantitative risk factors, the clinical decision may not depend on whether or not the result is 'normal'. For example, higher total cholesterol is associated with a higher risk of myocardial infarction within the normal population, and cholesterol-lowering therapy may benefit people with values within the normal range. Similar arguments may apply for blood pressure, blood glucose, bone mineral density, etc.

Each test in a member of the normal population carries a 5% (1 in 20) chance of a result outside the 'normal range'. Indiscriminate repeat testing increases the chance of such 'abnormal' results and should be avoided.

Normal ranges defined either by test manufacturers or local laboratories are often established in small numbers of young healthy people who are not necessarily representative of the patient population.

If a substantial proportion of the normal population have an unrecordably low result (e.g. serum troponin), the distribution cannot be described by mean and SD. In these circumstances, results from normal and abnormal people are used to identify 'cut-off' values associated with a certain risk of disease.

SENSITIVITY AND SPECIFICITY

All diagnostic tests can produce false positives (an abnormal result in the absence of disease) and false negatives (a normal test in a patient with disease). The diagnostic accuracy of a test can be expressed in terms of its sensitivity and its specificity (Box 1.3). In interpreting results there is a trade-off between sensitivity and specificity. For example, defining an exercise ECG as abnormal if there is ≥0.5 mm ST depression ensures that very few cases of coronary disease are missed, but will generate many false positive tests. Conversely, a cut-off of ≥2.0 mm ST depression will detect most important coronary disease with far fewer false positive results.

1.3 THE ACCURACY OF DIAGNOSTIC TESTS

	Affected	Unaffected
Positive test	True +ve (a)	False +ve (b)
Negative test	False –ve (c)	True –ve (d)
Sensitivity (%) = a × 100/(a + c)		Specificity (%) = d × 100/(b + d)
Positive predictive value = a/(a + b)		Negative predictive value = d/(c + d)

PREDICTIVE VALUE

The value of a test is determined by the prevalence of the condition in the test population. Bayes' theorem allows the probability that a subject has a particular condition (the post-test probability) to be calculated if the pre-test probability and the sensitivity and specificity of the test are known. The positive predictive value (see Box 1.3) is the probability that a patient with a positive test has the condition. The negative predictive value is the probability that a patient with a negative test does not have the condition.

Thus the interpretation of a test is critically dependent on clinical context. For example, 2 mm ST elevation in ECG leads V_2 and V_3 is likely to represent myocardial infarction in a 54-yr-old Caucasian male with multiple risk factors and typical chest pain, but will probably be a normal variant in an asymptomatic 18-yr-old Afro-Caribbean man.

ESTIMATING AND COMMUNICATING RISK

Medical management decisions are usually made by balancing the anticipated benefits of a particular procedure or treatment against the potential risks. Providing relevant biomedical facts is seldom sufficient to communicate risk because a patient's perception of risk is often coloured by emotional, and sometimes irrational, factors. The clinician must recognise that patients receive information from multiple, potentially conflicting sources (e.g. internet, books, magazines, self-help groups, other health-care professionals, friends and family).

The next step in decision-making is to present the evidence base. Statistics and probabilities can be confusing and data can be presented in many ways (Box 1.4).

Relative risk describes the proportional increase in risk: a useful measure of the size of an effect. In contrast, absolute risk describes the actual

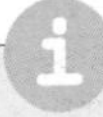

1.4 EXPLAINING THE RISKS AND BENEFITS OF THERAPY

Would you take a drug once a day for a year to prevent stroke if:

- it reduced your risk of having a stroke by 47%?
- it reduced your chance of suffering a stroke from 0.26% to 0.14%?
- there was 1 chance in 850 that it would prevent you from having a stroke?
- 849 out of 850 patients derived no benefit from the treatment?
- there was a 99.7% chance that you would not have a stroke anyway?

All these statements are derived from the same data* and describe an equivalent effect.

*MRC trial of treatment of mild hypertension (bendroflumethiazide vs placebo). BMJ 1985; 291:97–104.

chance of an event, and is what matters to most patients. Whenever possible, clinicians should quote numerical information using consistent denominators (e.g. '90 of every 100 patients who have this operation feel much better, 1 will die during the operation and 2 will suffer a stroke').

CLINICAL ETHICS

The four key principles of clinical ethics are often abbreviated to:
• Autonomy. • Beneficence. • Non-maleficence. • Justice.

RESPECT FOR PERSONS AND THEIR AUTONOMY

Patients seek a physician in order to prevent disability or disease from limiting their autonomy (the power or right of self-determination). The physician must therefore respect the patient's autonomy, including the right to refuse therapy, while empowering the patient with adequate information. Respect for autonomy has important implications for truth-telling, informed consent and confidentiality.

TRUTH-TELLING

Telling the truth is essential for doctor–patient trust. This includes providing information about the illness, prognosis and therapeutic alternatives, and answering questions honestly and with sensitivity to the patient's capacity to cope with bad news. There are two rare situations where the truth may sometimes be withheld:
• If it will cause real harm to patients (e.g. depressed patients likely to commit suicide if told they have cancer). • If patients make it clear that they do not want to hear the bad news (bearing in mind that this may be a stage in the patient's adjustment to the condition).

INFORMED CONSENT

To engage a patient in health-care decisions, the clinician must provide an adequate explanation, with details of the relevant risks, benefits and uncertainties of each option. The amount of information will depend on the patient's condition, the complexity of proposed treatment, and the physician's assessment of the patient's understanding. Legally and ethically, the patient retains the right to decide what is in his or her best interests. If patients make choices that seem irrational or are at variance with professional advice, that does not mean they lack capacity. In this context, capacity means the patient is able (with appropriate help) to understand the key information, consider the relevant options and communicate a decision.

When the patient does lack capacity, the clinician must always act in the patient's best interests.
• In an emergency, consent may be presumed for treatment that is immediately necessary to preserve life and health, provided there is no clear

evidence that this would be against the patient's previous wishes when competent (e.g. blood transfusion in an adult Jehovah's Witness). • If the patient has a legally entitled surrogate decision-maker, that person's consent should be sought wherever possible. • It is good practice to involve close relatives in decision-making, depending on local laws and culture.

CONFIDENTIALITY

Confidentiality concerning patient-specific information is important in maintaining trust between patients and doctors. Health-care teams must prevent unauthorised access to patient records, and may disclose information only when the patient has given consent or when required by law. Where such information is shared, it should be done on a strictly 'need-to-know' basis.

BENEFICENCE

This is the principle of doing good, or acting in another person's best interests. It means considering patients' views of their own best interests, as well as their medical best interests. If there is a conflict between what is good for the individual and what is best for society, the traditional approach is that 'The health of my patient will be my first consideration.'

NON-MALEFICENCE

This is the principle of doing no harm: *primum non nocere*.

JUSTICE

In order to distribute health resources justly, the concept of utility—'the greatest good for the greatest number'—must be considered. In the case of individual patients, however, justice is also equated with being 'fair' and 'even-handed'. Three perspectives apply:

Respect for the needs of the individual: Health care is given first to those who need it most.

Respect for the rights of a person: Everyone who needs health care is entitled to a fair share of the available resources.

Respect for merit: Health care is delivered on the basis of financial, political or social value judgements relating to the value of the individual to society. In the health-care setting these value judgements are difficult to make and to defend ethically.

COMPLEMENTARY AND ALTERNATIVE MEDICINE (CAM)

CAM refers to medical and health-care practices and products that are outside conventional medicine. It covers an enormous range of activities, from well-established physical therapies such as osteopathy to spiritual measures such as prayer specifically for health. Several complementary therapies (e.g. aromatherapy and massage) are inherently pleasurable, contributing to their therapeutic benefit. Proponents maintain that CAM focuses on the whole person as well as the physical complaints.

• 'Complementary medicine' describes the use of these treatments in conjunction with conventional medicine (e.g. acupuncture to reduce post-operative pain). • 'Alternative medicine' describes their use in place of conventional medicine (e.g. reflexology instead of anti-inflammatory drugs for arthritis). • 'Integrative medicine' describes the use of conventional therapy together with complementary therapies for which there is evidence of efficacy and safety.

EVIDENCE

In an era where evidence-based medicine is the norm, advocates of CAM are increasingly challenged to justify these treatments through independent, well-conducted, randomised controlled clinical trials. In some cases this may be difficult (e.g. the placebo arm of a double-blind trial of acupuncture). In addition, it may be argued that different types and standards of evidence, focusing on patient satisfaction and subjective benefit rather than measurable clinical outcomes, are more appropriate for CAM. The literature in this area is growing rapidly but, at present, only a small minority of CAM therapies are supported by evidence that would be acceptable for conventional medicine. Moreover, where evidence does exist, it is often limited to a small subset of the clinical conditions for which the treatment is used.

REGULATION

The 'big five' CAM therapies (homeopathy, osteopathy, chiropractic, acupuncture and herbal medicine) have professional regulatory frameworks in place; some others are following suit. Nevertheless, for many CAM therapies, there is no established structure of training, certification and accreditation, and practice is effectively open to all. Set against the demanding training and life-long continuous professional development required in conventional medicine, this constitutes an important barrier to integrative medicine.

2 Ageing and disease

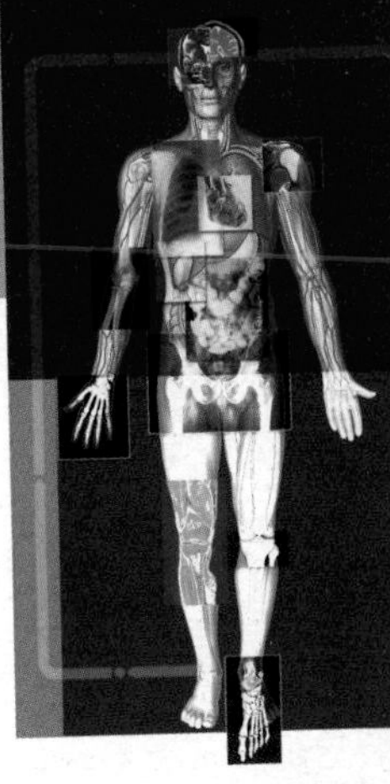

Over the last 100 years the proportion of people in the UK aged >65 yrs has risen from 5% to 16%, and is projected to increase steadily to 24% in 2061. This increase has been particularly apparent in people aged >85. Life expectancy in the developed world is now substantial, even in old age. Although the proportion of the population aged >65 is greater in developed countries, most older people live in the developing world. Two-thirds of the world population of people aged >65 live in developing countries at present, and this is projected to rise to 75% in 2025.

Geriatric medicine applies the knowledge and clinical skills of the organ-based specialties to a complex group: frail older people. This group is defined by the reduction in physiological capacity that makes them more susceptible to disease and mortality. As a result they frequently have multiple pathology, and illness often presents in atypical ways with confusion, falls, or loss of mobility and day-to-day functioning. Frail older people are also prone to adverse drug reactions, partly because of polypharmacy and partly because of age-related changes in responses to drugs and their elimination. Disability is common in old age but patients' function can often be improved by the interventions of the multidisciplinary team (Box 2.1), which includes nurses as well as physiotherapy, occupational and speech therapy, and medical staff.

COMPREHENSIVE GERIATRIC ASSESSMENT

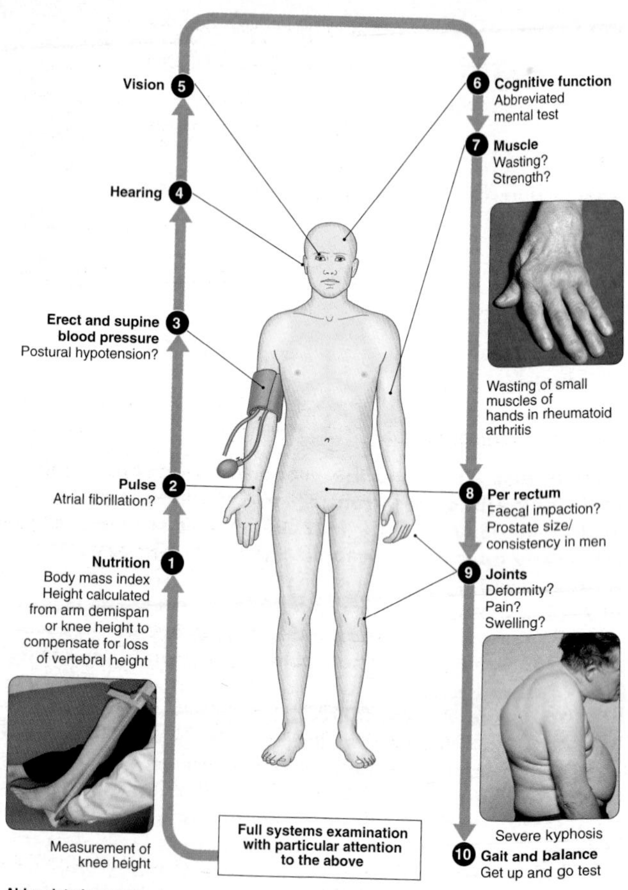

Wasting of small muscles of hands in rheumatoid arthritis

Measurement of knee height

Severe kyphosis

Abbreviated mental test

Each correct answer scores 1 mark

1 What time is it? (to the nearest hour)
2 What year is it
3 What is the name of this place/hospital?
4 How old are you? (exact year)
5 What is your date of birth

Please memorise the following address: 42 West Street

6 When did the First World War begin?
7 Who is the present monarch
8 Please count backwards from 20 down to 1
9 Can you recognise two people (e.g. relative or photograph)
10 Can you tell me the address I asked you to memorise a few minutes ago?

Mini Mental State Examination used for more deatiled assessmant

2.1 MULTIDISCIPLINARY TEAM (MDT) AND FUNCTIONAL ASSESSMENT	
Team member	**Activity assessed and promoted**
Physiotherapist	Mobility, balance and upper limb function
Occupational therapist	Activities of daily living, e.g. dressing, cooking; (assessment of home environment)
Dietitian	Nutrition
Speech and language therapist	Communication and swallowing
Social worker	Care needs
Nurse	Motivation and initiation of activities; feeding; continence

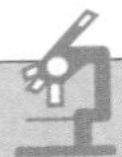

2.2 INVESTIGATIONS TO IDENTIFY ACUTE ILLNESS

- FBC
- U&Es, LFTs, calcium and glucose
- CXR
- ECG
- Urinalysis for leucocytes and nitrites; if positive, urine culture
- CRP: useful marker for occult infection
- Blood cultures if pyrexial

PRESENTING PROBLEMS

For the sake of clarity the common presenting problems are described individually here, but in real life, older patients often present with several at the same time, particularly confusion, incontinence and falls. These share some underlying causes and may precipitate each other.

The approach to most presenting problems in old age can be summarised as follows:

The telephone test: Find out the patient's usual status (e.g. mobility, cognitive state) from a relative or carer.

Check medication: Have there been any recent changes?

Search for and treat any acute illness: See Box 2.2.

Identify and reverse predisposing risk factors: These depend on the presenting problem.

FALLS

Falls and unsteadiness are very common in older people. Although only 10–15% of falls result in serious injury, they are the principal cause of fractured neck of femur in this age group. Falls also lead to loss of confidence and fear, and are frequently the 'final straw' that makes an older person decide to move to institutional care. The approach to the patient varies according to the underlying cause of falls, as follows.

Accidental trip

Those who have simply tripped may not require detailed assessment unless they are doing so frequently or have sustained an injury.

Blackouts

A proportion of older people who 'fall' have in fact had a syncopal episode. It is important to ask about loss of consciousness and, if this is a possibility, to perform appropriate investigations (pp. 211 and 617). Recent research suggests that in small numbers of patients, carotid sinus hypersensitivity (p. 212) may be the cause of otherwise unexplained falls.

Acute illness

Falling is one of the classical atypical presentations of acute illness in the frail. The reduced reserves in older people's integrative neurological function mean that they are less able to maintain their balance when challenged by an acute illness. Suspicion should be especially high when falls have occurred suddenly over a period of a few days. Common underlying illnesses include infection, stroke, metabolic disturbance and heart failure. Thorough examination and investigation are required to identify these (Box 2.2). It is also important to establish whether any drug has been started recently, as this may precipitate falls. Once an underlying acute illness has been treated, falls may no longer be a problem.

Multiple risk factors

Many patients, especially those with recurrent falls, are frail with multiple medical problems and chronic disabilities. Their tendency to fall is associated with risk factors that have been well established from prospective

2.3 RISK FACTORS FOR FALLS

- Muscle weakness
- History of falls
- Gait or balance abnormality
- Use of a walking aid
- Visual impairment
- Arthritis
- Impaired activities of daily living
- Depression
- Cognitive impairment
- Age >80 yrs
- Drugs
  - Polypharmacy (four or more drugs)
  - Digoxin
  - Diuretics
  - Drugs associated with sedation: benzodiazepines, phenothiazines, antidepressants
  - Type I anti-arrhythmics

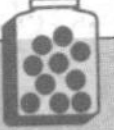

2.4 MULTIFACTORIAL INTERVENTIONS TO PREVENT FALLS

- Balance and exercise training
- Rationalisation of medication, especially sedative drugs
- Correction of visual impairment
- Home environmental hazard assessment and safety education
- Treatment of cardiovascular disorders, including carotid sinus hypersensitivity and postural hypotension

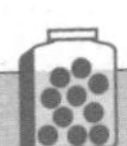

2.5 MANAGEMENT OF POSTURAL HYPOTENSION

- Correction of dehydration
- Tilting the head of the bed upwards
- Support stockings (older patients may struggle to get these on)
- NSAIDs (increase circulating volume due to salt and water retention; gastric side-effects limit use)
- Fludrocortisone (causes salt and water retention but poorly tolerated due to cardiac failure)

studies (Box 2.3). The annual risk of falling increases linearly with the number of risk factors present: from 8% with no risk factors to 78% in those with four or more. Obviously, such patients may present with a fall resulting from an acute illness or syncope as above, but they will remain at risk of further falls even when the acute illness has resolved.

It has been shown that an effective way of preventing further falls in this group is multiple risk factor intervention. Examples of such interventions are shown in Box 2.4 and require a multidisciplinary approach. The most effective is balance and exercise training by physiotherapists. Rationalising medication may help to reduce sedation, although many older patients are reluctant to stop their hypnotic. It will also help reduce postural hypotension, defined as a drop in BP of >20 mmHg systolic or >10 mmHg diastolic pressure on standing from supine. Other measures to reduce postural hypotension are shown in Box 2.5.

Bone protection

Osteoporosis prophylaxis should be considered in all older patients who have recurrent falls, particularly if they have already sustained a fracture. In female patients in institutional care, calcium and vitamin D_3 have been shown to reduce fracture rates and may also reduce falls due to improvements in muscle function.

ACUTE CONFUSION

The presentation, diagnosis and management of acute confusion are described on page 635. It is very important to establish the patient's usual cognitive function with a relative or carer, remembering that dementia is a risk factor for acute confusion so they may coexist. Almost any acute illness may present with confusion in old age, but the most common are infection and stroke. The recent addition of a drug is a further common precipitant. Predisposing factors include visual or hearing impairment, alcohol misuse and poor nutrition.

In addition to the investigations shown in Box 2.2, CT is indicated if there is a history of injury or focal neurological signs, and in those who fail to improve despite appropriate treatment. If confusion puts patients or others at risk, sedation with low-dose haloperidol or lorazepam may be required.

URINARY INCONTINENCE

Urinary incontinence is defined as the involuntary loss of urine, sufficiently severe to cause a social or hygiene problem. It occurs in all age groups but becomes more prevalent in old age. While age-dependent changes in the lower urinary tract predispose older people to incontinence, it is not an inevitable consequence of ageing and always requires investigation. Urinary incontinence is frequently precipitated by acute illness in old age and is commonly multifactorial (Box 2.6; see also p. 170).

POLYPHARMACY

Polypharmacy is defined as the inappropriate use of multiple drugs and is common in old age. Older people receive many more prescribed drugs than younger people and this is increasing in the UK. Even when appropriate—many cardiovascular conditions such as hypertension, myocardial infarction and heart failure dictate the use of several drugs—multiple drugs put older patients at increased risk of adverse drug reactions and interactions, falls and acute confusion. The clinical presentations of polypharmacy are extremely diverse, so for *any* presenting problem in old age the possibility that the patient's medication is a contributory factor should *always* be considered.

2.6 CAUSES OF TRANSIENT INCONTINENCE

- Restricted mobility
- Acute confusional state
- Urinary tract infection
- Severe constipation
- Drugs, e.g. diuretics, sedatives
- Hyperglycaemia
- Hypercalcaemia

DIZZINESS

Dizziness is very common, affecting at least 30% of those aged >65 yrs, according to community surveys. Acute dizziness is relatively straightforward and common causes include:

• Hypotension due to arrhythmia, acute myocardial infarction, gastrointestinal bleed or pulmonary embolism etc. • Acute posterior fossa stroke. • Vestibular neuronitis.

Older people, however, more commonly present with recurrent dizzy spells. They often find it difficult to describe the sensation they experience, so assessment can be very frustrating. Nevertheless, the most effective way of establishing the cause(s) of the problem is to determine which of the following is the predominant symptom, even if more than one is often present:

• Lightheadedness suggestive of presyncope. • Vertigo suggestive of labyrinthine or brain-stem disease. • Unsteadiness/poor balance suggestive of joint or neurological disease.

Investigation can then be focused on the specific symptom. For example, a 24-hr ambulatory ECG may be helpful in some patients with presyncope, but not in those with vertigo or unsteadiness. The most common underlying diagnoses in this age group include:

• Cerebrovascular disease, either stroke or small-vessel disease, which may cause unsteadiness and/or lightheadedness. • Degenerative joint disease, especially of weight-bearing joints and cervical spine. • Hypotensive medication, which often also exacerbates postural hypotension. • Benign paroxysmal positional vertigo (p. 619).

Most symptoms are provoked by activity, although if a patient is experiencing symptoms at rest, arrhythmia should be excluded. Anxiety and poor vision are frequent concomitants of dizziness in old age but are rarely the only cause. If the patient is falling as a result of dizziness, the interventions for falls described above should be applied.

HYPOTHERMIA

Hypothermia occurs when the body's core temperature falls below 35°C. The very young are susceptible because they have poor thermoregulation and a high body surface area to weight ratio, but the elderly are at highest risk.

Clinical assessment

Diagnosis is dependent on recognition of the environmental circumstances and measurement of core (rectal) body temperature. Measurement of tympanic membrane, cutaneous or oral temperatures can be misleading. Clinical features depend on the degree of hypothermia:

• Mild hypothermia: shivering, confusion, dehydration, ataxia. • Severe hypothermia: depressed conscious level, muscle stiffness, failed vasocon-

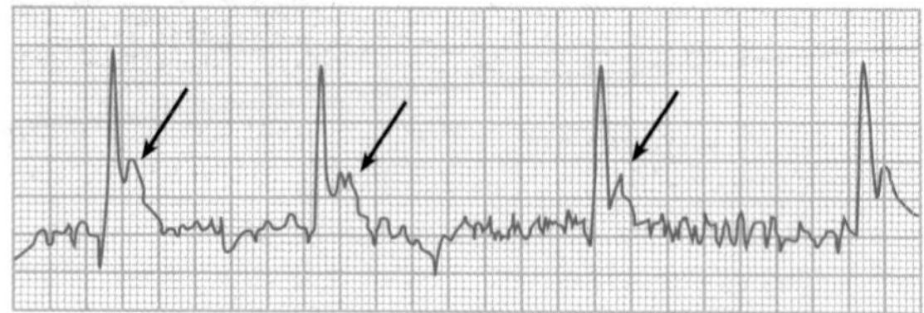

Fig. 2.1 ECG showing J waves (arrows) in a hypothermic patient.

striction/shivering, bradycardia, hypotension, ECG J waves, dysrhythmias. • Below 28°C: coma, absent pupillary reflexes, appears dead, absent corneal reflex (<23°C), cardiac standstill.

It is very difficult to diagnose death reliably by clinical means in a cold patient. Resuscitative measures should continue until the core temperature is normal and only then should a diagnosis of brain death be considered.

Investigations

• Haemoconcentration and metabolic acidosis are common. • J waves, which occur at the junction of the QRS complex and the ST segment, may be seen on the ECG (Fig. 2.1). • Cardiac dysrhythmias, including ventricular fibrillation, may occur. • Serum aspartate aminotransferase and creatine kinase may be elevated secondary to muscle damage; serum amylase is often high due to subclinical pancreatitis. • If the cause of hypothermia is not obvious, additional tests should identify thyroid and pituitary dysfunction, hypoglycaemia and the possibility of drug intoxication.

Management

Mild hypothermia (32–35°C): In a conscious patient this is treated with passive rewarming. Patients should be maintained in a warm room, with additional thermal insulation (blankets and/or space film blanket). They should be given warm fluids to drink and an adequate calorie intake. Core temperature rises slowly due to normal metabolic heat production.

Severe hypothermia (<32°C): Is associated with metabolic disturbance and cardiac dysrhythmias. Immersion victims (rapid fall in core temperature) can be rewarmed in a bath of water at 40°C. When temperature has fallen more gradually, rewarming should take place more slowly. The patient should be warmed by 1°C/hr, preferably in an ICU. Surface rewarming may cause reperfusion and vasodilatation of surface tissues, precipitating hypotension, increasing oxygen demand and worsening acidosis. In addition to supplementary oxygen, warm i.v. fluids should be given and acidosis corrected. Monitoring of cardiac rhythm and ABGs is essential.

REHABILITATION

Rehabilitation aims to improve the ability of people of all ages to perform day-to-day activities and to restore their physical, mental and social capabilities as far as possible.

THE PROCESS

Rehabilitation is a problem-solving process focused on improving a patient's function. This includes not only physical capacities, but also psychological and social functioning. It covers:

Assessment: The nature and extent of the patient's problems are identified from a comprehensive assessment using the framework in Box 2.7.

Goal-setting: Goals are specific to the patient's problems, realistic and agreed by the patient with the rehabilitation team.

Intervention: This includes active treatments to achieve the set goals and to maintain the patient's health and quality of life.

Reassessment: There is ongoing re-evaluation of the patient's function and progress towards the set goals, with modification of the interventions if necessary. This requires regular review by all members of the rehabilitation team, the patient and the carer.

2.7 INTERNATIONAL CLASSIFICATION OF FUNCTIONING AND DISABILITY

Factor	Intervention required
Health condition The underlying disease, e.g. stroke, osteoarthritis	Medical or surgical treatment
Impairment The symptoms or signs of the condition, e.g. hemiparesis, visual loss	Medical or surgical treatment
Activity limitation The resultant loss of function, e.g. walking, dressing	Rehabilitation, assistance, aids
Participation restriction The resultant loss of social function, e.g. cooking, shopping	Adapted accommodation Social services

3

Critical care and emergency medicine

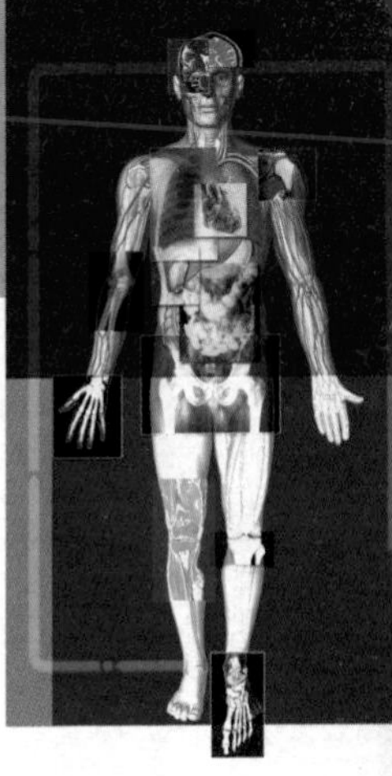

A critically ill patient is one at imminent risk of death. The approach required in managing the critically ill patient differs from that required in less severely ill patients, with immediate resuscitation and stabilisation of the patient's condition taking precedence. Intensive care units (ICUs) are for patients with potential or established organ failure. Initially established for the provision of mechanical ventilation for patients with respiratory failure, ICUs now monitor and support all the major organ systems. High-dependency care provides an intermediate level between intensive care and general ward care; it is appropriate for patients who have had major surgery and for those with single-organ failure.

Rigid rules to determine admission to ICU/HDU are destined to fail because every case must be evaluated on its own merits. The guiding principle when considering ICU/HDU admission should be the timely use of this resource in patients who have a realistic prospect of recovering to achieve a reasonable quality of life. Early identification and admission of critically ill patients improves survival and reduces the length of stay on the ICU (Box 3.1).

MONITORING

On entering an ICU, relatives, students and even clinicians may be intimidated by the numerous tubes and cables attaching each patient to a battery of 'alarming' machines. Trends in data collected provide an important guide to a patient's progress.

CLINICAL EXAMINATION OF THE CRITICALLY ILL PATIENT

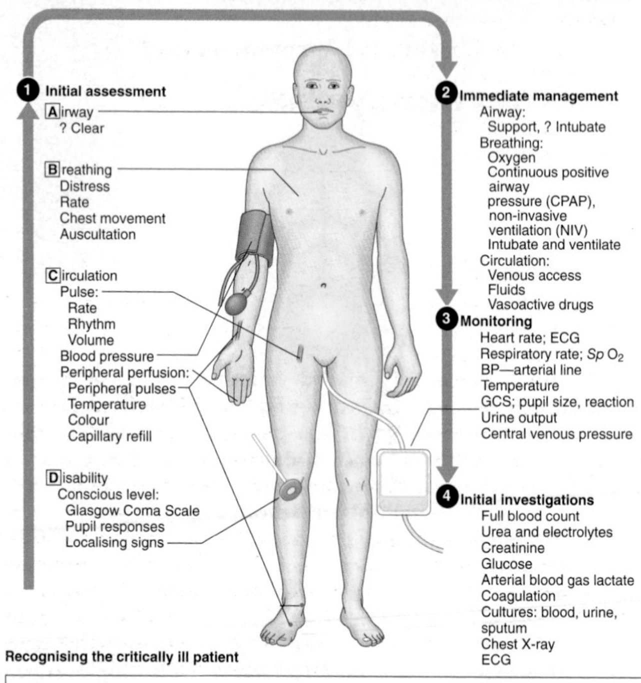

Recognising the critically ill patient

Cardiovascular signs
- Cardiac arrest
- Pulse rate < 40 or > 140 bpm
- Systolic blood pressure (BP) < 100 mmHg
- Tissue hypoxia
  - Poor peripheral perfusion
  - Metabolic acidosis
  - Hyperlactataemia
- Poor response to volume resuscitation
- Oliguria: < 0.5 ml/kg/hr (check urea, creatinine, K^+

Respiratory signs
- Threatened or obstructed airway
- Stridor, intercostal recession
- Respiratory arrest
- Respiratory rate < 8 or > 35/min
- Respiratory 'distress': use of accessory muscles; unable to speak in complete sentences
- SpO_2 < 90% on high-flow O_2
- Rising $PaCO_2$ > 8 kPa (> 60 mmHg), or > 2 kPa (> 15 mmHg) above 'normal' with acidosis

Neurological signs
- Threatened or obstructed airway
- Absent gag or cough reflex
- Failure to maintain normal PaO_2 and $PaCO_2$
- Failure to obey commands
- Glasgow Coma Scale (GCS) < 10
- Sudden fall in level of consciousness (GCS fall > 2 points)
- Repeated or prolonged seizures

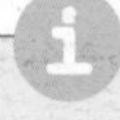

3.1 FACTORS IN THE ASSESSMENT OF A POSSIBLE ICU ADMISSION

- Primary diagnosis and other active medical problems
- Prognosis of underlying condition
- Severity of physiological disturbance—is recovery still possible?
- Life expectancy and anticipated quality of life post-discharge (age alone should not be a contraindication to admission)
- Wishes of the patient and/or relatives
- Availability of the required treatment/technology

MONITORING THE CIRCULATION

• ECG monitoring records changes in heart rate and rhythm. • Arterial BP is measured continuously using an arterial line placed in the radial artery. • Central venous pressure (CVP) is monitored using a catheter placed in the right internal jugular vein or the subclavian vein with the distal end sited in the upper right atrium. If the CVP is low in the presence of a low BP, fluid resuscitation is necessary. However, a raised CVP does not necessarily mean that the patient is adequately volume-resuscitated, as pulmonary hypertension or right ventricular dysfunction can also lead to a raised CVP. • If CVP interpretation is difficult, it may be appropriate to insert a pulmonary artery flotation catheter so that pulmonary artery pressure and pulmonary artery 'wedge' pressure (PAWP), which approximates to left atrial pressure, can be measured and used to guide fluid resuscitation. • Cardiac output can be assessed with the thermodilution technique using a PA catheter. Less invasive alternative methods include oesophageal Doppler USS. • Urine output is a sensitive measure of renal perfusion, provided that the kidneys are not damaged (e.g. acute tubular necrosis) or affected by drugs (e.g. diuretics, dopamine), and can be monitored accurately if a urinary catheter is in place. • Fluid balance should be accurately assessed. The insensible loss from skin, respiration etc. is normally 500–1000 ml/day but can exceed 2 litres/day in a pyrexial patient with open wounds. • A metabolic acidosis with base deficit >5 mmol/l often indicates increased lactic acid production in poorly perfused, hypoxic tissues. Serial lactate measurements may help in monitoring response to treatment.

MONITORING RESPIRATORY FUNCTION

• Oxygen saturation (SpO_2) is measured continuously. • ABGs are measured several times a day in a ventilated patient so that inspired oxygen and minute volume can be adjusted to achieve the desired PaO_2 and $PaCO_2$. • Capnography measures CO_2 in expired air continuously and helps to assess the adequacy of alveolar ventilation in intubated patients.

PRESENTING PROBLEMS

CIRCULATORY FAILURE: 'SHOCK'

Circulatory failure or 'shock' exists when the oxygen delivery fails to meet the metabolic requirements of the tissues. 'Shock' is often considered to be synonymous with hypotension, although hypotension may be a late manifestation of circulatory failure. The causes of 'shock' may be classified into:

Hypovolaemic: Any condition provoking a major reduction in blood volume, e.g. haemorrhage, severe burns, dehydration.

Cardiogenic: Any form of severe heart failure, e.g. myocardial infarction, acute mitral regurgitation.

Obstructive: Obstruction to blood flow around the circulation, e.g. major pulmonary embolism, cardiac tamponade, 'tension' pneumothorax.

Neurogenic: Caused by major brain or spinal injury producing disruption of brain-stem and neurogenic vasomotor control; may be associated with neurogenic pulmonary oedema.

Anaphylactic: Inappropriate vasodilatation triggered by an allergen (e.g. bee sting).

Septic/SIRS: Infection or other causes of a systemic inflammatory response syndrome (SIRS) that produce widespread endothelial damage with vasodilatation, arteriovenous shunting, microvascular occlusion and tissue oedema, resulting in organ failure.

General features of shock are shown in Box 3.2.

Hypovolaemic, cardiogenic and obstructive causes of circulatory failure produce the 'classical' image of shock, with cold peripheries, weak central pulses and evidence of a low cardiac output. In contrast, neurogenic, anaphylactic and septic shock is usually associated with warm peripheries, bounding pulses and features of a high cardiac output.

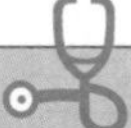

3.2 GENERAL FEATURES OF SHOCK

- Hypotension (systolic BP <100 mmHg)
- Tachycardia (>100/min)
- Cold, clammy skin
- Rapid, shallow respiration
- Drowsiness, confusion, irritability
- Oliguria (urine output <30 ml/hr)
- Elevated or reduced CVP
- Multi-organ failure

RESPIRATORY FAILURE, INCLUDING ARDS

The majority of patients admitted to ICU/HDU will have respiratory problems either as the primary cause of their admission or secondary to pathology elsewhere. Attempts should be made to reduce the work of breathing, e.g. by treating bronchoconstriction or using continuous positive airways pressure (CPAP). The patient's appearance (tachypnoea, difficulty speaking in complete sentences, laboured breathing, exhaustion, agitation or increasing obtundation) is more important than measurement of ABGs in deciding when to intubate and ventilate.

Acute respiratory distress syndrome (ARDS): This describes the acute, diffuse pulmonary inflammatory response to either direct (via airway or chest trauma) or indirect blood-borne insults from extrapulmonary pathology. It is characterised by neutrophil sequestration in pulmonary capillaries, increased capillary permeability and protein-rich pulmonary oedema. If this early phase does not resolve with treatment of the underlying cause, a fibroproliferative phase ensues and causes pulmonary fibrosis. It is frequently associated with other organ dysfunction as part of multiple organ failure. The term ARDS is often limited to patients requiring ventilatory support on the ICU, but less severe forms, conventionally referred to as acute lung injury (ALI) and with similar pathology, occur on acute medical and surgical wards. The clinical picture is non-specific and shares features that are common in other conditions (diffuse bilateral shadowing on CXR in the absence of raised left atrial pressure, hypoxaemia, impaired lung compliance).

ANAPHYLAXIS

Anaphylaxis is a life-threatening, systemic allergic reaction caused by the release of histamine and other vasoactive mediators. Clinical features are wheeze, stridor, angioedema, urticaria and a feeling of impending doom. Potential allergen triggers should be ascertained. The most common are:

• Foods (peanut, shellfish, eggs). • Latex. • Insect venom (bee and wasp). • Drugs (penicillin, anaesthetic agents).

The route of allergen exposure influences the features of the reaction; e.g. an inhaled allergen leads to wheezing.

Investigations: Measurement of acute and convalescent serum mast cell tryptase concentrations may be useful to confirm the diagnosis. Anaphylactoid reactions result from the non-specific degranulation of mast cells by drugs (opiates, aspirin), chemicals (radiocontrast media) or other triggers (exercise, cold), and do not involve IgE antibodies. The clinical presentations are indistinguishable, and in the acute situation discriminating between them is unnecessary. Specific IgE tests may be preferable to skin prick tests when investigating patients with a history of anaphylaxis.

Management: Anaphylaxis is an acute medical emergency. The immediate management includes:

• Preventing further allergen exposure (e.g. removal of bee sting). • Ensuring airway patency. • Administration of oxygen. • Restoration of blood pressure (laying the patient flat, i.v. fluids). • Prompt administration of adrenaline (epinephrine).

Adrenaline reverses the action of histamine within minutes. It should be given i.m. (adult dose 0.3–1.0 ml 1 : 1000 solution) and repeated if needed.

This should be followed by i.v. antihistamines (chlorphenamine 10–20 mg i.m. or slow i.v. injection). Corticosteroids (hydrocortisone 100–300 mg) prevent late-phase symptoms. Nebulised β_2-agonists are indicated for wheeze.

Patients should be referred for specialist assessment. The aims are to: • Identify the trigger factor. • Educate the patient regarding avoidance and management of subsequent episodes. • Identify whether immunotherapy is indicated.

Patients should be prescribed self-injectable adrenaline and should wear a MedicAlert bracelet. If the trigger factor cannot be identified (~30%), recurrence is common.

RENAL FAILURE

Oliguria is frequently an early sign of systemic problems in critical illness and successful resuscitation is associated with restoration of good urine output, an improving acid–base balance and correction of plasma potassium, urea and creatinine. Acute renal failure (ARF; p. 176) in the context of critical illness is usually due to pre-renal factors such as uncorrected hypovolaemia, hypotension or ischaemia causing acute tubular necrosis (ATN). Sepsis is frequently a compounding factor and may be associated with disseminated intravascular coagulation (DIC). In the presence of pre-existing chronic renal impairment or nephrotoxic drugs, ARF may result from relatively minor ischaemic or hypotensive insults. Obstruction must always be excluded early by abdominal USS.

NEUROLOGICAL FAILURE (COMA)

Impaired consciousness or coma is often an early feature of severe systemic illness. Prompt assessment and management of airway, breathing and circulation are essential to prevent further brain injury, to allow diagnosis and for definitive treatment to be instituted. Impaired conscious level is graded according to the Glasgow Coma Scale (GCS; p. 636), which is also used to monitor progress. Although limited, careful neurological examination is very important in the unconscious patient. Pupil size and reaction to light, presence or absence of neck stiffness, focal neurological signs and evidence of other organ impairment should be noted.

SEPSIS

Any or all of the features of SIRS (Box 3.3) may be present, together with an obvious focus of infection such as purulent sputum from the chest with

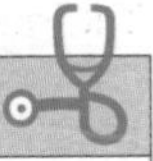

3.3 SYSTEMIC INFLAMMATORY RESPONSE SYNDROME (SIRS)	
• Encompasses inflammatory response to both infective and non-infective causes such as pancreatitis, trauma, cardiopulmonary bypass, vasculitis etc.	
• Defined by presence of two or more of:	
Temperature >38.0°C or <36.0°C	Respiratory rate >20/min
$P\text{a}CO_2$ <4.3 kPa (<32 mmHg) or ventilated	WCC >12 × 10^9/l or <4 × 10^9/l
Heart rate >90/min	

shadowing on CXR or erythema around an i.v. line. However, severe sepsis may present as unexplained hypotension and the speed of onset may simulate major pulmonary embolism or myocardial infarction.

A distinction should be made between community-acquired and hospital-acquired infections as the likely causative microorganism may be different and this will direct the initial choice of antibiotics. The aim of management is to identify and treat the underlying cause.

Nosocomial infections are an increasing problem on critical care units; cross-infection is a major concern, particularly with regard to MRSA and multidrug-resistant Gram-negative organisms. The most important practice in preventing cross-infection is thorough hand-washing after every patient contact. Limiting the use of antibiotics helps to prevent the emergence of multidrug-resistant bacteria.

DISSEMINATED INTRAVASCULAR COAGULATION (DIC)

DIC is common in critically ill patients and often heralds the onset of multiple organ failure.

It is characterised by an increase in prothrombin time, partial thromboplastin time and fibrin degradation products, and a fall in platelets and fibrinogen. It may manifest as widespread bleeding from vascular access points, GI tract, bronchial tree and surgical wound sites, or widespread evidence of thrombosis. Management is supportive with infusions of fresh frozen plasma and platelets while the underlying cause is treated.

MANAGEMENT OF MAJOR ORGAN FAILURE

Assessing critically ill patients requires a systematic approach. An integrated management plan should be made, specifying goals for each organ system.

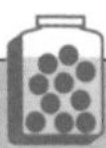

3.4 INITIAL MANAGEMENT OF CIRCULATORY COLLAPSE

- Correct hypoxaemia: Oxygen therapy
- Consider ventilation: Intractable hypoxaemia
  Hypercapnia: $PaCO_2$ >6.5 kPa
  Respiratory distress
  Impaired conscious level
- Assess circulation: Heart rate
  BP: direct arterial pressure
  CVP
  Peripheral perfusion
- Optimise volume status: Fluid challenge(s)
  CVP <6 mmHg: 250 ml normal saline or colloid
  CVP >6 mmHg or poor ventricular function suspected: 100 ml boluses
  Consider PA catheter
- Optimise haemoglobin concentration: 70–90 g/l; 100 g/l if ischaemic heart disease. Red cells as required
- Achieve target BP: Use vasopressor/inotrope only after hypovolaemia corrected
- Achieve adequate CO and DO_2: inotropic agent if fluid alone inadequate
- Monitor trend in haemodynamics, ABG H^+, base deficit, lactate

CIRCULATORY SUPPORT

The primary goals are to:
• Restore global oxygen delivery by ensuring an adequate cardiac output. • Maintain a BP that ensures adequate perfusion of vital organs. • Avoid levels of left atrial pressure that produce pulmonary oedema.

The initial management of circulatory collapse is shown in Box 3.4. If cardiac output is poor despite an adequate preload, the therapeutic options are to provide inotropic support or reduce the afterload with vasoactive drugs (Box 3.5), or to control the heart rate and rhythm if this is abnormal.

RESPIRATORY SUPPORT

Respiratory support is indicated to maintain the patency of the airway, correct hypoxaemia and hypercapnia, and reduce the work of breathing.

Oxygen therapy: Ensure adequate arterial oxygenation (SpO_2 >90%). If a patient remains hypoxaemic on high-flow oxygen, other measures are required. Common modes of ventilatory support are summarised in Box 3.6.

Non-invasive respiratory support: If the patient has respiratory failure associated with decreased lung volume, application of CPAP will improve

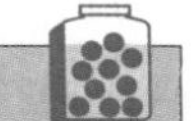

3.5 CIRCULATORY EFFECTS OF COMMONLY USED VASOACTIVE DRUG INFUSIONS

Drug (receptors)	Cardiac contractility	Heart rate	BP	Cardiac output	Splanchnic blood flow	SVR	PVR
Dopamine							
(<5 μg/kg/min) **(DA$_1$,β$_1$,α)**	↑	→/↑	→/↑	↑	→/↑	→/↑	→/↑
(>5 μg/kg/min) **(β$_1$,α,DA$_1$,β$_2$)**	↑↑	↑	↑	↑↑	→	↑	↑
Adrenaline (epinephrine) (β$_1$,α,β$_2$)	↑↑	↑	↑↑	↑↑↑	↓	↑	↑
Noradrenaline (norepinephrine) (α,β$_1$)	→/↑	→/↓	↑↑	→/↓	→/↓	↑↑	↑↑
Isoprenaline (β$_1$,β$_2$)	↑	↑↑	→/↓	↑	→/↑	→/↓	↓
Dobutamine (β$_1$,β$_2$,α)	↑	↑	→/↓	↑↑	→	↓	↓
Dopexamine (β$_2$,DA$_1$,DA$_2$)	↑	↑↑	→/↓	↑	↑	↓	↓
Glyceryl trinitrate (NO)	→	↑	↓	↑	↑	↓	↓

Receptors through which these vasoactive drugs work are given in parentheses and listed in order of the extent of receptor stimulation produced. Note that dopamine acts more like adrenaline at high doses.
(α = α-adrenoceptor; β$_1$, β$_2$ = β-adrenoceptors 1 and 2; DA$_1$, DA$_2$ = dopaminergic receptors 1 and 2; NO = acts via local nitric oxide release.)

3.6 MECHANICAL VENTILATION	
Intermittent positive pressure ventilation (IPPV)	Generic term for all types of positive pressure ventilation
Controlled mandatory ventilation (CMV)	Most basic classic form of ventilation; pre-set rate and tidal volume (V_T)
Synchronised intermittent mandatory ventilation (SIMV)	Pre-set rate of mandatory breaths with pre-set V_T; allows spontaneous breaths (may be pressure-supported) between mandatory breaths
Pressure-controlled ventilation (PCV)	Pre-set rate and inspiratory pressure; used in management of severe acute respiratory failure to avoid high airway pressure, often with prolonged inspiratory to expiratory ratio (pressure-controlled inverse ratio ventilation, PCIRV)
Pressure support ventilation (PSV)	Provides positive pressure to augment patient's breaths; useful for weaning
Positive end-expiratory pressure (PEEP)	Applied during expiration; improves oxygenation by recruiting atelectatic or oedematous lung; may impair venous return and reduce cardiac output
Continuous positive airways pressure (CPAP)	Positive airway pressure applied throughout the respiratory cycle, via either an endotracheal tube or a tight-fitting facemask
Bi-level positive airway pressure (BiPAP)	Two levels of positive airway pressure (higher level in inspiration); in fully ventilated patients, BiPAP is essentially the same as PCV with PEEP; in partially ventilated patients, and especially if used non-invasively, BiPAP is essentially PSV with CPAP
Non-invasive intermittent positive pressure ventilation (NIPPV)	Ventilation applied using a facemask or nasal mask; BiPAP is the usual mode, typically with 15–20 cmH_2O on inspiration and 3–5 cmH_2O on expiration, often with a back-up mandatory rate; indications include acute exacerbations of COPD

oxygenation by recruitment of under-ventilated alveoli and reduce the work of breathing. CPAP is most successful when alveoli are readily recruited (e.g. pulmonary oedema, post-operative atelectasis). Patients should be cooperative, be able to protect their airway and have the strength to breathe spontaneously and cough effectively. Non-invasive positive pressure ventilation (NIPPV) may avoid the need for endotracheal intubation in patients with type 2 respiratory failure (e.g. exacerbations of COPD; p. 288), and is also used during weaning from conventional ventilation.

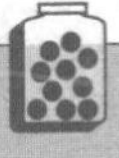

3.7 INDICATIONS FOR TRACHEAL INTUBATION AND MECHANICAL VENTILATION

- Protection of airway
- Removal of secretions
- Hypoxaemia (PaO_2 <8 kPa (<60 mmHg); SpO_2 <90%) despite CPAP with FiO_2 >0.6
- Hypercapnia if conscious level impaired or risk of raised intracranial pressure
- Vital capacity <1.2 litres in neuromuscular disease
- Removing the work of breathing in exhausted patients

Endotracheal intubation and mechanical ventilation: Over 60% of patients admitted to ICU require intubation and mechanical ventilation. Indications for intubation are summarised in Box 3.7. In the conscious patient, intubation requires induction of anaesthesia and muscle relaxation, while in more obtunded patients sedation alone may be adequate. Hypotension commonly follows sedation or anaesthesia because of direct cardiovascular effects of the drugs and loss of sympathetic drive; positive pressure ventilation may compound this problem by increasing intrathoracic pressure, which reduces venous return.

The selection of ventilator mode and settings for tidal volume, respiratory rate, positive end-expiratory pressure (PEEP) and inspiratory to expiratory ratio is dependent on the cause of the respiratory failure.

Weaning from respiratory support: The majority of patients require mechanical ventilatory support for only a few days and do not need a process of weaning. In contrast, patients who have required long-term ventilatory support for severe lung disease, e.g. ARDS, may initially be unable to sustain even a modest degree of respiratory work due to reduced lung compliance and muscle weakness and hence require a programme of gradual weaning from ventilation.

Tracheostomy: Usually performed electively when endotracheal intubation is likely to be prolonged (>14 days). Tracheostomies help patient comfort, aid weaning from ventilation, and allow access for tracheal toilet and intermittent respiratory support.

RENAL SUPPORT

Oliguria requires explanation and early intervention to correct renal hypoperfusion. Renal tract obstruction should be excluded by USS, and underlying sepsis diagnosed and treated. If renal function cannot be restored following resuscitation, renal replacement therapy is indicated (p. 185). There is little evidence that low-dose dopamine, furosemide or mannitol (aimed at inducing a diuresis) have any additional beneficial value in restoring renal function beyond that achieved by adequate fluid resuscitation.

GASTROINTESTINAL AND HEPATIC SUPPORT

The GI tract and liver play an important role in the evolution of multiple organ failure, even when the primary diagnosis is unrelated.

Early institution of enteral nutrition is the most effective strategy for protecting the gut mucosa and providing nutrition. Total parenteral nutrition (TPN) should be started if attempts at enteral feeding have failed. Recent evidence suggests that tight glycaemic control (often requiring i.v. insulin) can improve outcomes in the critically ill.

Hepatic ischaemia leads to impaired filtering of endotoxin from the portal circulation and, as SIRS develops, inflammatory mediators are released from activated hepatic macrophages into the systemic circulation, increasing the risk of ARF developing.

NEUROLOGICAL SUPPORT

The aim of management in acute brain injury is to optimise cerebral oxygen delivery by maintaining a normal arterial oxygen content and a cerebral perfusion pressure >70 mmHg. A rise in intracranial pressure (ICP) as a result of haematoma, contusions or ischaemic swelling is damaging both directly to the cerebral cortex and by producing downward pressure on the brain stem, and indirectly by reducing cerebral perfusion pressure.

Complex neurological monitoring must be combined with frequent clinical assessment. The motor response to pain is a particularly important prognostic sign. No response or extension of the upper limbs is associated with severe injury, and unless there is improvement within a few days, prognosis is very poor. A flexor response is encouraging and indicates that a good outcome is still possible.

Critical illness polyneuropathy is another potential complication in patients with sepsis and multiple organ failure. It can result in areflexia, gross muscle-wasting and failure to wean from the ventilator, thus prolonging the duration of intensive care.

MANAGEMENT OF SEPSIS

Prompt administration of broad-spectrum antibiotics which cover probable causative organisms (based on the site of infection, previous antibiotic therapy and local resistance patterns) is essential. The early stages of septic shock are often dominated by hypotension with relative volume depletion due to marked arteriolar and particularly venular dilatation. Sufficient i.v. fluid should be given to ensure that the intravascular volume is not the limiting factor in determining oxygen delivery.

Vasoactive drugs are often used in the ICU. The choice of the most appropriate vasoactive drug to use should be based on a full analysis of the circulation and knowledge of the different inotropic, dilating or constricting properties of these drugs (see Box 3.5). In most cases a vasoconstrictor such as noradrenaline (norepinephrine) is necessary to increase SVR and BP, while an inotrope (dobutamine) may be necessary to maintain cardiac output and prevent regional ischaemia.

SPECIFIC THERAPIES

Corticosteroids: Assessment of the pituitary–adrenal axis is difficult in the critically ill but up to 30% of patients may have adrenal insufficiency. Corticosteroid replacement therapy is controversial; early studies using short-term, high-dose methylprednisolone showed no benefit, but recent studies using lower-dose infusions of hydrocortisone have demonstrated an improvement in outcome measures.

Activated protein C: Administration of activated protein C (levels of which frequently fall in critical illness) has recently been shown to produce a substantial reduction in mortality in patients with SIRS.

WITHDRAWAL OF CARE

Withdrawal of support is appropriate when it is clear that the patient has no realistic prospect of recovery or of surviving with a quality of life that he or she would value. In these situations intensive care will only prolong the dying process and is therefore both futile and an inhumane waste of resources. Nevertheless, when active support is withdrawn, management should remain positive and be directed towards allowing the patient to die with dignity and as free from distress as possible.

4

Poisoning

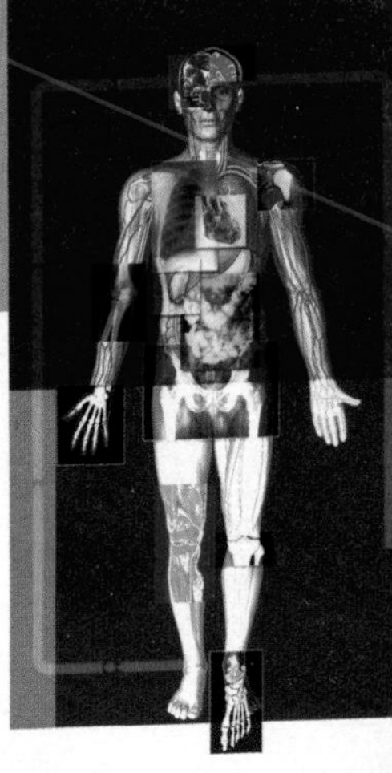

Acute poisoning accounts for 10–20% of acute medical admissions in the UK. There is wide geographical variation in the substances involved in poisoning. In the UK, paracetamol poisoning is common, but it accounts for only 7% of overdoses in the USA. Poisoning with tricyclic antidepressants (TCAs), selective serotonin re-uptake inhibitors (SSRIs) and drugs of misuse is very common in the UK and USA. In Southeast Asia, pesticide ingestion is endemic, and constitutes the most common cause of death by poisoning.

GENERAL APPROACH TO THE POISONED PATIENT

The diagnosis of poisoning is usually apparent from the history. Occasionally, the ingested substance is unknown or patients deliberately mislead doctors (e.g. drug misusers). Full details of the type of substance, quantity and timing of ingestion should be sought. Remaining pills or empty packets may help to corroborate the substance taken. Commercially available databases (e.g. TICTAC®; http://tictac.vhn.net/home/) can be used to identify unlabelled pills from their visual appearance. Establishing the source of the drug (i.e. over the counter/prescription/belonging to a relative) is important in the prevention of future poisoning.

Ask the patient why the overdose was taken and take time to listen to the explanation. Reasons often include relationship difficulties, work- or school-related difficulties, drug addiction, psychiatric illness or bereavement. Details of the past medical history, particularly a history of asthma, jaundice, drug misuse, head injury, epilepsy, cardiovascular problems,

CLINICAL EXAMINATION OF THE POISONED PATIENT

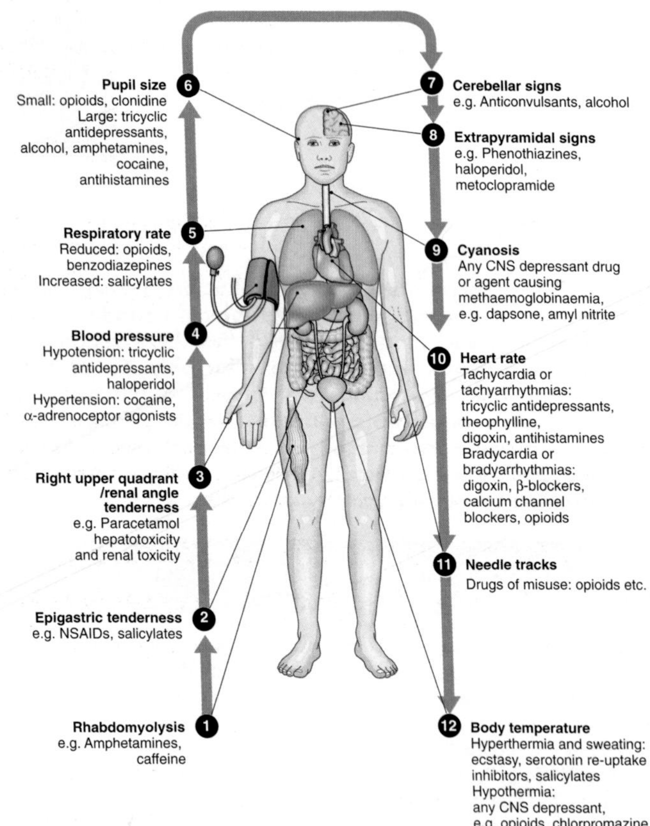

previous psychiatric illness and self-harm, should be taken. It is also important to ask about allergies and alcohol history.

CLINICAL FEATURES (p. 34)

• Look for needle marks or evidence of previous self-harm, e.g. razor marks on forearms. • Pupil size, respiratory rate and heart rate may help to narrow down the potential list of toxins. • The Glasgow Coma Scale (GCS, p. 636) is most frequently used to assess the degree of impaired consciousness. • The patient's weight helps to determine whether toxicity is likely to occur, given the dose ingested. • When patients are unconscious and no history is available, other causes of coma must be excluded (especially meningitis, intracerebral bleeds, hypoglycaemia, diabetic ketoacidosis, uraemia and encephalopathy).

INVESTIGATIONS

The diagnosis is usually made on the history and clinical signs alone. Paracetamol, aspirin or iron poisoning require serum levels to guide treatment. In unconscious patients, a urinary drug screen can confirm recent use of drugs such as benzodiazepines, cocaine, ecstasy, opioids and cannabis.

PSYCHIATRIC ASSESSMENT

To determine appropriate placement and supervision for a patient, an initial assessment of suicidal intent must be made. Suicide attempts were once much more common in women than in men but now the ratios are more equal. Risk factors for suicide are shown in Box 4.1.

MANAGEMENT OF THE POISONED PATIENT

Most patients admitted with poisoning require only general care. Up-to-date information on diagnosis and management of overdoses of specific substances can be found on TOXBASE® (www.toxbase.org). Eye or skin

4.1 RISK FACTORS FOR SUICIDE

- Psychiatric illness (depression, schizophrenia)
- Male sex
- Living alone
- Recent bereavement, divorce or separation
- Suicide note written
- Age >45
- Unemployment
- Chronic physical ill health
- Drug or alcohol misuse
- Previous attempts (violent method)

contamination should be treated with appropriate washing or irrigation. Only patients who have ingested significant overdoses need further measures to prevent absorption or increase elimination:

• Activated charcoal (50 g p.o.) can be given, if a potentially toxic amount of poison has been ingested <1 hr before presentation. Agents that do not bind to activated charcoal include ethylene glycol, iron, lithium and methanol. • Whole bowel irrigation with polyethylene glycol can be used for toxic ingestions of iron, lithium and theophylline. • Urinary alkalinisation using i.v. sodium bicarbonate enhances elimination of salicylates and the herbicide 2,4-D. • Haemodialysis is occasionally used for serious poisoning with salicylates, theophylline, ethylene glycol, methanol or carbamazepine.

In the seriously poisoned patient, meticulous supportive care, including the treatment of seizures, coma and cardiovascular complications, along with ventilatory support where required, is critical to good outcome. Despite popular misconceptions, specific antidotes are only available for a small number of poisons (Box 4.2).

4.2 ANTIDOTES AVAILABLE FOR THE TREATMENT OF SPECIFIC POISONINGS

Poison	Antidote
Anticoagulants (e.g. warfarin)	Vitamin K, fresh frozen plasma
β-adrenoceptor antagonists (β-blockers)	I.v. glucagon, adrenaline (epinephrine)
Calcium channel blockers	Calcium gluconate, calcium chloride, glucagon
Cyanide	Oxygen, dicobalt edetate, nitrites, sodium thiosulphate, hydroxocobalamin
Ethylene glycol/methanol	Ethanol, 4-methylpyrazole
Lead	DMSA, DMPS, disodium calcium edetate
Mercury	DMPS
Iron salts	Desferrioxamine
Opioids	Naloxone
Organophosphorus insecticides, nerve agents	Atropine, oximes (pralidoxime, obidoxime salts, HI-6, HLo-7)
Paracetamol	N-acetylcysteine, methionine
Cardiac glycosides, e.g. digoxin	Digoxin-specific antibody fragments (F_{ab})

POISONING BY SPECIFIC PHARMACEUTICAL AGENTS

PARACETAMOL

This causes hepatic damage in overdose and can occasionally cause renal failure. The antidote of choice is i.v. N-acetylcysteine (NAC), which provides complete protection against toxicity if given <10 hrs after overdose (Fig. 4.1). A patient presenting >8 hrs after ingestion should have immediate NAC administration, which can later be stopped if the paracetamol level is below the treatment line. If a patient presents >15 hrs after ingestion, LFTs, PTR (or INR) and renal function tests should be performed, the antidote started, and a poisons information centre or local liver unit contacted for advice. Liver transplantation should be considered in individuals who develop acute liver failure due to paracetamol poisoning. If multiple ingestions of paracetamol have taken place over several hours or days (a staggered overdose), plasma paracetamol concentration will be uninterpretable. Such patients should be given NAC if the paracetamol dose exceeds 150 mg/kg body weight in any one 24-hr period (75 mg/kg in 'high-risk groups').

SALICYLATES (ASPIRIN)

Doses >150, 250 and 500 mg aspirin/kg body weight produce mild, moderate and severe poisoning respectively. Common symptoms are nausea, vomiting, tinnitus and deafness. Direct stimulation of the respiratory centre produces hyperventilation. Signs of serious salicylate poisoning include metabolic acidosis, renal failure and CNS effects such as agitation, confusion, coma and fits. Death can occur as a consequence of CNS depression and cardiovascular collapse. Plasma salicylate concentration is most accurately measured >6 hrs after ingestion because of continued absorption of the drug. Any significant metabolic acidosis should be treated with sufficient i.v. sodium bicarbonate (8.4%) to normalise [H^+]. Patients are often very dehydrated, and fluid loss from vomiting and sweating must be replaced. Urinary alkalinisation is indicated for adult patients with salicylate concentrations of 600–800 mg/l. It is critical to check that urine pH has increased to >8. Haemodialysis should be considered if serum salicylate is >800 mg/l; if there is resistant metabolic acidosis; or if there are severe CNS effects (coma, convulsions).

NON-STEROIDAL ANTI-INFLAMMATORY DRUGS (NSAIDS)

Overdose of most NSAIDs usually causes little more than minor GI upset, including mild abdominal pain, vomiting and diarrhoea. However, 10–20% of patients have convulsions; these are usually self-limiting and seldom need treatment other than airway protection and oxygen.

CARDIOTOXIC DRUGS

The main categories are β-blockers, digoxin, calcium channel blockers and TCAs.

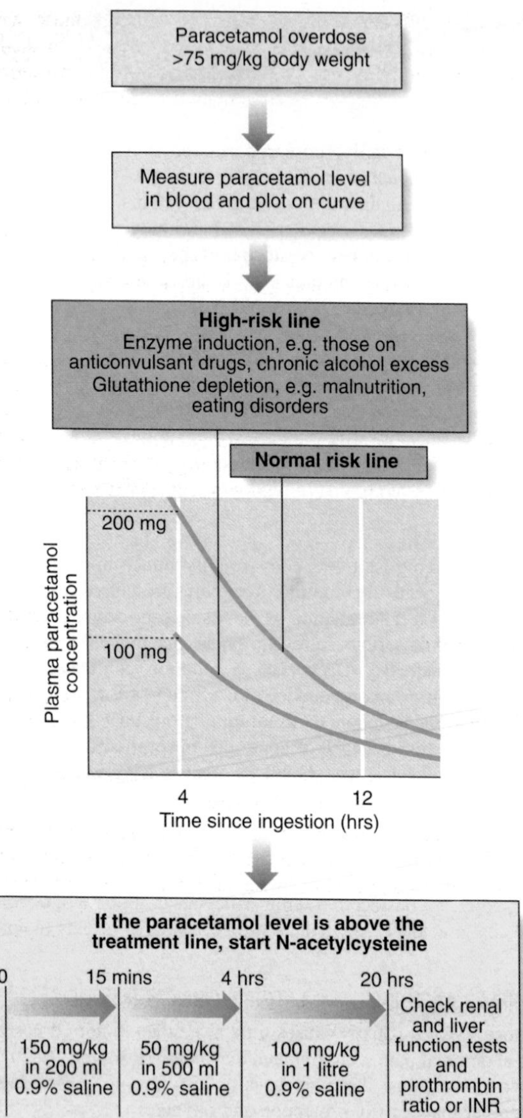

Fig. 4.1 The management of a paracetamol overdose patient.

• An individual's response to overdose is highly variable; those with cardiac disease are more at risk of toxicity, such as pulmonary oedema. Toxicity can be delayed and prolonged with modified-release preparations.
• Myocardial suppression with hypotension is treated with volume replacement and inotropes.
• Bradycardia responds to atropine or pacing.
• Tachyarrhythmias are treated by pacing, cardioversion or i.v. magnesium, as appropriate.

In many countries, the more cardiotoxic TCAs are being replaced with the less cardiotoxic SSRIs for the treatment of depression. However, in large doses SSRIs can still cause hypotension and arrhythmias.

QUININE

The average fatal dose in an adult is 8 g, although deaths have been reported with as little as 1.5 g in an adult and 900 mg in a child. Quinine causes retinal vasoconstriction and has a direct toxic effect on retinal photoreceptor cells; it can cause blindness. Other features include nausea, vomiting, tinnitus, deafness, headache and tremor. In large overdoses, ataxia, drowsiness, coma, respiratory depression, haemolysis and cardiac effects can occur (hypotension, arrhythmias). Treatment is with activated charcoal and ventilatory support, as required.

ANTIDIABETIC AGENTS

These include the sulphonylureas (e.g. gliclazide, glipizide), biguanides (metformin) and insulins. All can cause hypoglycaemia in overdose, although insulin is non-toxic if ingested.
• The onset and duration of hypoglycaemia vary, but can last for several days with the longer-acting agents such as isophane and lente insulins.
• Metformin overdose can cause lactic acidosis, particularly in elderly patients and those with renal or hepatic impairment, or if co-ingested with ethanol, when there is a significant mortality rate.

• Hypoglycaemia should be corrected urgently with 50 ml i.v. 50% dextrose, or with a sugary drink if the patient is conscious. This should be followed by an infusion of 10% or 20% dextrose titrated to the patient's blood glucose to prevent further hypoglycaemia. Blood glucose and U&Es should be checked regularly. Octreotide may be of value in severe sulphonylurea overdose.

DRUGS OF MISUSE

CANNABIS

Cannabis (grass, pot, ganja, spliff, reefer) is commonly smoked with tobacco or eaten.
• In low doses, cannabis produces euphoria, perceptual alterations and conjunctival injection, followed by relaxation and drowsiness, hypertension, tachycardia, slurred speech and ataxia. • High doses can produce an

acute paranoid psychosis. • Cannabis rarely results in serious poisoning, although cannabis extract injected intravenously can cause acute renal failure and pulmonary oedema.

BENZODIAZEPINES

In general, lone benzodiazepine overdoses are remarkably safe and near-full recovery takes place within 24 hrs. Polydrug abusers commonly misuse these drugs and difficulties occur when other CNS depressants, such as TCAs, opioids or alcohol, are also taken.

Common symptoms are drowsiness, ataxia, dysarthria, nystagmus and confusion. Respiratory arrest is rare, unless shorter-acting drugs, such as midazolam, are taken. Patients should be observed for ≥6 hrs post-ingestion, or for 24 hrs in more serious cases, with particular attention to maintenance of the airway in those with impaired consciousness.

Flumazenil is a specific benzodiazepine antagonist but is not used in the vast majority of benzodiazepine overdoses. In patients with a history of convulsions or toxin-induced cardiotoxicity, or in those who have co-ingested TCAs, flumazenil may precipitate seizures or ventricular arrhythmias.

COCAINE

Cocaine is usually purchased as a white crystalline powder or colourless crystals. It may be sniffed/snorted into the nose, from which it is rapidly absorbed, or injected intravenously. After intranasal use, effects are experienced within minutes and tend to last 20–90 mins. With i.v. use the peak 'high' occurs within 10 mins.

• Mild to moderate intoxication with cocaine causes euphoria, agitation, aggression, cerebellar signs, dilated pupils, vomiting, pallor, headache, cold sweats, twitching, pyrexia, tachycardia, hallucinations and hypertension.

• Features of severe intoxication include convulsions, coma, muscular paralysis, severe hypertension and stroke. A toxic psychosis may occur with high levels of consumption, and tactile hallucinations (formication) may be prominent. Coronary artery spasm may result in myocardial ischaemia or infarction, even in patients with normal coronary arteries. All patients should be observed with ECG monitoring for ≥2 hrs. Aspirin and i.v. nitrates should be used to treat chest pain.

• In fatal poisoning, the onset and progression of symptoms are accelerated and death may occur in minutes.

ECSTASY/AMPHETAMINES

MDMA (3,4-methylenedioxymethamphetamine, ecstasy) is a 'designer' amphetamine, also known as E, Adam, white dove, white burger, or red and black. It produces feelings of euphoria and emotional intimacy, and distorted sensory perceptions. Tolerance is common, and most regular users need to take considerably higher doses.

Supraventricular and ventricular arrhythmias are common and may cause death. Agitation or drowsiness is also common. Whilst most patients who have taken ecstasy are profoundly dehydrated, a small proportion develop hyponatraemia, usually through drinking excessive amounts of water in the absence of sufficient exertion to sweat it out. Coma, convulsions, hyperthermia and rhabdomyolysis indicate severe toxicity. All symptomatic patients should have ECG, BP and temperature monitoring for ≥6 hrs.

GAMMAHYDROXYBUTYRATE (GHB)

GHB (liquid X, cherry meth, easy lay, scoop) is marketed illegally for body-building and weight loss and as a replacement for L-tryptophan. Many misusers simply 'guzzle' it until they reach an adequate high, which is often achieved shortly before becoming unconscious. Owing to the drowsiness that may occur, it is sometimes mixed with amphetamines to prolong the 'high' for several hours. Bizarrely, patients often recover quickly (within 1–2 hrs), and self-extubation and rapid reversal of coma are seen.

LSD

d-Lysergic acid diethylamide (LSD; acid, trips, dots, paper mushrooms or 'L') is a synthetic hallucinogen. It is usually ingested as small squares of impregnated absorbent paper, which are often printed with a distinctive design.

Vision is affected most often, with heightened visual awareness of objects, especially colours, image distortion and hallucinations. Patients presenting to hospital usually do so because of a 'bad trip', panic reaction, vivid visual hallucinations or aggression, or after a suicide attempt. LSD itself is of low acute toxicity; fatalities are a result of the behavioural changes it induces, which lead to accidents such as drowning.

OPIOIDS

These include heroin, morphine, methadone, codeine, pethidine, dihydrocodeine and dextropropoxyphene. They give a rapid, intensely pleasurable experience, often accompanied by heightened sexual arousal. Physical dependence occurs within a few weeks of regular high-dose injection; as a result, the dose is escalated and the addict's life becomes increasingly centred around obtaining and taking the drug.

Opioid poisoning: Accidental overdose is common. The hallmarks of opioid poisoning are depressed respiration, pinpoint or small pupils, and signs of i.v. drug misuse (e.g. needle track marks). Death can occur by respiratory arrest or from aspiration of gastric contents. Unconscious patients should always have their paracetamol concentration checked because of the wide use of combination opioid/paracetamol drugs.

Management of opioid poisoning: The airway should be cleared and breathing supported if necessary. High-flow oxygen should be administered. ABG should be performed to check the adequacy of ventilation.

Endotracheal intubation can often be avoided by prompt administration of the opioid antagonist naloxone. It should be used as a bolus dose (0.8–2 mg i.v.) in adults, repeated every 2 mins as necessary until the level of consciousness and respiratory rate increase and the pupils dilate. An infusion of naloxone may be needed because its half-life is much shorter than the half-lives of most opioids.

Opioid withdrawal

The withdrawal syndrome, which can start within 12 hrs, presents with intense craving, rhinorrhoea, lacrimation, yawning, perspiration, shivering, piloerection, vomiting, diarrhoea and abdominal cramps. Examination reveals tachycardia, hypertension, mydriasis and facial flushing.

ALCOHOL MISUSE AND DEPENDENCE

Alcohol consumption associated with social, psychological and physical problems constitutes harmful use. The criteria for alcohol dependence, a more restricted term, are shown in Box 4.3. Approximately one-quarter of male patients in general hospital medical wards in the UK have a current or previous alcohol problem. Availability of alcohol and social patterns of use appear to be the most important factors. Genetic factors may play some part in predisposition to dependence. The majority of alcoholics do not have an associated psychiatric illness, but a few drink heavily in an attempt to relieve anxiety or depression.

Alcohol misuse may emerge during the patient's history, although a history of alcohol intake may be misleading. Withdrawal symptoms in those admitted to hospital are a common presentation, as high alcohol intake cannot be sustained in this setting. Social problems include absenteeism from work, unemployment, marital tensions, child abuse, financial difficulties and problems with the law, such as violence and traffic offences.

Consequences of chronic alcohol misuse

Psychological problems: Depression is common and is usually reactive to the numerous social problems which heavy drinking creates. Alcohol

4.3 CRITERIA FOR ALCOHOL DEPENDENCE

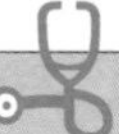

- Narrowing of the drinking repertoire (restriction to one type of alcohol, e.g. spirits)
- Priority of drinking over other activities (salience)
- Tolerance of effects of alcohol
- Repeated withdrawal symptoms
- Relief of withdrawal symptoms by further drinking
- Subjective compulsion to drink
- Reinstatement of drinking behaviour after abstinence

also has a direct depressant effect. Alcohol misuse is often implicated in suicide attempts. Anxiety is relieved by alcohol. People who are socially anxious may consequently use alcohol in this way and may develop dependence. Conversely, alcohol withdrawal increases anxiety.

Alcoholic hallucinosis is a rare condition in which alcoholic individuals experience auditory hallucination in clear consciousness. Alcohol withdrawal is described in Box 4.4. Symptoms usually become maximal 2 days after the last drink, and can include seizures. Delirium tremens is a form of delirium associated with severe alcohol withdrawal. It has a significant mortality and morbidity.

Effects on the brain: Established alcoholism may lead to alcoholic dementia, a global cognitive impairment resembling Alzheimer's disease, but which does not progress if the patient becomes abstinent.

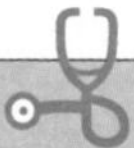

4.4 CONSEQUENCES OF CHRONIC ALCHOL MISUSE

Acute intoxication

- Emotional and behavioural disturbance; medical problems—hypoglycaemia, aspiration of vomit, respiratory depression; accidents, and injuries sustained in fights

Withdrawal phenomena

- Psychological symptoms—restlessness, anxiety, panic attacks; autonomic symptoms—tachycardia, sweating, pupil dilatation, nausea, vomiting; delirium tremens—agitation, hallucinations, illusions, delusions; seizures

Harmful use

MEDICAL CONSEQUENCES

- Neurological—peripheral neuropathy; cerebral haemorrhage; cerebellar degeneration; dementia
- Hepatic—fatty change and cirrhosis; liver cancer
- GI—oesophagitis, gastritis; Mallory–Weiss syndrome; pancreatitis; malabsorption; oesophageal cancer; oesophageal varices
- Respiratory—pulmonary TB; pneumonia
- Skin—spider naevi; Dupuytren's contractures; palmar erythema; telangiectasis
- Cardiac—cardiomyopathy; hypertension
- Musculoskeletal—myopathy; fractures
- Endocrine and metabolic—pseudo-Cushing's syndrome; gout; hypoglycaemia
- Reproductive—hypogonadism; infertility; fetal alcohol syndrome

PSYCHIATRIC AND CEREBRAL CONSEQUENCES

- Depression; alcoholic hallucinosis; alcoholic 'blackouts'; Wernicke's encephalopathy—nystagmus, ophthalmoplegia, ataxia, confusion; Korsakoff's syndrome—short-term memory deficits, confabulation

Indirect effects on behaviour can result from head injury, hypoglycaemia and portosystemic encephalopathy.

Wernicke–Korsakoff syndrome is an organic brain disorder caused by thiamine (vitamin B_1) deficiency that results from damage to the mamillary bodies, dorsomedial nuclei of the thalamus and adjacent areas of grey matter. The most common cause is long-standing heavy drinking and an inadequate diet. Without prompt treatment, the acute presentation of Wernicke's encephalopathy (nystagmus, ophthalmoplegia, ataxia and confusion) can progress to the irreversible deficits of Korsakoff's syndrome (severe short-term memory deficits and confabulation).

Effects on other organs: These are protean and virtually any organ can be involved (see Box 4.4); alcohol has replaced syphilis as the great mimic of disease.

Management and prognosis

• Advice about the harmful effects of alcohol and safe levels of consumption is often all that is needed. Altering leisure activities or changing jobs may help, if these are contributing to the problem. • Psychological treatment is used for patients who have recurrent relapses and is usually available at specialised centres. Support is also provided by voluntary organisations such as Alcoholics Anonymous (AA) in the UK. • Withdrawal syndromes can be prevented, or treated, with benzodiazepines. Large doses may be required (e.g. diazepam 20 mg 6-hourly), tailed off over a period of 5–7 days as symptoms subside. • Prevention of the Wernicke–Korsakoff complex requires the immediate use of high doses of thiamine (i.v. Pabrinex). There is no treatment for Korsakoff's syndrome once it has arisen. • Disulfiram can be given as a deterrent to patients who have difficulty resisting the impulse to drink after becoming abstinent. It blocks the metabolism of alcohol, causing acetaldehyde to accumulate, and leads to an unpleasant reaction if alcohol is consumed (headache, flushing and nausea). • Acamprosate has recently been introduced to maintain abstinence by reducing the craving for alcohol. • Many but not all who become dependent on alcohol relapse after treatment.

CHEMICALS AND PESTICIDES

CARBON MONOXIDE AND SMOKE

Carbon monoxide (CO) is a major cause of death by poisoning, and is particularly dangerous because it is colourless, non-irritant and odourless. CO binds to haemoglobin to form carboxyhaemoglobin (COHb), reducing the oxygen-carrying capacity of the blood. It also acts as a chemical asphyxiant, as it impairs the function of cytochrome oxidases and thus utilisation of oxygen by tissues.

Clinical features

• Headache, nausea and vomiting, ataxia and nystagmus, drowsiness, hyperventilation, hyper-reflexia and shivering can occur. • Late features include lethargy, coma, convulsions, hypotension, respiratory depression and cardiovascular collapse. • ECG abnormalities (ST segment depression, T-wave abnormalities, ventricular tachycardia or ventricular fibrillation) are often seen. • The COHb concentration is of value in confirming exposure to CO, although it does not correlate well with the severity of poisoning. • Pulse oximetry is misleading, as this measures both COHb and oxyhaemoglobin.

Management

• High-flow oxygen should be given as soon as possible (it reduces the half-life of COHb). It should be continued until the COHb is <5% and for at least 6 hrs after exposure. • Hyperbaric oxygen can reduce the half-life of COHb further, although the logistical difficulties of transporting sick patients to hyperbaric chambers should not be underestimated.

ORGANOPHOSPHORUS INSECTICIDES/NERVE AGENTS

Organophosphorus (OP) compounds are widely used as pesticides in agriculture, for eradication of vectors of malaria and filariasis (e.g. malathion, fenthion), and as chemical warfare agents (e.g. sarin). OPs inactivate acetylcholinesterase (AChE) by phosphorylation, leading to the accumulation of acetylcholine (ACh) at cholinergic synapses. The fatality rate following deliberate ingestion of OP pesticides in developing countries in Asia is ~20% and may reach 70% during certain seasons and at rural hospitals. A sequential triphasic illness follows OP intoxication:

Acute cholinergic syndrome: Occurs within 1 hr of exposure and lasts 48–72 hrs. Clinical features are miosis and muscle fasciculation, followed by paralysis of limb, respiratory and sometimes extraocular muscles.

Intermediate syndrome (IMS): Occurs >48 hrs after poisoning. Progressive muscle weakness due to receptor dysfunction at the neuromuscular junction causes respiratory failure. The onset of the IMS is often rapid, but complete recovery is possible with adequate ventilatory care.

Organophosphate-induced delayed polyneuropathy (OPIDN): Occurs ~1–3 wks after acute exposure or following chronic exposure. Degeneration of long myelinated nerve fibres leads to paraesthesiae and progressive limb weakness. Recovery from OPIDN is often incomplete.

Management (Fig. 4.2)

• Cholinesterase (ChE) estimations (plasma butyryl cholinesterase and red cell AChE) are the only useful biochemical tool for confirming exposure to OPs, but are a poor guide to management and prognosis. • Following removal of contaminated clothing, activated charcoal is given. • Atropine is used to reverse ACh-induced bronchospasm, bronchorrhoea, bradycardia and hypotension. • The role of the oximes, which reactivate phosphorylated AChE, is contentious and dosage and duration of therapy are uncertain. Cost and lack of availability restrict the use of oximes in developing countries.

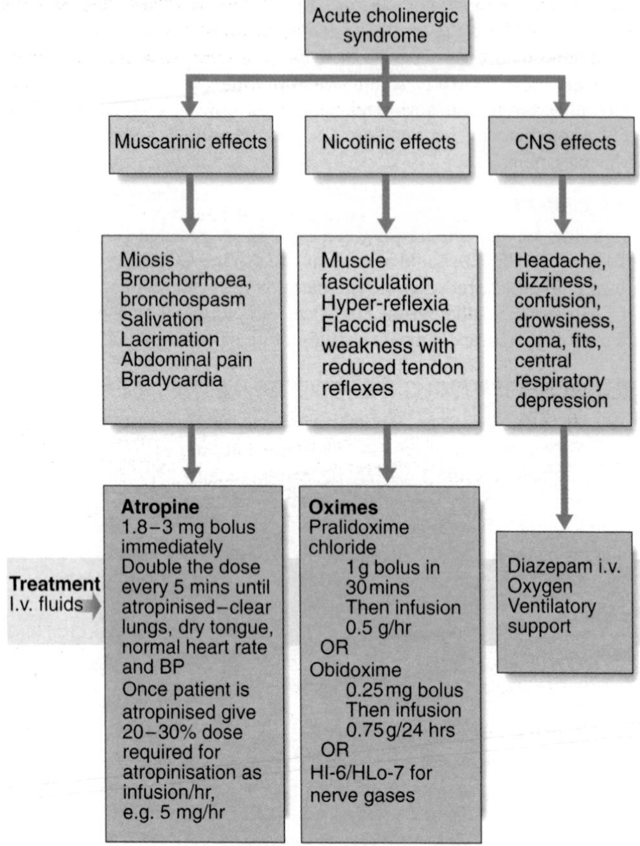

Fig. 4.2 Management of poisoning with organophosphorus compounds.

ENVENOMING

SNAKE BITES

Snake bite is a common life-threatening condition in many tropical countries; farmers, hunters and rice-pickers are at particular risk and prompt medical treatment is vital. The virtually global presence of venomous snakes explains the world-wide estimates of 3–5 million victims/yr, with nearly 50 000 deaths. Snake venoms are complex mixtures of proteins and small polypeptides with enzymatic activity that can produce diverse effects. The classification of snake venoms into neurotoxins, haematotoxins (haemorrhagic or coagulopathic) or cardiotoxins is misleading, as these effects often occur in combination. Management involves:

• Immobilisation of the bitten area to minimise venom spread. • Identification of the snake. • Timely administration of the species-appropriate antivenin. • Cardiovascular, respiratory and renal support may be needed, as may treatment for disseminated intravascular coagulation.

SPIDER BITES

Although nearly all spiders are venomous and bite, most species are not associated with severe envenoming. Factors affecting the clinical features of a spider bite include:

• Species, size, maturity and sex of the spider. • Quantity of venom injected.
• Bacterial flora on the mouthparts. • Number and duration of bites.

For the victim, the severity of envenoming depends on:

• Age. • Pre-existing health. • Size and site of the bite.

The majority of spider bites cause only minor effects (local swelling, pain, erythema and pruritus). Most bites require no first aid measures, but a few species can cause severe systemic effects, in which case an appropriate antivenin is used (e.g. Australian funnel-web spider; the efficacy of this antivenin is such that there have been no published deaths since its introduction).

SCORPION STINGS

In many tropical regions of the world, scorpions are the most important venomous animals after snakes. Most scorpion species produce venom, which causes only minor local reactions in humans, but in Mexico, Tunisia, Algeria, Morocco and Libya scorpion stings are a serious health hazard, and some species produce a venom that contains neurotoxins. More severe envenoming may necessitate airway support and i.v. antivenin.

5

Infectious diseases

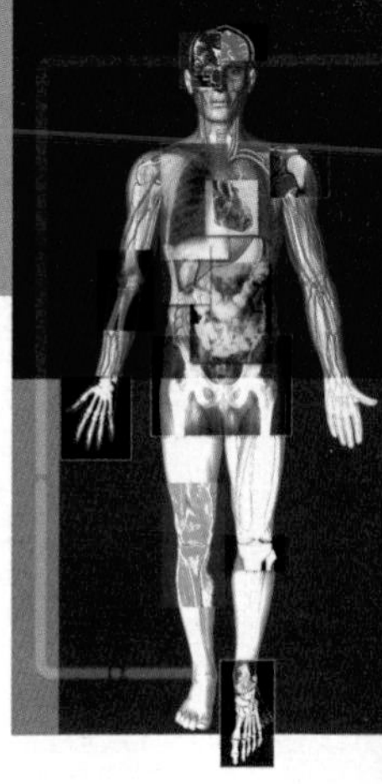

Infectious diseases remain the greatest killers of humankind. Infection differs from other disease processes in that it comprises an interaction between the human body and another organism. Infection has been part of our evolution, evident by the development of a complex immune system. All body systems are susceptible to infection, and understanding infection and its management is integral to clinical care in every medical subspecialty.

PRINCIPLES OF INFECTIOUS DISEASE

The interaction of viruses, bacteria, fungi and protozoa with the human body is:

- Symbiotic (mutually advantageous coexistence). This relationship is the most common, e.g. the numerous colonising bacteria in the human gut. Often the body benefits from this colonisation, as in the prevention of infection with *Clostridium difficile* by normal gut flora.
- Saprophytic (organisms colonise dead material without causing disease). Fungal skin infections are saprophytic, with minimal local damage and systemic upset.
- Parasitic (organisms are detrimental to the host). True infection occurs when organisms breach physiological barriers and enter normally sterile environments such as blood, bones, joints, internal organs or the central nervous system.

CLINICAL EXAMINATION OF THE PYREXIAL PATIENT

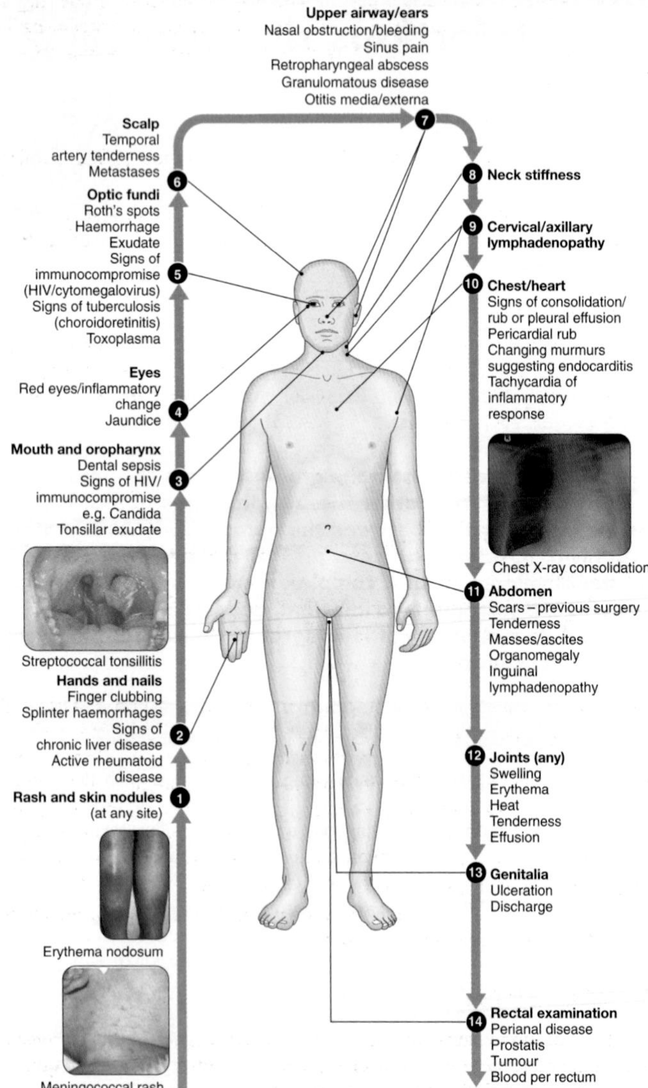

RESERVOIRS OF INFECTION

HUMAN RESERVOIRS

Infection may originate from the skin, nasopharynx or bowel, or from outside sources, often another person who may be infected or carrying a pathogen. Carriers are usually healthy and may harbour the organism in the throat (e.g. meningococci), bowel (e.g. *Salmonella*) or blood (e.g. hepatitis B).

ANIMAL RESERVOIRS

Animals are a significant source of human infections (zoonoses). Examples are:

• Contaminated meat/poultry (*Salmonella*). • Milk (TB, brucellosis). • Body fluids, e.g. saliva (rabies), urine (leptospirosis, Lassa fever). • Bird faeces/ secretions (psittacosis).

ENVIRONMENTAL RESERVOIRS

Environmental infective pathogens include *Legionella* in air conditioning or domestic water pipes, and enteropathogens (typhoid, cholera, *Cryptosporidia* or hepatitis A) in water supplies. The soil may harbour spores of *Clostridia* (tetanus) or anthrax.

TRANSMISSION OF INFECTION

This occurs by several routes:

Endogenous infection: May result from local spread, e.g. from bowel to peritoneum, or via the blood stream.

Exogenous infection: May be acquired by direct contact, aerosol inhalation, needlestick injury or a bite from an animal vector.

HEALTH CARE-ACQUIRED INFECTION (HAI)

Although community-acquired infection predominates, the transmission of infection during health care has become extremely important. HAIs affect approximately 10% of all hospital admissions and create a significant clinical and economic burden. The close proximity of compromised patients in hospitals, coupled with the concentrated use of antibiotics and the ease of transmission by health-care workers, has led to the selection of multidrug-resistant organisms such as MRSA and vancomycin-resistant enterococci (VRE). In addition, the easy spread of these organisms, plus infections such as *Clostridium difficile* and norovirus, may lead to outbreaks of infection necessitating ward or hospital closure.

MANAGEMENT OF INFECTION

Infectious disease results from the interaction between the microorganism and the immune system. The management of infection therefore requires both action to inhibit the microorganism and limitation of the host's inflammatory response. This may involve more than simple antimicrobial therapy; indeed, antibiotics are not required for all infections.

PREVENTION OF INFECTION

• Reduction in the reservoirs of infection will reduce the incidence of disease produced by these organisms. Endogenous reservoirs may be reduced by chemoprophylaxis or by isolation of infective cases. • Separation of animal sources from human hosts and rapid treatment will reduce zoonoses. Blockage of transmission by isolation and vector control will also halt the spread of infection. • Public health measures control spread of infection and vaccination may improve 'herd immunity' in communities. • Prophylactic treatment may help some individuals at high risk of infection.

VACCINATION

The potential to prevent disease by inducing immunity through vaccination remains important. There is a need both to generate new vaccines (e.g. for HIV and malaria), and to improve the efficacy of current vaccines, e.g. influenza.

The world-wide eradication of smallpox (declared by the WHO in 1980) is the best example of how successful vaccination can be in controlling infection. Vaccination becomes successful once the 'herd immunity' of the population reaches the required level to prevent continued spread of the wild-type virus. For example, measles requires >90% vaccination in susceptible persons before this can be achieved. Significant reductions in notifications of both measles and mumps have followed the introduction of effective vaccination schedules. From the mid-1990s in the UK, public concern about possible links of measles, mumps and rubella (MMR) vaccine to autism and inflammatory bowel disease (IBD) reduced vaccine uptake to levels that allowed reappearance of wild virus activity. The UK Medical Research Council expert group and the Commission on Human Medicines both concluded that there is no scientific evidence to link MMR to autism or IBD.

INFECTION CONTROL

HAIs have to be managed by comprehensive antibiotic policies and careful adherence to strict infection control protocols. Although environmental cleanliness and clean clothing are cosmetically important, recent evidence has confirmed the absolute importance of hand hygiene in the control of HAI. The use of alcohol hand lotion by all health-care workers between every patient contact is an effective alternative to soap and water in prevention of most HAI, but not *Clostridium difficile*.

OUTBREAK CONTROL

An outbreak of infection is defined as two or more linked cases of an infectious disease occurring simultaneously or unexpectedly, or the occurrence of any disease clearly in excess of normal expectancy. Many countries have systems of compulsory notification of contagious conditions to public health authorities so that outbreaks can be recognised and appropriate measures put in place to control the further spread of the condition. These measures may include:

• Source isolation. • Quarantine of sufferers or those incubating the condition. • Mass treatment or vaccination.

PRESENTING PROBLEMS IN INFECTIOUS DISEASES

PYREXIA OF UNKNOWN ORIGIN (PUO)

PUO is a common presenting problem and may be defined as a consistently elevated body temperature of >37.5°C persisting for >2 wks with no diagnosis after initial investigation. Many causes of PUO are listed in Box 5.1. Two or more causes of fever may coexist.

5.1 AETIOLOGY OF PUO IN DEVELOPED COUNTRIES
Infections (30%)
• Sepsis: abscess at any site, cholecystitis/cholangitis, urinary tract infection, prostatitis, dental, sinus, bone and joint infections • Imported infections, e.g. malaria, dengue, brucellosis • Occult Bacterial infections; enteric fever, infective endocarditis, TB (particularly extrapulmonary) • Enteric fevers; infective endocarditis; TB (particularly extrapulmonary) • Viral infections (cytomegalovirus (CMV), Epstein–Barr virus (EBV), HIV); toxoplasmosis; fungal infections
Malignancy (20%)
• Lymphoma, myeloma and leukaemia; solid tumours (renal, liver, colon, stomach, pancreas)
Connective tissue disorders (15%)
• Vasculitic disorders; temporal arteritis/polymyalgia rheumatica • Systemic lupus erythematosus (SLE); Still's disease; polymyositis • Rheumatic fever
Miscellaneous (20%)
• Inflammatory bowel disease; liver disease: cirrhosis, granulomatous hepatitis • Sarcoidosis; drug reactions; atrial myxoma; thyrotoxicosis; hypothalamic lesions • Familial Mediterranean fever
No diagnosis or resolves spontaneously (15%)

5.2 FEVER IN OLD AGE
• **Temperature measurement**: fever may be missed because oral temperatures are unreliable in older people. Rectal measurement may be needed but core temperature is increasingly measured using eardrum reflectance.
• **Associated acute confusion**: frequent with fever, especially in those with underlying cerebrovascular disease or other causes of dementia.
• **Prominent causes of PUO**: include endocarditis, TB and intra-abdominal sepsis. Non-infective causes include polymyalgia rheumatica and temporal arteritis.
• **Common infective causes in the very frail** (e.g. nursing home residents): include pneumonia, urinary infection, soft tissue infection and gastroenteritis.

The following account applies to immunocompetent individuals in developed countries with community-acquired PUO. Infection will account for a higher percentage of PUO in developing countries. Fever in old age merits special attention (Box 5.2).

Ask about:

Travel abroad and countries of origin: Malaria, respiratory infections, viral hepatitis, typhoid and dengue are the most common causes of imported fever in the UK.

Personal and social history: Exposure to sexually transmitted infection, illicit drug use.

Occupational or recreational history: Animal exposure, consumption of unpasteurised milk.

Investigations and management

• Measure temperature and vital signs 4-hourly. • Regularly review and expand history-taking. • Repeat physical examination regularly for emerging signs such as cardiac murmurs, lymphadenopathy and rashes. • Investigations should be ordered in a stepwise fashion, in order of increasing complexity and invasiveness (Boxes 5.3 and 5.4).

The role of biopsies in investigation

Liver biopsy: A low-yield investigation, with an estimated mortality of ~0.01%, this may reveal TB, lymphoma or granulomatous disease including sarcoidosis. Biopsies should always be sent for culture, including for TB. Liver biopsy is unlikely to be helpful in patients with normal LFTs and normal liver parenchyma on imaging.

Bone marrow biopsy: Overall, the diagnostic yield of a bone marrow biopsy in PUO is ~15%, the most commonly detected diseases being myelodysplasia, other haematological malignancies and TB. More rarely, brucellosis, enteric fever or visceral leishmaniasis may be detected, underlining the importance of sending samples for culture as well as microscopy.

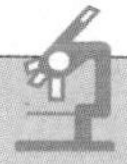

5.3 EARLY TESTS IN THE INVESTIGATION OF PUO IN DEVELOPED COUNTRIES

- FBC and differential white cell count
- ESR and CRP
- Urea, creatinine and electrolytes
- LFTs, including γ-glutamyl transferase
- Blood glucose; serum ferritin; bone biochemistry; creatine phosphokinase
- Malaria blood films (if travel history)
- Urinalysis; MSU for microscopy and culture
- Faeces culture
- Sputum microscopy and culture for common pathogens and for mycobacteria
- Blood cultures × 3
- CXR; USS of abdomen
- ECG

5.4 USEFUL SEROLOGICAL INVESTIGATIONS IN THE MANAGEMENT OF PUO IN DEVELOPED COUNTRIES

Viral	CMV, hepatitis A, B and C, infectious mononucleosis, erythrovirus, HIV, if travel history: Arbovirus
Bacterial	Chlamydia, leptospirosis, Q fever, Lyme disease, brucellosis, *Yersinia*, *Mycoplasma, Streptococcus*, syphilis
If travel history	Rickettsia, relapsing fever, melioidosis, bartonellosis
Fungal	Cryptococcosis (antigen detection)
If travel history	Histoplasmosis, coccidioidomycosis
Protozoal and parasitic	Toxoplasmosis
If travel history	Schistosomiasis, leishmaniasis, amoebiasis, trypanosomiasis

Temporal artery biopsy: Should be considered in patients over the age of 50, even if the ESR is not significantly elevated. Since arteritis is patchy, diagnostic yield is increased if a 5 cm section of artery is biopsied.

Prognosis in PUO

The overall mortality of PUO is 30–40% (5% in patients aged <55 yrs, 40% in those aged >55 yrs), though if no cause is found on exhaustive investigation, the mortality is low. Older patients are more likely to have a malignancy.

FEVER IN THE RETURNING TRAVELLER/ TROPICAL RESIDENT

Presentation of illness as fever is common both in patients returning from the tropics and in tropical residents. Both tropical and non-tropical infection may present after tropical travel. The most common final diagnoses in febrile patients returning from the tropics are:

• Malaria. • Typhoid fever. • Viral hepatitis. • Dengue fever.

Ask about:

• Countries visited. • Arrival and departure dates. • Exposure to animals while abroad. • Food/water consumed. • Freshwater swimming. • Sexual exposure. • Drug use. • Any local medicines/remedies taken.

Vaccinations and prophylaxis

• Ask about vaccinations and their validity; those against yellow fever and against hepatitis A and B virtually rule out these infections. Oral and injectable typhoid vaccinations are 70–90% effective. • Enquire about malaria prophylaxis and establish precisely which tablets, if any, were being taken. Determine malarial resistance levels to the medicine in the country in question.

Examination

A careful examination is vital and must be repeated regularly (Fig. 5.1).

Investigations

Initial investigations in all settings should start with thick and thin blood films for malaria parasites, FBC, urinalysis and CXR if indicated. Box 5.5 gives the diagnoses that should be considered in acute fever with no localising signs, grouped according to differential WCC.

FEVER ASSOCIATED WITH A RASH

Many infective processes produce skin manifestations, either as a result of infection or a toxin or as part of an immune reaction. Different patterns of rash associated with fever are summarised in Box 5.6. Although the combination of fever and rash frequently indicates infection in the mind of the patient, there are many non-infectious causes of this combination, such as the autoimmune vasculitides.

FEVER IN THE INJECTION DRUG-USER

Ask about:

Duration: The risk of contracting hepatitis B/hepatitis C increases with each year of i.v. drug use.

Site: I.v. injection may cause DVT with infection; arterial injection may cause false aneurysm formation and compartment syndrome. Psoas abscess and septic arthritis also occur. *Clostridium* infection has been recorded with i.m. injection of heroin.

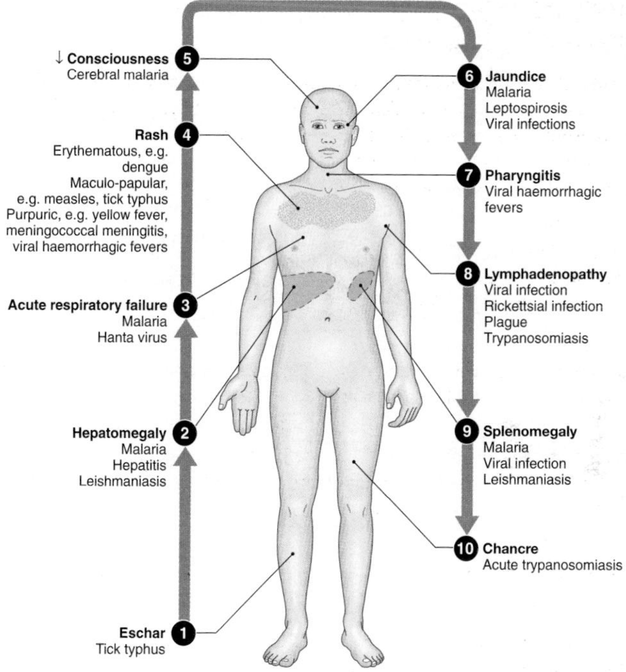

Fig. 5.1 Acute fever in/from the tropics: clinical examination.

Technical details: Sharing of needles and spoons, and use of contaminated drugs or solvents increase the risk of infection.

Clinical assessment

Symptoms are as follows:

Breathlessness: May represent opportunistic infection secondary to HIV/immunosuppression (p. 137). Acute onset with or without pleuritic pain may indicate septic emboli from a distant injection site or from a right-sided (tricuspid or pulmonary valve) endocarditis.

Myalgia and muscle pains: May represent i.m. abscess formation; for example, flexion at the hip eliciting back pain is indicative of ilio-psoas abscess.

Abdominal pain: Opiate-induced constipation, capsular swelling in acute viral hepatitis, splenic infarct secondary to infective endocarditis.

Signs are as follows:

Skin: Necrotising infection, rashes.

Joints: Pain and redness suggest seeding from bacteraemia or direct injection into the joint space. Frequently there is associated osteomyelitis.

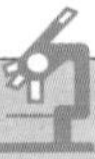

5.5 DIFFERENTIAL WCC: ACUTE FEVER IN THE ABSENCE OF LOCALISING SIGNS		
WCC differential	**Potential diagnoses**	**Further investigations**
Neutrophil leucocytosis	Bacterial sepsis	Blood culture
	Leptospira and *Borrelia*	
	Leptospirosis	Culture of blood and urine, serology
	Tick-borne relapsing fever	Blood film
	Louse-borne relapsing fever	Blood film
	Amoebic liver abscess	USS
Normal WCC and differential	Typhoid fever	Blood, stool and culture
	Typhus	Serology
	Arboviral infection	Serology (PCR and viral culture)
Lymphocytosis	Viral fevers	Serology
	Infectious mononucleosis	Monospot test
	Rickettsial fevers	Serology

New murmurs or evidence of cardiac decompensation: May suggest either right- or left-sided endocarditis (check nails for splinter haemorrhages), or the cardiomyopathy of generalised sepsis. The JVP may show V waves in tricuspid endocarditis. Pleural rub or effusion is seen in DVT with PE, or septic emboli from endocarditis or infected DVT.

Neurological features: Stupor in drug overdose or hepatic encephalopathy, agitation with drug withdrawal, headache and drowsiness in meningitis or encephalitis, local paralysis or spasms with tetanus or botulism.

Legs: Groin injection sites may show abscess, false aneurysm, sinuses or haematoma. DVT or compartment syndrome may be seen in the legs. Hip flexor spasm with back pain suggests an ilio-psoas abscess.

Management

Management is that of the underlying condition. Appropriate sedative medicines should be provided for those suffering withdrawal symptoms after a long period of dependency.

FEVER IN THE NEUTROPENIC PATIENT

Neutropenia is defined as a neutrophil count of $<1.5 \times 10^9$/l.

Patients with neutropenia, particularly $<1.0 \times 10^9$/l, either from drug toxicity (including chemotherapy for cancer) or from marrow invasion or failure, are particularly prone to bacterial infections. Gram-positive organisms have now superseded Gram-negative infections as the most common pathogens in this condition, particularly where any line infection or indwell-

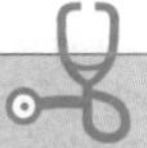

5.6 PATTERNS OF RASH ASSOCIATED WITH INFECTION
Macular or maculo-papular
• Measles*, CMV, rubella, HIV seroconversion illness, enteroviral infection, typhoid and paratyphoid fevers, herpes virus type 6 infections, rickettsial infections, infectious mononucleosis, dengue fever, toxoplasmosis, secondary syphilis, drug rashes
Haemorrhagic
• Meningococcal infection, septicaemia with DIC, viral haemorrhagic fevers, rickettsial infections, leptospirosis
Urticarial
• Toxocariasis, strongyloidiasis, fascioliasis, schistosomiasis
Vesicular/pustular
• Chickenpox*, hand, foot and mouth disease, shingles*, herpangina (mouth), herpes simplex infections*, poxviruses (monkey pox)
Nodular
• Erythema nodosum (primary TB and leprosy, streptococcal infection, *Mycoplasma*)
Erythematous
• Scarlet fever*, Lyme disease, toxic shock syndrome*, drug rashes, human erythrovirus 19 infection*, dengue fever
Chancres (ulcerating nodules)
• Syphilis, typhus (tick and mite), trypanosomiasis, anthrax, rat-bite fever
*Rash is illustrated later in this chapter.

ing catheter is present. Specimens such as blood cultures, swabs and urine samples should be taken and empirical antibiotic therapy started, commonly with a broad-spectrum penicillin and an aminoglycoside (e.g. piperacillin/tazobactam + gentamicin). Any potential nidus of infection such as a urinary or vascular catheter should be removed and, if necessary, replaced.

ACUTE DIARRHOEA

Acute diarrhoea is an extremely common presenting problem, and may result from both infectious and non-infectious causes (Box 5.7). Infectious diarrhoea is caused by faecal–oral transmission of bacterial toxins, viruses, bacteria or protozoal organisms. Psychological or physical stress may also

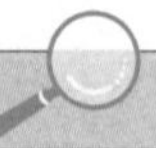

5.7 CAUSES OF ACUTE DIARRHOEA
Infectious
• **Toxin-mediated:** *Bacillus cereus*, clostridial spp., enterotoxin, staphylococcal enterotoxin, scombrotoxic • **Infective food poisoning:** Rotavirus gastroenteritis, *Shigella*, *Campylobacter*, *Clostridium difficile*, *Salmonella*, norovirus, verocytotoxigenic *E. coli*, cholera, other *E. coli* (e.g. travellers' diarrhoea) • **Protozoal:** Giardiasis, isosporiasis, amoebic dysentery, microsporidiosis, *Cryptosporidium* • **Systemic illness:** Sepsis (+ sepsis syndrome), pneumonia (especially 'atypical disease'), meningococcal sepsis, malaria
Non-infectious
• **GI:** Acute diverticulitis, pelvic inflammatory disease, ulcerative colitis, Crohn's disease, overflow from constipation, bowel malignancy • **Metabolic:** Ketosis (e.g. diabetic decompensation), carcinoid syndrome, vasoactive intestinal peptide release, uraemia • **Drugs and toxins:** NSAIDs, dinoflagellates, cytotoxic agents, plant toxins, antibiotics, heavy metals, ciguatera fish poisoning

precipitate diarrhoea. Occasionally, diarrhoea may be the presenting feature of another systemic illness, such as a lobar pneumonia.

FOOD POISONING AND GASTROENTERITIS

Acute gastroenteritis is a major cause of morbidity and mortality in both developing and developed countries. Causative organisms are listed in Boxes 5.7 and 5.8. The clinical features of food-borne disease depend on the organism; for example, enterotoxic organisms produce vomiting and 'secretory' watery diarrhoea. Organisms that invade the mucosa, such as *Shigella* and *Salmonella*, have longer incubation periods and may cause systemic upset and blood in the stool.

ASSESSMENT OF THE PATIENT WITH ACUTE DIARRHOEA

Box 5.9 shows markers of severity and coexisting conditions which increase the likelihood that intensive treatment (e.g. antimicrobials) will be needed.

Ask about:

• Duration and frequency of diarrhoea. • Presence of blood, abdominal pain and tenesmus. • Suspect foods. • Other family members affected.

Examination

• Record 4-hourly temperature and vital signs. • Assess degree of dehydration by skin turgor and BP measurement. • Measure urine output and ongoing stool losses. • Carry out regular full abdominal examination.

5.8 CAUSES OF BLOODY DIARRHOEA
Infectious
• *Campylobacter* spp., *Shigella* dysentery, non-typhoidal salmonellae, enterohaemorrhagic or entero-invasive *E. coli*, *Clostridium difficile*, *Vibrio parahaemolyticus*, *Entamoeba histolytica*
Non-infectious
• Diverticular disease, rectal or colonic malignancy, inflammatory bowel disease, bleeding haemorrhoids, anal fissure, ischaemic colitis, intussusception

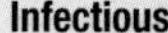

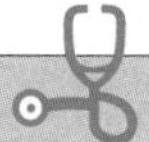

5.9 SEVERITY MARKERS IN ACUTE GASTROENTERITIS
Chronic conditions
• Age >65, diabetes mellitus, rheumatoid or other autoimmune disease, chronic renal disease, valvular heart disease (esp. with valve replacements), acquired or secondary immunodeficiency, any internal prostheses
Current drug therapy
• Diuretics, ACE inhibitors, corticosteroids, cytotoxics, proton pump or H_2-receptor blockers
Current illness
• No. of stools/24 hrs, presence of blood p.r., abdominal pain, associated systemic toxicity

Investigations

• Stool microscopy and culture. • FBC and serum electrolytes. • Blood film for malaria if patient has been in an affected area.

MANAGEMENT OF ACUTE DIARRHOEA

Isolation: All patients with acute, potentially infective diarrhoea should be appropriately isolated to minimise person-to-person spread of infection.

Fluid replacement: Replace established losses and ongoing losses, as well as normal daily requirements. This may be done with i.v. fluid or with oral rehydration solution (ORS).

Antibiotics/antimicrobial therapy: Not generally used, except in severe cases (Box 5.9). Have a high threshold for their use and discuss with the infectious diseases department.

Adjunctive antidiarrhoeal therapy: Anti-motility drugs are not generally recommended and may indeed prolong or worsen the course of an acute infective gastroenteritis.

CHRONIC DIARRHOEA

This is defined as diarrhoea persisting for >14 days. The differential diagnosis can be wide, and parasitic and bacterial causes, tropical malabsorption, inflammatory bowel disease and neoplasia should all be considered. Causes of chronic diarrhoea in the tropics include giardiasis, strongyloidiasis, HIV enteropathy, intestinal flukes and chronic intestinal schistosomiasis. The key signs and symptoms are:

• Diarrhoea with pale, bulky stools. • Abdominal symptoms with distension and flatulence. • Nutritional deficiencies. • General ill health.

Specific causes should be treated as described later in this chapter.

EOSINOPHILIA

Eosinophilia is associated both with parasite infections (particularly helminths) and with allergic reactions. Eosinophils have an important role in mediating antibody-dependent damage to helminths. Anybody with an eosinophil count $>0.4 \times 10^9$ should be investigated for both parasitic and non-parasitic causes of eosinophilia (Box 5.10). Eosinophilia is not a typical feature in malaria, amoebiasis, leishmaniasis, leprosy or tapeworm infections other than cysticercosis.

Ask about:

• Travel and activity abroad, e.g. freshwater bathing in sub-Saharan Africa. • Any rashes or itching (schistosomiasis, strongyloidiasis). • Haematuria (schistosomiasis). • Subcutaneous swellings (loiasis, cutaneous larva migrans).

Clinical assessment

See Box 5.11.

5.10 CAUSES OF EOSINOPHILIA

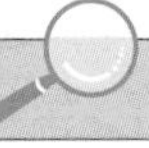

• Metazoan parasite infections	• Atopy and allergic drug reactions
• Skin diseases	• Pulmonary eosinophilia
• HIV	• Human T-cell lymphotropic virus 1 (HTLV 1)
• Lymphomas	• Leukaemias
• Polyarteritis nodosa	• Sarcoidosis
• Hypereosinophilic syndrome	

5.11 CLINICAL FEATURES ASSOCIATED WITH HELMINTHIC INFECTIONS AND EOSINOPHILIA	
Urticarial rashes	Strongyloidiasis, onchocerciasis, fascioliasis, hydatid disease, trichinosis
Cutaneous larva migrans	*Ancylostoma braziliense*
Dermatitis	Onchocerciasis
Migratory subcutaneous swellings	Loiasis, gnathostomiasis
Lymphangitis, orchitis	Lymphatic filariasis
Myositis	Trichinosis, cysticercosis
Febrile hepatosplenomegaly	Schistosomiasis, toxocariasis
Pneumonitis	Migratory stage of larval helminths (Löffler's syndrome), lymphatic filariasis (tropical pulmonary eosinophilia), systemic strongyloidiasis
Enteritis and colitis	Strongyloidiasis, capillariasis, trichinosis
Meningitis	Angiostrongyliasis, strongyloidiasis

5.12 INITIAL INVESTIGATION OF EOSINOPHILIA

Investigation	Pathogens sought
Stool microscopy	Ova, cysts and parasites
Terminal urine	Ova of *Schistosoma haematobium*
Duodenal aspirate	Filariform larvae of *Strongyloides*, liver fluke ova
Day bloods	Microfilariae *Brugia malayi, Loa loa*
Night bloods	Microfilariae *Wuchereria bancrofti*
Skin snips	*Onchocerca volvulus*
Serology	*Schistosoma*, *Filaria*, *Strongyloides*, hydatid, trichinosis etc.

Investigations

Direct visualisation of adult worms, larvae or ova provides the best evidence. Box 5.12 lists the initial investigations for eosinophilia.

SKIN CONDITIONS IN THE RETURNING TRAVELLER/TROPICAL RESIDENT

CUTANEOUS LARVA MIGRANS (CLM)

CLM is the most common linear lesion seen in travellers. Intensely pruritic, linear, serpiginous lesions result from the larval migration of the dog hookworm (*Ancylostoma caninum*). The track migrates across the skin at a rate of 2–3 cm/day. Most patients have recently visited a beach where the affected part (foot, elbows, buttocks or breast) was exposed. The diagnosis is clinical, and treatment consists of topical application of 15% tiabendazole cream 12-hourly, or a single systemic dose of albendazole or ivermectin.

TROPICAL ULCER

Tropical ulcer occurs in hot humid regions and most commonly starts with a papule on the lower legs that rapidly breaks down to a sharply defined, painful ulcer with a foul slough at the base. It is due to a synergistic bacterial infection caused by the anaerobe *Fusobacterium ulcerans* and *Treponema vincentii*. Penicillin and metronidazole are useful in the early stages but rest, elevation and dressings are the mainstays of treatment.

JIGGERS (TUNGIASIS)

This is widespread in tropical America and Africa, and is caused by the sand flea *Tunga penetrans,* which burrows into the skin around toes depositing large numbers of eggs. The burrows are intensely irritating and the whole inflammatory nodule should be removed with a sterile needle. Secondary infection is common.

MYIASIS

Myiasis is due to larvae of the South American botfly, *Dermatobia hominis*, and the African Tumbu fly, *Cordylobia anthropophaga*, infesting the subcutaneous space. Patients with myiasis feel movement within the larval burrow and experience intermittent sharp, lancinating pains. The larva may be extruded by squeezing gently on the burrow and catching it with tweezers. Alternatively, it may be suffocated by blocking the respiratory orifice with petroleum jelly. Rapid healing follows removal of intact larvae.

VIRAL INFECTIONS

Viruses are simple infectious agents consisting of a portion of genetic material, RNA or DNA, enclosed in a protein coat which is antigenically unique for that species. They cannot exist in a free-living state, needing to infect host cells to survive. Once inside cells, they utilise host material for protein synthesis and genetic reproduction. All viral infections must therefore originate from an infected source by either direct or vector-mediated spread. Viruses affecting humans are summarised in Boxes 5.13 and 5.14.

COMMON VIRAL INFECTIONS AND CHILDHOOD EXANTHEMS

The term 'exanthem' describes the rash that characterises an eruptive fever. Although the incidence of exanthems has diminished as a result of vaccina-

5.13 DNA VIRUSES INVOLVED IN HUMAN DISEASE	
Classification/viruses involved	**Clinical syndromes**
Adenoviruses	Upper respiratory tract infection/pharyngitis, acute diarrhoea
Herpes viruses	
Herpes simplex types 1 and 2	Acute/recurrent vesicular rash
Varicella zoster	Chickenpox/shingles
Cytomegalovirus	Acute/recurrent hepatorenal infection
Human herpes virus 6 and 7	Roseola infantum
Epstein–Barr virus	Infectious mononucleosis, Burkitt's lymphoma
Human herpes virus 8	Nasopharyngeal carcinoma, Kaposi's sarcoma
Papovaviruses	
Human papillomavirus	Common wart
Polyoma (human BK and JC)	Progressive multifocal leucoencephalopathy
Human erythrovirus 19	Erythema infectiosum
Poxviruses	
Variola	Smallpox
Monkey pox	
Cowpox	
Vaccinia	Smallpox vaccination
Orf virus	
Molluscum contagiosum	

tion programmes, they still represent an important cause of morbidity and mortality world-wide.

MEASLES

This paramyxovirus infection is endemic world-wide. It is probably the most infectious of all microbial agents. Maternal antibody gives protection for the first 6 mths of life. With live attenuated vaccine, the condition is potentially completely controllable by immunisation. Incomplete vaccination of only 70–80% of the population may lead to outbreaks in older children and adults, in whom complications are more frequent. This necessitates repeat mass immunisation campaigns or second dosing of vaccine in an older age group.

Clinical features and complications

Infection is by droplet spread with an incubation period of 14 days to onset of rash. A prodromal illness 1–3 days before the rash appears heralds the most infectious, 'catarrhal' stage with upper respiratory symptoms, conjunctivitis and the presence of 'Koplik's spots' (small white spots sur-

5.14 RNA VIRUSES INVOLVED IN HUMAN DISEASE

Classification/viruses involved	Clinical syndromes
Picornaviruses	
Poliovirus, echoviruses, Coxsackie, enteroviruses 68–72	Gut/neurological illness
Hepatitis A	
Rhinoviruses	Upper respiratory tract infection
Rheoviruses	
Rheovirus	Mild upper respiratory tract infection/ gut disease
Rotavirus	Gastroenteritis
Togaviruses	
Rubella	German measles
Alphaviruses	Mosquito-borne encephalitides
Flaviviruses	
Yellow fever	Yellow/haemorrhagic fever
Dengue, other arboviruses	Haemorrhagic fevers
Hepatitis C	Chronic hepatitis
Bunyaviruses	
Congo–Crimean fever	Acute hepatitis
Hantavirus	Gastroenteritis
Calicivirus	
Hepatitis E, norovirus	Acute gastroenteritis
Astrovirus	Acute epidemic lower respiratory tract infection
Orthomyxoviruses	
Influenza A, B	Influenza
Paramyxoviruses	
Measles, mumps, respiratory syncytial virus	
Rhabdoviruses	Rabies
Retroviruses	
HIV-1 and 2	HIV infection syndrome/AIDS
Arenaviruses	
Lassa	Lassa fever
Lymphocytic choriomeningitis	
Filoviruses	
Marburg and Ebola viruses	
Hepadnavirus	
Hepatitis B	

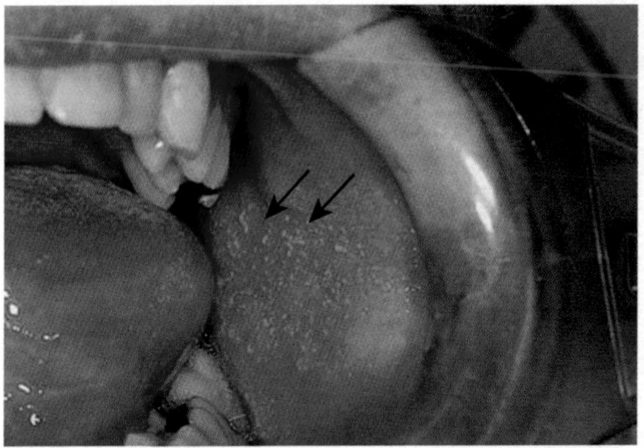

Fig. 5.2 Koplik's spots (arrows) seen on buccal mucosa in the early stages of clinical measles.

rounded by erythema) on the internal buccal mucosa (Fig. 5.2). At this stage the patient is miserable, irritable and photophobic, corresponding to the peak of a second viraemia. As natural antibody develops, the rash appears (Fig. 5.3), lasting 5–6 days and gradually fading with 'staining' in the pale-skinned. Lymphadenopathy and diarrhoea are common.

Complications include:

• Encephalitis/convulsions. • Bacterial pneumonia. • Otitis media. • Subacute sclerosing panencephalitis.

Management

• In the immunocompetent, the disease is self-limiting and confers life-long immunity. • Pregnant women should be considered for treatment with immunoglobulin. • All children should be vaccinated against measles. • Antibiotics are only indicated for superinfection.

RUBELLA (GERMAN MEASLES)

Rubella is a viral illness transmitted by aerosol, with infectivity from up to 1 wk before to 1 wk after the onset of the rash. Outbreaks occur in spring and early summer, with epidemics every 7–10 yrs. Many childhood cases are subclinical, and the greatest significance of rubella is for the pregnant woman, as rubella infection in the early stages of pregnancy may result in profound congenital abnormalities.

Infection presents with lymphadenopathy and a maculo-papular non-confluent rash which starts on the face and moves to the trunk. Petechial lesions ('Forchheimer spots') appear on the soft palate, associated with a mild coryza/conjunctivitis. Fever occurs only on the first day of the rash. Arthralgia and mild hepatitis can occur. Encephalitis can rarely complicate rubella. If infection is suspected in a pregnant woman, it is important to

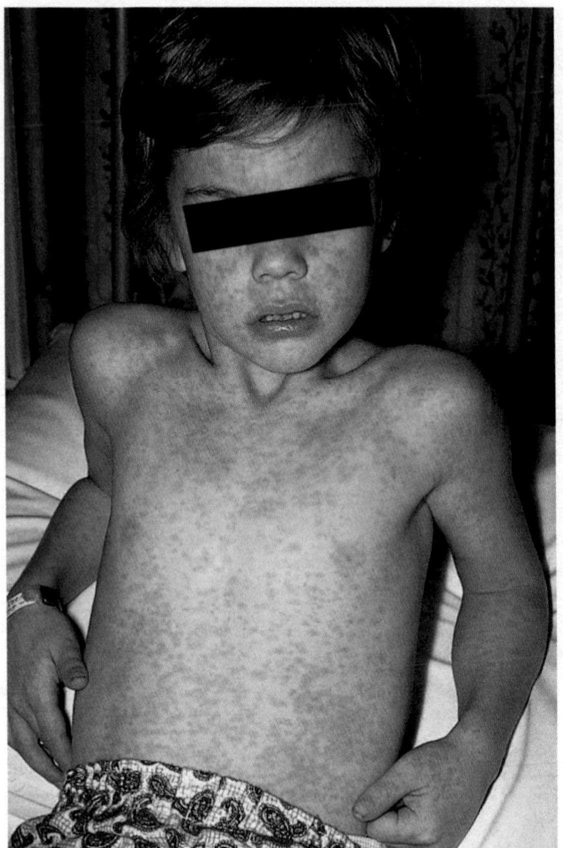

Fig. 5.3 Typical measles rash.

establish immune status. Detection of rubella-specific IgG indicates past infection and thus immunity. Children should be immunised against rubella as part of standard vaccination programmes.

HUMAN ERYTHROVIRUS 19 (PARVOVIRUS B19) (Fig. 5.4)

This air-borne virus occurs world-wide and produces a mild or subclinical infection in normal hosts. In addition to the clinical manifestations summarised in Box 5.15, there may be a transient bone marrow suppression resulting in a mild thrombocytopenia, lymphopenia and neutropenia. Erythrovirus 19 DNA may be detected in the serum by PCR; however, as illness

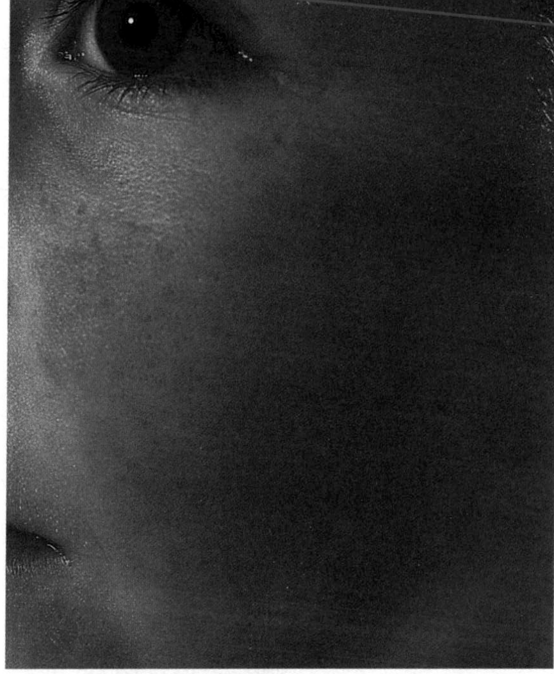

Fig. 5.4 Slapped cheek syndrome. The typical facial rash of human erythrovirus 19 infection.

is usually mild or subclinical, confirmatory blood tests are not always required. If infection occurs during pregnancy, the fetus should be monitored closely for signs of hydrops.

MUMPS

This paramyxovirus is endemic world-wide. In non-vaccinated populations, it occurs in epidemics every 2–3 yrs, primarily infecting 5–9-yr-old children. If vaccination has been employed without complete eradication of the disease, there is increased susceptibility in older teenagers. Infection is by droplets or direct salivary spread and initial infection is through the upper respiratory tract. A primary viraemia seeds the virus to target organs: parotid glands, other exocrine glands, meninges and sites of gametogenesis. The incubation period lasts 14–21 days and the patient is infectious from day 12 to day 25 after exposure. Classical tender parotid enlargement, which is bilateral in 75%, follows a prodrome of pyrexia and malaise. Other salivary glands are involved in ~10% of cases.

5.15 CLINICAL FEATURES OF HUMAN ERYTHROVIRUS 19 INFECTION		
Disease caused by erythrovirus 19	**Affected age group**	**Clinical manifestations**
Fifth disease (erythema infectiosum)	Small children	Three clinical stages: a 'slapped cheek' appearance, reticulate eruption on the body and limbs, then resolution. Often the child is quite well throughout
Gloves and socks syndrome	Young adults	Fever and an acral purpuric eruption with a clear margin at the wrists and ankles. Mucosal involvement also occurs
Arthropathies	Adults, occasionally children	Polyarthropathy of small joints. In children it tends to involve the larger joints in an asymmetrical distribution
Red cell aplasia	Adults, those with haematological disease, the immunosuppressed	Can cause a mild anaemia but in an individual with underlying haematological abnormality can precipitate an aplastic crisis
Hydrops fetalis	Transplacental fetal infection	Asymptomatic or symptomatic maternal infection can cause fetal anaemia with aplastic crisis leading to non-immune hydrops fetalis and spontaneous abortion

Complications

• Oophoritis and orchitis (only occur post-pubertally). • Testicular atrophy—though sterility is most unlikely. • Mumps meningitis—three times more common in males than females. • Encephalitis. • Transient hearing loss and labyrinthitis—uncommon. • Spontaneous abortion.

Management

• Mumps vaccine, given as part of the MMR combined vaccine, has markedly reduced the incidence of natural infection and, if used widely, abolishes the epidemic pattern of disease. • Short-course oral steroids may be of use in orchitis.

HUMAN HERPES VIRUS 6 AND 7 (HHV-6 AND HHV-7)

These viruses were only identified in the 1990s. They are associated with a benign febrile illness of children with a maculo-papular erythematous rash: 'roseola infantum'/'exanthem subitum'. In the immunocompromised they cause lymphadenopathy.

VIRAL INFECTIONS OF THE SKIN

A number of viral infections produce manifestations predominantly in the skin. The herpes virus group consists of at least eight organisms causing different pathologies (see Box 5.13).

HERPES SIMPLEX VIRUS (HSV)

Types 1 and 2 of this common virus affect humans.

• Type 1 HSV produces mucocutaneous lesions, predominantly of the head and neck. • Type 2 disease is a sexually transmitted anogenital infection.

The source of infection is a case of primary or active recurrent disease (HSV is reactivated from latency in the dorsal root ganglion). Primary infection normally occurs as a vesiculating gingivostomatitis. It may also present as a keratitis (dendritic ulcer), viral paronychia, vulvovaginitis, cervicitis (often unrecognised), balanitis or rarely as encephalitis. Diagnosis is by PCR, electron microscopy or culture of vesicular fluid.

Complications

• Dendritic ulcers: may produce corneal ulcers and scarring. • Encephalitis: preferentially affects the temporal lobe. • Eczema herpeticum (Fig. 5.5): HSV infection in patients with eczema can result in a serious infection and

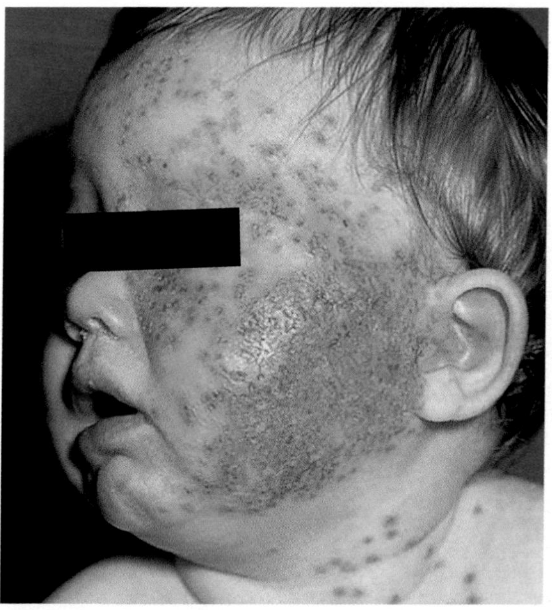

Fig. 5.5 Eczema herpeticum. HSV-1 infection spreads rapidly in eczematous skin.

needs urgent investigation and empirical antiviral treatment. • Neonatal HSV infection: may be disseminated and potentially fatal.

Management

Treatment is with antiviral agents such as aciclovir or famciclovir.

CHICKENPOX

Varicella zoster virus (VZV) is spread by the aerosol route and is highly infectious. Disease in children is usually better tolerated than in adults, pregnant women and the immunocompromised.

The incubation period is 14–21 days, after which a vesicular eruption begins (Fig. 5.6), often on mucosal surfaces first, followed by rapid dissemination in a centripetal fashion. New lesions occur in crops every 2–4 days, accompanied by fever. The rash progresses from small pink macules to vesicles and pustules within 24 hrs, which then crust. Infectivity lasts until crusts separate. Diagnosis is clinical but may be confirmed by PCR of vesicular fluid. Antiviral agents such as aciclovir and famciclovir have a role only in the immunosuppressed or those with pneumonitis. Human VZV immunoglobulin may attenuate infection in highly susceptible contacts of chickenpox sufferers such as the immunosuppressed and pregnant women. VZV vaccine, now in use in the USA, offers effective protection.

Complications

• Secondary bacterial infection of rash (due to scratching). • Self-limiting cerebellar ataxia. • Congenital abnormalities if maternal disease is contracted in the first trimester. • Severe life-threatening pneumonitis.

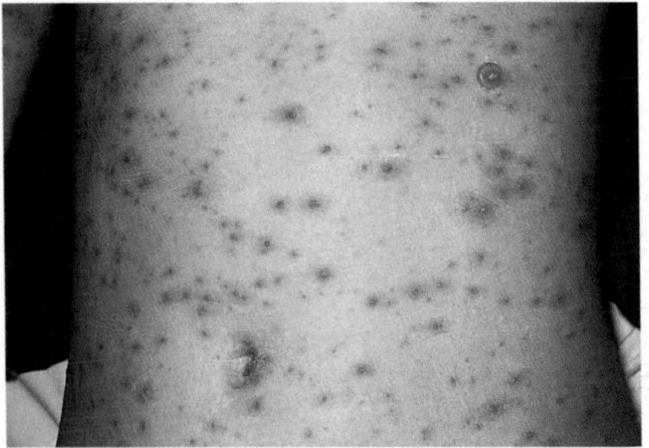

Fig. 5.6 Chickenpox.

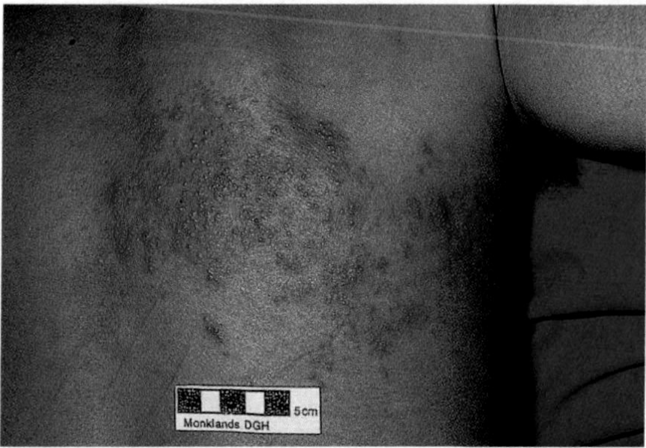

Fig. 5.7 Typical 'shingles' varicella zoster virus infection reactivating in a thoracic dermatome: 'a band of roses from Hell'.

SHINGLES (HERPES ZOSTER)

This is produced by reactivation of latent VZV from the dorsal root ganglion of sensory nerves and most commonly involves the thoracic dermatomes and the ophthalmic division of the trigeminal nerve (Fig. 5.7).

Shingles starts with a prodromal burning discomfort, followed by a vesicular rash. There may be systemic flu-like symptoms. Commonly seen in the elderly, it may present in younger patients with immune deficiency or after intrauterine infection. The diagnosis is clinical but may be confirmed by PCR of vesicular fluid. Early therapy with aciclovir or valaciclovir is indicated, and may prevent the development of post-herpetic neuralgia.

Complications

• Ramsay Hunt syndrome: facial palsy, ipsilateral loss of taste and buccal ulceration, and a rash in the external auditory canal. • Post-herpetic neuralgia: can be difficult to treat but may respond to amitriptyline or gabapentin. • Myelitis/encephalitis: rare.

HUMAN HERPES VIRUS 8 (HHV-8)

This virus (see Box 5.13) has been linked to Kaposi's sarcoma tumour cells in both AIDS-related and endemic non-AIDS-related forms.

HAND, FOOT AND MOUTH DISEASE/HERPANGINA

These are largely diseases of childhood, caused by Coxsackie viruses. Hand, foot and mouth disease is a relatively mild illness with fever, lymphadenopathy, mouth ulceration and a vesicular eruption on the hands and feet. Herpangina causes discrete vesicles on the palate associated with high fever, sore throat and headache. Both conditions are self-limiting without treatment.

POXVIRUS INFECTIONS

These DNA viruses are potentially important pathogens but nowadays rarely cause significant human disease. They include smallpox, monkey pox and cow pox, as well as orf and molluscum contagiosum (p. 722).

Smallpox (variola): This severe disease, with a 30% mortality in the unvaccinated and no current effective therapy, was eradicated world-wide in 1980 following a successful international vaccination campaign. The classical form is characterised by a typical centrifugal vesicular/pustular rash, worst on the face and extremities, with no cropping (i.e. unlike chickenpox) and accompanied by fever, severe myalgia and odynophagia.

SYSTEMIC VIRAL INFECTIONS

INFLUENZA

See page 292.

INFECTIOUS MONONUCLEOSIS (IM)

IM is caused by the Epstein–Barr virus (EBV), a herpes virus usually acquired from asymptomatic excreters. Saliva is the main means of spread, either by droplet infection or environmental contamination in childhood, or by kissing among adolescents and young adults, the age group in which infection is most common. There is a good correlation between sexual maturity and IM, and the age/sex distribution of the disease resembles that of gonorrhoea. IM is not highly contagious, isolation is unnecessary and documented outbreaks seldom occur.

Clinical features

• Lymphadenopathy, especially posterior cervical. • Pharyngeal inflammation or exudates. • Fever. • Splenomegaly. • Palatal petechiae. • Periorbital oedema. • Clinical or biochemical evidence of hepatitis. • A non-specific rash.

Complications

• Common complications include an antibiotic-induced rash (classically amoxicillin), severe laryngeal oedema and chronic fatigue syndrome. • Less common sequelae include cranial nerve palsies, meningoencephalitis, haemolytic anaemia, thrombocytopenia, glomerulonephritis, pericarditis, pneumonitis and splenic rupture.

Diagnosis

• Monospot test (heterophile antibody absorption test): may initially be negative so should be repeated if clinical suspicion is high. • Atypical lymphocytes (>20%) on blood film.

Management

• Treatment is symptomatic, e.g. aspirin gargles to relieve a sore throat. • Oral prednisolone may be required to relieve laryngeal oedema. • Chronic fatigue is difficult to treat but may respond to graded exercise programmes. • Contact sports should be avoided until splenomegaly has resolved to avoid splenic rupture.

ACQUIRED CYTOMEGALOVIRUS (CMV) INFECTION

CMV is a herpes virus which usually causes asymptomatic infection in children and young adults. The infection is transferred by contact with an excreter, who sheds virus in saliva, urine and genital secretions.

CMV infection may occasionally produce a flu-like illness resembling IM. Lymphadenopathy, pharyngitis and tonsillitis are found less often than in IM. Unusual complications include neurological involvement, autoimmune haemolytic anaemia, pericarditis, pneumonitis and arthropathy. CMV retinitis is an AIDS-defining illness important in immunosuppressed patients. Gestational CMV infection may result in congenital neurological damage to the fetus, as the virus can cross the placenta.

Monospot test will be negative in CMV infection. Atypical lymphocytes may be seen on blood film but are less common than in IM. Detection of CMV-specific IgM antibody confirms the diagnosis and treatment is symptomatic.

DENGUE

The dengue flavivirus is spread by the vector mosquito *Aedes aegypti* in South-east Asia, India and Africa. There have been recent large epidemics in the Caribbean and Americas.

The incubation period following an infected mosquito bite is 2–7 days, with a prodrome of malaise and headache, followed by a morbilliform rash, arthralgia, pain on eye movement, headache, nausea, vomiting, lymphadenopathy and fever. The rash spreads centrifugally, spares the palms and the soles, and may desquamate on resolution. The disease is self-limiting but convalescence is slow.

Dengue haemorrhagic fever or dengue shock syndrome: Occasionally, patients may have a more severe manifestation of the infection, characterised by fever, circulatory failure and features of a capillary leak syndrome. Disseminated intravascular coagulation (DIC) may occur, followed by major and minor haemorrhagic complications such as petechiae, ecchymoses, epistaxis or GI bleeding. There may also be a hepatitis. Case fatality with this aggressive form of the disease may be as high as 10%.

Investigations

• Amplification of dengue RNA by PCR. • Detection of a rise in anti-dengue IgG antibody titres.

Management and prevention

• Management is supportive, with treatment of haemorrhage, shock and pain as required. • Insecticides which control mosquito levels help to limit transmission. • There is currently no vaccine; a tetravalent one would be required to cover the four serotypes.

YELLOW FEVER

Yellow fever is caused by a flavivirus and is normally a zoonosis of monkeys that inhabit tropical rainforests in West and Central Africa and South and Central America. It is transferred to humans by infected *Aedes* mosquitoes and is a major public health problem, causing 200 000 to 300 000 deaths a year, mainly in sub-Saharan Africa.

The incubation period is 3–6 days, and the acute phase is usually characterised by a mild febrile illness lasting less than a week. In severe cases the disease starts suddenly with rigors and high fever, severe backache, headache and bone pains. Nausea and vomiting then develop. The face is flushed and the conjunctivae are injected. Bradycardia and leucopenia are characteristic of this phase of the illness, which lasts 3 days and is followed by a period of remission lasting a few hours or days. The fever then returns with acute hepatic and renal failure. There is jaundice and a haemorrhagic diathesis with petechiae, haemorrhages into the mucosa and GI bleeding plus oliguria. Patients commonly die in the third stage, often after a period of coma.

Management

• Treatment is supportive, with meticulous attention to fluid and electrolyte balance, urine output and BP. • Blood transfusions, plasma expanders and peritoneal dialysis may be necessary. • A vaccination effective for at least 10 yrs is available.

VIRAL HAEMORRHAGIC FEVERS

The viral haemorrhagic fevers are zoonoses caused by several different viruses, and are endemic world-wide. They are summarised in Box 5.16. Management is supportive, with the addition of i.v. ribavirin. Patients should be isolated and infection control measures implemented in order to prevent spread.

GASTROINTESTINAL VIRAL INFECTIONS

NOROVIRUS (NORWALK AGENT)

Norovirus has been identified both in outbreaks related to infected food handlers and in endemic person-to-person gastroenteritis. Seroprevalence surveys suggest that many adults are susceptible to this infection. These viruses spread by faeco-oral transmission, or by aerosol spread if susceptible individuals are in the vicinity of a sufferer actively vomiting. After a 48-hr incubation period there is a brisk 2–3-day illness with marked nausea, predominant vomiting and little diarrhoea. Stepwise transmission of illness through nurseries and families remains very common. Norovirus outbreaks in health-care facilities are becoming a major problem.

ROTAVIRUS

Rotaviruses are the major cause of diarrhoeal illness in young children, accounting for 30–50% of cases admitted to hospital in developed coun-

5.16 COMMON VIRAL HAEMORRHAGIC FEVERS

Disease	Reservoir	Transmission	Geography	Mortality	Clinical features[1]
Lassa fever	Multimammate rats Patient	Urine Body fluids	W. Africa	Up to 50%	Encephalopathy, ARDS (responds to ribavirin)
Marburg/Ebola virus	? Monkeys	Body fluids	Central Africa	25–90%	Thrombocytopenia, blood oozing
Yellow fever	Monkeys	Mosquitoes	Tropical Africa, S. and Central America	10–60%	Hepatic failure, blood oozing
Dengue	Humans	*Aedes aegypti*	Tropical and subtropical coasts	Nil–10%[2]	Joint and bone pain, petechiae
Crimean–Congo	*Ixodes* tick	*Ixodes* tick	Africa, Asia, E. Europe	15–70%	Thrombocytopenia, blood oozing, petechiae
Bolivian and Argentinean	Rodents (*Calomys* spp.)	Urine	South America	?	Thrombocytopenia, petechiae
Haemorrhagic fever with renal syndrome (Hantan fever)	Rodents	Faeces	N. Asia, N. Europe	30%	Petechiae, renal failure, ARDS

[1] All potentially have circulatory failure.
[2] Mortality of uncomplicated and haemorrhagic dengue fever, respectively.

tries, and 10–20% of deaths due to gastroenteritis in developing countries. Infection is endemic in developing countries. There are winter epidemics in developed countries, particularly in hospitals. The virus infects enterocytes, causing decreased surface absorption and loss of enzymes on the brush border. The incubation period is 48 hrs and patients present with watery diarrhoea, vomiting, fever and abdominal pain. Diagnosis is aided by commercially available enzyme immunoassay kits which simply require fresh or refrigerated stool for effective demonstration of the pathogens. The disease is self-limiting but dehydration needs appropriate management.

OTHER VIRUSES

Adenoviruses are frequently identified from stool culture and implicated as a cause of diarrhoea. Two serotypes (40 and 41) appear to be more frequently found in association with diarrhoea than the more common upper respiratory types 1–7.

BACTERIAL INFECTIONS

BACTERIAL INFECTIONS OF THE SKIN AND SOFT TISSUES

STAPHYLOCOCCAL INFECTIONS

Staphylococci are normal commensals of human skin, which do not normally cause infection unless there is a break in the integument, either induced by a foreign body such as a cannula or a surgical incision, or as a result of a primary skin condition such as eczema when skin barrier function is impaired. Ecthyma, folliculitis, furuncles and carbuncles represent superficial skin infection with this ubiquitous organism (p. 720).

Wound infections and cannula-related infections caused by *Staph. aureus* are important causes of inpatient morbidity. Their incidence may be lessened by good infection control techniques. In cases where there is evidence of spreading infection such as a surrounding cellulitis, anti-staphylococcal antimicrobial therapy, e.g. flucloxacillin and benzylpenicillin, should be instituted. I.V. drug-users who share injecting equipment are susceptible to skin and subcutaneous tissue infections, and may also develop thrombosis in the affected limb. If staphylococcal infection reaches the blood stream (staphylococcal septicaemia), this may cause severe sepsis and needs to be treated aggressively. Secondary spread to the heart valves causing endocarditis is possible in any superficial staphylococcal infection.

Meticillin-resistant Staph. aureus (MRSA)

Resistance to meticillin due to the production of an additional penicillin-binding protein has been recognised in *Staph. aureus* for over 30 yrs. MRSA is a major health care-acquired pathogen, and the recent recognition of resistance to vancomycin/teicoplanin (glycopeptides) in either glycopeptide intermediate *Staph. aureus* (GISA) or, rarely, vancomycin-resistant (VRSA) strains threatens our ability to manage serious infections produced by such organisms. MRSA now accounts for up to 40% of staphylococcal bacteraemia in developed countries, requiring care in both control and specific therapy of these infections. Clinicians must be aware of the potential danger and take whatever appropriate infection control measures are advised locally.

Staphylococcal toxic shock syndrome (TSS)

This serious and life-threatening disease is associated with infection by *Staph. aureus* which is producing toxic shock syndrome toxin 1 (TSST1). It is most commonly seen in young women during, or immediately after, menstruation and is associated with the use of highly absorbent tampons. The toxin acts as a 'super-antigen', triggering significant T-helper cell activation and very high peripheral polymorphonuclear leucocyte numbers.

TSS has an abrupt onset with high fever, generalised systemic upset (myalgia, headache, sore throat and vomiting), a generalised erythematous blanching rash resembling scarlet fever, and hypotension. It rapidly progresses over a matter of hours to multisystem involvement with cardiac, renal and hepatic compromise, leading to death in 10–20%. The diagnosis is clinical, supported by Gram stain of menstrual fluid demonstrating typical staphylococci. Treatment is with anti-staphylococcal antibiotics such as flucloxacillin or vancomycin. Recovery is accompanied at 7–10 days by desquamation (Fig. 5.8).

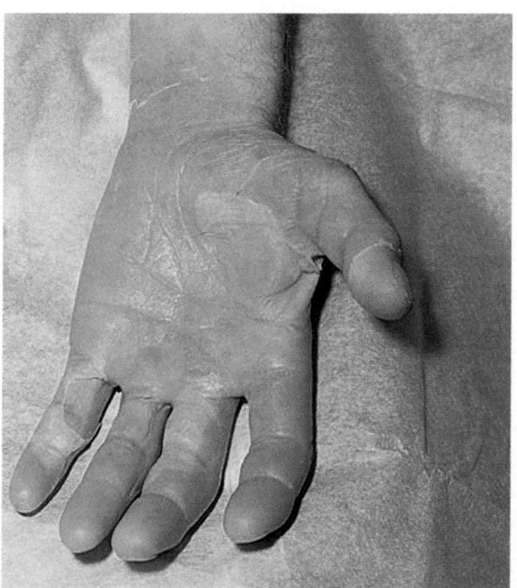

Fig. 5.8 Full-thickness desquamation after toxic shock syndrome.

STREPTOCOCCAL INFECTIONS

Streptococcal scarlet fever

Group A and occasionally group C and G streptococci are implicated. The source is often a relatively uncomplicated streptococcal pharyngitis or tonsillitis. Common in school-age children, scarlet fever can occur in young adults who have contact with young children.

A diffuse erythematous rash occurs, which blanches on pressure (Fig. 5.9), classically with circumoral pallor. The tongue, initially coated, becomes red and swollen ('strawberry tongue'). The disease lasts about 7 days, the rash disappearing in 7–10 days followed by a fine desquamation. Residual petechial lesions in the antecubital fossa may be seen. Treatment involves active therapy for the underlying infection (benzylpenicillin or orally available penicillin) plus symptomatic measures.

Streptococcal toxic shock syndrome

This is associated with severe group A streptococcal skin infections producing pyogenic exotoxin A.

Initially, an influenza-like illness occurs with, in 50% of cases, signs of necrotising fasciitis (see below). A faint erythematous rash, mainly on the

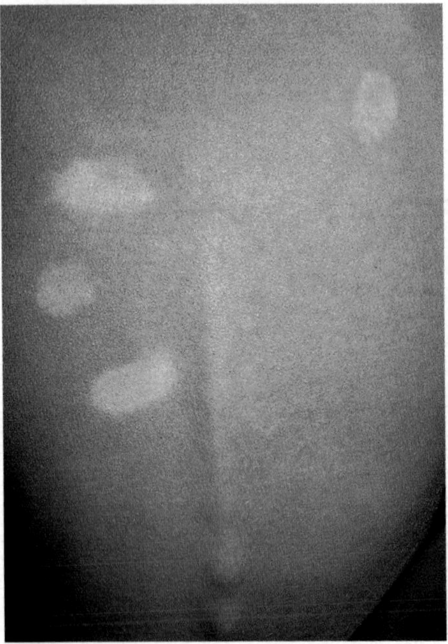

Fig. 5.9 Scarlet fever. Note blanching on pressure.

5.17 STREPTOCOCCAL AND RELATED INFECTIONS	
Strep. pyogenes	
• Skin and soft tissue infection (incl. erysipelas, impetigo, necrotising fasciitis) • Streptococcal toxic shock syndrome • Bone and joint infection	• Puerperal sepsis • Scarlet fever • Glomerulonephritis • Rheumatic fever • Tonsillitis
Alpha-haemolytic streptococci (*Strep. mitis, sanguis, mutans, salivarius*)	
• Endocarditis	• Septicaemia in immunosuppressed
Group B streptococci	
• Neonatal infections, incl. meningitis	• Female pelvic infections
Enterococcus faecalis	
• Endocarditis	• Urinary tract infection
Anaerobic streptococci (*Peptostreptococcus* spp.)	
• Peritonitis • Dental infections	• Liver abscess • Pelvic inflammatory disease
N.B. All streptococci can cause septicaemia.	

chest, rapidly progresses to a toxic multisystem shock-like state. Fluid resuscitation must be undertaken, linked to parenteral antistreptococcal antibiotic therapy, usually with benzylpenicillin ± clindamycin.

Cellulitis, erysipelas and impetigo

See pages 718–720.
Other streptococcal infections are shown in Box 5.17.

SEVERE NECROTISING SOFT TISSUE INFECTIONS

Cellulitis may progress rapidly to extensive necrosis of subcutaneous tissue and overlying skin. Treatment should be aggressive, with broad-spectrum antibiotic therapy in the first instance. Surgical débridement should subsequently be considered if control is not achieved.

Necrotising fasciitis

There are two major categories of necrotising fasciitis, both of which produce a severe, rapidly progressive and destructive inflammation of the dermis, subcutaneous tissues, subcutaneous fat and tissue planes, including the deep fascia. This leads to profound toxaemia and multisystem failure.

Type 1 is a polymicrobial infection with Enterobacteriaceae and anaerobic organisms. It often occurs following surgery or in diabetic or immunocompromised patients. *Type 2* (sometimes known as streptococcal gangrene) is caused by pure growth of *Strep. pyogenes* Lancefield group A.

Necrotising fasciitis is associated with profound toxaemia and multisystem failure. The whole process is hyperacute, often arising from an apparently minor breach in skin integrity. The affected area is erythematous, hot and shiny. Central anaesthesia (due to cutaneous nerve damage), surrounded by exquisitely tender erythematous skin, is pathognomonic.

Management is as follows:

• Urgent and extensive surgical débridement and empirical antibiotic therapy against Gram-positive, anaerobic and Gram-negative organisms (e.g. benzylpenicillin and a quinolone, + either clindamycin or metronidazole). • Material debrided should be sent for Gram stain and culture in order to identify the causative organism. • Mortality is high (30–80%) and up to 50% may require amputation of affected limbs and/or plastic surgical management.

CLOSTRIDIAL SOFT TISSUE INFECTIONS

Anaerobic cellulitis

Although *Clostridia* may colonise or contaminate wounds, no action is required unless evidence of spreading infection is present. In anaerobic cellulitis, usually due to *Cl. perfringens*, gas forms locally and extends along tissue planes, but bacteraemia and invasion of healthy tissue are not found. Prompt surgical débridement of devitalised tissue, along with penicillin or clindamycin therapy, usually results in an excellent outcome.

Gas gangrene or myonecrosis

This is defined as acute invasion of healthy living muscle undamaged by previous trauma. It develops following deep penetrating injury sufficient to create an anaerobic environment and allow clostridial introduction and proliferation. *Cl. perfringens* accounts for the majority of these infections.

• Severe pain at the site of the injury progresses rapidly over 18–24 hrs. • Skin colour changes from pallor to bronze/purple discoloration and the skin is tense and exquisitely tender. • Gas in tissues may be obvious with crepitus on clinical examination or visible on X-ray, CT or USS. • Signs of systemic toxicity develop rapidly with high leucocytosis, multi-organ dysfunction, raised creatine kinase and evidence of disseminated intravascular haemolysis. • Antibiotic therapy with high-dose i.v. penicillin, clindamycin, cephalosporins and metronidazole is very effective, and should be coupled with aggressive surgical débridement of affected tissues. • Use of hyperbaric oxygen is controversial.

TREPONEMATOSES

Syphilis

This disease is described on page 129.

Endemic treponematoses

Yaws: This granulomatous disease, caused by *Treponema pertenue*, is morphologically indistinguishable from the causative organisms of syphilis and pinta. The three infections induce similar serological changes and possibly some degree of cross-immunity. Organisms are transmitted by bodily contact from a patient with infectious yaws through minor abrasions of the skin, producing the primary lesion usually on the leg or buttock. The secondary eruption usually follows a few weeks or months later, as crops of papillomas covered with a whitish-yellow exudate, especially in the flexures and around the mouth. Phalanges, nasal bones and tibiae swell and become distorted. The tertiary lesions of 'late yaws' are nodules or ulcers in the skin, hyperkeratotic lesions of palms or soles ('dry crab yaws') and gummatous lesions of bone. They may occur 10–15 yrs after the disease is contracted.

Pinta and bejel: These two treponemal infections occur in poor rural populations with low standards of domestic hygiene, but are found in separate parts of the world (pinta: South and Central America; bejel: Middle East, Central Asia). They have features in common, notably that they are transmitted by contact, usually within the family and not sexually, and in the case of bejel, through common eating and drinking utensils. Diagnosis is by microscopic detection of spirochaetes and serology; treatment involves a single i.m. dose of benzylpenicillin.

SYSTEMIC BACTERIAL INFECTIONS

SEPSIS

Sepsis is the systemic invasion of microbes and/or the effects of their toxins resulting in a diseased state, characterised by high fever, rigors, tachypnoea and with or without localising signs.

Clinical features

Sepsis has a clear definition of the suspected presence of infection associated with a systemic inflammatory response syndrome (SIRS) (see p. 25). Sepsis syndrome occurs when sepsis is present with evidence of organ hypoperfusion involving lungs (hypoxaemia), liver (DIC/bleeding, lactate and acidosis), kidney (oliguria/renal impairment), brain (altered mentation, Glasgow Coma Scale) and myocardium (cardiac failure, acute myocarditis).

Hypotension unresponsive to fluids complicates organ dysfunction. It is often difficult to implicate the causative organism from the clinical features; however, generalised erythroderma suggests toxic shock syndrome (*Staph. aureus, Strep. pyogenes*) and petechial or haemorrhagic rash suggests meningococcus (*N. meningitidis*).

Investigations

• FBC: polymorphonuclear leucocytosis, thrombocytopenia. • U&Es, LFT: renal/liver failure. • ABG: metabolic acidosis. • CXR: features of ARDS. • Blood cultures: vital for identifying the causative organism.

Management

• Empirical broad-spectrum antibiotic cover should be commenced following blood cultures and culture of material from other potentially septic foci. • Ventilatory, circulatory and other organ support should be provided as required. • Corticosteroids and activated protein C have been shown to improve survival in some studies.

BRUCELLOSIS

Brucellosis is an intracellular organism endemic in animals. Although six species of *Brucella* are known, only four are important to humans:

• *B. melitensis* (goats, sheep and camels). • *B. abortus* (cattle). • *B. suis* (pigs). • *B. canis* (dogs).

B. melitensis causes the most severe disease.

Infected animals may excrete brucellae in their milk for long periods and human infection is acquired by ingesting contaminated milk, cheese, yoghurt, butter and uncooked meat.

Clinical features

Acute illness is characterised by a high swinging temperature, rigors, sweating, lethargy, headache, and joint and muscle pains. Occasionally, there is delirium, abdominal pain and constipation. Physical signs are non-specific, e.g. a palpable spleen or enlarged lymph nodes. Enlargement of the spleen may lead to hypersplenism and thrombocytopenia. Other features are shown in Box 5.18.

Diagnosis

• Serum agglutination test: the most commonly used method of detecting infection world-wide. • Blood cultures: prolonged incubation may be required. *B. melitensis* is the most readily cultured species. • CSF culture in neurobrucellosis: positive in about ~30% of cases.

Management

• Aminoglycosides show synergistic activity with tetracyclines when used against brucellae. Standard therapy therefore consists of doxycycline with

5.18 FOCAL MANIFESTATIONS OF BRUCELLOSIS	
Musculoskeletal	Suppurative arthritis, synovitis, bursitis; spinal spondylitis; osteomyelitis; paravertebral or psoas abscess
CNS	Meningitis; stroke; cranial nerve palsies; myelopathy; intracranial or subarachnoid haemorrhage; radiculopathy
Ocular	Uveitis; retinal thrombophlebitis
Cardiac	Myocarditis; endocarditis

streptomycin for the first 2 wks. • Treatment should be given for at least 3 mths. • The relapse rate after treatment is ~5%.

LYME BORRELIOSIS

The causative agent of Lyme disease (named after the town of Old Lyme in Connecticut, USA) is the spirochaete *Borrelia burgdorferi*. The reservoir of infection is maintained in ixodid (hard) ticks that feed on a variety of large mammals, particularly deer. The organism is transmitted to humans via the bite of infected ticks. Lyme disease is found in the USA, Europe, Russia, China, Japan and Australia.

Clinical features

Clinical features can be classified into three stages: early localised, early disseminated and late disease. Progression may be arrested at any stage.

Early localised disease: The characteristic feature is a skin reaction around the site of the tick bite, known as erythema chronica migrans. Initially, a red macule or papule appears 2–30 days after the bite. It then enlarges peripherally with central clearing, and may persist for months. The rash may be accompanied by fever, headache and regional lymphadenopathy.

Early disseminated disease: During this stage the organism seeds to other organs via the blood stream and lymphatics. There may be a pronounced systemic reaction with malaise, arthralgia and occasionally metastatic areas of erythema migrans. Neurological involvement may follow weeks or months after infection. Common features include lymphocytic meningitis, cranial nerve palsies (especially unilateral or bilateral facial palsy) and peripheral neuropathy. Radiculopathy, often painful, may present a year or more after initial infection. Carditis, sometimes accompanied by atrioventricular conduction defects, is not uncommon in the USA but is rarer in Europe.

Late disease: Late manifestations include arthritis, polyneuritis and encephalopathy. Prolonged arthritis, particularly affecting large joints, is a well-described feature but is rare in the UK. Brain parenchymal involvement causing neuropsychiatric abnormalities may also be encountered, but is again very rare in the UK. Acrodermatitis chronica atrophicans is an uncommon late complication seen more frequently in Europe than North America. Doughy, patchy discoloration occurs on the peripheries, eventually leading to shiny atrophic skin. The lesions are easily mistaken for those of peripheral vascular disease.

Diagnosis

• The diagnosis of Lyme borreliosis is primarily clinical. • Anti-*Borrelia* antibody detection is the best means of detecting disease, but titres may not be positive in the early stages. • Culture from biopsy material is not generally available, has a low yield and may take >6 wks. • PCR positivity in CSF is useful in confirming the diagnosis of neuroborreliosis but has low sensitivity.

Management

Standard therapy consists of a 14-day course of doxycycline or amoxicillin; disseminated disease will require more prolonged treatment. Some 15% of patients with early disease will develop a mild Jarisch–Herxheimer reaction during the first 24 hrs of therapy. Neuroborreliosis is treated with parenteral β-lactam antibiotics for 3–4 wks. Preventative measures (such as protective clothing and insect repellents) should be used in tick-infested areas.

RELAPSING FEVER

This term applies to two distinct types of relapsing fever due to systemic infection by borrelial spirochaetes: louse-borne relapsing fever and tick-borne relapsing fever, both characterised by recurrent febrile illnesses following an initial amelioration of symptoms.

Louse-borne relapsing fever

The human body louse, *Pediculus humanus*, causes itching. Borreliae (*B. recurrentis*) are liberated from the infected lice when they are crushed during scratching, which also inoculates the borreliae into the skin.

The borreliae invade most tissues of the body, including liver, spleen and meninges, causing hepatosplenomegaly, jaundice and meningism, accompanied by high fever. Marked thrombocytopenia results in petechial rash and epistaxis. The acute illness lasts between 4 and 10 days. A proportion of patients may relapse. Thick and thin blood films or dark field microscopy allow diagnosis. Treatment is with procaine penicillin followed by tetracycline. A severe Jarisch–Herxheimer reaction is seen with successful chemotherapy.

Tick-borne relapsing fever

Soft ticks (*Ornithodoros* spp.) transmit *B. duttoni* (and several other *Borrelia* species) through saliva while feeding on their host. Rodents are the reservoir in all parts of the world, except in East Africa where humans are the reservoir.

Clinical manifestations are similar to the louse-borne disease but spirochaetes are detected in fewer patients on dark field microscopy. A 7-day course of treatment with either tetracycline or erythromycin is needed.

LEPTOSPIROSIS

Leptospires are tightly coiled, thread-like organisms, about 5–7 microns in length, which are actively motile by rotating and bending. In reservoir species they persist in the convoluted tubules of the kidney without causing apparent disease, and are shed into the urine in massive numbers. Particular leptospiral serogroups are associated with characteristic animal hosts:

• *L. ictero-haemorrhagica* is the classical parasite of rats. • *L. canicola*: dogs. • *L. hebdomadis*: cattle. • *L. pomona*: pigs.

Leptospires can enter their human hosts through intact or injured skin or mucous membranes, for example following immersion in contaminated water.

Clinical features

The incubation period averages 1–2 wks. Four main clinical syndromes can be discerned:

Bacteraemic leptospirosis: A non-specific illness in which there is high fever accompanied by weakness, muscle pain and tenderness (especially of the calf and back), intense headache and photophobia, and sometimes diarrhoea and vomiting. Conjunctival congestion is the only notable physical sign. The illness comes to an end after ~1 wk, or else merges into one of the other forms of infection.

Aseptic meningitis: Very difficult to distinguish from viral meningitis. The conjunctivae may be congested but there are no other differentiating signs.

Icteric leptospirosis (Weil's disease): A dramatic life-threatening event, accounting for <10% of symptomatic infections. It is characterised by fever, haemorrhages, jaundice and renal impairment. Conjunctival hyperaemia is a frequent feature. The patient may have a transient macular erythematous rash, but the characteristic skin changes are those of purpura, with large areas of bruising. In severe cases there may be epistaxis, haematemesis and melaena, or bleeding into the pleural, pericardial or subarachnoid spaces. Thrombocytopenia is present in 50% of cases. Jaundice is deep and the liver is enlarged, but there is usually little evidence of hepatic failure or encephalopathy. Renal failure, primarily caused by impaired renal perfusion and acute tubular necrosis, becomes manifest as oliguria or anuria, with the presence of albumin, blood and casts in the urine. Weil's disease may also be associated with myocarditis, encephalitis and aseptic meningitis. Uveitis and iritis may appear months after apparent clinical recovery.

Pulmonary syndrome: This is characterised by haemoptysis, patchy lung infiltrates on CXR and respiratory failure. Total bilateral lung consolidation and ARDS develop in fatal cases. This is particularly recognised in the Far East.

Diagnosis

Non-specific results of routine laboratory tests include polymorphonuclear leucocytosis, thrombocytopenia and elevated creatine phosphokinase. In jaundiced patients LFTs are mildly hepatitic in pattern, with moderately raised transaminases; the prothrombin time may be a little prolonged. A lumbar puncture may show moderately elevated protein level and a normal glucose content in the CSF. Definitive diagnosis requires detection of the organism, its DNA, or a rising antibody titre:

• Blood culture: most likely to be positive if taken before the 10th day of illness. • Urine culture: leptospires are present in the urine from the 2nd week of illness. • Microscopic agglutination test (MAT): seroconversion or a fourfold rise in titre between acute and convalescent sera is confirmatory.

• PCR: can detect leptospiral DNA in blood in early symptomatic disease, and is positive in urine from the 8th day and for many months afterwards.

Management and prevention

Doxycycline and i.v. benzylpenicillin have been reported to be effective but evidence is insufficient to provide clear guidelines for practice. A Jarisch–Herxheimer reaction may occur during treatment but is usually mild. Supportive management, including the transfusion of blood and platelets, along with dialysis, is critical.

PLAGUE

Epidemics of plague, such as the 'Black Death', have attacked humans since ancient times, with a high fatality rate. The causative organism, *Yersinia pestis*, is a small Gram-negative bacillus that is spread between rodents by their fleas, which may also bite humans. In the late stages of human plague, *Y. pestis* may be expectorated and spread between humans by droplets. The incubation period is 3–6 days, and three distinct forms are recognised.

Bubonic plague: In this, the most common form of the disease, the onset is usually sudden with a rigor, high fever, dry skin and severe headache. Soon, aching and swelling at the site of the affected lymph nodes begin. The groin is the most common site of the 'bubo' (the swollen lymph nodes and surrounding tissue). A rapid pulse, hypotension, mental confusion and splenomegaly develop rapidly.

Septicaemic plague: The patient is toxic and may have GI symptoms such as nausea, vomiting, abdominal pain and diarrhoea. DIC may occur, manifested by bleeding from various orifices or puncture sites, along with ecchymoses. Hypotension, shock, renal failure and ARDS may lead to further deterioration. Meningitis, pneumonia and expectoration of blood-stained sputum may complicate the picture. There is a high mortality.

Pneumonic plague: The onset is very sudden with cough and dyspnoea. The patient soon expectorates copious blood-stained, frothy, highly infective sputum, becomes cyanosed and dies. X-rays of the lung show a lobar opacity.

Investigations

• A high index of clinical suspicion is required. • An aspirate from a bubo, sputum or the buffy coat (leucocyte fraction) of blood is used to show the characteristic bipolar staining organisms by staining with methylene blue or by immunofluorescence. • Blood, sputum and aspirate should be cultured. • DNA diagnosis through PCR and rapid diagnostic tests (RDTs) has been developed to improve on the sensitivity of the existing methods. • Plague is a notifiable disease.

Management

• Streptomycin or gentamicin is the drug of choice. • Tetracycline and chloramphenicol are alternatives. • Treatment may also be needed for acute circulatory failure, DIC and hypoxia. • Those treating the patient should wear protective clothing, and inadvertent exposure should prompt prophylactic treatment with doxycycline.

LISTERIOSIS

Listeria monocytogenes is an environmental bacterium which can contaminate food, including cheese and undercooked meats. It is of particular importance in pregnancy when, in addition to systemic symptoms like fever and myalgia, listeriosis causes chorioamnionitis, fetal deaths, abortions and neonatal infection. Gastroenteritis and meningitis are the other common manifestations. Diagnosis is made by blood and CSF culture. The most effective treatment is a combination of i.v. penicillin or ampicillin + an aminoglycoside. A sulfamethoxazole/trimethoprim combination can be used in those with penicillin sensitivity. Good food hygiene practices help to prevent infection.

TYPHOID AND PARATYPHOID (ENTERIC) FEVERS

In developing countries typhoid and paratyphoid fevers, which are transmitted by the faecal–oral route, are important causes of fever. Elsewhere they are relatively rare. The causative organisms are *Salmonella typhi* and *S. paratyphi* A and B (see also p. 91). High levels of transmission continue in India, sub-Saharan Africa and Latin America. The incubation period of typhoid fever is about 10–14 days; that of paratyphoid is somewhat shorter.

Clinical features

Typhoid fever: The onset may be insidious. The temperature rises in a stepladder fashion for 4 or 5 days. There is malaise, with increasing headache, drowsiness and aching in the limbs. Constipation may be present, although in children diarrhoea and vomiting may be prominent early in the illness. There is a relative bradycardia. At the end of the first week a rash may appear on the upper abdomen and on the back as sparse, slightly raised, rose-red spots, which fade on pressure. Cough and epistaxis occur. Around the 7th–10th day the spleen becomes palpable. Constipation is then succeeded by diarrhoea and abdominal distension with tenderness. Bronchitis and delirium may develop. By the end of the 2nd week the patient may be profoundly ill unless the disease is modified by antibiotic treatment. Without treatment, in the 3rd week toxaemia increases and the patient may pass into coma and die. Following recovery, up to 5% of patients become chronic carriers of *S. typhi*.

Paratyphoid fever: The course tends to be shorter and milder than that of typhoid fever and the onset is often more abrupt with acute enteritis. The rash may be more abundant and the intestinal complications less frequent.

Complications

• Haemorrhage from, or a perforation of, the ulcerated Peyer's patches, where the bacilli localise, may occur at the end of the 2nd week or during the 3rd week of the illness. • Additional complications include cholecystitis, pneumonia, myocarditis, arthritis, osteomyelitis and meningitis. • Bone and joint infection, especially in children with sickle-cell disease.

Investigations

• Blood culture is the most important diagnostic method in a suspected case. • The faeces will contain the organism more frequently during the 2nd and 3rd weeks. • The Widal reaction detects antibodies to the causative organisms; however, it is not a reliable diagnostic test.

Management

• Ciprofloxacin (or another fluoroquinolone antibiotic) is the drug of choice. • Treatment should be continued for 14 days; pyrexia may persist for up to 5 days after the start of specific therapy. • Improved sanitation and living conditions reduce the incidence of typhoid.

TULARAEMIA

Tularaemia is caused by a highly infectious Gram-negative bacillus, *Francisella tularensis,* and is a zoonotic disease of the northern hemisphere. Wild rabbits, domestic dogs or cats are the reservoirs and ticks are the vectors.

Infection is introduced through the bite of ticks, resulting in the most common ulceroglandular variety of the disease (70–80%), characterised by skin ulceration with regional lymphadenopathy. Inhalation of the infected aerosols may result in pulmonary tularaemia, presenting as pneumonia. Rarely, the portal of entry of infection may be the conjuctiva, leading to a nodular, ulcerated conjunctivitis with regional lymphadenopathy (an 'oculoglandular' form). Demonstration of a single high titre (≥1 : 160) or a fourfold rise in 2–3 wks in the tularaemia tube agglutination test confirms the diagnosis. PCR has been developed for reliable and rapid diagnosis. Treatment consists of a 7–10-day course of parenteral aminoglycosides, streptomycin or gentamicin.

GASTROINTESTINAL BACTERIAL INFECTIONS

FOOD POISONING

Bacterial causes of acute gastroenteritis are listed in Box 5.7.

STAPHYLOCOCCAL FOOD POISONING

Staph. aureus is a common commensal of the anterior nares and is readily transferred to foodstuffs such as dairy products, including cheese, and cooked meats where there are poor hygiene practices.

Nausea and vomiting develop within 6 hrs of ingestion of contaminated food, caused by enterotoxins produced by the organism. Most cases settle rapidly but severe dehydration and rare fatalities have occurred due to acute fluid loss and shock. The mainstays of treatment are antiemetics and fluid replacement. Public Health authorities should be notified if the source was a food vendor.

BACILLUS CEREUS

Rapid onset of vomiting within hours of food consumption is caused by the ingestion of the pre-formed enterotoxins of *B. cereus*. Fried rice or freshly made vanilla sauces are frequent sources. 1–4 hrs after ingestion, brisk vomiting and some diarrhoea occur, with rapid resolution within 24 hrs.

In some cases, viable organisms are ingested, and the toxin is produced in the gut. In these cases, the incubation period is 12–24 hrs and watery diarrhoea and cramps are the predominant symptoms. The disease is self-limiting. Management simply consists of fluid replacement and public health notification.

CLOSTRIDIUM PERFRINGENS

Spores of *Cl. perfringens* are widespread in the guts of large animals and in soil. In anaerobic conditions, *Cl. perfringens* spores in contaminated meat germinate and viable organisms multiply to give large numbers. Subsequent reheating of the food causes heat-shock sporulation of the organisms, during which they elute an enterotoxin. Symptoms (diarrhoea and cramps) occur some 6–12 hrs following ingestion.

'Point source' outbreaks, in which a number of cases all become symptomatic following ingestion, classically occur after school or canteen lunches where meat stews are served. Clostridial enterotoxins are potent and most people who ingest them will be symptomatic. The illness is usually self-limiting.

CAMPYLOBACTER JEJUNI

This infection is a zoonosis carried in the gut of cattle and poultry, and is the most common cause of bacterial gastroenteritis in the UK. The most common source of the infection is meat, such as chicken, or contaminated milk products.

The incubation period is 2–5 days. Colicky abdominal pain ensues, along with nausea, vomiting and quite significant diarrhoea, the latter frequently becoming blood-stained. The majority of *Campylobacter* infections affect fit young adults and are self-limiting after 5–7 days. Prolonged symptomatology merits treatment with antibiotics such as ciprofloxacin or a macrolide. About 1% of cases will develop bacteraemia and possible distant foci of infection. *Campylobacter* spp. have been clearly linked to Guillain–Barré syndrome and post-infectious reactive arthritis.

SALMONELLA SPECIES

These Gram-negative organisms produce two distinct clinical entities:

The serotypes *S. typhi* and *S. paratyphi* A, B, C have a purely human reservoir and produce the septicaemic illness 'enteric fever'. Other *Salmonella* serotypes are subdivided into five distinct subgroups which produce gastroenteritis, widely distributed among the animal kingdom.

Transmission is by contaminated water or food, particularly poultry, egg products and related fast foods.

The incubation period of *Salmonella* gastroenteritis is 12–72 hrs and the predominant feature is diarrhoea. Vomiting may be present at the outset and blood is quite frequently noted in the stool. ~5% of cases will be bacteraemic. Reactive (post-infective) arthritis occurs in ~2% of cases. Evidence of bacteraemia is a clear indication for antibiotic therapy, as salmonellae are notorious for persistent infection and often colonise endothelial surfaces such as an atherosclerotic aorta or a major blood vessel.

ESCHERICHIA COLI

E. coli is a major member of the Enterobacteriaceae and may be present without causing disease in the human gut at any given time. There are five different clinico-pathological patterns of disease, all associated with diarrhoea.

Enterotoxigenic E. coli (ETEC): These cause most cases of travellers' diarrhoea in developing countries, although other causes are possible (Box 5.19). The organisms produce either a heat-labile or a heat-stable enterotoxin, causing marked secretory diarrhoea and vomiting after 1–2 days' incubation. The illness is usually mild and self-limiting after 3–4 days. Antibiotics have been used to limit the duration of symptoms and prophylaxis may help to prevent this disease.

Entero-invasive E. coli (EIEC): This illness is very similar to *Shigella* dysentery and is caused by invasion and destruction of colonic mucosal cells. No enterotoxin is produced. Acute watery diarrhoea, abdominal cramps and some scanty blood-staining of the stool are common. The symptoms are rarely severe and are usually self-limiting.

Enteropathogenic E. coli (EPEC): These are very important in infant diarrhoea. Ability to attach to the gut mucosa is the basis of their pathogenicity. This causes destruction of microvilli and disruption of normal absorptive capacity. The symptoms vary from mild non-bloody diarrhoea to quite severe illness.

Entero-aggregative E. coli (EAEC): These strains also adhere to the mucosa and produce a locally active enterotoxin. A 'stacked brick' aggregation is seen in the small bowel. They have been associated with prolonged diarrhoea in children in South America, South-east Asia and India.

Enterohaemorrhagic E. coli (EHEC): A number of distinct 'O' serotypes of *E. coli* produce two distinct enterotoxins (verocytotoxin) which are identical to toxins produced by *Shigella* ('shiga-toxins 1 and 2'). *E. coli* O157:H7 is perhaps the best known of these verocytotoxigenic *E. coli* (VTEC), but others, including types O126 and O11, are also implicated. The reservoir of infection is in the gut of herbivores. Contaminated meat products, such as hamburgers, have long been recognised as a source of

5.19 MOST COMMON CAUSES OF TRAVELLERS' DIARRHOEA

- Enterotoxigenic *E. coli* (ETEC)
- *Shigella* spp.
- *Campylobacter jejuni*
- *Salmonella* spp.
- *Plesiomonas shigelloides*
- Non-cholera *Vibrio* spp.
- *Aeromonas* spp.

this infection. The organism has an extremely low infecting dose (10–100 organisms).

• The incubation period is between 1 and 7 days. • Initial watery diarrhoea becomes frankly and uniformly blood-stained in 70% of cases and is associated with severe and often constant abdominal pain. • There is little systemic upset, vomiting or fever. • Enterotoxins, if produced, have both a local effect on the bowel and a distant effect on particular body tissues such as glomerular apparatus, heart and brain. • The potentially life-threatening haemolytic uraemic syndrome (HUS—p. 192) occurs in 10–15% of sufferers from this infection, arising 5–7 days after the onset of symptoms. It is most likely at the extremes of age, is heralded by a high peripheral leucocyte count and may be induced, particularly in children, by antibiotic therapy. HUS is treated by dialysis if necessary and may be averted by active intervention with processes such as plasma exchange.

ANTIBIOTIC-ASSOCIATED DIARRHOEA (*CL. DIFFICILE* INFECTION)

A history of any antibiotic therapy in the 6 wks prior to the onset of diarrhoea can be linked to the finding of *Cl. difficile* or its toxins in the stool. This organism, through its toxin mediation, is a potent cause of diarrhoea, particularly in the elderly, and has become a very significant cause of health-care acquired infection in recent years. A number of different ribo types of the organism exist but the emergence of the 027 ribo type, producing very severe disease and significant mortality, requires vigilance and concerted action involving careful infection control, hand-washing (alcohol gel does not remove clostridial spores) and careful attention to antibiotic prescription. The acute illness can be treated with metronidazole orally for 10 days or, in severe cases, oral vancomycin.

YERSINIA ENTEROCOLITICA

This organism, commonly found in pork, causes mild to moderate gastroenteritis and can produce significant mesenteric adenitis after an incubation period of 3–7 days. It predominantly causes disease in children but adults may also be affected. The illness resolves slowly, with 10–30% of cases complicated by persistent arthritis or Reiter's syndrome.

VIBRIO CHOLERAE

Cholera, caused by *Vibrio cholerae* serotype 01, is the archetypal bacterial cause of acute watery diarrhoea. Infection spreads via the stools or vomit of symptomatic patients or of the much larger number of subclinical cases. It survives for up to 2 wks in fresh water and 8 wks in salt water. Transmission is normally through infected drinking water, shellfish and food contaminated by flies, or on the hands of carriers.

Clinical features

Severe diarrhoea without pain or colic begins suddenly and is succeeded by vomiting. Following the evacuation of normal gut faecal contents, typical 'rice-water' material is passed consisting of clear fluid with flecks of mucus, resulting in enormous loss of fluid and electrolytes. Shock and oliguria ensue, necessitating fluid and electrolyte replacement.

Diagnosis and management

The diagnosis should be confirmed by visualisation of the organism on stool dark field microscopy (shows the 'shooting star' motility of *V. cholerae*). Rectal swab or stool cultures allow identification. Cholera is notifiable under international health regulations. Replacement of fluid and electrolyte losses is paramount. Oral rehydration solution (ORS) is ideal for this purpose. Treatment with tetracycline or ciprofloxacin reduces the duration of excretion of *Vibrio.* Strict personal hygiene, a clean piped water supply and good food hygiene practices prevent the spread of disease.

VIBRIO PARAHAEMOLYTICUS

This marine organism produces a disease similar to enterotoxigenic *E. coli.* It is acquired from raw seafood and is very common where ingestion of such food is widespread (e.g. Japan). After an incubation period of ~20 hrs, explosive diarrhoea, abdominal cramps and vomiting occur. Systemic symptoms of headache and fever are frequent but the illness is self-limiting, taking 4–7 days to resolve.

BACILLARY DYSENTERY (SHIGELLOSIS)

Shigellae are Gram-negative rods, closely related to *E. coli*, that invade the colonic mucosa. They are often multi-resistant to antibiotics. The organism only infects humans and its spread is facilitated by its low infecting dose of ~10 organisms. Transmission by unwashed hands after defaecation is by far the most common. Outbreaks occur in mental hospitals, residential schools and other closed institutions.

Symptoms include diarrhoea, which may be bloody, colicky abdominal pain and tenesmus. Arthritis or iritis may occasionally complicate bacillary dysentery (Reiter's syndrome; p. 590), and may be associated with HLA-B27. Disease severity varies with serotype; cases due to *Sh. sonnei* are mild, while those due to *Sh. dysenteriae* may be fulminating and cause death within 48 hrs. Oral rehydration therapy to replace water and electrolyte loss is necessary. Antibiotic therapy with ciprofloxacin for 3 days is effective in known shigellosis and appropriate in epidemics. Hand-washing is important to prevent faecal contamination of food and milk.

NON-INFECTIOUS CAUSES OF FOOD POISONING

Whilst acute food poisoning and gastroenteritis are frequently caused by bacteria or their toxins, a number of non-infectious causes must be considered in the differential diagnosis. These include plant toxins such as alkaloids found in potato tubers, or hallucinogens found in certain fungi. Chemical toxins may also cause food poisoning; these include paralytic shellfish poisoning, ciguatera fish poisoning, scombrotoxic fish poisoning, or poisoning from food contaminated with heavy metals such as thallium.

RESPIRATORY BACTERIAL INFECTIONS

Pneumonia, bronchitis and pulmonary TB are dealt with in Chapter 9.

DIPHTHERIA

Diphtheria was eradicated from much of the developed world by mass vaccination in the mid-20th century but remains an important cause of illness in some countries, which has prompted the WHO to issue guidelines for the management of infection. *Corynebacterium diphtheriae* is the causative organism and the average incubation period is 2–4 days. It is highly contagious.

Clinical features

Acutely, the disease presents as membranous tonsillitis, nasal infection or laryngeal infection. The diagnostic feature is the 'wash-leather' elevated greyish-green membrane on the tonsils. There may be swelling of the neck ('bull-neck') and tender enlargement of the lymph nodes, as well as a blood-stained nasal discharge. Late complications occur as a result of toxin action on the heart or nervous system, and include myocarditis and peripheral neuropathy. Laryngeal obstruction or paralysis may occur and is life-threatening.

Management

This should take place in a hospital for infectious diseases. Treatment should begin once appropriate swabs have been taken rather than waiting for microbiological confirmation. Three main areas of management are:

• Administration of diphtheria antitoxin: neutralises any toxin not fixed to tissue. • Administration of antibiotics: penicillin or amoxicillin. • Strict isolation procedures: cases must be isolated until cultures from three daily nose and throat swabs are negative.

Prevention

Active immunisation should be given to all children. If diphtheria occurs in a closed community, contacts should be given erythromycin, which is more effective than penicillin in eradicating the organism in carriers. All contacts should also be immunised or given a booster dose of toxoid. Booster doses are required every 10 yrs to maintain immunity.

ANTHRAX

There are three recognised forms of infection with *Bacillus anthracis*:

Cutaneous anthrax: Spores are inoculated into exposed skin, producing an irritated papule on an oedematous haemorrhagic base. This develops into a black eschar.

GI anthrax: The caecum is the seat of infection, producing nausea, vomiting, anorexia and fever, followed 2–3 days later by abdominal pain and bloody diarrhoea.

Inhalational (pulmonary) anthrax: Fever, dyspnoea, cough and headache develop 3–14 days after exposure. This form of the disease is very rare and carries a mortality of >90%. It is a potential weapon for bioterrorists.

Management

• *B. anthracis* can be cultured from lesional skin swabs. • Skin lesions are readily curable with early antibiotic therapy. Treatment is with ciprofloxacin until penicillin susceptibility is confirmed; the regimen can then be changed to benzylpenicillin i.m. • Aggressive fluid resuscitation and the addition of an aminoglycoside may improve the outlook. • Ventilatory assistance will be required in inhalational disease. • Prophylaxis with ciprofloxacin is recommended for anyone at high risk of exposure to biological warfare.

BACTERIAL INFECTIONS WITH NEUROLOGICAL INVOLVEMENT

Bacterial meningitis and tetanus are dealt with in Chapter 16.

BOTULISM

Botulism is a syndrome of paralysis and neurological dysfunction produced by the neurotoxins of *Cl. botulinum*. Common contaminated sources include canned meat and salmon, home-preserved vegetables and honey. Wound botulism is a growing problem in injection drug-users. Ingestion of this extremely potent neurotoxin in even picogram amounts causes predominately bulbar and ocular palsies (difficulty in swallowing, blurred or double vision, ptosis), progressing to limb weakness and respiratory paralysis. Management includes assisted ventilation and general supportive measures until the toxin eventually dissociates from nerve endings at 6–8 wks following ingestion.

MYCOBACTERIAL INFECTIONS

LEPROSY

Leprosy (Hansen's disease) is a chronic granulomatous disease affecting skin and nerve caused by *Mycobacterium leprae*. The clinical form of the disease is determined by the degree of cell-mediated immunity (CMI) expressed by that individual towards *M. leprae*. High levels of CMI with elimination of leprosy bacilli produce tuberculoid leprosy, whereas absent CMI results in lepromatous leprosy. The medical complications of leprosy are due to nerve damage, immunological reactions and bacillary infiltration. Nerve damage accompanying leprosy is a serious complication causing considerable morbidity. It affects 4 million people world-wide, 70% of whom live in India, with the remainder in Brazil, Indonesia, Mozambique, Madagascar, Tanzania and Nepal.

Untreated lepromatous patients discharge bacilli from the nose. Infection occurs through the nose, followed by haematogenous spread to skin and nerve. The incubation period is 2–5 yrs for tuberculoid cases and 8–12 yrs for lepromatous cases.

Clinical features

Skin: The most common skin lesions are macules or plaques. In lepromatous leprosy, papules, nodules or diffuse infiltration of the skin occur. Tuberculoid patients have few, hypopigmented lesions whilst lepromatous patients have numerous, sometimes confluent lesions.

Anaesthesia: Occurs in skin lesions when dermal nerves are involved or in the distribution of a large peripheral nerve. In skin lesions the small dermal sensory and autonomic nerve fibres are damaged, causing local sensory loss and loss of sweating within that area.

Peripheral neuropathy with thickened peripheral nerves: Sites of predilection include the ulnar (elbow), median (wrist), radial (humerus, causing wrist drop), radial cutaneous (wrist), common peroneal (knee), posterior tibial and sural nerves at the ankle, facial nerve as it crosses the zygomatic arch, and great auricular in the posterior triangle of the neck. All these nerves should be examined for enlargement and tenderness and tested for motor and sensory function. The CNS is not affected.

Eye involvement: Blindness due to leprosy is a devastating complication for a patient with anaesthetic hands and feet. Eyelid closure is impaired when the facial (7th) nerve is affected. Damage to the trigeminal (5th) nerve causes anaesthesia of the cornea and conjunctiva. The cornea is then susceptible to trauma and ulceration.

The following clinical variants are recognised:

• Tuberculoid leprosy (TT): has a good prognosis; it may self-heal and peripheral nerve damage is limited.

• Borderline tuberculoid (BT): the skin lesions are similar to those in tuberculoid leprosy but are more numerous. Damage to peripheral nerves may be widespread and severe. These patients are prone to type 1 reactions (see below) with consequent nerve damage.

• Borderline leprosy (BB): unstable. Patients have numerous skin lesions varying in size, shape and distribution. Annular lesions with a broad, irregular edge and a sharply defined, punched-out centre are characteristic. Nerve damage is variable.

• Borderline lepromatous leprosy (BL): characterised by widespread small macules. Patients may experience both type 1 and type 2 reactions. Peripheral nerve involvement is widespread.

• Lepromatous leprosy (LL): the earliest lesions are ill defined; gradually, the skin becomes infiltrated and thickened. Facial skin thickening leads to the characteristic leonine facies (Fig. 5.10). Dermal nerves are destroyed, sweating is lost, and a 'glove and stocking' neuropathy is common. Nerve damage to large peripheral nerves occurs late in the disease. Nasal collapse occurs secondary to bacillary destruction of the bony nasal spine. Testicular atrophy is caused by diffuse infiltration and the acute orchitis that occurs with type 2 reactions. This results in azoospermia and gynaecomastia.

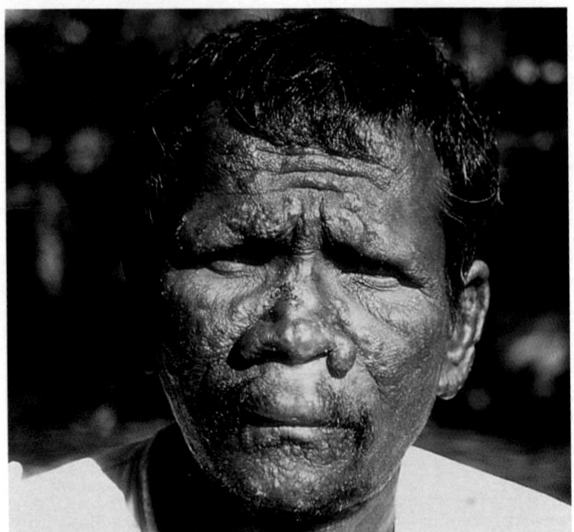

Fig. 5.10 Lepromatous leprosy. Widespread nodules and infiltration with loss of the eyebrows. This man also has early collapse of the nose.

Leprosy reactions

Leprosy reactions are clinical events superimposed on the cardinal features described above.

Type 1 (reversal) reactions: Occur in 30% of borderline patients (BT, BB, BL) and are delayed hypersensitivity reactions caused by increased recognition of *M. leprae* antigens in skin and nerve sites. Skin lesions become erythematous; peripheral nerves become tender and painful. Loss of nerve function can be sudden, with foot drop occurring overnight. Reversal reactions may occur spontaneously, after starting treatment or after completion of multidrug therapy.

Type 2 (erythema nodosum leprosum—ENL) reactions: Are partly due to immune complex deposition and occur in BL and LL patients who produce antibodies and have a high antigen load. They manifest with malaise, fever and crops of small pink nodules on the face and limbs. Iritis and episcleritis are common. Other signs are acute neuritis, lymphadenitis, orchitis, bone pain, dactylitis, arthritis and proteinuria. ENL may continue intermittently for several years.

Investigations

• Slit skin smears: dermal material is scraped on to a glass slide and acid-fast bacilli may be seen on microscopy. • Skin biopsy: histological examination may aid diagnosis. • Neither serology nor PCR testing for *M. leprae* DNA is sensitive or specific enough for diagnosis.

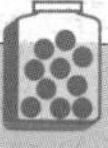

5.20 MODIFIED WHO-RECOMMENDED MULTIDRUG THERAPY REGIMENS IN LEPROSY

Type of leprosy*	Monthly supervised drug treatment	Daily self-administered drug treatment	Duration of treatment
Paucibacillary	Rifampicin 600 mg	Dapsone 100 mg	6 mths
Multibacillary	Rifampicin 600 mg Clofazimine 300 mg	Clofazimine 50 mg Dapsone 100 mg	12 mths

*WHO classification for field use when slit skin smears are not available:

- paucibacillary (1–5 skin lesions; includes old 'single-lesion' category)
- multibacillary (>5 skin lesions).

In this field classification WHO recommends treatment of multibacillary patients for 12 mths only.

Differential diagnosis

Skin: Pityriasis versicolor, vitiligo, post-inflammatory hypopigmentation, psoriasis, eczema, onchocercosis.

Nerves: Amyloidosis, HIV infection, diabetes, alcoholism, vasculitis, Charcot–Marie–Tooth disease.

Management

All leprosy patients should be given an appropriate multidrug combination (Box 5.20). Patients can be classified into paucibacillary (skin smear-negative tuberculoid and BT) and multibacillary (skin smear-positive BT, all BB, BL and LL). The first-line anti-leprosy drugs are rifampicin, clofazimine and dapsone. Rifampicin is a potent bactericidal for *M. leprae* but there are some problems with resistance and so it should always be given as part of MDT. Dapsone is bacteriostatic. It commonly causes mild haemolysis but rarely anaemia. Clofazimine is a red, fat-soluble crystalline dye, weakly bactericidal for *M. leprae*. • Skin discoloration (red to purple-black) and ichthyosis are troublesome side-effects, particularly on pale skins (see Box 5.20). Clinical improvement with MDT is rapid and toxicity rare. Relapse after MDT is uncommon, the WHO reporting 1.07% for paucibacillary leprosy and 0.77% for multibacillary leprosy at 9 yrs after completion of MDT.

Treatment of reactions

The principles of treating immune-mediated reactions are to:
• Control the acute inflammation and ease the pain. • Treat the neuritis.
• Halt eye damage.

Control of these reactions is most readily achieved with high-dose oral prednisolone. Thalidomide may also be used but its teratogenicity limits its use in women of child-bearing potential.

Prevention of disability

The morbidity and disability associated with nerve damage in leprosy are considerable. Priorities include:

• Scrupulous attention to skin care is required if patients are to avoid damage to their anaesthetic limb. • Appropriate footware should help to protect pressure points. • Ulceration should be treated seriously, the cause of the injury identified, and the patient advised not to weight-bear until the ulcer has healed. • Physiotherapy can help prevent contractures and atrophy of muscles.

Prognosis

The majority of patients, especially those who have no nerve damage at the time of diagnosis, do well on MDT, with resolution of skin lesions. Borderline patients are at risk of developing type 1 reactions which may result in devastating nerve damage.

Prevention and control

Programmes aimed at case detection and provision of MDT are now in place in many of the countries affected by leprosy. BCG vaccination has been shown to give good but variable protection against leprosy; adding killed *M. leprae* to BCG does not give enhanced protection.

BURULI ULCER

This ulcer is caused by *Mycobacterium ulcerans* and occurs world-wide in tropical rainforests. The ulcer starts with acute necrosis. Clumps of acid-fast bacilli are present on the ulcer floor. Later, healing occurs with granuloma formation.

Clinical features

The initial lesion is a small subcutaneous nodule on the arm or leg. This breaks down to form a shallow, necrotic ulcer with deeply undermined edges, which extends rapidly. Healing may occur after 6 mths but the accompanying fibrosis causes contractures and deformity.

Management

• A combination of rifampicin and streptomycin can cure the infection. • Infected tissue should be removed surgically. • In Ghana, a campaign prioritising early removal of pre-ulcerative nodules has had a positive impact on the incidence of Buruli ulcers.

RICKETTSIAL FEVERS

These are caused by Gram-negative organisms which parasitise the intestines of arthropods, and are the most common tick-borne infections. Following an inoculating tick bite, patients present acutely with headache, rash and sometimes neurological disturbance. There are two main groups of rickettsial fevers: spotted fever group and the typhus group.

SPOTTED FEVER GROUP

Rocky Mountain spotted fever: *Rickettsia rickettsii* is transmitted by tick bites, largely in western and south-eastern states of the USA and also in South America. The incubation period is about 7 days. The rash appears on about the 3rd or 4th day, looking at first like measles, but in a few hours the typical maculo-papular eruption develops. Within 24–48 hrs the rash spreads in a centripetal fashion from wrists, forearms and ankles to the back, limbs and chest, and then to the abdomen where it is least pronounced. Larger cutaneous and subcutaneous haemorrhages may appear in severe cases. The liver and spleen become palpable. At the extremes of life the mortality is 5–10%.

TYPHUS GROUP

Scrub typhus fever: Caused by *R. tsutsugamushi*, transmitted by mites. It occurs in the Far East, Myanmar, Pakistan, Bangladesh, India, Indonesia, the South Pacific islands and Queensland. Initially the patient develops one eschar or more, surrounded by an area of cellulitis and enlargement of regional lymph nodes. The incubation period is ~9 days. Mild or subclinical cases are common. The onset of symptoms is usually sudden with headache, often retro-orbital, fever, malaise, weakness and cough. An erythematous maculo-papular rash appears on about the 5th–7th day and spreads to the trunk, face and limbs including the palms and soles, with generalised painless lymphadenopathy. The rash fades by the 14th day. The patient develops a remittent fever which falls by the 12th–18th day. In severe infection the patient is prostrate with cough, pneumonia, confusion and deafness. Cardiac failure, renal failure and haemorrhage may develop. Convalescence is often slow and tachycardia may persist for some weeks.

Epidemic (louse-borne) typhus: Caused by *R. prowazekii* and prevalent in parts of Africa, especially Ethiopia and Rwanda, and in the South American Andes and Afghanistan. Overcrowding facilitates spread. The incubation period is usually 12–14 days. The onset is usually sudden, with rigors, fever, frontal headaches, pains in the back and limbs, constipation and bronchitis. The face is flushed and cyanotic, the eyes are congested and the patient becomes dull and confused. A petechial, mottled rash appears on the 4th–6th day, first on the anterior folds of the axillae, sides of the abdomen or backs of hands, then on the trunk and forearms sparing the head and neck. During the 2nd week symptoms increase in severity. Sores develop on the lips. The tongue becomes dry, brown, shrunken and tremulous. The spleen is palpable, the pulse feeble and the patient stuporous and delirious. The temperature falls rapidly at the end of the 2nd week and the patient recovers gradually. The mortality rate of 40% is usually due to toxaemia, cardiac or renal failure, or pneumonia.

Endemic (flea-borne) typhus: Flea-borne or 'endemic' typhus caused by *R. mooseri* is endemic world-wide. Humans are infected when the faeces or contents of a crushed flea which has fed on an infected rat (the reservoir for the disease) are introduced into the skin. The incubation period is 8–14 days. The symptoms resemble those of a mild louse-borne typhus. The rash may be scanty and transient.

Investigation of rickettsial infection

The diagnosis of rickettsial infection is essentially clinical, although species-specific antibodies may be detected by complement fixation, micro-agglutination and fluorescence in specialised laboratories.

Differential diagnosis

• Malaria. • Typhoid. • Meningococcal septicaemia. • Leptospirosis.

Management of the rickettsial diseases

The different rickettsial fevers vary greatly in severity but all respond to tetracycline antibiotics, such as doxycycline, or chloramphenicol. Reservoirs of the disease, such as fleas, ticks and mites, need to be controlled with insecticides.

Q FEVER

Q fever occurs world-wide and is caused by the rickettsia-like organism *Coxiella burnetii*, an obligate intracellular organism that can survive in the extracellular environment. Cattle, sheep and goats are important reservoirs and the organism is transmitted by inhalation of aerosolised particles derived from products of conception or animal excreta.

Clinical features

The incubation period is 3–4 wks. • The initial symptoms are non-specific with fever, headache and chills; in 20% of cases a maculo-papular rash occurs. Other presentations include pneumonia and hepatitis. Chronic Q fever may present with osteomyelitis, encephalitis and endocarditis.

Investigations

Diagnosis is usually serological and the stage of the infection can be distinguished by isotype tests and phase-specific antigens. Acute phase II IgM titres peak at 4–6 wks. In chronic infections IgG titres to phase I and II antigens may be raised.

Management

• Doxycycline is the treatment of choice. • Rifampicin is added in cases of Q fever endocarditis, which can be recalcitrant to treatment, even when two antimicrobial agents are used.

BARTONELLOSIS

This group of diseases is caused by intracellular Gram-negative rods closely related to the rickettsia. The principal human pathogens are *Bartonella quintana* and *B. henselae*. *Bartonella* infections are associated with the following clinical conditions:

Trench fever: This is a relapsing fever with severe leg pain, which is debilitating but not fatal.

Bacteraemia and endocarditis in the homeless: The endocarditis is associated with severe damage to the heart valves.

Cat scratch disease: *B. henselae* causes this common benign lymphadenopathy in children and young adults. A vesicle or papule develops on the head, neck or arms after a cat scratch. The lesion resolves spontaneously but lymphadenopathy may persist for up to 4 mths.

Bacillary angiomatosis: This is an HIV-associated disease.

Investigations

• Blood cultures: require prolonged incubation and enriched media. • Serological testing: haemagglutination, indirect immunofluorescence, ELISA.

Management

• *Bartonella* isolates are susceptible to β-lactams, rifampicin, erythromycin and tetracyclines. • Antibiotic use is guided by clinical need. • Cat scratch disease usually resolves spontaneously but *Bartonella* endocarditis requires valve replacement and combination antibiotic therapy.

CHLAMYDIAL INFECTIONS

Chlamydia trachomatis: Causes trachoma (see below), lymphogranuloma venereum and sexually transmitted genital infections (p. 130).

Chlamydia psittaci: Causes psittacosis (p. 292).

Chlamydia pneumoniae: A cause of atypical pneumonia (p. 292).

TRACHOMA

Trachoma is a chronic keratoconjunctivitis caused by *Chlamydia trachomatis*, and is the most common cause of avoidable blindness. Transmission occurs through flies, on fingers and within families. In endemic areas the disease is most common in children.

Clinical features

The onset is usually insidious and infection may not be apparent to the patient. Early symptoms include conjunctival irritation and blepharospasm, and it may be difficult to distinguish these from viral forms of conjunctivitis. The problem may not be detected until vision begins to fail.

Investigations

Intracellular inclusions may be demonstrated in conjunctival scrapings by staining with iodine or immunofluorescence.

Management

• A single dose of azithromycin (20 mg/kg) is first choice of treatment, being more effective than tetracycline eye ointment. • Deformity and scarring of the lids, and corneal opacities, ulceration and scarring require surgical treatment after control of local infection. • The WHO is promoting the SAFE strategy for trachoma control (**s**urgery, **a**ntibiotics, **f**acial cleanliness and **e**nvironmental improvement). • Proper eye care of newborns and young children is essential.

PROTOZOAL INFECTIONS

BLOOD AND TISSUE PARASITES

MALARIA

Malaria is a disease transmitted to humans by the bite of female anopheline mosquitoes and occurs throughout the tropics and subtropics at altitudes below 1500 m. There are up to 250 million clinical cases per year, caused by one of the four malarial organisms: *Plasmodium falciparum*, *P. vivax*, *P. ovale* and *P. malariae*. Chloroquine resistance has now become problematic, notably in Asia and Africa. Due to increased travel and neglect of chemoprophylaxis, over 2000 cases are imported annually into Britain. Most are due to *P. falciparum*, usually from Africa, and of these 1% die because of late diagnosis. Immigrants returning home after a long residence in the UK are particularly at risk. They have lost their partial immunity and do not realise that they should be taking malaria prophylaxis. A few people living near airports in Europe have acquired malaria from accidentally imported mosquitoes.

Life cycle

The female anopheline mosquito becomes infected by feeding on human blood containing malarial parasite gametocytes. Human infection starts when an infected mosquito inoculates sporozoites into the skin during feeding; these disappear from human blood within half an hour and enter the liver. After some days merozoites leave the liver and invade red blood cells, where further cycles of multiplication take place, producing schizonts. Rupture of the schizont releases more merozoites into the blood and causes fever, the periodicity of which depends on the species of parasite.

P. vivax and *P. ovale* may persist in liver cells as dormant forms, hypnozoites, capable of developing into merozoites months or years later. Thus the first attack of clinical malaria may occur long after the patient has left the endemic area, and the disease may relapse after treatment with drugs that kill only the erythrocytic stage of the parasite. *P. falciparum* and *P. malariae* have no persistent exo-erythrocytic phase but recrudescences of fever may result from multiplication in the red cells of parasites which have not been eliminated by treatment and immune processes.

Clinical features

The pathology in malaria is due to haemolysis of infected red cells and adherence of infected red blood cells to capillaries.

P. falciparum infection: This is the most dangerous of the malarias. The onset is often insidious, with malaise, headache and vomiting, and is often mistaken for influenza. Cough and mild diarrhoea are also common. The fever has no particular pattern. Jaundice is common due to haemolysis and hepatic dysfunction. The liver and spleen enlarge and become tender. Anaemia develops rapidly. Complications of falciparum malaria are as follows:

• Cerebral malaria: the most grave complication, causing either confusion or coma, usually without localising signs. • Convulsions. • Hypoglycaemia. • Severe anaemia. • Acute pulmonary oedema. • Acute renal failure. • Coagulopathy/spontaneous bleeding. • Metabolic acidosis. • Aspiration pneumonia.

Splenectomy increases the risk of severe malaria.

P. vivax and P. ovale infection: In many cases the illness starts with several days of continued fever before the development of classical bouts of fever on alternate days. Fever starts with a rigor. The patient feels cold and the temperature rises to about 40°C. After half an hour to an hour the hot or flush phase begins. It lasts several hours and gives way to profuse perspiration and a gradual fall in temperature. The cycle is repeated 48 hrs later. Gradually the spleen and liver enlarge and may become tender. Anaemia develops slowly. Herpes simplex is common. Relapses are frequent in the first 2 yrs after leaving the malarious area.

P. malariae infection: This is usually associated with mild symptoms and bouts of fever every 3rd day. Parasitaemia may persist for many years with the occasional recrudescence of fever, or without producing any symptoms. *P. malariae* causes glomerulonephritis and the nephrotic syndrome in children.

Diagnosis

Both thick and thin blood films should be taken.

In the thick film erythrocytes are lysed, releasing all blood stages of the parasite. This facilitates the diagnosis of low-level parasitaemias. A thin film is essential to confirm the diagnosis, to identify the species of parasite and, in *P. falciparum* infections, to quantify the parasite load (by counting the percentage of infected erythrocytes).

Immunochromatographic 'dipstick' tests for *P. falciparum* antigen are now marketed and provide a useful non-microscopic means of diagnosing this infection. They should be used in parallel with blood film examination but are ~100 times less sensitive than a carefully examined blood film.

Management

Chemotherapy of mild P. falciparum malaria: *P. falciparum* is now resistant to chloroquine almost world-wide, so quinine is the drug of choice. Quinine dihydrochloride or sulphate 600 mg *salt* (10 mg/kg) 8-hourly by mouth is given until the patient is clinically better and the blood is free of parasites (usually 3–5 days). This regimen should be followed by a single dose of sulfadoxine 1.5 g combined with pyrimethamine 75 mg, i.e. 3 tablets of Fansidar. In pregnancy a 7-day course of quinine alone should be given. If sulphonamide sensitivity is suspected, quinine may be followed by doxycycline 100 mg daily for 7 days.

Management of complicated P. falciparum malaria: Severe malaria is a medical emergency and cerebral malaria is the most common presentation and cause of death in adults with malaria. Cerebral malaria is assumed when asexual parasites are present in the blood film, the patient has impaired consciousness and other encephalopathies have been excluded, particularly bacterial meningitis and locally occurring viral encephalitides. Complications of severe malaria include hypoglycaemia, severe anaemia, renal failure and metabolic acidosis. Severe malaria should be considered in any non-immune patient with a parasite count >2%. Management should include:

• Early and appropriate antimalarial chemotherapy. • Active treatment of complications. • Correction of fluid, electrolyte and acid–base balance. • Quinine is given as an i.v. infusion over 4 hrs. • The patient should have ECG monitoring during the infusion for arrhythmias. • *P. vivax*, *P. ovale* and *P. malariae* infections should be treated with chloroquine: 600 mg chloroquine *base* followed by 300 mg *base* in 6 hrs, then 150 mg *base* 12-hourly for 2 more days.

Radical cure of malaria due to P. vivax and P. ovale: Relapses can be prevented by taking one of the antimalarial drugs in suppressive doses. Radical cure is achieved in most patients with a course of primaquine, which destroys the hypnozoite phase in the liver. Haemolysis may develop in those who are glucose-6-phosphate dehydrogenase (G6PD)-deficient. Cyanosis due to the formation of methaemoglobin in the red cells is more common but not dangerous.

Prevention

Choice of prophylactic agent is determined by the risk of malaria in the area being visited and the degree of chloroquine resistance. Chemoprophylaxis is begun 1 wk before departure and is continued for 4 wks after leaving the area. Chloroquine ± proguanil may be used in areas where resistance is low to moderate; mefloquine, malarone or doxycycline are alternatives in areas where chloroquine resistance is high. Use of mosquito nets, insect repellents and protective clothing are also important means of reducing infection.

BABESIOSIS

This is caused by a tick-borne intra-erythrocytic protozoon parasite. Patients present with fever 1–4 wks after a tick bite. Severe illness is seen in splenectomised patients. The diagnosis is made by blood film examination. Treatment is with quinine and clindamycin.

LEISHMANIASIS

Leishmaniasis is caused by unicellular flagellate intracellular protozoa belonging to the genus *Leishmania*. It comprises three broad groups of disorder:

• Visceral leishmaniasis (VL, kala-azar). • Cutaneous leishmaniasis (CL). • Mucosal leishmaniasis (ML).

Although most clinical syndromes are caused by zoonotic transmission of any one of 21 species of parasite from animals (chiefly canine and rodent reservoirs) to humans through phlebotomine sandfly vectors, humans are the only known reservoir (anthroponotic) in major VL foci in India and Sudan. The disease occurs in 88 countries around the world, with an estimated annual incidence of 2 million new cases.

Life cycle

Flagellar promastigotes (10–20 μm) are introduced by the feeding female sandfly (*Phlebotomus* in the eastern hemisphere, *Lutzomyia* and *Psyodopygus* in the western hemisphere). Sandfly saliva helps *Leishmania* evade immunity. The promastigotes are taken up by macrophages where they lose their flagellae and transform into amastigotes (2–4 μm). These multiply, ultimately causing lysis of the macrophages and infection of another cell. Sandflies pick up amastigotes when feeding on infected patients or animal reservoirs. In the sandfly, the parasite transforms into a flagellar promastigote which multiplies by binary fission in the gut of the vector and migrates to the proboscis to infect a new host.

VISCERAL LEISHMANIASIS (KALA-AZAR)

VL is caused by the protozoon *Leishmania donovani* complex and transmitted by the phlebotomine sandfly. Rarely, a dermatotropic species (e.g. *Leishmania tropica*) may cause visceral disease. India, Sudan, Bangladesh and Brazil account for 90% of cases of VL, while other affected regions include the Mediterranean, East Africa, China, Arabia, Israel and other South American countries. The disease can present unexpectedly in immunosuppressed patients: e.g. after renal transplantation and in AIDS.

Clinical features

The great majority of people infected with flagellar promastigotes remain asymptomatic and control the infection. Immunosuppression and malnutrition predispose to infection. The incubation period ranges from weeks to months (occasionally several years). Features are as follows:

• Fever: accompanied initially by rigor and chills; frequency decreases over time. • Splenomegaly: develops quickly in the first few weeks and may become massive. • Hepatomegaly. • Lymphadenopathy. • Skin: a blackish discoloration of the skin ('kala azar' is Hindi for 'black skin') is a feature of advanced disease now rarely seen. • Haematological abnormalities: severe anaemia, thrombocytopenia, pancytopenia. • Oedema and ascites: secondary to low albumin. • Secondary infection: profound immunosuppression may result in TB, amoebic dysentery, herpes zoster and chickenpox. Skin infections, cellulites and scabies are common.

Investigations

• FBC: pancytopenia, with granulocytopenia and monocytosis. • LFTs: hypoalbuminaemia. • Immunology: hypergammaglobulinaemia (IgG first, then IgM). • Splenic biopsy: a smear will demonstrate amastigotes (Leishman–Donovan bodies) with 98% sensitivity as a diagnostic test. • PCR: performed on peripheral blood; the investigation used most in developed countries. • Serodiagnosis by indirect immunofluorescence: also used in developed countries. • In developing countries, a highly sensitive and specific direct agglutination test of stained promastigotes and an equally efficient rapid immunochromatographic k39 strip test have been developed.

Differential diagnosis

This includes malaria, typhoid, TB, schistosomiasis and many other infectious and neoplastic conditions, some of which may coexist with VL. Fever, splenomegaly, pancytopenia and non-response to antimalarial therapy may provide the clue before specific laboratory diagnosis is made.

Management

Pentavalent antimonials: Antimony (Sb) compounds such as sodium stibogluconate and meglumine antimoniate are the mainstay of treatment in most parts of the world. Treatment is given for 28 days. Side-effects are common and include arthralgias, myalgias, raised hepatic transaminases and pancreatitis, especially in patients co-infected with HIV. Severe cardiotoxicity, manifested by concave ST segment elevation, prolongation of QT_c >0.5 msec, ventricular ectopics, runs of ventricular tachycardia, torsades de pointes, ventricular fibrillation and sudden death, is not uncommon. The incidence of cardiotoxicity and death can be very high with improperly manufactured Sb.

Amphotericin B: Approximately two-thirds of cases of kala-azar in India are resistant to antimonial treatment. The antifungal drug, amphotericin B, may be used as an alternative. It has a cure rate of nearly 100%. Infusion-related side-effects, e.g. high fever with rigor, thrombophlebitis, diarrhoea and vomiting, are extremely common. Serious (occasionally fatal) adverse events, such as renal or hepatic toxicity, hypokalaemia, thrombocytopenia and myocarditis, are not uncommon. Lipid formulations (amphotericin B lipid complex—Abelcet) and liposomal amphotericin B (AmBisome) are less toxic and have been tested widely for the treatment of VL. High daily doses of the lipid formulations are well tolerated, thus reducing hospital stay and cost. The high price of lipid formulations may preclude their use in some endemic regions.

Miltefosin, paromomycin, pentamidine: These agents have also been used to treat VL.

Response to treatment

A good response results in abatement of fever, a feeling of well-being, gradual decrease in splenic size, weight gain and recovery of blood counts. Patients should be followed regularly for a period of 6–12 mths, as a small minority may relapse. Relapse is indicated by enlargement of the spleen, return of fever, weight loss and decline in blood counts. Relapse may be retreated with either Sb or conventional or lipid amphotericin B.

HIV-visceral leishmaniasis co-infection

A high index of suspicion is required to make the diagnosis of VL with the atypical clinical presentations of the disease in patients co-infected with HIV.

The clinical triad of fever, splenomegaly and hepatomegaly is found in less than half the patients with a CD4 count <50 cells/mm^3. VL may present with GI involvement (stomach, duodenum or colon), ascites, pleural or pericardial effusion, or involvement of lungs, tonsil, oral mucosa or skin. Diagnostic principles remain the same as those in non-HIV patients, based on the detection of amastigotes in body fluids or PCR of the blood. Treatment of VL in a setting of HIV co-infection remains essentially the same as in immunocompetent patients, using amphotericin B or Sb, but there are some differences in outcome. Highly active antiretroviral therapy (HAART) has led to a remarkable decline in the incidence of VL co-infection.

Post-kala-azar dermal leishmaniasis (PKDL)

After treatment and recovery from the visceral disease in India and Sudan, some patients develop dermatological manifestations. In India, dermatological changes occur in a small minority of patients (usually adults) 6 mths to ≥3 yrs after the initial infection in contrast to Sudan where 50% of patients (usually children) develop PKDL rapidly (within 6 mths). The diagnosis is clinical, based on the characteristic appearance of macules, papules, nodules (most frequently) and plaques on the face, especially the area around the chin. The face often appears erythematous. Hypopigmented macules can occur and are highly variable in extent and location. There are no systemic symptoms but such patients are a human reservoir for disease. Treatment of Indian PKDL is difficult—Sb for 120 days or several courses of amphotericin B infusions are required. In Sudan, spontaneous healing occurs in about three-quarters of cases within 1 yr.

Prevention and control

Insecticides, as well as physical barriers such as mosquito nets and protective clothing, help prevent the transmission of the disease to humans. Dogs and other animals known to be infected should be destroyed. Early detection and adequate treatment of cases reduce the human reservoir of the disease.

CUTANEOUS AND MUCOSAL LEISHMANIASIS

Cutaneous leishmaniasis

CL (oriental sore) occurs in both the Old World and the New World, causing two distinct types of leishmaniasis:

Old World CL: Caused by *L. major*, *L. tropica* and *L. aethiopica*; it is found around the Mediterranean basin, throughout the Middle East and Central Asia as far as Pakistan, and in sub-Saharan West Africa and Sudan.

New World CL: Caused by the *L. mexicana* complex, composed of *L. mexicana*, *L. amazonensis* and *L. venezuelensis*, and by the *Viannia* subgenus *L. (V.) brasiliensis* complex constituted by *L. (V.) guyanensis*, *L. (V.) panamensis*, *L. (V.) brasiliensis* and *L. (V.) peruviana*. This form of the disease is largely found in Central and South America.

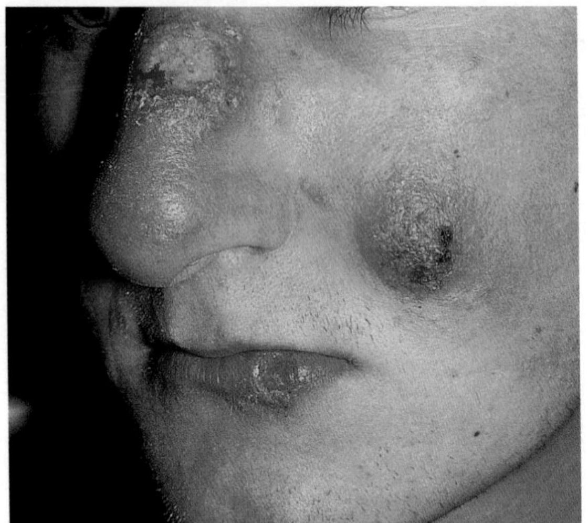

Fig. 5.11 Cutaneous leishmaniasis.

All forms of CL are characterised by ulcerated papules which form at the site of a vector bite. They may be single or multiple, and may measure up to 10 cm in diameter (Fig. 5.11). The incubation period is 2–3 mths (range 2 wks to 5 yrs). There can be satellite lesions, especially in *L. major* and occasionally in *L. tropica* infections. Regional lymphadenopathy, pain, pruritus and secondary bacterial infections may occur. Lesions on the pinna of the ear are more common in New World CL. *L. mexicana* is responsible for chiclero ulcers, self-healing sores seen in Mexico. If immunity is good, there is usually spontaneous healing in *L. tropica*, *L. major* and *L. mexicana* lesions. In some patients with anergy to *Leishmania*, the skin lesions of *L. aethiopica*, *L. mexicana* and *L. amazonensis* infections progress to the development of diffuse CL; this is characterised by spread of the infection from the initial ulcer, usually on the face, to involve the whole body in the form of non-ulcerative nodules. Occasionally, in *L. tropica* infections, sores that have apparently healed relapse persistently (recidivans or lupoid leishmaniasis).

Mucosal leishmaniasis

The *Viannia* subgenus (New World CL) extends from the Amazon basin to Paraguay and Costa Rica and is responsible for deep sores and mucosal leishmaniasis. Young men with chronic lesions are particularly at risk, and between 2% and 40% of infected persons develop 'espundia', metastatic lesions in the mucosa of the nose or mouth. This is characterised by thickening, erythema and later ulceration of the nasal mucosa, typically starting at the junction of the nose and upper lip. The lips, soft palate, fauces and larynx may also be invaded and destroyed. There is no spontaneous healing, and death may result from severe respiratory tract infections due to massive destruction of the pharynx.

Investigations in CL and ML

• Slit skin smear: amastigotes identified using Giemsa stain. • Culture: material obtained from sores or fine needle aspiration. • PCR: increasingly used for diagnosis and speciation.

Management of CL and ML

Treatment of CL should be individualised on the basis of the causative organism, severity of the lesions, availability of drugs, tolerance of the patient for toxicity, and local resistance patterns.

• Small lesions: may self-heal or be treated by freezing with liquid nitrogen or curettage. • Topical application of paromomycin 15% plus methylbenzethonium chloride 12% is beneficial in both Old and New World CL. • Parenteral Sb should be used for multiple lesions. • Intralesional Sb and intralesional antimony have also been used with encouraging results in both Old and New World CL. • ML is treated with 28 days' systemic Sb. • Refractory CL or ML should be treated with conventional or liposomal amphotericin B.

Prevention of CL and ML

Personal protection against sandfly bites is important. No effective vaccine is yet available.

AFRICAN TRYPANOSOMIASIS (SLEEPING SICKNESS)

African sleeping sickness is caused by trypanosomes conveyed to humans by the bites of infected tsetse flies and is unique to sub-Saharan Africa. Two trypanosomes affect humans in Africa: *Trypanosoma brucei gambiense* and *T. rhodesiense. Gambiense* trypanosomiasis has a wide distribution in West and Central Africa; *rhodesiense* trypanosomiasis is found in parts of East and Central Africa.

Clinical features

A bite by a tsetse fly is painful and commonly becomes inflamed, but if trypanosomes are introduced, the site may again become painful and swollen about 10 days later ('trypanosomal chancre') and the regional lymph nodes enlarge ('Winterbottom's sign'). Within 2–3 wks of infection the trypanosomes invade the blood stream.

Rhodesiense infections: Acute and severe. Within days or a few weeks the patient is usually severely ill and may have developed pleural effusions and signs of myocarditis or hepatitis. There may be a petechial rash. The patient may die before there are signs of involvement of the CNS. If the illness is less acute, drowsiness, tremors and coma develop.

Gambiense infection: More indolent, with irregular bouts of fever and firm, discrete, rubbery and painless enlargement of lymph nodes. These are particularly prominent in the posterior triangle of the neck. The spleen and

5.21 TREATMENT OF AFRICAN TRYPANOSOMIASIS		
	First-line	**Second-line**
***Gambiense* trypanosomiasis**		
Stage 1	Pentamidine	Eflornithine or melarsoprol
Stage 2	Melarsoprol	Eflornithine
***Rhodesiense* trypanosomiasis**		
Stage 1	Suramin	Melarsoprol
Stage 2	Melarsoprol	Nifurtimox with melarsoprol

liver may become palpable. After some months, in the absence of treatment, the CNS is invaded. This is shown clinically by headache and changed behaviour, blunting of higher mental functions, insomnia by night and sleepiness by day, mental confusion and eventually tremors, pareses, wasting, coma and death.

Investigations

• Thick and thin blood films: stained as for the detection of malaria, these will reveal trypanosomes. • Card agglutination trypanosomiasis test (CATT): may demonstrate parasitaemia simply and quickly. • Lumbar puncture: in cases of CNS involvement, CSF will reveal raised protein and WCC, with diminished glucose.

Management

Unfortunately, therapeutic options for African trypanosomiasis are limited and most of the antitrypanosomal drugs are toxic and expensive. The prognosis is good if treatment is begun early before the brain has been invaded. Treatments are summarised in Box 5.21.

AMERICAN TRYPANOSOMIASIS (CHAGAS DISEASE)

Chagas disease occurs widely in South and Central America. The cause is *Trypanosoma cruzi*, transmitted to humans from the faeces of a reduviid (triatomine) bug in which the trypanosomes develop before becoming infective to humans. Infected faeces from the bugs are rubbed in through the conjunctiva, mucosa of mouth or nose, or abrasions of the skin in humans. Blood transfusions are responsible for up to 5% of infections and vertical spread may also occur.

Clinical features

Acute phase: The acute phase is seen in only 1–2% of infected individuals before the age of 15 yrs. Young children (1–5 yrs) are most commonly affected. The entrance of *T. cruzi* through an abrasion produces a dusky-red firm swelling and enlargement of regional lymph nodes. A conjunctival lesion, although less common, is more characteristic; the unilateral firm reddish swelling of the lids may close the eye and constitutes 'Romaña's sign'. In a few patients an acute generalised infection soon appears, with a transient morbilliform or urticarial rash, fever, lymphadenopathy and enlargement of the spleen and liver. In a small minority of patients acute myocarditis and heart failure or neurological features, including personality changes and signs of meningoencephalitis, may be seen. The acute infection may be fatal to infants.

Chronic phase: About 50–70% of infected patients become seropositive and develop an indeterminate form when no parasitaemia is detectable. They have a normal lifespan with no symptoms but are a natural reservoir for the disease and maintain the life cycle of parasites. After a latent period of several years, 10–30% of chronic cases develop low-grade myocarditis, and damage to conducting fibres causing a cardiomyopathy. In nearly 10% of patients damage to Auerbach's plexus results in dilatation of various parts of the alimentary canal, especially the colon and oesophagus, so-called 'mega' disease. Dilatation of the bile ducts and bronchi is also a recognised sequela. Reactivation of Chagas disease can occur in patients with AIDS if the CD4 count falls <200 cells/mm^3 (p. 134).

Investigations

• Blood film: *T. cruzi* is easily detectable in the acute illness. • Xenodiagnosis: infection-free, laboratory-bred reduviid bugs are allowed to feed on the patient and the bugs' faeces are subsequently examined for parasites. • PCR: parasite DNA detection by PCR is highly sensitive. • ELISA and indirect immunofluorescence allow diagnosis serologically.

Management

• Nifurtimox and benznidazole are both parasiticidal drugs used in the acute phase for 60–90 days. • Adverse reactions to both drugs are frequent (30–55%). • Cure rates of up to 80% may be achieved. • Surgery may be required for 'mega' disease. • Rates of infection may be reduced by destruction of the reduviid bugs with insecticides.

ACQUIRED TOXOPLASMOSIS

Toxoplasma gondii is a coccidian intracellular parasite ubiquitous in mammals. It is acquired by humans via the consumption of contaminated soil on salads and vegetables, or from undercooked meat. It is the most common protozoal infection in developed countries, and 22% of adults in the UK are seropositive. Up to 60% of pregnant women in India and Brazil are seropositive. Most infections in humans are subclinical. Congenital infection or that occurring in HIV-positive patients may cause considerable morbidity and may be fatal.

Life cycle

The sexual phase of the parasite's life cycle occurs in the small intestinal epithelium of the cat. Oöcysts shed in cat faeces are spread to intermediate hosts (pork, lamb), including humans, through widespread contamination of soil. Once they are ingested by the intermediate host the parasite undergoes transformation, inside the intestinal epithelium, into rapidly dividing tachyzoites through cycles of asexual multiplication, and then infects other tissues. This leads to the formation of microscopic tissue cysts containing bradyzoites which persist for the lifetime of the host. Cats become infected or reinfected by ingesting tissue cysts in their prey.

Clinical features

In most immunocompetent individuals, including children and pregnant women, the infection goes unnoticed. In ~10% of patients it causes a self-limiting illness. The peak incidence of clinical illness is in adults aged 25–35 yrs.

The most common presenting feature is painless lymphadenopathy, which may be localised or generalised. Systemic symptoms, which are flu-like, are infrequent. Complete resolution usually occurs within a few months, although symptoms and lymphadenopathy tend to fluctuate unpredictably and some patients do not recover completely for a year or more. Very infrequently, encephalitis, myocarditis, polymyositis, pneumonitis or hepatitis may develop. Retinochoroiditis is nearly always the result of congenital infection. Toxoplasmosis acquired in utero by vertical spread can also cause hydrocephalus and microcephaly.

Investigations

• Indirect serology: used in immunocompetent patients. Avidity tests for IgG are used to distinguish between past and recent infection; this is important in pregnancy. • Sabin–Feldman dye test: indirect fluorescent antibody test. • Double sandwich IgM ELISA and IgM immunosorbent agglutination assay (ISAGA): may be useful in confirming acute infection. • Lymph node tissue: may be used as a source of *T. gondii* DNA to be amplified by PCR, or be stained with *T. gondii* antisera to demonstrate treponemes histochemically.

Management

As the disease is usually self-limiting, treatment is reserved for rare cases of severe or progressive disease, and for infection in immunocompromised patients *T. gondii* infection responds poorly to antimicrobial therapy but pyrimethamine, sulfadiazine and folinic acid may be used.

GASTROINTESTINAL PROTOZOAL INFECTIONS

AMOEBIASIS

Amoebiasis is caused by *Entamoeba histolytica*; it is common throughout the tropics and occasionally acquired in the UK. Infection can give rise to amoebic dysentery or extra-intestinal amoebiasis, e.g. amoebic liver abscess.

Clinical features

Intestinal amoebiasis or amoebic dysentery: Cysts of *E. histolytica* are ingested in water or uncooked food contaminated by human faeces. The parasite invades the mucous membrane of the large bowel, producing ulceration. The incubation period of amoebiasis ranges from 2 wks to many years, followed by a chronic course with grumbling abdominal pains and two or more unformed stools a day. Diarrhoea alternating with constipation is common, as is mucus, sometimes with streaks of blood; the stools often have an offensive odour. There may be tenderness along the line of the colon, especially over the caecum (which may simulate acute appendicitis) and pelvic colon.

Diagnosis

• Fresh stool sample: may reveal motile trophozoites on microscopy. • Sigmoidoscopy: typical flask-shaped ulcers may be seen and should be scraped for microscopy. • Antibodies are detectable by immunofluorescence in 95% of patients with hepatic amoebiasis and intestinal amoeboma but in only ~60% of dysenteric amoebiasis.

Management

• Intestinal amoebiasis responds quickly to oral metronidazole. • Diloxanide furoate should be given orally for 10 days after treatment to eliminate luminal cysts.

AMOEBIC LIVER ABSCESS

An amoebic liver abscess occurs when a trophozoite enters the portal venous circulation by burrowing through the large bowel mucosa. The trophozoites are carried to the liver, where they multiply and rapidly destroy the parenchyma, forming an amoebic abscess. It is common in the tropics and an important cause of imported fever in Britain.

Clinical features

Local symptoms of an enlarged, tender liver, cough and pain in the right shoulder are characteristic, but symptoms may remain vague and signs minimal. The absence of toxicity in the presence of a high swinging fever is noticeable. A large liver abscess may penetrate the diaphragm and rupture into the lung, from where its contents may be coughed up. Rupture into the pleural cavity, the peritoneal cavity or pericardial sac is less common but more serious.

Investigations

• FBC: neutrophil leucocytosis. • USS of abdomen: visualisation of the abscess. • Aspiration of pus from the amoebic abscess: can occasionally allow visualisation on microscopy. • Detectable antibodies in 95% of patients.

Management

• Metronidazole: used as per intestinal amoebiasis. • Diloxanide furoate: to eliminate the intestinal infection. • Drainage/aspiration: may be required when the abscess threatens to burst.

GIARDIASIS

Infection with *Giardia intestinalis*, also known as *G. lamblia*, is found world-wide and is common in the tropics. It particularly affects children, tourists and immunosuppressed individuals, and is the parasite most commonly imported into the UK. The cysts remain viable in water for up to 3 mths and infection usually occurs by ingesting contaminated water.

The parasites attach to the duodenal and jejunal mucosa, causing inflammation. After an incubation period of 1–3 wks, there is diarrhoea, abdominal pain, weakness, anorexia, nausea and vomiting. On examination there may be abdominal distension and tenderness. Diagnosis is made on stool microscopy demonstrating cysts. Treatment is with a single dose of tinidazole 2 g, or metronidazole 2 g once daily for 3 days or 400 mg 8-hourly for 10 days.

CRYPTOSPORIDIOSIS

Cryptosporidium parvum is a coccidian protozoal parasite of humans and domestic animals. Infection is acquired by the faecal–oral route through contaminated water supplies. The incubation period is approximately 7–10 days, and is followed by watery diarrhoea and abdominal cramps. The illness is usually self-limiting, but in immunocompromised patients, especially those with AIDS, the illness can be devastating, with persistent severe diarrhoea and substantial weight loss (p. 136).

INFECTIONS CAUSED BY HELMINTHS

Helminths (from the Greek *helmins*, meaning worm) include several classes of parasitic worm, large multicellular organisms with complex tissues and organs. Three groups of helminths parasitise humans:

• Annelids (segmented worms), including leeches. • Nematodes (roundworms): intestinal (e.g. *Ancylostoma*, *Strongyloides*, *Ascaris*) or tissue-dwelling (e.g. *Wuchereria bancrofti* (filaria)). • Platyhelminths (flatworms), including trematodes (flukes) and cestodes (tapeworms).

INTESTINAL HUMAN NEMATODES

ANCYLOSTOMIASIS (HOOKWORM)

The causative organism is *Ancylostoma duodenale* or *Necator americanus*. It is one of the main causes of anaemia in the tropics. The life cycle involves the passage of the hookworm from the soil through the skin via the blood stream to the lungs. The worms ascend the bronchi and are swallowed, the adult worm inhabiting the duodenum and jejunum. Eggs are passed in faeces, and develop through the larval stage to the filariform infective stage in the soil. Geographic distribution is as follows:

• *A. duodenale*: Far East, Mediterranean coastal regions, Africa. • *N. americanus*: West, East and Central Africa, Central and South America, Far East.

Clinical features

• Cutaneous: dermatitis of the feet at the time of infection. • Pulmonary: paroxysmal cough, blood-stained sputum. • GI: vomiting, epigastric pain, diarrhoea. • Systemic: symptoms of iron deficiency anaemia such as tiredness, malaise.

Investigations

• Stool sample: culture and microscopy. FOB testing may be positive. • FBC: eosinophilia. • CXR: patchy consolidation.

Management

• Mebendazole for 3 days is the treatment of choice. • Albendazole can be used if a single-dose treatment is required. • Oral iron supplementation should be used in patients who are anaemic.

STRONGYLOIDIASIS

Strongyloides stercoralis is the causative organism (2 mm × 0.4 mm). The life cycle involves the passage of the filariform larvae in the soil through the skin to the upper part of the small intestine where the adult worms live. Eggs produced by the female hatch in the bowel and are passed in the larval stage in the faeces. Autoinfection may lead to a chronic form of the disease. It is found in the tropics, subtropics and Far East.

Clinical features

• Cutaneous: itchy rash, urticarial papules and plaques, larva currens (linear urticarial weals on buttocks and abdomen). • GI: diarrhoea, abdominal pain, steatorrhoea, weight loss. • Pulmonary symptoms (wheeze, cough) and neurological symptoms (meningoencephalitis) may occur in disseminated infection.

Investigations

• Stool sample: microscopy (motile larvae may be seen) and culture. • Jejunal aspirate/string test. • Blood: eosinophilia and antibodies by ELISA.

Management

• Ivermectin is first choice. • Albendazole is an alternative.

ASCARIS LUMBRICOIDES (ROUNDWORM)

Disease is caused by a pale yellow nematode (20–35 cm long) and is an important cause of intestinal obstruction in the tropics. The life cycle begins with ingestion of mature ova in contaminated food. *Ascaris* larvae hatch in the duodenum, migrate through the lungs, ascend the bronchial tree, are swallowed and mature in the small intestine.

Clinical features

• GI: abdominal pain, severe obstructive complications (particularly at the terminal ileum), intussusception, volvulus, haemorrhagic infarction and perforation, weight loss. • Hepatobiliary: blockage of the bile or pancreatic duct with worms. • Symptoms due to a generalised hypersensitivity reaction caused by tissue migration: pneumonitis, bronchial asthma, urticaria.

Investigations

• Stool sample: adult worms visible; microscopy reveals ova. • FBC: eosinophilia. • Barium enema: may occasionally demonstrate worms.

Management

• Mebendazole for 3 days is the treatment of choice; alternatively, single-dose treatment with albendazole or piperazine. • Patients should be warned they may expel numerous large worms.

ENTEROBIUS VERMICULARIS (THREADWORM)

This helminthic infection is common throughout the world, especially in children. The life cycle begins with the ingestion of ova which develop in the small intestine. Adult worms live in the colon. The adult female lays eggs around the anus, causing intense itching; eggs may be carried on the fingers to the mouth, causing autoinfection.

Clinical features

Intense itch in the perianal or genital area is the most common presenting symptom.

Investigations

Ova may be collected on a strip of adhesive tape applied in the morning to the perianal skin.

Management

• Single dose of mebendazole 100 mg, albendazole 400 mg or piperazine 4 g. Dosing should be repeated at 2 wks to prevent auto-reinfection. • If infection is recurrent, all family members should be treated. • General hygiene measures help to prevent spread: laundering of bed clothes, keeping nails short and clean.

TRICHURIS TRICHIURA (WHIPWORM)

This is common all over the world under unhygienic conditions. The life cycle begins with ingestion of ova in contaminated food. Adult worms 3–5 cm in length live in the caecum, lower ileum, appendix, colon and anal canal.

• Infection is usually asymptomatic; intense infections may cause persistent diarrhoea or rectal prolapse. • Diagnosis is by stool microscopy for ova. • Treatment involves mebendazole for 3 days or albendazole if single-dose treatment is required.

TISSUE-DWELLING HUMAN NEMATODES

FILARIASES

Filarial worms are tissue-dwelling nematodes. The larval stages are inoculated by biting mosquitoes or flies. The larvae develop into adult worms

(2–50 cm long) which, after mating, produce millions of microfilariae (170–320 microns long) that migrate in blood or skin. Worms live 10–15 yrs and microfilariae 2–3 yrs. The life cycle is completed when the vector takes up microfilariae while feeding on humans, normally the only host.

LYMPHATIC FILARIASIS

The causative organisms are *Wuchereria bancrofti* and *Brugia malayi*, which have different geographic distribution:
• *W. bancrofti* occurs in tropical Africa, coastal areas of North Africa, Asia, Indonesia and northern Australia, the South Pacific islands, the West Indies and North and South America. • *B. malayi* affects Indonesia, Borneo, Malaysia, Vietnam, South China, South India and Sri Lanka.

Clinical features

Acute: Filarial lymphangitis presents with fever, pain, tenderness and erythema along the course of inflamed lymphatic vessels. Inflammation of the spermatic cord, epididymitis and orchitis are common. The whole episode lasts a few days but may recur several times a year.

Chronic: Oedema becomes persistent and regional lymph nodes enlarge. Progressive enlargement, coarsening, corrugation and fissuring of the skin and subcutaneous tissue develop gradually, causing irreversible 'elephantiasis'. The scrotum may reach an enormous size. Chyluria and chylous effusions are milky and opalescent.

Tropical pulmonary eosinophilia: May develop when filariae enter pulmonary capillaries, causing a massive allergic response. This presents with cough, wheeze and fever, and may progress to chronic interstitial lung disease.

Investigations

• FBC: massive eosinophilia (the highest of all the helminthic infections). • Indirect immunofluorescence on serum to detect filarial antibodies. • Wet blood film from a sample drawn at night (microfilariae circulate in large numbers at night). • Radiology: calcified filariae may be detected on X-ray.

Management

Diethylcarbamazine (DEC) kills microfilariae and adult worms. In the first 24–36 hrs of therapy, a severe allergic response to dying microfilariae, characterised by fever, headache, nausea, vomiting, arthralgia and prostration, may be seen, and severity is proportional to the filarial load. Antihistamines and oral steroid may be used to control the symptoms. Chronic lymphoedema should be managed with physiotherapy, tight bandaging and elevation, as well as scrupulous attention to skin care to prevent infection. DEC can also be used for prophylaxis in endemic area with a once-yearly dose. Surgery is useful in selected cases.

LOIASIS

The causative organism is the filaria *Loa loa*. The adults, 3–7 cm × 4 mm, chiefly parasitise the subcutaneous tissue of humans.

Clinical features

The infection is often symptomless. The first sign is usually a Calabar swelling, an irritating, tense, localised swelling up to a few centimetres in diameter that develops around an adult worm. The swelling is generally on a limb, and may be particularly painful if near a joint. It usually disappears after a few days but may persist for 2 or 3 wks. Other cutaneous signs include urticaria or, rarely, a visible worm wriggling under the skin (especially that of an eyelid).

Investigations

• Blood: direct visualisation of filariae, eosinophilia. • Immunology: indirect immunofluorescence showing antibodies to filariae. • X-rays: may demonstrate a calcified worm.

Management

• DEC for 3 wks. • Protective clothing and insect repellent to prevent inoculation.

ONCHOCERCIASIS (RIVER BLINDNESS)

The causative organism is *Onchocerca volvulus*; it is transmitted to humans by a bite from the *Simulium* fly. It is a major cause of blindness in sub-Saharan Africa, Yemen, and parts of Central and South America. The worms live for up to 17 yrs in human tissue. Live microfilariae are poorly immunogenic, but dead ones elicit severe allergic inflammation. When this process occurs in the eye, conjunctivitis, sclerosing keratitis, 'snowflake' deposits on the cornea, choroidoretinitis and optic neuritis may result.

Clinical features

• May be symptomless in the early stages of disease. • Itchy papular urticaria: excoriated papules, patchy hyperpigmentation, thickened, wrinkled skin. • Superficial lymph node enlargement: may become pendulous in the groin area. • Firm subcutaneous nodules (onchocercomas) resulting from fibrosis around adult worms. • Eyes: itch, lacrimation, conjunctival injection progressing to the changes listed above.

Investigations

• Direct microscopy of skin snip/shaving: demonstrates microfilariae. • FBC: eosinophilia. • Immunology: indirect immunofluorescence of serum may demonstrate filarial antibodies.

Management

• Ivermectin in a single dose is the treatment of choice, as it is non-toxic and, unlike DEC, does not trigger severe reactions. • Prevention takes the form of protective clothing, population prophylaxis with ivermectin, and insecticides to kill the *Simulium* fly.

DRACUNCULIASIS (GUINEA WORM)

The Guinea worm (*Dracunculus medinensis*) is another tissue-dwelling nematode that is transmitted to humans by the ingestion of the crustacean *Cyclops*, now found only in sub-Saharan Africa. Management is by extraction of the protruding worm (which is over a metre long), by winding it out gently over several days on a matchstick. The worm must not be broken.

ZOONOTIC NEMATODES

TRICHINOSIS (TRICHINELLOSIS)

Trichinella spiralis is a nematode that parasitises rats and pigs and is transmitted to humans by consumption of partially cooked infected pork or bear meat. Symptoms result from invasion of intestinal submucosa by ingested larvae, which develop into adult worms, and the secondary invasion of tissues, particularly striated muscle, by fresh larvae produced by these adult worms. Outbreaks have occurred in the UK as well as in other countries where pork is eaten.

Clinical features

• Infection may be asymptomatic. • GI symptoms such as nausea and diarrhoea develop within 24–48 hrs coincident with invasion of the intestinal mucosa. • Larval invasion on day 4–5 produces fever and oedema of the face, eyelids and conjunctivae. • Larval invasion of muscle produces myositis. • Larval migration may cause acute myocarditis and encephalitis.

Investigations

• Muscle biopsy: microscopy may reveal encysted larvae. • Public health investigations: may reveal a cluster of cases who have eaten infected pork from a common source.

Management

• Albendazole kills newly formed adult worms. • Corticosteroids are required to counteract the effects of acute inflammation.

TREMATODES (FLUKES)

These leaf-shaped worms are parasitic to humans and animals. Their complex life cycles may involve one or more intermediate hosts, often freshwater molluscs.

SCHISTOSOMIASIS

Schistosomiasis (bilharziasis) is a major cause of morbidity in the tropics and is being spread by irrigation schemes. There are three species of the genus *Schistosoma* which commonly cause disease in humans: *S. haematobium*, *S. mansoni* and *S. japonicum*. The life cycle of *S. haematobium* is illustrated in Figure 5.12. The human is the definitive host, and the freshwater snail the intermediate host.

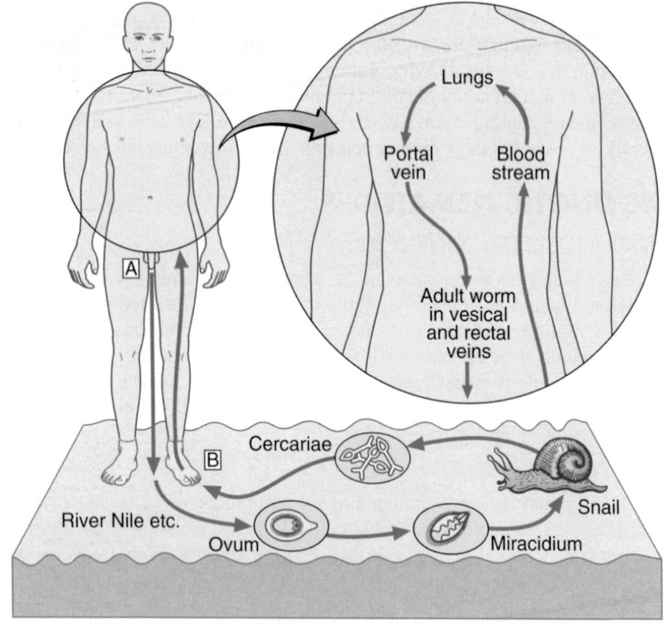

Fig. 5.12 Life cycle of *Schistosoma*. A Ova are passed into fresh water in urine and faeces. B Cercariae in fresh water penetrate the skin of bathers, infecting a new host.

Clinical features

These vary between species and are dependent on the stage of infection. The eggs of *S. haematobium* mainly pass through the wall of the bladder, but may also involve the rectum, seminal vesicles, vagina, cervix and Fallopian tubes. Painless terminal haematuria is the most common symptom. *S. mansoni* and *S. japonicum* mainly pass through the wall of the bowel and are deposited in the liver. Hepatosplenomegaly is a common sign in these infections. A summary of the symptoms of cercarial infection as they correlate to the stage of infection is illustrated in Box 5.22. Chronic schistosomiasis may also occur, with the intensity of symptoms related to the helminthic load.

Investigations

S. haematobium: Dipstick urine testing shows blood and albumin. Microscopy of terminal urine sample shows spined eggs. USS may demonstrate bladder wall thickening, hydronephrosis and bladder calcification. Cystoscopy reveals 'sandy' patches, bleeding mucosa and later distortion.

S. mansoni/S. japonicum: Stool microscopy demonstrates the characteristic egg with its lateral spine. Rectal biopsy may demonstrate schistosomes. USS of the liver may reveal calcified schistosomes. Blood tests

5.22 CLINICAL PATHOLOGY OF SCHISTOSOMIASIS			
Stage	**Time**	***S. haematobium***	***S. mansoni* and *S. japonicum***
Cercarial penetration	Days	Papular dermatitis at site of penetration	As for *S. haematobium*
Larval migration and maturation	Weeks	Pneumonitis; myositis; hepatitis; fever; 'serum sickness'; eosinophilia; seroconversion	As for *S. haematobium*
Early egg deposition	Months	Cystitis; haematuria; ectopic granulomatous lesions: skin, CNS; immune complex glomerulonephritis	Colitis; granulomatous hepatitis; acute portal hypertension; ectopic lesions as for *S. haematobium*
Late egg deposition	Years	Fibrosis and calcification of ureters, bladder: bacterial infection, calculi, hydronephrosis, carcinoma; pulmonary granulomas and pulmonary hypertension	Colonic polyposis and strictures; periportal fibrosis; portal hypertension; pulmonary features as for *S. haematobium*

show eosinophilia. Serology (ELISA) aids screening but remains positive after cure.

Management

• Praziquantel is the drug of choice for all forms of schistosomiasis, producing parasitological cure in 80% of individuals. • Side-effects are uncommon but include nausea and abdominal pain. • Surgical intervention for ureteric stricture or bladder thickening may be required.

LIVER FLUKES

Liver flukes infect at least 20 million people and remain an important public health problem in many endemic areas. They are associated with abdominal pain, hepatomegaly and relapsing cholangitis. *Clonorchis sinensis* is a major aetiological agent of bile duct cancer.

CESTODES (TAPEWORMS)

Cestodes are ribbon-shaped worms which inhabit the intestinal tract of humans who have ingested undercooked infected beef, pork or fish. The causative organisms in each of these foods are respectively *Taenia saginata*, *T. solium and Diphyllobothrium latum*. *T. solium* is common in central

Europe, South Africa, South America and parts of Asia, while infection with *T. saginata* occurs in all parts of the world. The adult worm may be several metres long. Diagnosis is by finding ova on examination of the stool. Praziquantel is the drug of choice, and prevention depends on efficient meat inspection and the thorough cooking of beef.

CYSTICERCOSIS

Human cysticercosis is acquired either by ingesting *T. solium* ova on contaminated fingers (faeco-oral route) or by eating undercooked, contaminated pork (Fig. 5.13). The larvae are liberated from eggs in the stomach, penetrate the intestinal mucosa and are carried to many parts of the body where they develop and form cysticerci, 0.5–1 cm cysts that contain the

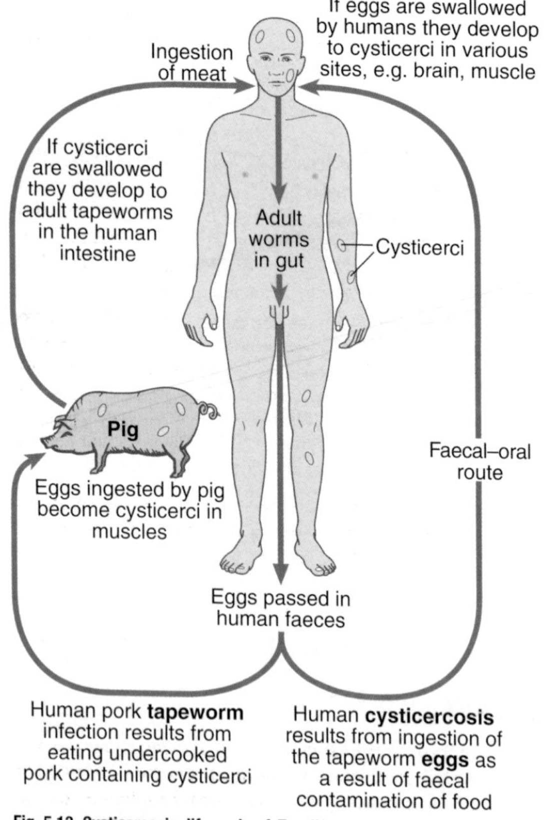

Fig. 5.13 Cysticercosis: life cycle of *T. solium*.

head of a young worm. Common locations are the subcutaneous tissue, skeletal muscles and brain.

Clinical features

• There are palpable cutaneous nodules which may calcify. • Infection of the cerebral tissue may cause personality change, epilepsy, hydrocephalus or encephalitis.

Investigations

• Biopsy of a cutaneous nodule: may demonstrate cysticerci. • CT/MRI: will demonstrate calcified cysts. • Immunology: cysticercosis antibodies may be detected by indirect immunofluorescence on serum.

Management and prevention

• Praziquantel is the drug of choice for cerebral cysticercosis. • Albendazole is the drug of choice for parenchymal neurocysticercosis. • Seizures should be controlled with appropriate anti-epileptic medicines. • Good food handling and hygiene practices will reduce transmission.

ECHINOCOCCUS GRANULOSUS (*TAENIA ECHINOCOCCUS*) AND HYDATID DISEASE

Dogs are the definitive hosts of the tiny tapeworm *E. granulosus*; ova produced by the adult worms inhabiting the dog are ingested by intermediate hosts, which include sheep, cattle, camels and humans. The embryo is liberated from the ovum in the small intestine and gains access to the blood stream and thus to the liver. The resultant cyst grows very slowly, sometimes intermittently, and may outlive the patient. It may calcify or rupture, giving rise to multiple cysts. The disease is common in the Middle East, North and East Africa, Australia and Argentina. Foci of infection persist in rural Wales and Scotland.

Clinical features

Hydatid disease is typically acquired in childhood; it causes cysts in the liver (75% of cases), lung, bone or brain, in order of frequency. Symptoms are slow to develop and are a result of local pressure.

Investigations

• USS or CT usually demonstrates the cyst. • Serology is positive in 70–90%.

Management and prevention

• Surgical excision is the treatment of choice, with praziquantel administered peri-operatively to kill protoscolices. • Albendazole may be used for inoperable disease. • Good personal hygiene and animal handling practices, and regular deworming of dogs can reduce disease prevalence.

FUNGAL INFECTIONS

Superficial fungal infections of the skin (ringworm, dermatophytosis) are described in Chapter 17.

DEEP FUNGAL INFECTIONS OF THE SKIN AND SUBCUTANEOUS TISSUES

SPOROTRICHOSIS

The causative organism is *Sporothrix schenckii*. The clinical presentation is usually a localised subcutaneous nodule that develops at the site of infection, which subsequently ulcerates with a pustular discharge (fixed cutaneous). The disease may then spread along the cutaneous lymphatic channels, resulting in multiple cutaneous nodules along their route, which ulcerate and produce a pustular discharge (lymphocutaneous). Pulmonary involvement occurs but is rare.

Diagnosis

Biopsy: tissue should be sent for microscopy and culture.

Management

• Oral itraconazole for cutaneous and lymphocutaneous disease. • Amphotericin B for systemic life-threatening illness.

MYCETOMA

Mycetoma is a chronic suppurative infection of the deep soft tissues and bones, occurring mainly in the tropics. The limbs are most commonly affected. It is caused either by anaerobic filamentous bacteria, *Actinomycetes* (60%—actinomycetoma), or by true fungi, *Eumycetes* (40%—eumycetoma). Both groups produce characteristically coloured grains, the colour depending on the organism.

Clinical features

The causative organism is usually introduced by a thorn and the infection is most common on the foot (Madura foot). The mycetoma begins as a painless swelling at the site of implantation, which grows and spreads steadily within the soft tissues, causing further swelling and eventually penetrating bones. Nodules develop under the epidermis and these rupture, revealing sinuses through which grains (fungal colonies) are discharged. Deeper tissue invasion and involvement of bone are rapid and greater in actinomycetoma than eumycetoma. There is little pain and usually no fever or lymphadenopathy, but there is progressive disability.

Investigations

Biopsy/aspiration of pus: send for microscopy, culture and determination of sensitivity.

Management

• *Eumycetes*: ketoconazole or itraconazole. • *Actinomycetes*: streptomycin/amikacin plus dapsone/co-trimoxazole. • Surgical: resection of lesions, amputation in severe cases.

CHROMOMYCOSIS (CHROMOBLASTOMYCOSIS)

Chromomycosis is a tropical fungal disease of the cutaneous and subcutaneous tissue. The causative organism is most commonly *Fonsecaea pedrosoi*, and the disease is inoculated by trauma, particularly in those walking barefoot. Lesions may start several months after the injury in the form of a papule which later turns into a painless, itchy, scaly nodule or plaque. Later there may be hypertrophy of the tissue, leading to a verrucous and cauliflower-like appearance.

Diagnosis

Biopsy shows brown, rounded sclerotic bodies. • Culture confirms the aetiological agent.

Management

• Oral itraconazole or terbinafine. • Cryosurgery with liquid nitrogen.

SYSTEMIC FUNGAL INFECTIONS

CANDIDIASIS

Of the 200 species of *Candida,* only 10% are involved in human disease, most commonly *C. albicans*. Other species increasingly implicated are *C. tropicalis*, *C. glabrata* and *C. krusei*. Infection is most common in the immunosuppressed, particularly neutropenic patients, as neutrophils form the body's main defence against *Candida*. The source of infection is usually endogenous, originating in flora in the patient's oropharyngeal and genital areas, most commonly producing oropharyngeal or vaginal candidiasis or 'thrush'.

Clinical features

There are three typical manifestations of systemic candidiasis:

Ophthalmic involvement: 'Cotton wool' exudates on the retina, progressing to vitreous haze. This can result in blindness.

Skin lesions: Non-tender pink/red nodules that occasionally coalesce.

Chronic disseminated hepatosplenic candidiasis: Presents in leukaemic patients as persistent fever in neutropenia despite antibacterial therapy. The alkaline phosphatase is elevated and multiple lesions are seen in liver and spleen on imaging. This infection may last for months despite therapy.

Management

• Infection detected on blood culture must be treated aggressively. • Amphotericin B is the treatment of choice. • Fluconazole is useful if the causative organism is *C. albicans.*

HISTOPLASMOSIS

Histoplasmosis is caused by *Histoplasma capsulatum* and is found in all parts of the USA, especially in the east central states. A variant, *H. duboisii*, is found in parts of tropical Africa. *H. capsulatum* multiplies in soil enriched by the droppings of birds and bats. Infection is by inhalation of infected dust.

Clinical features

• *Histoplasma* infection is usually asymptomatic or self-limiting. • Pulmonary symptoms are common, with non-productive cough, pleuritic pain and an influenza-like illness. • On examination lymphadenopathy, rashes and pulmonary crackles may be found.

Investigations

• Biopsy: tissue should be sent for smear, histology and culture. • CXR/USS: may show calcified lesions in lungs/spleen. • Complement-fixating and precipitin tests.

Management

• Amphotericin B i.v. in severe infection. • Itraconazole for chronic infection. • Prednisolone: may be used for dyspnoea.

COCCIDIOIDOMYCOSIS

This is caused by the air-borne organism *Coccidioides immitis* and is found in Central America. The infection behaves like TB or histoplasmosis. Carriage may be asymptomatic (40%), or may affect the lungs, lymph nodes and skin. Pulmonary coccidioidomycosis has two forms:

Primary coccidioidomycosis: Behaves like primary TB or histoplasmosis and is often asymptomatic.

Progressive coccidioidomycosis: Associated with marked systemic upset and features of lobar pneumonia.

Diagnosis is by complement fixation and precipitin tests, and treatment is with systemic anti-fungals (e.g. amphotericin, fluconazole).

PARACOCCIDIOIDOMYCOSIS

This is caused by *Paracoccidioides brasiliensis* and occurs in South America. Mucocutaneous lesions occur early. Involvement of lymphatic nodes and the lungs is prominent and the GI tract may also be attacked. Treatment is with systemic antifungal agents.

BLASTOMYCOSIS

North American blastomycosis is caused by *Blastomyces dermatitidis*. It also occurs in Africa. Systemic infection begins in the lungs and mediastinal lymph nodes and resembles pulmonary TB. Bones, skin and the genitourinary tract may also be affected. Treatment is with systemic antifungal agents.

CRYPTOCOCCOSIS

This is found world-wide and is caused by *Cryptococcus neoformans*. It causes local gumma-like tumours and granulomatous lesions of the lung, bones, brain and meninges. Immunocompromised individuals are at special risk, including those with HIV infection.

The diagnosis is made by culture or recognition of spores in the CSF (India ink stain). The CSF shows a lymphocytosis and is often at high pressure (consequently, the condition may be complicated by raised intracranial pressure). Biopsy and serological detection of antigen may also be useful. Treatment is with i.v. antifungal agents such as amphotericin B. Recovery may be monitored by a fall in the antigen titres.

SEXUALLY TRANSMITTED BACTERIAL INFECTIONS

SYPHILIS

Syphilis is caused by infection, through abrasions in the skin or mucous membranes, with the spirochaete *Treponema pallidum*. In adults the infection is usually sexually acquired; however, transmission by kissing, blood transfusion and percutaneous injury has been reported. Transplacental infection of the fetus can occur.

Primary syphilis: The incubation period is usually between 14 and 28 days with a range of 9–90 days. The primary lesion or chancre develops at the site of infection, usually in the genital area. A dull red macule develops, becomes papular and then erodes to form an indurated, painless ulcer (chancre). Without treatment, the chancre will resolve within 2–6 wks to leave a thin atrophic scar.

Secondary syphilis: This occurs 6–8 wks after the development of the chancre when treponemes disseminate to produce a multisystem disease. Constitutional features such as mild fever, malaise and headache are common. Over 75% of patients present with a rash on the trunk and limbs that may later involve the palms and soles. Generalised non-tender lymphadenopathy is present in >50% of patients. Mucosal lesions, known as mucous patches, may affect the genitalia, mouth, pharynx or larynx and are essentially modified papules, which become eroded. Rarely, confluence produces characteristic 'snail track ulcers' in the mouth.

Tertiary syphilis: This may develop between 3 and 10 yrs after infection. The characteristic feature is a chronic granulomatous lesion called a gumma, which may be single or multiple and can affect skin, mucosa, bone, muscles or viscera. Resolution of active disease should follow treatment, though some tissue damage may be permanent.

After several years, cardiovascular syphilis, particularly aortitis, and neurosyphilis, which may present as meningovascular disease, tabes dorsalis or general paralysis of the insane, may develop (see page 673).

Congenital syphilis: This is rare where antenatal serological screening is practised. Antisyphilitic treatment in pregnancy treats the fetus, if infected, as well as the mother. Treponemal infection in pregnancy may result in:

• Miscarriage or stillbirth. • A syphilitic baby (a very sick baby with hepatosplenomegaly and a bullous rash). • A baby who develops signs of congenital syphilis (condylomata lata, oral/anal/genital fissures, 'snuffles', lymphadenopathy and hepatosplenomegaly).

Adults with congenital syphilis may display the following classic features:

• Hutchinson's incisors (anterior–posterior thickening with notch on narrowed cutting edge). • Mulberry molars (imperfectly formed cusps/deficient dental enamel). • High arched palate. • Maxillary hypoplasia. • Rhagades (radiating scars around mouth, nose and anus). • Sabre tibia (from periostitis). • Bossing of frontal and parietal bones.

The treatment of choice is penicillin by injection.

GONORRHOEA

Gonorrhoea is caused by infection with *Neisseria gonorrhoeae* and may involve columnar epithelium in the lower genital tract, rectum, pharynx and eyes. Transmission is usually the result of vaginal, anal or oral sex. The incubation period is usually 2–10 days.

In men the anterior urethra is commonly infected, causing urethral discharge and dysuria, but symptoms are absent in ~10% of cases. Epididymo-orchitis may occur. In women, the urethra, para-urethral glands/ducts, Bartholin's glands/ducts or endocervical canal may be infected. Acute pelvic inflammatory disease (PID, see below) is a rare complication. The rectum may also be involved, either due to contamination from a urogenital site or as a result of anal sex. Gramnegative intracellular diplococci are seen on direct smears from infected sites. Uncomplicated gonorrhoea responds to a single adequate dose of a suitable antimicrobial, e.g. oral cefixime 400 mg.

CHLAMYDIAL INFECTION

Chlamydia is transmitted and presents in a similar way to gonorrhea:

In men, urethral symptoms are usually mild and occur in <50% of cases. Epididymo-orchitis may occur. In women, the cervix and urethra are commonly involved. Infection is asymptomatic in ~80% of women but may cause vaginal discharge, dysuria, intermenstrual and/or postcoital bleeding. Lower abdominal pain, dyspareunia and intermenstrual bleeding suggest complicating pelvic inflammatory disease (PID). Examination may reveal mucopurulent cervicitis, contact bleeding from the cervix, evidence of PID or no obvious clinical signs. PID, with the risk of tubal damage and subsequent infertility or ectopic pregnancy, is an important long-term complication. Treatment options for chlamydia include a single 1 g oral dose of azithromycin although PID requires more prolonged treatment.

SEXUALLY TRANSMITTED VIRAL INFECTIONS

Herpes simplex: Genital herpes simplex transmission is usually sexual (vaginal, anal, orogenital or oro-anal), but perinatal infection of the neonate may also occur. The manifestations of herpes simplex infection are covered on page 71.

Human papillomavirus (HPV): Of the many subtypes of HPV, genotypes 6, 11, 16 and 18 most commonly infect the genital tract through sexual transmission.

Genotypes HPV-6 and 11 cause benign anogenital warts. • Genotypes such as 16 and 18 are associated with dysplastic conditions and cancers, but not benign warts. Anogenital warts are the result of HPV-driven hyperplasia and usually develop after an incubation period of between 3 mths and 2 yrs. Local treatment with cryotherapy or podophyllotoxin may help; condoms offer some protection and vaccines are now in use in some countries.

HUMAN IMMUNODEFICIENCY VIRUS INFECTION

The acquired immunodeficiency syndrome (AIDS) is caused by the human immunodeficiency virus (HIV-1) and was first recognised in 1981. HIV-2 causes a similar but less aggressive illness occurring mainly in West Africa. AIDS has become the second leading cause of disease world-wide and the leading cause of death in Africa (causing >20% of deaths). Immune deficiency arises from continuous HIV replication leading to virus- and immune-mediated destruction of CD4 lymphocytes.

GLOBAL EPIDEMIC AND REGIONAL PATTERNS

In 2004, the WHO estimated that there were 39.4 million people living with HIV/AIDS, 4.9 million new infections and 3.1 million deaths. The cumulative death toll since 1981 exceeds 20 million, the vast majority in sub-Saharan Africa where over 13 million children have been orphaned. In Botswana, South Africa, Swaziland and Zimbabwe, 25–40% of adults are infected. Since 2002, the steepest increases (50%) have been seen in East Asia (principally in China), and in Eastern Europe and Central Asia (40%), particularly in the Ukraine, Latvia and Russia.

In the USA and northern Europe, the epidemic has until now predominantly affected men who have sex with men (MSM), whereas in southern and Eastern Europe, Vietnam and China the incidence has been greatest in injection drug-users. In Africa, the Caribbean and much of South-east Asia most transmission is heterosexual and many additional cases arise from mother to child transmission (vertical).

In industrialised nations, heterosexual transmission has recently become the dominant route, with racial and ethnic minorities representing an increasing fraction. Around 58% of infections in the UK in 2003 were acquired heterosexually and 75% of these were acquired abroad in countries with a high prevalence of HIV, mainly in sub-Saharan Africa.

MODES OF TRANSMISSION

HIV is present in blood, semen and other body fluids such as breast milk and saliva. Exposure to infected fluid leads to a risk of infection, which is dependent on the integrity of the exposed site, the type and volume of body fluid, and the viral load. HIV can enter either as free virus or within cells. The modes of spread are:

• Sexual (man to man, heterosexual and oral). • Parenteral (blood or blood products, injection drug-users and those experiencing occupational injury). • Vertical.

The transmission risk after exposure is:

• >90% for blood or blood products. • 15–40% for the vertical route. • 0.5–1.0% for injection drug use. • 0.2–0.5% for genital mucous membrane spread. • <0.1% for non-genital mucous membrane spread.

World-wide, the major route of transmission (>75%) is heterosexual. Between 5 and 10% of new HIV infections are in children and >90% of these are infected during pregnancy, birth or breastfeeding.

Around 70% of patients with haemophilia A and 30% of those with haemophilia B had been infected through contaminated blood products by the time HIV antibody screening was adopted in the USA and Europe in 1985. In developed nations, because of routine antibody screening, the likelihood of acquiring HIV from blood products is now <1 : 500 000 and arises from donors in the seroconverting phase of infection. However, the WHO estimates that because of the lack of adequate screening facilities in resource-poor countries, 5–10% of blood transfusions globally are with HIV-infected blood. There have been ~100 definite and 200 possible cases of HIV acquired occupationally in health-care workers.

VIROLOGY AND IMMUNOLOGY

HIV is a single-stranded RNA retrovirus. The different stages of the viral replication process offer opportunities for drug therapy (Box 5.23). A minority of T cells (<0.01%) either produce small quantities of virus or enter a post-integration latent phase and represent the main reservoir of HIV. Within these cells, low-level replication continues even when plasma levels of HIV are undetectable as a result of antiretroviral treatment. Viral half-life is:

• 1–2 hrs in plasma. • 1.5 days in productively infected CD4 cells. • >12 mths in latently infected CD4 cells.

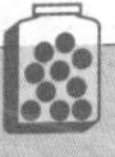

5.23 STAGES OF VIRAL REPLICATION AND CORRESPONDING DRUG TARGETS

Stage	Steps in replication	Drug targets
1	Attachment to CD4 receptor	CCR5/CXCR4 receptor inhibitors
2	Binding to co-receptor CCR5 or CXCR4	
3	Fusion	Fusion inhibitors
4	Reverse transcription	Nucleoside and non-nucleoside reverse transcription inhibitors (NRTIs and NNRTIs)
5	Integration	Integrase inhibitors
6	Transcription	
7	Translation	
8	Cleavage of polypeptides and assembly	Protease inhibitors (PIs)
9	Viral release	

NATURAL HISTORY AND CLASSIFICATION OF HIV

PRIMARY INFECTION

Primary infection is symptomatic in 70–80% of cases and usually occurs 2–6 wks after exposure. The major clinical manifestations are:

• Fever with rash. • Pharyngitis with cervical lymphadenopathy. • Myalgia/arthralgia. • Headache. • Mucosal ulceration.

Rarely, presentation may be neurological (aseptic meningitis, encephalitis, myelitis, polyneuritis). Symptomatic recovery normally takes 1–2 wks but may take up to 10 wks, and parallels the return of the CD4 count and the fall in viral load. In many patients the illness is mild and is only identified by retrospective enquiry.

Diagnosis is made by detecting HIV-RNA in the serum, or antibodies to early proteins. The differential diagnosis of primary HIV includes:

• Acute Epstein–Barr virus (EBV). • Cytomegalovirus (CMV). • Streptococcal pharyngitis. • Toxoplasmosis. • Secondary syphilis.

ASYMPTOMATIC INFECTION

This lasts for a variable period, during which the infected individual remains well with no evidence of disease, except for the possible presence of persistent generalised lymphadenopathy (PGL, defined as enlarged glands at ≥2 extra-inguinal sites). There is sustained viraemia with a decline in CD4 count dependent on the height of the viral load but usually between 50 and 150 cells/yr (Fig. 5.14).

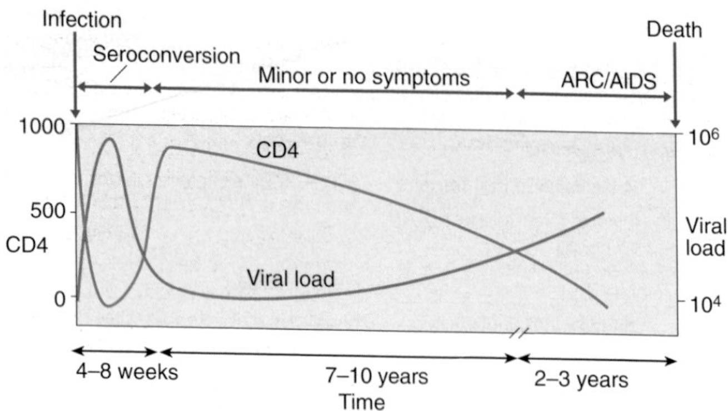

Fig. 5.14 Virological and immunological progression of HIV infection. (ARC = AIDS-related complex)

MILDLY SYMPTOMATIC DISEASE

The majority of patients then develop a variety of problems, indicating impairment of the cellular immune system (AIDS-related complex (ARC)):

• Oral hairy leucoplakia. • Recurrent oropharyngeal or vaginal candidiasis. • Severe PID. • Bacillary angiomatosis. • Cervical dysplasia. • Idiopathic thrombocytopenic purpura. • Weight loss. • Chronic diarrhoea. • Herpes zoster. • Peripheral neuropathy. • Low-grade fever/night sweats.

The median interval from infection to the development of symptoms is 7–10 yrs, although subgroups of patients exhibit 'fast' or 'slow' rates of progression.

AIDS

AIDS is defined by the development of specified opportunistic infections, tumours and other clinical features (Box 5.24). This is accomparied by a fall in CD4 count to <200 cells/mm^3, and a change in the spectrum of associated infections (Box 5.25).

PRESENTING PROBLEMS IN HIV INFECTION

SPECIFIC SKIN CONDITIONS

Fungal infections

Early HIV-associated skin diseases include:

• Xerosis with pruritus. • Seborrhoeic dermatitis. • An itchy folliculitic rash which may be fungal, staphylococcal or eosinophilic in aetiology.

Viral infections

• Herpes simplex (type 1 or 2) may affect the lips, mouth, skin or anogenital area and is seen in 20% of cases. • Varicella zoster usually presents with a

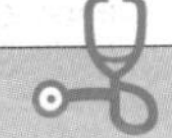

5.24 AIDS-DEFINING DISEASES

- Oesophageal candidiasis
- Chronic cryptosporidial diarrhoea
- Chronic mucocutaneous herpes simplex
- Pulmonary or extrapulmonary TB
- Progressive multifocal leucoencephalopathy
- Recurrent non-typhi *Salmonella* septicaemia
- Invasive cervical cancer
- Kaposi's sarcoma
- HIV-associated wasting
- Primary cerebral lymphoma
- Cryptococcal meningitis
- CMV retinitis or colitis
- *Pneumocystis jirovecii* pneumonia
- Disseminated *Mycobacterium avium intracellulare* (MAI)
- Cerebral toxoplasmosis
- Extrapulmonary coccidioidomycosis
- Extrapulmonary histoplasmosis
- Non-Hodgkin lymphoma
- HIV-associated dementia

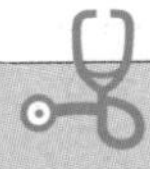

5.25 CORRELATIONS BETWEEN CD4 COUNT AND HIV-ASSOCIATED DISEASES

>500 cells/mm^3

- Acute primary infection, persistent generalised lymphadenopathy, recurrent vaginal candidiasis

<500 cells/mm^3

- Pulmonary TB, pneumococcal pneumonia, Herpes zoster, oropharyngeal candidiasis, oral hairy leucoplakia, extra-intestinal salmonellosis, Kaposi's sarcoma, HIV-associated idiopathic thrombocytopenic purpura, cervical intra-epithelial neoplasia II–III, lymphoid interstitial pneumonitis

<200 cells/mm^3

- *Pneumocystis jirovecii* pneumonia (PCP), oesophageal candidiasis, mucocutaneous herpes simplex, miliary/extrapulmonary TB, cryptosporidiosis, HIV-associated wasting, microsporidiosis, peripheral neuropathy

<100 cells/mm^3

- Cerebral toxoplasmosis, HIV-associated dementia, cryptococcal meningitis, progressive multifocal leucoencephalopathy, primary CNS lymphoma, non-Hodgkin lymphoma

<50 cells/mm^3

- CMV retinitis/GI disease, disseminated MAI

dermatomal vesicular rash on an erythematous base and may be the first sign of HIV infection. • HPV infection is frequent amongst HIV patients, usually takes the form of anogenital disease and may be difficult to manage.

Bacterial and parasitic infections

• These include *Staphylococcus aureus* (folliculitis, cellulitis and abscesses), syphilis and scabies. • Bacillary angiomatosis is a bacterial infection due to the cat-scratch bacillus, *Bartonella henselae*, which may become disseminated with fevers, lymphadenopathy and hepatosplenomegaly.

SPECIFIC ORAL CONDITIONS

Candidiasis

Candida infection in HIV is almost exclusively mucosal, affects nearly all patients with CD4 counts <200 cells/mm^3, and in early disease is nearly always caused by *C. albicans*. Treatment is with an oral azole drug.

Oral hairy leucoplakia

Oral hairy leucoplakia has the appearance of corrugated white plaques running vertically on the side of the tongue and is virtually pathognomonic of HIV disease in the context of HIV risk factors. It is usually asymptomatic and does not require treatment.

GASTROINTESTINAL DISEASE

Cytomegalovirus (CMV)

Gastrointestinal CMV occurs in up to one-third of patients with AIDS and is only seen if the CD4 count is <100 cells/mm^3 (usually <50). It may affect any part of the GI tract, liver and biliary tree, but is most commonly found in the oesophagus and colon. CMV colitis occurs in up to 5% of patients and causes watery diarrhoea, often with blood, colicky abdominal pain, weight loss and fever.

Cryptosporidium

Cryptosporidium is a highly contagious protozoan that infects a range of animals. It accounts for 15–20% of cases of diarrhoea, producing large-volume watery stools and abdominal pain.

Microsporidium

Microsporidia are a group of intracellular protozoa carried by a range of animals, birds and fish. Like *Cryptosporidia*, they account for 10–20% of cases of diarrhoea in HIV patients, leading to weight loss and malabsorption.

Other infections

• *Isospora* (Africa and Latin America) and *Cyclospora* (Asia) cause watery diarrhoea, weight loss and malabsorption, accounting overall for 2–4% of cases in the UK. • HIV enteropathy is a term given to a complex of chronic diarrhoea and partial villous atrophy for which no other cause can be found (10–20% of cases).

Mycobacterium avium intracellulare (MAI)

This environmental mycobacterium is commonly found in water and food. It causes disseminated infection in advanced HIV, with heavy infiltration of organisms and little inflammatory response. Clinical features include:

• Fevers and sweats. • Loss of weight/appetite. • Chronic diarrhoea and abdominal pain. • Hepatosplenomegaly. • Intra-abdominal/mediastinal lymphadenopathy. • Raised alkaline phosphatase. • Anaemia.

Mycobacterial disease is confirmed by identifying acid-fast bacilli on Ziehl–Neelsen staining of induced sputum, bone marrow, or liver or duodenal biopsy. MAI is confirmed by cultures.

LIVER DISEASE

Hepatitis C (HCV)

The major determinant of HIV/HCV co-infection rate is the mode of acquisition (>80% for haemophiliacs, 70–80% for injection drug-users, 10–15% for MSM and 3–5% for heterosexuals). Only 15–20% of patients ever clear their initial infection. Co-infected patients have:

• A higher HCV viral load. • Accelerated progression to cirrhosis (5–8 yrs after infection). • An increased risk of complications.

Hepatitis B (HBV)

The majority of persons with HIV have evidence of HBV exposure. Co-infected patients have:

• Higher DNA levels. • More aggressive disease, although in more advanced disease the immunosuppression affords some protection because hepatic damage is immune-mediated.

For both HBV and HCV, therapy may be associated with a flare of hepatitis as immunity recovers.

RESPIRATORY DISEASE

Pneumocystis jirovecii

Pneumocystis jirovecii (formerly *carinii*) pneumonia is the most common AIDS-defining illness.

Non-specific clinical features include: • fever, • exercise-induced O_2 desaturation, • hypoxaemia on ABGs, • impaired carbon monoxide transfer factor and • raised LDH (from lung damage). Auscultation is unremarkable and the CXR may be normal in early disease (15–20%) but classically shows perihilar ground-glass changes. Co-trimoxazole is used for treatment and prophylaxis.

Mycobacterium tuberculosis

Globally, approximately one-third of HIV-infected persons are co-infected with *M. tuberculosis*. The clinical presentation depends on immune function.

When the CD4 count is >200 cells/mm^3, disease is more likely to be reactivated, upper-lobe, open cavitatory disease. As immunosuppression increases, miliary, atypical pulmonary and extrapulmonary (especially pericardial, abdominal and meningeal) TB become progressively more common, as does mycobacteraemia (present in 50% of those with CD4 <200 cells/mm^3).

Multidrug-resistant TB (MDRTB) is a serious threat and requires combination therapy with multiple agents.

Bacterial infections

Bacterial pneumonia (p. 292) is common in HIV.

NERVOUS SYSTEM DISEASE

Neurological disease is common in HIV. It may be a direct consequence of HIV infection or an indirect result of CD4 cell depletion. Presentation may be as:

• A space-occupying lesion. • Encephalitis. • Meningitis. • Myelitis. • Spinal root disease. • Neuropathy.

Toxoplasma gondii

Toxoplasma infection (p. 113), results in a mild or subclinical illness in immunocompetent individuals, with the formation of latent tissue cysts that persist for life, commonly in brain tissue. The infection rate, as judged by seroconversion, is 0.5–1%/yr. In the presence of advanced HIV-induced immunosuppression, there is a >30% chance that these dormant cysts will reactivate, leading to cerebral toxoplasmosis.

Patients present with a short history of headache, fever and drowsiness, followed by confusion, seizures and focal signs. Cerebral CT or MRI typically shows multiple ring-enhancing lesions with marked surrounding oedema and mass effect. The response to a trial of anti-*Toxoplasma* therapy is usually diagnostic, with clinical improvement within 1 wk.

Primary CNS lymphoma (PCNSL)

PCNSL usually complicates late-stage HIV (CD4 <50 cells/mm^3), occurring in ~5% of AIDS patients and accounting for 20% of all focal CNS lesions. Tumours are nearly always high-grade, diffuse, B-cell neoplasms.

Characteristically, imaging demonstrates a large, single, homogeneously enhancing periventricular lesion with mild to moderate surrounding oedema and mass effect. Treatment is usually palliative with dexamethasone and symptomatic relief. Life expectancy is measured in months.

Progressive multifocal leucoencephalopathy (PMFL)

PMFL is a fatal demyelinating disease caused by the JC papovavirus that occurs in ~2–3% of AIDS patients at very low CD4 counts.

Patients present with focal deficits (80%), slow-onset visual field defects (25%) and ataxia. The presence of JC-DNA in CSF is diagnostic. Treatment with highly active antiretroviral therapy (HAART) and/or cidofovir occasionally induces prolonged clinical remission but most patients die in 3–12 mths.

HIV-associated dementia

HIV infects the CNS early during infection. Dementia occurs in late disease, with global deterioration of cognitive function, severe psychomotor retardation, paraparesis, ataxia, and urinary and faecal incontinence. The incidence has fallen dramatically as a result of HAART.

Cryptococcosis

Cryptococcus neoformans is the most common cause of meningitis associated with late-stage HIV (CD4 <50 cells/mm^3).

Patients usually present with a 2–3-wk history of headache, fever, vomiting and mild confusion; neck stiffness is often absent (<25%). Protein, cell counts and glucose may be normal in the CSF, although numerous organisms are present on India ink stain (60–80%), cultures are usually positive (>95%), and the CSF and serum cryptococcal antigen are strongly positive (95%).

Sensory neuropathy

A predominantly distal HIV-related sensory neuropathy of the lower limbs affects up to 30% of patients. It results from axonal degeneration, unmyelinated nerve fibres bearing the brunt. The nucleoside reverse transcriptase inhibitor (NRTI) drugs can produce an identical picture, but with remission if the offending agent is withdrawn early.

NEOPLASMS

Kaposi's sarcoma (1000-fold higher rate than in non-HIV-infected; Fig. 5.15) and non-Hodgkin lymphoma (100-fold greater) are the most common opportunistic malignancies associated with HIV and are AIDS-defining diagnoses. Increased incidence rates are also seen with Hodgkin lymphoma.

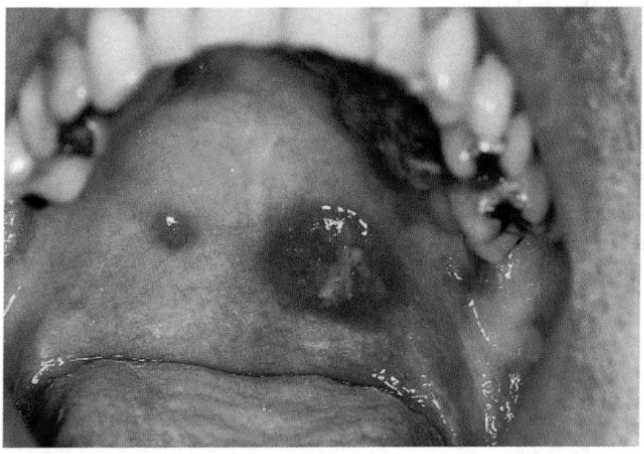

Fig. 5.15 Oral Kaposi's sarcoma. A full examination is important to detect disease that may affect the palate, gums, fauces or tongue.

MANAGEMENT OF HIV

Management of HIV involves both treatment of the virus and prevention of opportunistic infections. The targets of HIV treatment are to:

• Prolong life. • Prevent transmission. • Reduce the viral load to an undetectable level (<50 copies/ml) for as long as possible. • Improve the CD4 count (above a level of 200 cells/mm^3 significant HIV-related events rarely occur).

THE NAÏVE PATIENT

The decision to start therapy is influenced by the patient's symptom status, CD4 count and wishes. Comorbidity, side-effects and likely compliance should also be considered. Treatment should usually be commenced when the CD4 count falls below 350 cells/mm^3 or the patient is symptomatic. A potent combination (HAART) should always be used (Boxes 5.26 and 5.27). A viral resistance test should be performed before treatment as there is a 5–10% incidence of primary resistance.

With appropriate HAART, the chance of a VL of <50 copies/ml at 24 wks is >80%. Treatment failure suggests:

5.26 INDICATIONS TO START HAART

CD4 count (cells/mm^3)	Decision
Seroconversion	Consider[1]
>350	Monitor 3-monthly
200–350	Recommend treatment[2]
<200	Strongly recommend treatment[2]

[1] If severely symptomatic.

[2] Strongest recommendation for those with low CD4 counts, hepatitis B or C infection or high viral load.

5.27 RECOMMENDED COMBINATION TREATMENTS FOR THE NAÏVE PATIENT[1]

Regimen	A	B	C
Preferred	Efavirenz	Abacavir Tenofovir Zidovudine Didanosine	Emtricitabine Lamivudine
Alternative	Lopanivir/Ritonavir Fosamprenavir/Ritonavir, saquinavir/ritonavir, Nevirapine[2]		

[1] One drug from columns A, B and C.

[2] Only when CD4 <250 cells/mm^3 in females or <400 cells/mm^3 in males.

• Suboptimal drug regimen. • A high baseline VL. • Poor adherence. • Prior exposure to antiretroviral drugs. • Drug interaction or toxicity. • Primary acquisition or development of resistant virus.

THE 'TREATMENT-EXPERIENCED' PATIENT

A change in treatment may be necessitated by side-effects, difficulties in adherence or virus rebound in a patient with a previously undetectable VL. Treatment failure is associated with rising VL, falling CD4 count and clinical progression. Most early failures are due to adherence difficulties and most late failures occur because of virological resistance. A resistance test should be obtained before switching the failing regimen, and used to guide any change. Therapeutic drug monitoring can confirm that virological failure is not related to inadequate PI or NNRTI levels. As a rule, as many new agents as possible should be used.

PERINATAL TRANSMISSION

Reduction in perinatal transmission of HIV can be achieved by active treatment of the mother to reduce viral load coupled with short-course perinatal prophylaxis. Screening for HIV in the baby (RNA or proviral DNA) should be performed at birth (not on cord blood), 6 wks and 4–6 mths. If negative, vertical transmission has not occurred.

POST-EXPOSURE PROPHYLAXIS (PEP)

Combination therapy is now recommended for occupational PEP where the risk is deemed to be significant, although there is no evidence for this practice. The first dose should be given as soon as possible. Protection is not absolute and health-care workers have been reported to seroconvert despite taking a full course of three drugs started within hours of exposure. Approximately 77% of persons receiving PEP experience side-effects and only 40% complete therapy. Recommended PEP is ZDV, 3TC and indinavir or nelfinavir for 28 days.

6

Clinical biochemistry and metabolism

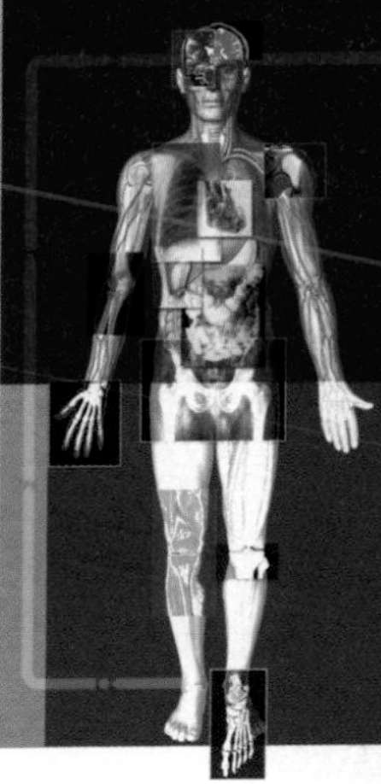

Between 60 and 70% of all critical decisions taken in regard to patients in health-care systems in developed countries involve a laboratory service or result. This chapter describes disorders whose primary manifestation is in abnormalities of biochemistry laboratory results, or whose underlying pathophysiology involves disturbance in specific biochemical pathways. Discussion of diabetes mellitus and other endocrine disorders is to be found in Chapters 10 and 11.

WATER AND ELECTROLYTE DISTRIBUTION

In a typical adult male, the 40 litres of total body water (TBW) constitute ~60% of the body weight. More than half is located inside cells (the intracellular fluid or ICF), while the remainder is in the extracellular fluid (ECF) compartment. Of the ECF, the plasma is itself a small fraction (some 3 litres), while the remainder is interstitial fluid within the tissues but outside the cells.

The dominant cation in the ICF is potassium, while in the ECF it is sodium (Fig. 6.1). Phosphates and negatively charged proteins constitute the major intracellular anions, while chloride and, to a lesser extent, bicarbonate dominate the ECF anions. An important difference between the plasma and interstitial ECF is that only plasma contains significant concentrations of protein.

The major force maintaining the difference in cation concentration between the ICF and ECF is the sodium–potassium pump (Na,K-activated ATPase) integral to all cell membranes. Maintenance of the cation gradients across cell membranes is essential for many cell processes, including the

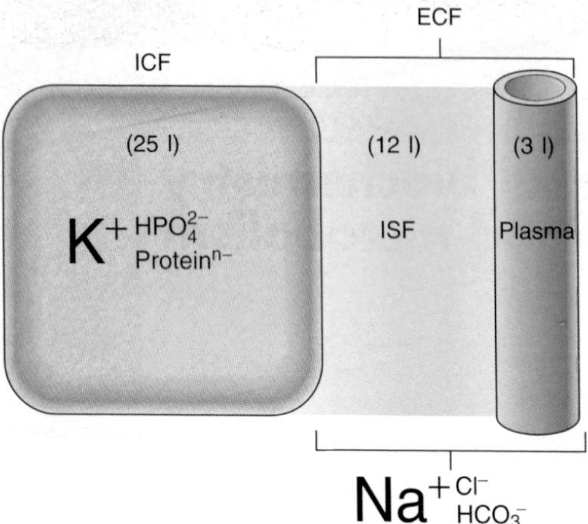

Fig. 6.1 Normal distribution of body water and electrolytes. Schematic representation of volume (l = litres) and composition (dominant ionic species only shown) of the intracellular fluid (ICF) and extracellular fluid (ECF) in a 70 kg male. Total body water (TBW) = ~60% of body weight. TBW = ICF + ECF = 40 litres. The main difference in composition between the plasma and interstitial fluid (ISF) is the presence of appreciable concentrations of protein in the plasma (not shown) but not the ISF. The sodium–potassium pump maintains the cation concentration difference between the ICF and ECF. The difference in protein content between the plasma and interstitial compartments is maintained by the permeability characteristics of the capillary wall.

excitability of conducting tissues such as nerve and muscle. The difference in protein content between the plasma and the interstitial fluid compartment is maintained by the protein permeability barrier at the capillary wall. This protein concentration gradient contributes to the balance of forces across the capillary wall favouring fluid retention within the capillaries (the colloid osmotic, or oncotic, pressure of the plasma), thus maintaining an adequate circulating plasma volume.

INVESTIGATION OF WATER AND ELECTROLYTES

Because the blood consists of both intracellular (red cell) and extracellular (plasma) components, it is important to avoid haemolysis of the sample, which causes contamination of the plasma by intracellular elements, particularly potassium. Blood should not be drawn from an arm into which an i.v. infusion is being given, to avoid contamination by the infused fluid.

Since the kidney maintains body fluid composition by adjusting urine volume and composition, it is often helpful to obtain a simultaneous sample of urine ('spot' specimen or 24-hr collection) at the time of blood analysis.

DISORDERS OF SODIUM BALANCE

When sodium balance is disturbed, as a result of imbalance between intake and excretion, any tendency for plasma sodium concentration to change is usually corrected by the osmotic mechanisms controlling water balance (see below). As a result, disorders in sodium balance present chiefly as altered ECF volume rather than altered sodium concentration.

SODIUM DEPLETION (USUALLY ASSOCIATED WITH HYPOVOLAEMIA)

Aetiology includes the following factors:

• Inadequate intake. • GI sodium loss: vomiting, diarrhoea, external fistula. • Skin sodium loss: excess sweating, burns. • Renal sodium loss: diuretics, mineralocorticoid deficiency. • Internal sequestration: bowel obstruction, pancreatitis.

Clinical features

Symptoms and signs of hypovolaemia are as follows:

• Thirst. • Dizziness on standing. • Weakness. • Low JVP. • Postural hypotension. • Tachycardia. • Dry mouth. • Confusion. • Weight loss.

Supportive biochemistry includes:

• Low plasma sodium (note that plasma sodium may be in the normal range if salt and water losses proceed in parallel). • High urea. • High urine osmolality. • Low urine sodium.

Management of sodium and water depletion

This has two main components:

• Treatment of the cause where possible, to stop ongoing salt and water losses. • Replacement of salt and water deficits, and provision of ongoing maintenance requirements, by i.v. infusion when depletion is severe.

I.v. fluid therapy: Box 6.1 shows the daily maintenance requirements for water and electrolytes in a typical adult, and Box 6.2 summarises the composition of some widely available i.v. fluids. The choice of fluid and the rate of administration will depend on the clinical circumstances, as assessed at the bedside and from laboratory data.

6.1 BASIC DAILY WATER AND ELECTROLYTE REQUIREMENTS

	Requirement per kg	Typical 70 kg adult
Water	35–45 ml/kg	2.5–3.0 l/day
Sodium	1.5–2 mmol/kg	100–140 mmol/day
Potassium	1.0–1.5 mmol/kg	70–100 mmol/day

NB for Na and K, mmol = meq

6.2 COMPOSITION OF SOME ISOTONIC I.V. FLUIDS (1 LITRE)*

Fluid	D-glucose	Kilojoules	Na^+	Cl^-	Other
5% dextrose	50 g	840	0	0	0
Normal saline	0	0	154	154	0
Hartmann's solution	0	0	131	111	K^+ 5 Ca^{2+} 2 $Lactate^-$ 29

*Electrolytes shown in mmol.

SODIUM EXCESS (USUALLY ASSOCIATED WITH HYPERVOLAEMIA)

In the presence of normal function of the heart and kidneys, an excessive intake of salt and water is compensated for by increased excretion and so is unlikely to lead to clinically obvious features of hypervolaemia.

Causes of sodium and water excess in clinical practice include:

• Impaired renal function: primary renal disease. • Primary hyperaldosteronism: Conn's syndrome. • Secondary hyperaldosteronism: congestive cardiac failure, cirrhotic liver disease, nephrotic syndrome.

Peripheral oedema is the most common physical sign associated with these conditions (p. 174) although it is not usually a feature of Conn's syndrome.

Management

The management of ECF volume overload involves:

• Specific treatment (where available) directed at the cause, e.g. ACE inhibitors in heart failure, corticosteroids in minimal change nephropathy. • Restriction of dietary sodium to match more closely the diminished excretory capacity, e.g. 50–80 mmol/day. • Treatment with diuretic drugs.

DISORDERS OF WATER BALANCE

Daily water intake can vary over a wide range, from 500 ml to several litres a day. While a certain amount of water is lost through the stool, sweat and the respiratory tract, the kidneys are chiefly responsible for adjusting water excretion to maintain a constant body water content and body fluid osmolality (normal range 280–300 mmol/kg).

Disturbances in body water metabolism, in the absence of changes in sodium balance, manifest principally as abnormalities of plasma sodium concentration, and hence of plasma osmolality. The main consequence of changes in plasma osmolality, especially when rapid, is altered cerebral function. This is because, when extracellular osmolality changes abruptly, water flows rapidly across cell membranes with resultant cell swelling (during hypo-osmolality) or shrinkage (during hyperosmolality). Cerebral cell function is very sensitive to such volume changes, particularly during cell swelling where an increase in intracerebral pressure occurs due to the constraints posed by the bony skull, resulting in impaired cerebral perfusion.

HYPONATRAEMIA

The causes of hyponatraemia (plasma Na <135 mmol/l) are best organised according to any associated change in ECF volume status, i.e. the total body sodium. In all cases, there is retention of water relative to sodium, and it is the clinical examination rather than the electrolyte test results which gives clues to the underlying problem.

Hypovolaemic (sodium deficit with a relatively smaller water deficit): Renal Na loss (diuretics), GI Na loss (vomiting, diarrhoea).

Euvolaemic (water retention alone, i.e. 'dilutional'): Primary polydipsia, SIADH (Box 6.3).

Hypervolaemic (sodium retention with relatively greater water retention): Heart failure, cirrhosis, chronic kidney disease (without water restriction).

Clinical features

When hyponatraemia develops gradually, it is relatively asymptomatic. More rapid changes in plasma osmolality and so plasma sodium may be associated with:

• Anorexia. • Nausea. • Vomiting. • Confusion. • Lethargy. • Seizures. • Coma.

6.3 SYNDROME OF INAPPROPRIATE ANTIDIURETIC HORMONE SECRETION (SIADH): CAUSES AND DIAGNOSIS
Causes
• Tumours, especially small-cell lung cancer • CNS disorders: stroke, trauma, infection, psychosis • Pulmonary disorders: pneumonia, TB • Drugs, e.g. carbamazepine, amitriptyline, morphine • Sustained pain, stress, nausea, e.g. post-operative state, acute porphyria • Idiopathic
Diagnosis
• Low plasma sodium concentration (typically <130 mmol/l) • Low plasma osmolality (<270 mmol/kg) • Urine osmolality not minimally low (>150 mmol/kg) • Urine sodium concentration not minimally low (>30 mmol/l) • Low–normal plasma urea, creatinine, uric acid • Exclusion of other causes of hyponatraemia • Appropriate clinical context (see above)
NB for Na and k, mmol = meq

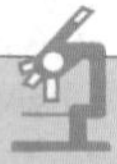

6.4 URINE Na AND OSMOLALITY IN THE DIFFERENTIAL DIAGNOSIS OF HYPONATRAEMIA*

Urine Na (mmol/l)	Urine osmolality (mmol/kg)	Possible diagnoses
Low (<30)	Low (<100)	Primary polydipsia, malnutrition
Low	High (>150)	Salt depletion, hypovolaemia
High (>40)	Low	Diuretic action (acute phase)
High	High	SIADH

*Note that intermediate urine results are of indeterminate significance and diagnosis depends on a comprehensive clinical assessment.

Investigations

Plasma and urine electrolytes and osmolality (Box 6.4) are usually the only tests required to classify the hyponatraemia.

Management

The treatment for hyponatraemia is critically dependent on the rate of development and severity, and on the underlying cause.

In general, if hyponatraemia has developed rapidly (over hours to days), morbidity will be high due to cerebral oedema, and it is generally safe to correct the plasma sodium relatively rapidly. This can include infusion of hypertonic (3%) sodium chloride solutions, especially when the patient is obtunded or convulsing.

Rapid correction of hyponatraemia that has developed slowly (over weeks to months) may lead to 'central pontine myelinolysis', which may cause permanent structural and functional cerebral changes and is generally fatal. The rate of plasma sodium correction in chronic asymptomatic hyponatraemia should not exceed 10 mmol/l/day, and an even slower rate would generally be safer.

Specific treatment should be directed at the underlying cause.

• For hypovolaemic patients, this will involve controlling sodium loss and giving i.v. saline if clinically warranted. • Patients with dilutional hyponatraemia usually respond to fluid restriction in the range of 600–1000 ml/day and removal of the precipitating stimulus (e.g. a drug causing SIADH). • Demeclocycline, or oral urea supplements, may be of use in SIADH.

HYPERNATRAEMIA

Just as hyponatraemia represents a failure of the mechanisms for diluting the urine during free access to water, so hypernatraemia (plasma Na > 150 mmol/l) reflects an inadequacy of the kidney in concentrating the urine in the face of relatively restricted water intake. Similar to hyponatraemia, the causes of hypernatraemia may be classified based on the volume state of the patient.

Hypovolaemic (sodium deficit with a relatively greater water deficit): Renal Na losses (diuretics), GI Na losses (colonic diarrhoea), skin Na losses (excessive sweating).

Euvolaemic (water deficit alone): Diabetes insipidus (central or nephrogenic, p. 377).

Hypervolaemic (sodium retention with relatively less water retention): Enteral or parenteral nutrition, oral salt administration, chronic kidney disease (during water restriction).

Clinical features

Patients with hypernatraemia generally have reduced cerebral function and cerebral dehydration. This triggers thirst and drinking, and if adequate water is obtained, is self-limiting. If adequate water is not obtained, dizziness, confusion, weakness and ultimately coma and death can result.

Management

Treatment of hypernatraemia depends on both the rate of development and the underlying cause.

If there is reason to think that the condition has developed rapidly, correction with appropriate volumes of i.v. hypotonic fluid may be attempted relatively rapidly.

In older institutionalised patients however, it is more likely that the disorder has developed slowly and extreme caution should be exhibited in lowering the plasma sodium rapidly, to avoid the risk of cerebral oedema.

DISORDERS OF POTASSIUM BALANCE

Potassium is the major intracellular cation (see Fig. 6.1), and the steep concentration gradient for potassium across the cell membrane of excitable cells plays an important part in generating the resting membrane potential and allowing the propagation of the action potential, which is crucial to normal functioning of nerve, muscle and cardiac tissues.

HYPOKALAEMIA

Aetiology includes the following factors:

Redistribution into cells: Alkalosis, insulin excess, β_2-agonists.

Reduced potassium intake: Dietary, i.v. therapy.

Excessive losses: These may be renal or gastrointestinal.

Renal losses may be caused by the following:

• If associated with hypertension: 1°/2° hyperaldosteronism, Cushing's syndrome, corticosteroids, ectopic ACTH. • With normal to low BP: diuretics, renal tubular acidosis, post-obstructive diuresis, recovery after acute tubular necrosis, inherited tubular disorders.

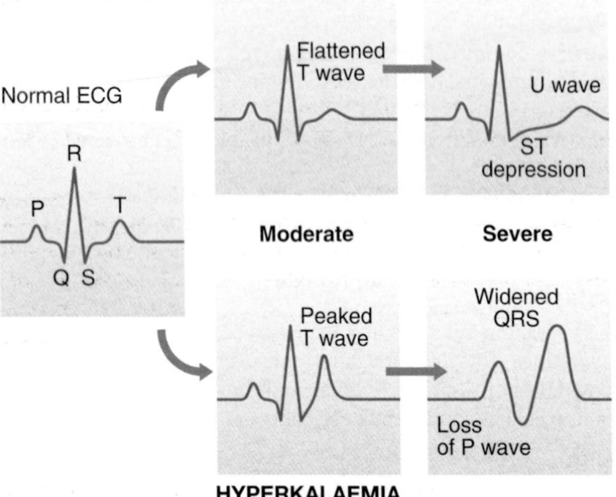

Fig. 6.2 The ECG in hypokalaemia and hyperkalaemia.

GI losses may be caused by:

• Vomiting. • Diarrhoea. • Bowel obstruction. • Laxative abuse.

Clinical features

• Muscular weakness. • Tiredness. • Cardiac effects: ventricular ectopics or more serious arrhythmias, potentiation of the adverse effects of digoxin. ECG shows typical T wave changes (Fig. 6.2). • Functional bowel obstruction due to paralytic ileus. • In long-standing hypokalaemia, damage to renal tubules (hypokalaemic nephropathy) and interference with the tubular response to ADH (acquired nephrogenic diabetes insipidus), causing polyuria and polydipsia.

Investigations

Measurement of plasma electrolytes, bicarbonate, urine potassium and sometimes of calcium and magnesium is usually sufficient to establish the diagnosis.

Plasma renin activity and aldosterone levels identify patients with primary hyperaldosteronism (p. 369) and other mineralocorticoid excess when renin is suppressed; in other causes of hypokalaemia renin is elevated.

Occasionally the cause of hypokalaemia is obscure, especially when the history is incomplete or unreliable, and the urine potassium is indeterminate. Many such cases are associated with metabolic alkalosis, and in this setting the measurement of urine chloride concentration can provide a helpful guide to diagnosis.

• A low urine chloride (<30 mmol/l) is characteristic of vomiting (spontaneous or self-induced). • A chloride >40 mmol/l suggests diuretic therapy (acute phase) or a tubular disorder.

Management

If the problem is redistribution of potassium into cells, reversal of the underlying cause (e.g. correction of alkalosis) may restore plasma potassium without supplements.

In most cases potassium replacement (oral or i.v.) will be required. The rate of administration depends on the severity of hypokalaemia and the presence of cardiac or neuromuscular complications, but should generally not exceed 10 mmol of potassium/hr. If higher rates are needed, the concentration of potassium infused may be increased to 40 mmol/l if a peripheral vein is used, but higher concentrations must be infused into a large 'central' vein with continuous cardiac monitoring.

HYPERKALAEMIA

Aetiology involves the following factors:

Redistribution out of cells: Acidosis, insulin deficiency, β-blockers, severe hyperglycaemia.

Increased intake: Exogenous (diet, i.v. therapy); endogenous (haemolysis, rhabdomyolysis).

Renal potassium retention: Renal failure (acute and chronic).

Tubular secretory failure: Drugs (NSAIDs, ACE inhibitors, spironolactone), tubulo-interstitial disease, Addison's disease.

Spurious result: in vitro haemolysis.

Clinical features

Patients typically present with progressive muscular weakness, but sometimes there are no symptoms until cardiac arrest occurs (caused by the marked slowing of action potential conduction in the presence of potassium levels >7 mmol/l).

Typical ECG changes are shown in Figure 6.2. Peaking of the T wave is an early ECG sign, but widening of the QRS complex presages a dangerous cardiac arrhythmia.

Investigations

Plasma electrolyte, creatinine and bicarbonate results, together with consideration of the clinical scenario, will usually provide the explanation for hyperkalaemia. Addison's disease should be excluded, unless there is an obvious alternative diagnosis, as described on page 366.

Management

Treatment of hyperkalaemia depends on the severity and the rate of development.

• In the absence of neuromuscular symptoms or ECG changes, reduction of potassium intake and correction of underlying abnormalities may be

6.5 TREATMENT OF HYPERKALAEMIA	
Mechanism	**Therapy**
Stabilise cell membrane potential[1]	I.v. calcium gluconate (10 ml of 10% solution)
Shift K into cells	Inhaled β_2-agonist, e.g. salbutamol I.v. glucose (50 ml of 50% solution) and insulin (5 U Actrapid) I.v. sodium bicarbonate[2] (100 ml of 8.4% solution)
Remove K from body	I.v. furosemide and normal saline[3] Ion exchange resin (e.g. Resonium) orally or rectally Dialysis

[1]If ECG changes suggestive of hyperkalaemia (K typically >7 mmol/l). [2]If acidosis present. [3]If adequate residual renal function.

sufficient. • In acute and/or severe hyperkalaemia, more urgent measures must be taken (Box 6.5).

DISORDERS OF ACID–BASE BALANCE

Patients with disturbances of acid–base balance may present clinically either with the effects of tissue malfunction due to disturbed pH (such as altered cardiac and CNS function), or with secondary changes in respiration as a response to the underlying metabolic change (e.g. Kussmaul respiration during metabolic acidosis). The clinical picture is often dominated by the cause of the acid–base change, such as uncontrolled diabetes or primary lung disease. Frequently the acid–base disturbance only becomes evident when the venous plasma bicarbonate concentration is noted to be abnormal, or when a full ABG analysis shows abnormalities in the pH, PCO_2 or bicarbonate.

The common patterns of abnormality in the blood gas parameters in acid–base disturbances are shown in Box 6.6. Interpretation of blood gas results is made easier by blood gas diagrams (e.g. Fig. 6.3), which indicate whether any acidosis or alkalosis is due to acute or chronic respiratory derangements of $PaCO_2$, or to metabolic causes.

In metabolic disturbances, respiratory compensation is almost immediate; i.e. the compensatory change in PCO_2 is achieved soon after the onset of the metabolic disturbance. In respiratory disorders, on the other hand, a small initial change in bicarbonate occurs as a result of chemical buffering of CO_2, largely within red blood cells, but further compensatory changes in bicarbonate occur via long-term adjustments in acid secretory capacity by the kidney, requiring days to weeks. When clinically obtained acid–base parameters do not accord with the predicted compensation shown, a mixed acid–base disturbance should be suspected.

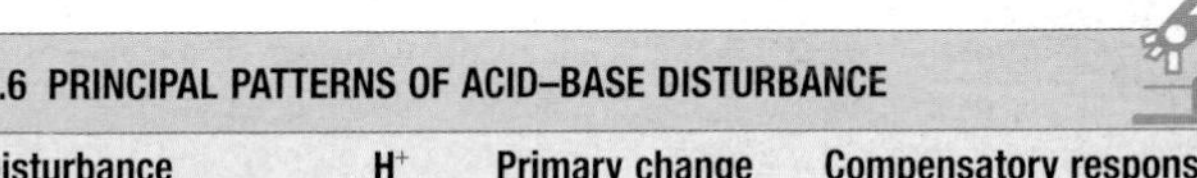

6.6 PRINCIPAL PATTERNS OF ACID–BASE DISTURBANCE

Disturbance	H^+	Primary change	Compensatory response
Metabolic acidosis	>40[1]	HCO_3^- <24 mmol/l	PCO_2 <5.33 kPa[2]
Metabolic alkalosis	<40[1]	HCO_3^- >24 mmol/l	PCO_2 >5.33 kPa[2,3]
Respiratory acidosis	>40[1]	PCO_2 >5.33 kPa[2]	HCO_3^- >24 mmol/l
Respiratory alkalosis	<40[1]	PCO_2 <5.33 kPa[2]	HCO_3^- <24 mmol/l

[1] H^+ of 40 nmol/l = pH of 7.40. [2] PCO_2 of 5.33 kPa = 40 mmHg. [3] PCO_2 does not rise above 7.33 kPa (55 mmHg); further hypoventilation prevents adequate oxygenation.

METABOLIC ACIDOSIS

Metabolic acidosis occurs when an acid other than carbonic acid (due to CO_2 retention) accumulates in the body, resulting in a fall in the plasma bicarbonate. The pH fall which would otherwise occur is blunted by hyperventilation, resulting in a reduced PCO_2. If the kidneys are intact (i.e. not the cause of the initial disturbance), renal excretion of acid can be gradually increased over days to weeks, raising the plasma bicarbonate and hence the pH towards normal in the new steady state.

Causes of a metabolic acidosis may be classified according to the anion gap, which is the difference between the main measured cations [$Na^+ + K^+$] and the main measured cations [$Cl^- + HCO_3^-$]. This is normally about 15 mmol/l but increases when an acid accumulates accompanied by a corresponding anion.

Metabolic acidosis with normal anion gap: GI base loss (loss of HCO_3^- in diarrhoea, small bowel fistula, urinary diversion procedure). Renal tubular acidosis (urinary loss of HCO_3^- in proximal RTA, impaired tubular acid secretion in distal RTA). Therapeutic infusion or poisoning with HCl or NH_4Cl.

Metabolic acidosis with increased anion gap: Diabetic ketoacidosis (accumulation of ketones with hyperglycaemia). Lactic acidosis (shock or liver disease). Renal failure. Poisoning (aspirin, methanol, ethylene glycol).

Management

Identify and correct the underlying cause. As metabolic acidosis is frequently associated with sodium and water depletion, resuscitation with appropriate i.v. fluids will often be needed. Use of i.v. bicarbonate in this setting is controversial.

METABOLIC ALKALOSIS

Metabolic alkalosis is characterised by an increase in the plasma bicarbonate concentration and the plasma pH (see Box 6.6). There is a compensatory rise in PCO_2 due to hypoventilation, but this is limited by the respiratory response to hypoxia.

Clinically, apart from manifestations of the underlying cause, there may be few symptoms or signs related to alkalosis itself. When the rise in systemic pH is abrupt, plasma ionised calcium falls and signs of increased neuromuscular irritability, such as tetany, may develop (p. 360).

The causes are best classified by the accompanying disturbance of ECF volume.

Hypovolaemic metabolic alkalosis (most common pattern): Sustained vomiting: acid-rich fluid is lost from the body; hypokalaemia stimulates renal H^+ excretion. Diuretics (not potassium-sparing diuretics) increase acid loss into the urine.

Normovolaemic (or hypervolaemic) metabolic alkalosis: Occurs when both bicarbonate retention and volume expansion are found together: • Corticosteroid excess (Conn's syndrome, Cushing's syndrome, corticosteroid therapy), • Overuse of antacids.

Management

• Metabolic alkalosis associated with hypovolaemia is treated with i.v. fluids, specifically isotonic sodium chloride. • Replacement of potassium helps correct the hypokalaemia and its consequences in the kidney. • In metabolic alkalosis associated with normal or increased volume, treatment should focus on correcting the underlying cause.

RESPIRATORY ACIDOSIS

Respiratory acidosis occurs when there is accumulation of CO_2 due to reduced effective alveolar ventilation. This results in a rise in the PCO_2, with a compensatory increase in plasma bicarbonate concentration, particularly when the disorder is of long duration and the kidney has fully developed its capacity for increased acid excretion.

The aetiology, clinical features and management of respiratory acidosis are covered in Chapter 9.

RESPIRATORY ALKALOSIS

Respiratory alkalosis develops when there is a period of hyperventilation resulting in a reduction of PCO_2 and increase in plasma pH. If the condition is sustained, renal compensation occurs such that tubular acid secretion is reduced and the plasma bicarbonate falls.

This acid–base disturbance is frequently of short duration, as in anxiety states or over-vigorous assisted ventilation. It can be prolonged in the context of pregnancy, pulmonary embolism, chronic liver disease, and ingestion of certain drugs which stimulate the brain stem respiratory centre (e.g. salicylates).

Clinical features of hyperventilation are described on p. 272; the characteristic perioral and digital tingling is due to a reduction in ionised calcium caused by increased binding of calcium to albumin in the alkalotic

ECF. In severe cases, Trousseau's sign and Chvostek's sign may be positive, and tetany or seizures may develop (p. 360). Clinical features of hyperventilation is discussed in Chapter 9 (p. 272).

MIXED ACID–BASE DISORDERS

In patients with complex illnesses, it is not uncommon for more than one independent disturbance of acid–base metabolism to be present at the same time. In these situations, the arterial pH will represent the net effect of all primary and compensatory changes. Indeed, the pH may be normal, but the presence of underlying acid–base disturbances can be gauged from concomitant abnormalities in the PCO_2 and bicarbonate concentration (see Fig. 6.3).

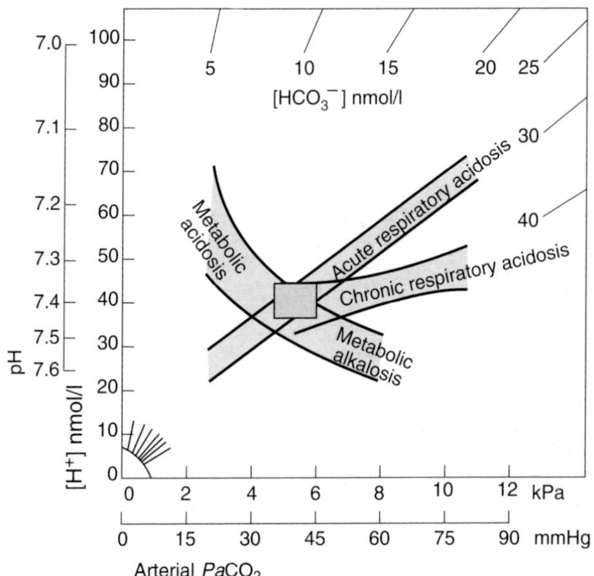

Fig. 6.3 Changes in blood [H^+], $PaCO_2$ and plasma [HCO_3^-] in acid–base disorders. The shaded rectangle indicates the limits of normal. The bands represent 95% confidence limits of single disturbances in human blood in vivo. The diagonal lines (top and right) indicate bicarbonate levels. For any measured value of [H^+], the corresponding value of $PaCO_2$ indicates whether the acidosis or alkalosis is primarily respiratory or metabolic in origin.

DISORDERS OF MAGNESIUM METABOLISM

Magnesium is mainly an intracellular cation, functionally important for many enzymes including the Na/K ATPase. It can also regulate potassium and calcium channels.

Free plasma magnesium (~70% of the total) is filtered at the glomerulus, with the majority of this reabsorbed in the loop of Henlé and tubules. Reabsorption is enhanced by parathyroid hormone (PTH). Disorders of calcium metabolism are covered in Chapter 10.

HYPOMAGNESAEMIA

Aetiology involves:

• Inadequate intake: starvation, parenteral nutrition. • Excessive losses: GI (vomiting, diarrhoea, fistulae), renal (diuretics, alcohol, acute tubular necrosis). • Complex formation: acute pancreatitis.

Clinical features

The clinical features of hypomagnesaemia and hypocalcaemia are similar: tetany, arrhythmias, especially torsades de pointes (p. 221), seizures. Hypomagnesaemia is associated with hypocalcaemia because magnesium is required for normal PTH secretion in response to a fall in serum calcium; also, hypomagnesaemia induces resistance to PTH in bone. Hypomagnesaemia is also associated with hyponatraemia and hypokalaemia, and these may mediate some of the clinical manifestations.

Management

• Treat the underlying cause. • Oral magnesium is poorly absorbed and may cause diarrhoea. • If disease is symptomatic, correct with i.v. magnesium. • If due to diuretic use, adjunctive use of a potassium-sparing diuretic will also reduce renal magnesium losses.

HYPERMAGNESAEMIA

Hypermagnesaemia is much less common than hypomagnesaemia. It may be due to:

• Acute and chronic renal failure. • Adrenocortical insufficiency. • Increased intake (antacids, laxatives, parenteral therapy).

Clinical features

• Bradycardia. • Hypotension. • Reduced consciousness. • Respiratory depression.

Management

• Restrict magnesium intake. • Optimise renal function. • Promote renal magnesium excretion with i.v. hydration and a loop diuretic. • Calcium gluconate may be used to reverse overt cardiac effects. • Ultimately, dialysis may be required.

DISORDERS OF PHOSPHATE METABOLISM

Inorganic phosphate is involved in cell metabolism, intracellular signalling and bone/mineral balance. It is freely filtered at the glomerulus, with ~65% reabsorbed in the proximal tubule and a further 10–20% reabsorbed in the distal tubules. Proximal reabsorption is reduced by PTH.

HYPOPHOSPHATAEMIA

Aetiology involves:

• Redistribution into cells: refeeding after starvation, respiratory alkalosis. • Inadequate intake or absorption: malabsorption, diarrhoea. • Increased renal excretion: hyperparathyroidism, volume expansion.

Clinical features

• Impaired function and survival of all blood cell lines. • Muscle weakness, respiratory failure, congestive cardiac failure, ileus. • Decreased consciousness, coma. • Osteomalacia.

Management

• Oral phosphate supplements. • I.v. sodium or potassium phosphate salts may be used in critical situations but there is a risk of hypocalcaemia and metastatic calcification.

HYPERPHOSPHATAEMIA

Aetiology involves:

• Reduced renal excretion: acute and chronic renal failure, hypoparathyroidism. • Redistribution from cells: tumour lysis syndrome. • All of the above will be aggravated when the patient is taking phosphate-containing preparations.

Clinical features

These relate to hypocalcaemia and metastatic calcification, especially in chronic renal failure and tertiary hyperparathyroidism where a high calcium phosphate product occurs.

Management

• Volume expansion with normal saline: this promotes renal phosphate excretion if renal function is normal. • Dietary phosphate restriction and phosphate binders in chronic renal failure.

DISORDERS OF LIPIDS

Abnormalities of lipid metabolism most commonly come to light following routine blood testing. A comprehensive lipid profile should include plasma cholesterol, triglyceride and HDL cholesterol obtained after a 12-hr fast. LDL cholesterol may be calculated based on these.

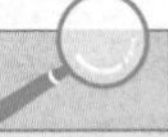

6.7 CAUSES OF SECONDARY HYPERLIPIDAEMIA	
Secondary hypercholesterolaemia	
• Hypothyroidism • Cholestatic liver disease • Anorexia nervosa • Pregnancy	• Drugs (diuretics, ciclosporin, corticosteroids, androgens) • Nephrotic syndrome • Hyperparathyroidism
Secondary hypertriglyceridaemia	
• Diabetes mellitus (type 2) • Chronic renal disease • Abdominal obesity	• Hepatocellular disease • Drugs (β-blockers, retinoids, corticosteroids) • Excess alcohol

Lipid measurements are usually performed for the following reasons:
• Screening for primary or secondary prevention of cardiovascular disease. • Investigation of patients with clinical features of lipid disorders. • Testing relatives of patients with one of the single gene defects causing dyslipidaemia.

Following the exclusion of secondary causes (Box 6.7), primary lipid abnormalities may be diagnosed.

PREDOMINANT HYPERCHOLESTEROLAEMIA

This may be dominant, recessive or polygenic. Familial hypercholesterolaemia is usually autosomal dominant and carries a high risk of cardiovascular disease.

Clinical features include:

• Xanthelasma. • Corneal arcus. • Tendon xanthomas.

PREDOMINANT HYPERTRIGLYCERIDAEMIA

If this is primary, it is most commonly polygenic, but many cases are secondary to alcohol, diabetes or insulin resistance syndrome (p. 386).

Clinical features in severe elevation include:

• Lipaemia retinalis. • Lipaemic blood and plasma. • Eruptive xanthomas (typically on trunk and buttocks). • Acute pancreatitis • Hepatosplenomegaly

MIXED HYPERLIPIDAEMIA

This is usually polygenic with no pathognomonic features unless caused by remnant lipoproteins.

MANAGEMENT OF DYSLIPIDAEMIA

Non-pharmacological treatment

Patients with lipid abnormalities should receive medical advice and, if necessary, dietary counselling to:

• Reduce intake of saturated and trans-unsaturated fat to <7–10% of total energy. • Reduce the intake of cholesterol to less than 250 mg/day. • Replace sources of saturated fat and cholesterol with alternative foods such as lean meat, low-fat dairy products, polyunsaturated spreads and low glycaemic index carbohydrates. • Reduce energy-dense foods such as fats and soft drinks, whilst increasing activity and exercise to achieve stable or negative energy balance (i.e. weight maintenance or weight loss). • Increase consumption of cardioprotective and nutrient-dense foods such as vegetables, unrefined carbohydrates, fish, nuts, pulses, legumes, fruit etc. • Adjust alcohol consumption, reducing intake if excessive or if associated with hypertension, hypertriglyceridaemia or central obesity. • Achieve additional benefits with supplementary intake of foods containing lipid-lowering nutrients such as n-3 fatty acids, dietary fibre and plant sterols.

Response to diet is usually apparent within 3–4 wks but dietary adjustment may need to be introduced gradually. Hyperlipidaemia in general, and hypertriglyceridaemia in particular, can be very responsive to these measures. Explanation, encouragement and other measures should be undertaken to reinforce patient compliance. Even minor weight loss can substantially reduce cardiovascular risk, especially in centrally obese patients.

All other modifiable cardiovascular risk factors should be assessed and treated. Where possible, intercurrent drug treatments that adversely affect the lipid profile should be replaced.

Pharmacological management

Drugs used to lower cholesterol fall into the following categories:

• HMG-CoA reductase inhibitors (statins). • Cholesterol absorption inhibitors. • Bile acid sequestering resins. • Nicotinic acid.

High triglyceride levels are treated with fibrates and fish oils. These are discussed further in Chapter 18.

OTHER BIOCHEMICAL DISORDERS

AMYLOIDOSIS

Amyloidosis is characterised by the extracellular deposition of insoluble proteins. These deposits consist of amyloid protein fibrils linked to glycosaminoglycans and proteoglycans, and serum amyloid P (SAP). The diagnosis should be considered in unexplained nephrotic syndrome, cardiomyopathy and peripheral neuropathy. Amyloid diseases are classified by aetiology and type of protein deposited:

Reactive (AA) amyloidosis: Increased production of serum amyloid A due to chronic infection (e.g. TB, bronchiectasis) or inflammation (e.g. rheumatoid arthritis). Around 90% of patients have proteinuria.

Light chain (AL) amyloidosis: Increased production of monoclonal light chains due to monoclonal gammopathies (myeloma, plasmacytoma). Clinical features include restrictive cardiomyopathy, neuropathy and macroglossia (pathognomonic). The condition has a poor prognosis.

Dialysis-associated (Aβ2M) amyloidosis: Accumulation of β_2-microglobulin due to dialysis. It occurs 5–10 yrs after starting dialysis, and presents with carpal tunnel syndrome, arthropathy and pathological fractures due to amyloid bone cysts.

Diagnosis

Biopsy of an affected organ, rectum or subcutaneous fat, when stained with Congo red dye, shows the pathognomonic apple-green birefringence of amyloid deposits under polarised light. Quantitative scintigraphy with radiolabelled SAP determines distribution of amyloid deposits.

Management

The aims of treatment are to support affected organs and, in acquired amyloidosis, to prevent further amyloid deposition through treatment of the primary cause. Liver transplantation may provide definitive treatment in selected patients with hereditary amyloidosis.

DISORDERS OF AMINO ACID METABOLISM

These usually present in the neonatal period and involve life-long treatment regimens.

PHENYLKETONURIA

This autosomal recessive condition causes deficiency of phenylalanine hydroxylase. Affected infants accumulate phenylalanine, causing mental retardation, which can be prevented by neonatal screening and dietary phenylalanine restriction.

HOMOCYSTINURIA

An autosomal recessive deficiency of cystathionine β-synthase results in increased urinary homocystine and methionine. Clinical manifestations involve:

• The eyes (displacement of the lens). • CNS mental retardation, seizures, psychiatric disturbances. • Skeleton (Marfan-like, with osteoporosis). • Vascular system (thrombosis). • Skin (hypopigmentation).

Treatment involves a methionine-restricted, cystine-supplemented diet and large doses of pyridoxine.

UNCOMMON DISORDERS OF CARBOHYDRATE METABOLISM

GALACTOSAEMIA

Galactosaemia is caused by an autosomal recessive mutation in the galactose-1-phosphate uridylyltransferase gene (GALT). The neonate is unable to metabolise galactose, leading to vomiting or diarrhoea after milk ingestion. Treatment involves life-long avoidance of galactose- and lactose-containing foods.

DISORDERS OF COMPLEX LIPID METABOLISM

These include the lysosomal storage disorders that have diverse clinical manifestations, typically including mental retardation. Some are now treatable using human enzyme replacement therapy, whilst others can be prevented through genetic screening.

DISORDERS OF HAEM METABOLISM: THE PORPHYRIAS

These are rare disorders due to inherited enzyme deficiencies of the haem biosynthetic pathway. They are divided into hepatic or erythropoietic, depending on the major site of excess porphyrin production. Inheritance is dominant with low penetrance, with environmental factors modifying disease expression.

Clinical features

Two patterns are recognised:

Photosensitive skin manifestations: Pain, erythema, bullae, erosions, hirsutism and hyperpigmentation are characteristic of the most common porphyria, porphyria cutanea tarda (PCT).

Acute relapsing and remitting neurological syndrome: Presents with acute abdominal pain and autonomic dysfunction (tachycardia, hypertension and constipation), and is characteristic of acute intermittent porphyria (AIP).

Attacks are often provoked by drugs such as anticonvulsants, sulphonamides, oestrogen and progesterone (oral contraceptive pill), or by alcohol and even fasting. In some cases, no precipitant can be identified.

Diagnosis

Measure porphyrins, their precursors and metabolites in blood, urine and faeces. It is now possible to measure some of the affected enzymes. Identification of the underlying gene mutations has made family testing possible for some variants.

Management

With neurovisceral attacks patients should avoid any known precipitants of acute porphyria. I.v. glucose can terminate acute attacks through a reduction in ALA synthetase activity. For photosensitive manifestations the primary goal is to avoid sun exposure and skin trauma. Barrier sun creams containing zinc or titanium oxide are the most effective products.

7

Kidney and urinary tract disease

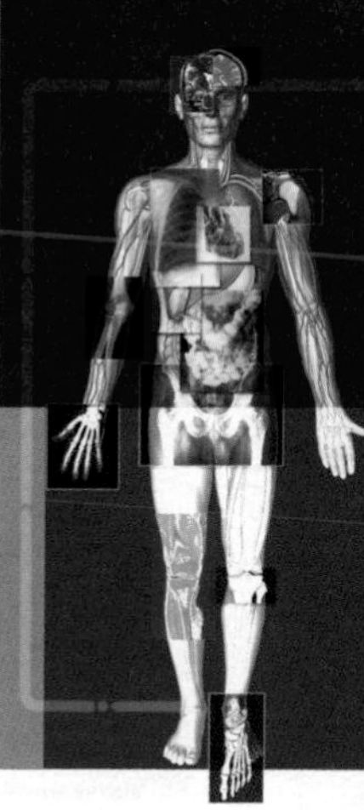

Renal medicine ranges from the management of common conditions (e.g. urinary tract infection) to the use of complex technology to replace renal function (e.g. dialysis and transplantation). There are close links with the surgical specialties of urology and transplantation. This chapter describes the common disorders of the kidneys and urinary tract which are encountered in everyday practice, as well as giving an overview of the highly specialised field of renal replacement therapy.

PRESENTING PROBLEMS

PATTERNS OF PRESENTATION

The broad categories of renal and urinary tract disease, and their typical manifestations, are shown in Figure 7.1.

CYSTITIS AND URINARY TRACT INFECTION

Urinary tract infection (UTI) is the most common bacterial infection managed in general medical practice and accounts for 1–3% of consultations. Up to 50% of women have a UTI at some time. UTI is defined as multiplication of organisms in the urinary tract. It is usually associated with the presence of neutrophils and $>10^5$ organisms/ml in a midstream sample of urine (MSU).

Organisms causing UTI in the community include:

• *Escherichia coli* derived from the GI tract (about 75% of infections). • *Proteus*. • *Pseudomonas* spp. • Streptococci. • *Staphylococcus epidermidis*.

CLINICAL EXAMINATION OF THE KIDNEY AND URINARY TRACT

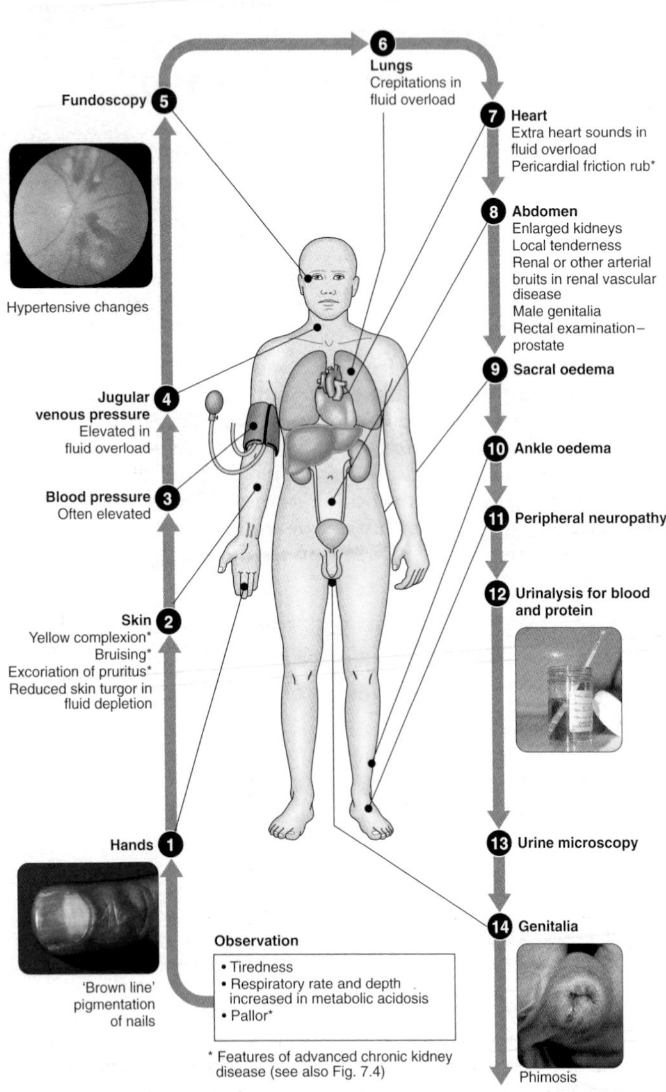

* Features of advanced chronic kidney disease (see also Fig. 7.4)

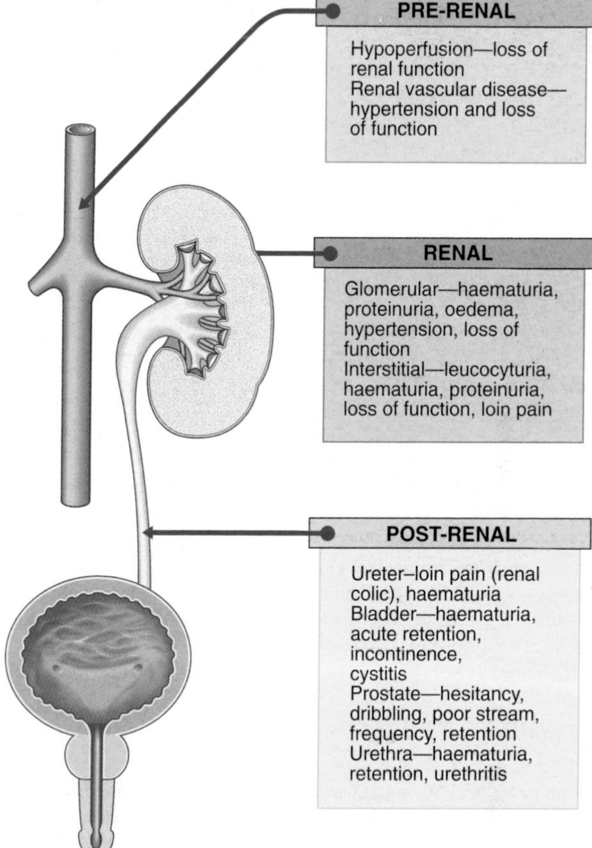

Fig. 7.1 Classification and manifestations of renal and urinary tract disease. Consequences of loss of renal function and effects on other organs are described on pages 181–185.

In hospital, *E. coli* still predominates, but *Klebsiella* or streptococci are more common than in the community. Certain strains of *E. coli* have a particular propensity to invade the urinary tract.

Clinical assessment

Typical features of cystitis and urethritis include:

• Abrupt onset of frequency of micturition. • Scalding pain in the urethra during micturition (dysuria). • Suprapubic pain during and after voiding. •

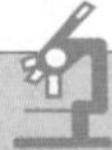

7.1 INVESTIGATION OF PATIENTS WITH UTI
All patients
• Urinalysis looking for blood/protein/nitrite • Urine microscopy and culture (MSU or urine obtained by suprapubic aspiration) • Blood tests: U&Es, FBC
Other investigations
• Blood culture: if evidence of sepsis • Pelvic examination: women with recurrent UTI • Rectal examination: men (to examine prostate) • Renal USS/CT/intravenous urogram (IVU): women who have acute pyelonephritis, recurrent UTI despite antibiotics, or UTI in pregnancy • Cystoscopy: patients with haematuria or suspected bladder lesion

Intense desire to pass more urine after micturition, due to spasm of the inflamed bladder wall (urgency). • Urine that may appear cloudy and have an unpleasant odour. • Microscopic or visible haematuria.

Systemic symptoms are usually slight or absent. However, infection in the lower urinary tract can spread; prominent systemic symptoms with fever and loin pain suggest the presence of acute pyelonephritis (p. 167) and may be an indication for hospitalisation.

The differential diagnosis includes urethritis due to an STD (p. 130) or Reiter's syndrome.

Investigations

An approach to investigation is shown in Box 7.1.

In an otherwise healthy woman with a single lower UTI and no indications of a complicated infection, urine culture prior to treatment is not mandatory. It is necessary, however, in patients with recurrent infection or after failure of initial treatment, during pregnancy, or in patients susceptible to serious infection (e.g. older people, those with diabetes, the immunocompromised or those with an indwelling catheter).

Management

• Antibiotics are recommended in all cases of proven UTI. If urine culture has been performed, treatment may be started while awaiting the result. • Treatment for 3 days is the norm and is less likely to induce antibiotic resistance than more prolonged therapy. • Trimethoprim is the usual choice for initial treatment. Between 10% and 40% of organisms causing UTI are resistant to trimethoprim, the lower rates being seen in community-based practice. • Nitrofurantoin, ciprofloxacin and cefalexin are also generally effective. • High fluid intake and urinary alkalinising agents are often recommended but are not evidence-based.

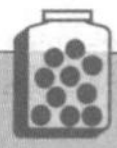

7.2 PROPHYLACTIC MEASURES TO BE ADOPTED BY WOMEN WITH RECURRENT UTI

- Fluid intake of at least 2 litres/day
- Regular complete emptying of bladder
- If vesico-ureteric reflux is present, practise double micturition (empty bladder then attempt micturition 10–15 mins later)
- Good personal hygiene
- Emptying of bladder before and after sexual intercourse
- Cranberry juice may be effective

PERSISTENT OR RECURRENT UTI

Treatment failure, with persistence of organisms on repeat culture, suggests an underlying cause, which should be investigated (Box 7.1) and treated. Reinfection with a different organism, or with the same organism after an interval, may also occur. In women, recurrent infections are common and further investigation is only justified if infections are severe or frequent (>2/yr).

If the cause cannot be removed, suppressive antibiotic therapy can be used to prevent recurrence and reduce the risk of septicaemia and renal damage. Regular urine culture and a regimen of two or three antibiotics in sequence, rotating every 6 mths, are used to reduce the emergence of resistant organisms. Other simple measures may help to prevent recurrence (Box 7.2).

ASYMPTOMATIC BACTERIURIA

This is defined as $>10^5$/ml organisms in the urine of apparently healthy asymptomatic patients. There is no evidence that this condition causes renal scarring in adults who are not pregnant and have a normal urinary tract, and in general, treatment is not indicated. Up to 30% of patients will develop symptomatic infection within 1 yr.

LOIN PAIN

Dull ache in the loin is rarely due to renal disease but may be caused by renal stone, renal tumour, acute pyelonephritis or obstruction of the renal pelvis.

ACUTE PYELONEPHRITIS

The kidneys are infected in a minority of patients with lower UTI or bacteriuria, although the exact proportion is unknown. Acute renal infection (pyelonephritis) presents as a classic triad of loin pain, fever and tenderness over the kidneys.

Clinical assessment

• Acute onset of pain in one or both loins, which may radiate to the iliac fossae and suprapubic area. • Associated lumbar tenderness and guarding.

• Dysuria due to associated cystitis in 30%. • Fever which may be associated with rigors, vomiting and hypotension. • Neutrophils, organisms, red cells and tubular epithelial cells in urine.

The differential diagnosis of acute pyelonephritis includes acute appendicitis, diverticulitis, cholecystitis and salpingitis. In perinephric abscess, there is marked pain and tenderness and often bulging of the loin on the affected side. Patients are extremely ill, with fever, leucocytosis and positive blood cultures. Urinary symptoms are absent, and urine contains neither pus cells nor organisms.

Investigations and management

• Bacteria and neutrophils in the urine with typical clinical features confirm the diagnosis. • Renal tract USS should be performed to exclude a perinephric collection and obstruction as a predisposing factor. • Adequate fluid intake must be ensured, if necessary i.v. • Antibiotics are continued for 7–14 days. Severe cases require initial i.v. therapy, with a cephalosporin, quinolone or gentamicin. • Urine should be cultured during and after treatment.

7.3 PREDISPOSING FACTORS FOR KIDNEY STONES

- Low urine volumes: high ambient temperatures, low fluid intake
- Diet: high protein intake, high sodium, low calcium
- High urinary sodium/oxalate/urate/citrate excretion
- Hypercalcaemia of any cause (p. 357)
- Ileal disease or resection (leads to increased oxalate absorption and urinary excretion)
- Renal tubular acidosis type I (distal, p. 198)
- Familial hypercalciuria
- Medullary sponge kidney
- Cystinuria

RENAL COLIC

Acute loin pain radiating to the groin ('renal colic'), together with haematuria, is typical of ureteric obstruction most commonly due to calculi.

Urinary calculi: These vary in frequency around the world, probably as a consequence of dietary and environmental factors, but genetic factors may also contribute. In Europe, 80% of renal stones contain crystals of calcium salts, about 15% contain magnesium ammonium phosphate, and small numbers of pure cystine or uric acid stones are found. In developing countries, bladder stones are common, particularly in children. In developed countries, the incidence of childhood bladder stones is low; renal stones in adults are more common. Several risk factors for renal stone formation are known (Box 7.3); however, in developed countries, most calculi occur in healthy young men with no clear predisposing cause.

Clinical assessment of impacted ureteric stone

• Renal colic: sudden pain in the loin, which radiates to the groin, testis or labium, in the first lumbar dermatome. Intensity steadily increases to reach a peak in a few minutes; the patient may groan in agony. • Pallor, sweating,

7.4 INVESTIGATIONS FOR RENAL STONES			
Sample	**Test**	**First stone**	**Recurrent stone**
Stone	Chemical composition—most valuable when possible	✓	✓
Blood	Calcium	✓	✓
	Phosphate	✓	✓
	Uric acid	✓	✓
	U&Es	✓	✓
	Parathyroid hormone (PTH)—only if calcium or calcium excretion high		(✓)
Urine	Dipstick test for protein, blood, glucose	✓	✓
	Amino acids		✓
24-hr urine	Urea		✓
	Creatinine clearance		✓
	Sodium		✓
	Calcium		✓
	Oxalate		✓
	Uric acid		✓

restlessness and often vomiting. • Frequency, dysuria and haematuria. • Intense pain which usually subsides within 2 hrs, but may continue for hours or days. It is usually constant during attacks, although slight fluctuations in severity may occur. A dull loin ache may follow.

Investigations

• Urinalysis: shows red cells. • AXR: about 90% of stones are radio-opaque. • IVU: may show delayed excretion of contrast from the kidney and a dilated ureter down to the stone. • USS and CT: may reveal more radiolucent stones.

Patients with a first renal stone should have a minimum set of investigations (Box 7.4); more detailed investigation is reserved for those with recurrent or multiple stones, or those with complicated or unexpected presentations. Since most stones pass spontaneously, urine should be sieved for a few days after an episode of colic to collect the calculus for chemical analysis.

Management

• Bed rest and application of warmth to the site of pain. • Powerful analgesia, e.g. morphine (10–20 mg), pethidine (100 mg) i.m. or diclofenac as a suppository (100 mg). • Fluid intake of 2 litres/day.

Around 90% of stones <4 mm in diameter will pass spontaneously, but only 10% of stones of >6 mm will pass and these may require active intervention. Immediate action is required if there is anuria or if severe infection occurs in the stagnant urine proximal to the stone (pyonephrosis). Most stones can be fragmented by extracorporeal shock wave lithotripsy in which shock waves generated outside the body are focused on the stone, breaking it into small pieces which can pass easily down the ureter. This requires free drainage of the distal urinary tract.

Endoscopic surgery is often required for stones, but open surgery is now very rarely needed except for large bladder stones. All stones are potentially infected and surgery should be covered with appropriate antibiotics.

EXCESSIVE MICTURITION

POLYURIA

Causes of an inappropriately high urine volume (>3 litres/day) are shown in Box 7.5. In the assessment of polyuria accurate documentation of intake is essential.

NOCTURIA

Waking up at night to void urine may be a consequence of polyuria but may also result from fluid intake or diuretic use in the late evening. Nocturia also occurs in chronic kidney disease, and in prostatic enlargement where it is associated with poor stream, hesitancy, incomplete bladder emptying, terminal dribbling and urinary frequency.

FREQUENCY

Frequency describes micturition more often than a patient's expectations. It may be a consequence of polyuria, often due to diuretic therapy, when volumes passed are normal or high. It is also a symptom of UTIs when urine volumes are low and associated with dysuria, urgency and a feeling of incomplete emptying.

URINARY INCONTINENCE

Urinary incontinence is defined as any involuntary leakage of urine. Urinary tract pathology causing incontinence is described below. It may also occur

7.5 CAUSES OF POLYURIA

- Excess fluid intake
- Osmotic, e.g. hyperglycaemia, hypercalcaemia
- Cranial diabetes insipidus (reduced ADH secretion)
- Idiopathic (50%), mass lesion, trauma, infection
- Nephrogenic diabetes insipidus (tubular dysfunction)
- Genetic tubular defects
- Drugs/toxins, e.g. lithium, diuretics
- Interstitial renal disease
- Hypokalaemia, hypercalcaemia

with a normal urinary tract, e.g. in association with poor cognition or poor mobility, or transiently during an acute illness or hospitalisation, especially in older people. Diuretics (medication, alcohol or caffeine) may worsen incontinence.

Clinical assessment and investigations

• A voiding diary is used to record the pattern of micturition, including the estimated volume voided, frequency of voiding, precipitating factors and associated features, e.g. urgency. • Cognitive function and mobility are assessed. • Neurological assessment reveals disorders such as MS that may affect the nervous supply of the bladder. Perineal sensation and anal sphincter tone should be examined since the same sacral nerve roots also supply the bladder and urethral sphincter. • The lumbar spine should be inspected for features of spina bifida occulta. • Rectal examination is needed to assess the prostate in men and to exclude faecal impaction. • Urinalysis and culture should be performed in all patients. • An assessment of post-micturition volume should be made, either by post-micturition USS or catheterisation. Urine flow rates and full urodynamic assessment may also be helpful in selected cases.

Incontinence syndromes

Stress incontinence: Leakage occurs because passive bladder pressure exceeds the urethral pressure, due to either poor pelvic floor support or a weak urethral sphincter, most often both. This is very common in women, especially following childbirth. It is rare in men, usually following prostate surgery. Urine leaks when abdominal pressure rises, e.g. when coughing or sneezing. In women, perineal inspection may reveal leakage of urine with coughs, and sometimes also a prolapse. Women often respond well to physiotherapy but if incontinence is persistent, surgical treatment is indicated.

Urge incontinence: Leakage usually occurs because of detrusor overactivity producing an increased bladder pressure which overcomes the urethral sphincter (motor urgency). Urgency with or without incontinence may also be driven by a hypersensitive bladder (sensory urgency) resulting from UTI or bladder stone. The incidence of urge incontinence increases with age, and is also seen in men with lower urinary tract obstruction; it most often remits after the obstruction is relieved. The diagnosis is made on the basis of symptoms after exclusion of urinary retention by bladder USS; confirmation requires urodynamic testing. Treatment is by bladder retraining, teaching patients to hold more urine voluntarily in their bladder, assisted by anticholinergic medication.

Overflow incontinence: This occurs when the bladder becomes chronically over-distended. It is most common in men with benign prostatic hyperplasia or bladder neck obstruction, but may occur in either sex as a result of detrusor muscle failure (atonic bladder). This may be idiopathic but more commonly results from pelvic nerve damage from surgery (e.g. hysterectomy or rectal excision), trauma or infection, or from compression of the cauda equina from disc prolapse, trauma or tumour. USS reveals a significant post-micturition volume (>100 ml). Obstructed bladders should be treated surgically. Unobstructed bladders need to be drained, preferably by intermittent self-catheterisation. Urodynamic testing helps clarify the aetiology.

Post-micturition dribble: This is very common in men, even in the relatively young. It is due to a small amount of urine becoming trapped in the U-bend of the bulbar urethra, which leaks out when the patient moves. It is more pronounced if associated with a urethral diverticulum or urethral stricture. It may occur in females with a urethral diverticulum and may mimic stress incontinence.

Neurological causes: Neurological disease resulting in abnormal bladder function is almost always associated with obvious neurological signs; these are described on page 646.

REDUCED MICTURITION

OLIGURIA/ANURIA

On a normal diet, between 300 and 500 ml/day of urine is required to excrete the solute load at maximum concentration. Volumes below this are termed oliguria. Anuria is the (almost) total absence of urine (<50 ml/day). A low measured urine volume is an important finding and is a consequence of reduced production, obstruction to urine flow or both.

HAEMATURIA

This indicates bleeding anywhere within the urinary tract, and may be visible (macroscopic) or only detectable on urinalysis (microscopic). Macroscopic haematuria is more likely to be caused by tumours, severe infections and renal infarction. Common causes are shown in Box 7.6.

Investigations and management of haematuria are outlined in Figure 7.2.

7.6 CAUSES OF HAEMATURIA	
Renal	Infection, infarction, interstitial disease, glomerular disease, vascular malformation, tumour, cysts, clotting disorders
Ureters	Stones, tumour
Bladder	Infection, tumour
Urethra	Trauma

PROTEINURIA

Proteinuria is usually asymptomatic, although large amounts may make urine froth easily.

Moderate amounts of low molecular weight protein do pass through the glomerular basement membrane (GBM). These are normally reabsorbed by tubular cells so that <150 mg/day appears in urine. Minor leakage of

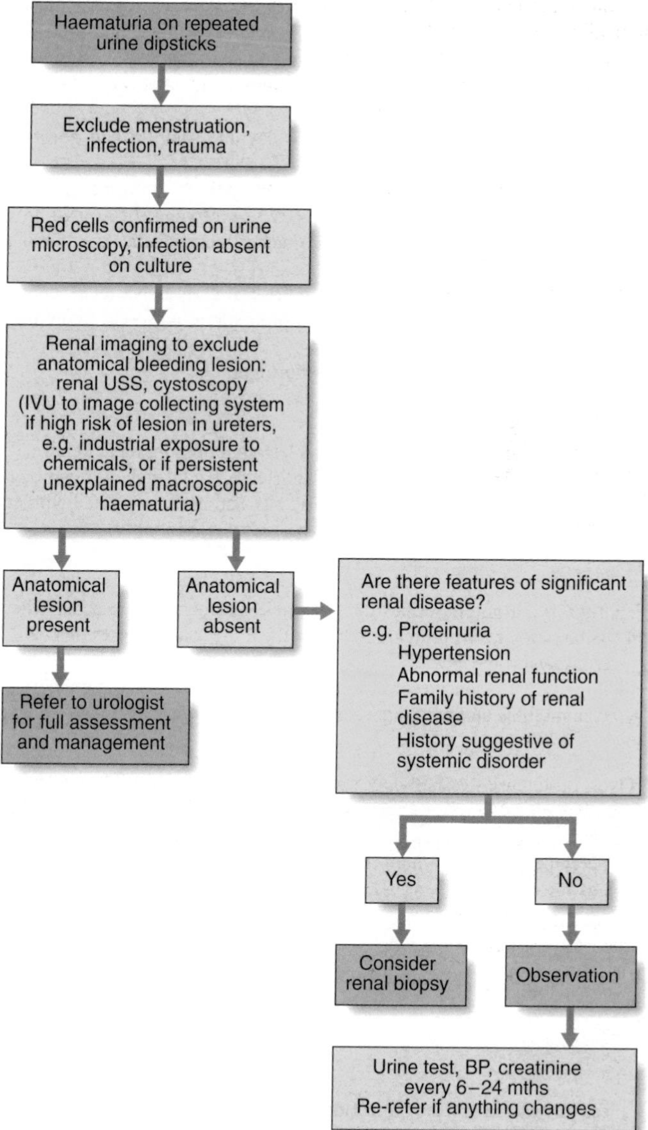

Fig. 7.2 Investigation and management of haematuria.

albumin into the urine may occur transiently after vigorous exercise, during fever or UTI, and in heart failure. Quantities do not reach nephrotic levels and tests should be repeated once the stimulus is no longer present.

Proteinuria >2.5 g/day indicates that a glomerular source is likely. Over 3.5 g/day is the nephrotic range.

'Orthostatic proteinuria', with positive daytime samples and negative morning samples, is usually benign.

Low molecular weight proteins may also appear in the urine in larger quantities than 150 mg/day (although rarely exceeding 1.5–2 g/24 hrs), indicating failure of reabsorption by damaged tubular cells, i.e. 'tubular proteinuria'.

Heavy proteinuria denotes an increased risk of progressive renal failure. Treatments that are effective at lowering proteinuria (e.g. ACE inhibitors) also lower this risk.

Investigation of proteinuria is shown in Figure 7.3.

MICROALBUMINURIA

Microalbuminuria (0.03–0.3 g/day) is a clear sign of glomerular abnormality and can identify very early glomerular disease, e.g. in diabetic nephropathy (p. 412). Persistent microalbuminuria has also been associated with an increased risk of atherosclerosis and cardiovascular mortality.

NEPHROTIC SYNDROME

Nephrotic syndrome describes the clinical consequences that occur when substantial amounts of protein are lost in the urine. The diseases that cause nephrotic syndrome always affect the glomerulus and tend to be non-inflammatory, or subacute examples of inflammatory glomerulonephritis. Diabetes mellitus and amyloidosis can also cause nephrotic syndrome.

Clinical assessment

• Overt proteinuria—usually >3.5 g/24 hrs (urine may be frothy). • Hypoalbuminaemia (<30 g/l). • Oedema and generalised fluid retention. • Intravascular volume depletion with hypotension, or expansion with hypertension. • Hypercholesterolaemia, high risk of atherosclerosis. • Hypercoagulability (venous thromboembolism). • Infection—hypogammaglobulinaemia.

Management

• Includes diuretics, low-sodium diet, statins, anticoagulation and vaccination against infection.

OEDEMA

Causes of oedema are shown in Box 7.7.

Investigations

The cause of oedema is usually apparent from the history and examination of the cardiovascular system and abdomen, combined with measurement

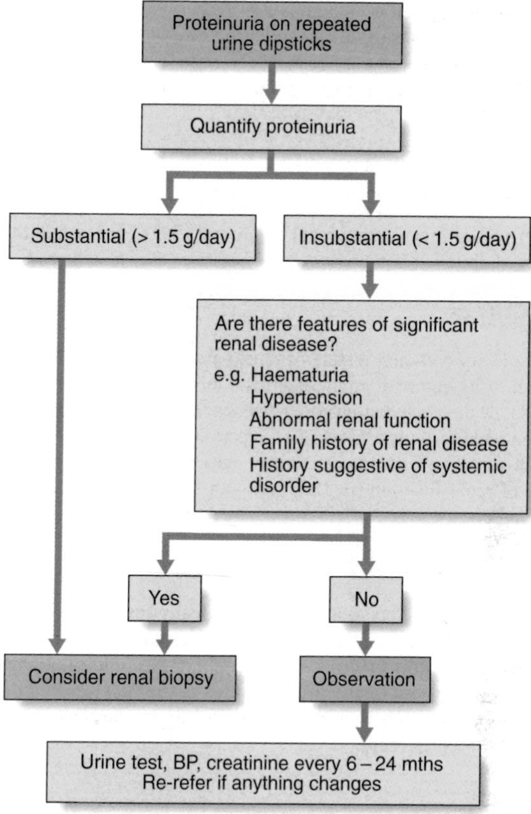

Fig. 7.3 Investigation of proteinuria.

7.7 CAUSES OF OEDEMA	
Low plasma oncotic pressure	Hypoalbuminaemia as seen in nephrotic syndrome, liver failure, malabsorption
Increased capillary permeability	Infection, drug-related (calcium channel blockers)
Increased hydrostatic pressure	High venous pressure/obstruction (congestive heart failure, DVT, pelvic tumour), lymphatic obstruction (malignancy, radiation injury, congenital abnormality)

of urinary protein and the serum albumin level. Where ascites or pleural effusions in isolation are causing diagnostic difficulty, aspiration of fluid with measurement of protein and glucose, and microscopy for cells, will usually clarify the diagnosis (p. 276).

Management

• Specific causes (e.g. venous thrombosis) should be treated. • Restrict sodium (and sometimes fluid) in generalised oedema. • Mild fluid retention will respond to a diuretic such as a thiazide or low-dose furosemide or bumetanide. • In nephrotic syndrome, renal failure and severe cardiac failure, very large doses of diuretics, sometimes in combination, may be required.

HYPERTENSION

Hypertension is a very common feature of renal parenchymal and vascular disease and is an early feature of glomerular disorders. As glomerular filtration rate (GFR) declines, hypertension becomes increasingly common, regardless of the renal diagnosis. Control of hypertension is very important in patients with renal impairment because of its close relationship with further decline of renal function (p. 183) and with the adverse cardiovascular risk in renal disease.

ACUTE RENAL FAILURE

Acute renal failure (ARF) refers to a sudden and usually reversible loss of renal function, which develops over a period of days or weeks and is usually accompanied by a reduction in urine volume. There are many possible causes (Box 7.8) and it is frequently multifactorial. If the cause cannot be rapidly corrected and renal function restored, temporary renal replacement therapy may be required (p. 185).

REVERSIBLE PRE-RENAL ARF

Because haemodynamic disturbances can initially produce acute renal dysfunction that has the potential to be rapidly reversed, prompt recognition and treatment are important.

7.8 CAUSES OF ARF	
Pre-renal	Systemic, e.g. heart failure, blood or fluid loss Local, e.g. renal artery occlusion/stenosis, disease affecting arterioles
Intrinsic renal disease	Acute tubular necrosis/toxic/septic renal failure (85%) Glomerular disease (5%) Interstitial disease (10%)
Post-renal	Obstruction, e.g. stones, tumour, prostatic enlargement

Clinical assessment

• There is hypotension with signs of poor peripheral perfusion (may be absent in those taking NSAIDs or ACE inhibitors). • Postural hypotension (>20/10 mmHg from lying to standing)—a useful sign of early hypovolaemia. • Although the cause of renal hypoperfusion may be obvious there may be concealed blood loss following trauma (e.g. pelvic fractures) or into a pregnant uterus. Also, large volumes of intravascular fluid may be lost following injuries and burns, and in severe inflammatory skin diseases or sepsis. • Metabolic acidosis and hyperkalaemia are present.

Management and prognosis

• Establish and correct the underlying cause. • If hypovolaemia is present, restore blood volume as rapidly as possible (with blood, plasma or isotonic saline (0.9%), depending on what has been lost). • Optimise systemic haemodynamics. Monitoring of the central venous pressure or pulmonary wedge pressure as an adjunct to clinical examination may aid in determining the rate of administration of fluid. Critically ill patients may require invasive haemodynamic monitoring to assess cardiac output and systemic vascular resistance, and the use of inotropic drugs to restore an effective BP (p. 27). • Correct metabolic acidosis. Restoration of blood volume will correct acidosis by restoring kidney function. Isotonic sodium bicarbonate (e.g. 500 ml of 1.26%) may be used. • Recent trials do not support the use of low-dose dopamine in severely ill patients at risk of ARF. • If treatment is given sufficiently early, renal function will usually improve rapidly; in such circumstances residual renal impairment is unlikely.

ESTABLISHED ARF

Established ARF with the histological pattern of acute tubular necrosis (ATN) may develop following severe or prolonged under-perfusion of the kidney (pre-renal ARF). In patients without an obvious cause of pre-renal ARF, alternative 'renal' and 'post-renal' causes must be considered (Boxes 7.8 and 7.9).

Clinical and biochemical assessment

These reflect the causal condition, together with features of renal failure.

Alterations in urine volume: Patients are usually oliguric (urine volume <500 ml daily). Anuria (complete absence of urine) is rare and usually indicates acute urinary tract obstruction or vascular occlusion. In about 20% of cases, the urine volume is normal or increased, but with a low GFR and a reduction of tubular reabsorption (non-oliguric ARF). Excretion is inadequate despite good urine output and the plasma urea and creatinine increase.

Disturbances of water, electrolyte and acid–base balance: Hyperkalaemia is common. Dilutional hyponatraemia occurs if the patient has continued to drink freely despite oliguria or has received inappropriate amounts of i.v. dextrose. Metabolic acidosis develops unless prevented by loss of hydrogen ions through vomiting or aspiration of gastric contents. Hypocal-

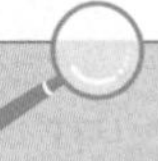

7.9 DIFFERENTIAL DIAGNOSIS OF ARF IN A HAEMODYNAMICALLY STABLE, NON-SEPTIC PATIENT

Urinary tract obstruction

- Suggested by a history of loin pain, haematuria, renal colic or difficulty in micturition but often clinically silent
- Can usually be excluded by renal USS—essential in any patient with unexplained ARF
- Prompt relief of obstruction restores renal function

Vascular event

- Due to major vascular occlusion or small-vessel diseases (p. 609)
- May be precipitated by ACE inhibitors in critical renal artery stenosis (p. 190)
- Urine usually shows minimal abnormalities but there may be haematuria in renal infarction

Rapidly progressive glomerulonephritis (RPGN) (p. 195)

- Typically, significant (dipsticks 3+) haematuria and proteinuria
- Sometimes associated with systemic features (e.g. systemic vasculitis, systemic lupus erythematosus)
- Useful blood tests include: ANCA, ANA, anti-GBM antibodies, complement, immunoglobulins
- Renal biopsy shows aggressive glomerular inflammation, usually with crescent formation

Acute interstitial nephritis (p. 195)

- Usually caused by an adverse drug reaction
- Characterised by small amounts of blood and protein in urine, often with leucocyturia
- Kidneys are normal size
- Requires cessation of drug and often prednisolone treatment

Drugs

For example:

- Haemodynamic effects (e.g. NSAIDs, ACE inhibitors)
- Direct toxicity to the tubule (e.g. aminoglycosides)

caemia, due to reduced renal production of 1,25-dihydroxycholecalciferol, is common.

Other features: 'Uraemic' features include initial anorexia, nausea and vomiting followed by drowsiness, apathy, confusion, muscle-twitching, hiccoughs, fits and coma. Respiratory rate may be increased due to acidosis, pulmonary oedema or respiratory infection. Anaemia is common, due to excessive blood loss, haemolysis or decreased erythropoiesis. Bleeding is more likely because of disordered platelet function and disturbances of the coagulation cascade. Severe infections may complicate ARF because immune mechanisms are depressed.

Management

Emergency resuscitation: Treat hyperkalaemia (a plasma K^+ concentration >6 mmol/l) immediately to prevent the development of life-threatening cardiac arrhythmias (p. 151). Circulating blood volume should be optimised to ensure adequate renal perfusion. Severe acidosis can be ameliorated with isotonic sodium bicarbonate (e.g. 500 ml of 1.26%) if volume status allows. In an anuric or volume-overloaded patient, renal replacement therapy may be required.

Addressing the underlying cause of the ARF: Investigations for established ARF are outlined in Box 7.10. In many cases, more than one factor contributes to the renal dysfunction. There is no specific treatment for ATN, other than restoring renal perfusion. Intrinsic renal disease may require specific therapy; for example, immunosuppressive drugs are of value in some causes of rapidly progressive glomerulonephritis (p. 195). 'Post-renal' obstruction should be relieved urgently. With rapid intervention, dialysis can usually be avoided.

Fluid and electrolyte balance: After initial resuscitation, daily fluid intake should equal urine output, plus an additional 500 ml to cover insensible losses; such losses are higher in febrile patients and in tropical climates. If abnormal losses occur, as in diarrhoea, additional fluid and electrolyte replacement is required. Since sodium and potassium are retained, intake of these substances should be restricted.

Nutrition: Parenteral or enteral tube feeding may be needed in hypercatabolic patients. Protein restriction (<40 g/day) may be needed in those not on dialysis.

Infection control: Patients with ARF are at risk of intercurrent infection, and prompt diagnosis and treatment are essential.

Drugs: Vasoactive drugs such as NSAIDs and ACE inhibitors may prolong ARF and temporary withdrawal should be considered. Many drugs are excreted renally and dose adjustment may be required in ARF.

Renal replacement therapy (p. 185)***:*** This may be required as supportive management in ARF.

Recovery and prognosis

A gradual return of urine output and a steady improvement in biochemistry accompany recovery.

Some patients, primarily those with ATN or in whom chronic urinary obstruction has been relieved, develop a 'diuretic phase'. Sufficient fluid to replace the urine output should be given. After a few days, urine volume falls to normal as the concentrating mechanisms recover.

In uncomplicated ARF, such as that due to simple haemorrhage or drugs, mortality is low even when renal replacement therapy is required. In ARF associated with serious infection and multiple organ failure, mortality is 50–70%. Outcome is usually determined by the underlying disorder and other complications, rather than by renal failure itself.

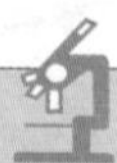

7.10 SUGGESTED SCREENING TESTS IN ARF	
Haematology	
• FBC • Blood film: in case of fragmentation of RBC	• Clotting screen
Biochemistry	
• U&Es, creatinine • Calcium	• Urinalysis • Proteinuria measurement
Microbiology	
• Blood cultures • CRP (ESR is misleading in ARF) • MSU	• Hepatitis and HIV serology: urgent if dialysis is needed (isolation of dialysis machine if positive) • Other cultures, e.g. wound, sputum, catheters
Imaging etc.	
• Renal USS: usually required urgently to confirm/refute two equal-sized, unobstructed kidneys • CXR	• ECG: if >40 yrs or there are risk factors for cardiac disease
If diagnosis is not known	
Consider: • Immunoglobulins and protein electrophoresis • Urinary Bence Jones protein • Complement • ANA and dsDNA: if ANA is positive • Extractable nuclear antigen (ENA): if a connective tissue disorder is suspected • Rheumatoid factor • ANCA and anti-GBM: in all possible inflammatory renal disease	• Cryoglobulins: if cryoglobulinaemia is clinically suspected • Myoglobin/creatine kinase: if rhabdomyolysis is possible • Anti-streptolysin O (ASO) titre: if post-streptococcal glomerulonephritis is possible • Other serology: if clinically suspected, e.g. leptospirosis, syphilis, Hantavirus • Pulmonary function: in systemic disease • Carbon monoxide transfer coefficient: if lung haemorrhage is suspected

CHRONIC KIDNEY DISEASE

Chronic kidney disease (CKD) refers to an irreversible deterioration in renal function which classically develops over a period of years (Box 7.11). Initially, it is manifest only as a biochemical abnormality. Eventually, loss of the excretory, metabolic and endocrine functions of the kidney leads to

7.11 STAGES OF CHRONIC KIDNEY DISEASE			
Stage	**Description**	**GFR (ml/min/1.73 m²)**	**Action**
1	Kidney damage* with normal or high GFR	≥90	Investigate, e.g. haematuria and proteinuria (see below)
2	Kidney damage with slightly low GFR	60–89	Renoprotection—BP control, dietary modifications
3	Moderately low GFR	30–59	
4	Severe low GFR	15–29	Prepare for renal replacement therapy (if appropriate)
5	Kidney failure	<15 or dialysis	

*Kidney damage means pathological abnormalities or markers of damage, including abnormalities in blood or urine tests or imaging studies or GFR <60 ml/min/1.73 m² for 3 months. Symptoms unusual until ≥ stage 3.

7.12 CAUSES OF CHRONIC KIDNEY DISEASE	
Diabetes mellitus	20–40%
Hypertension	5–25%
Glomerular diseases	10–20%
Interstitial diseases	5–15%
Renal artery stenosis	5%
Systemic inflammatory diseases	5%
Congenital and inherited	5%
Unknown	5–20%

the development of the clinical symptoms and signs of renal failure, which are referred to as uraemia. When death is likely without renal replacement therapy, it is called end-stage renal failure (ESRF).

CKD may be caused by any condition which destroys the normal structure and function of the kidney. Common causes are shown in Box 7.12.

Clinical assessment

Patients may remain asymptomatic until GFR falls below 30 ml/min (stage 4 or 5, Box 7.11). Thereafter, due to the widespread effects of renal failure, symptoms and signs may develop that are related to almost every body system (Fig. 7.4).

In ESRF (stage 5, Box 7.11) patients appear ill and anaemic. They do not necessarily retain fluid, and may show signs of sodium and water depletion. There may be unusually deep respiration related to metabolic acidosis

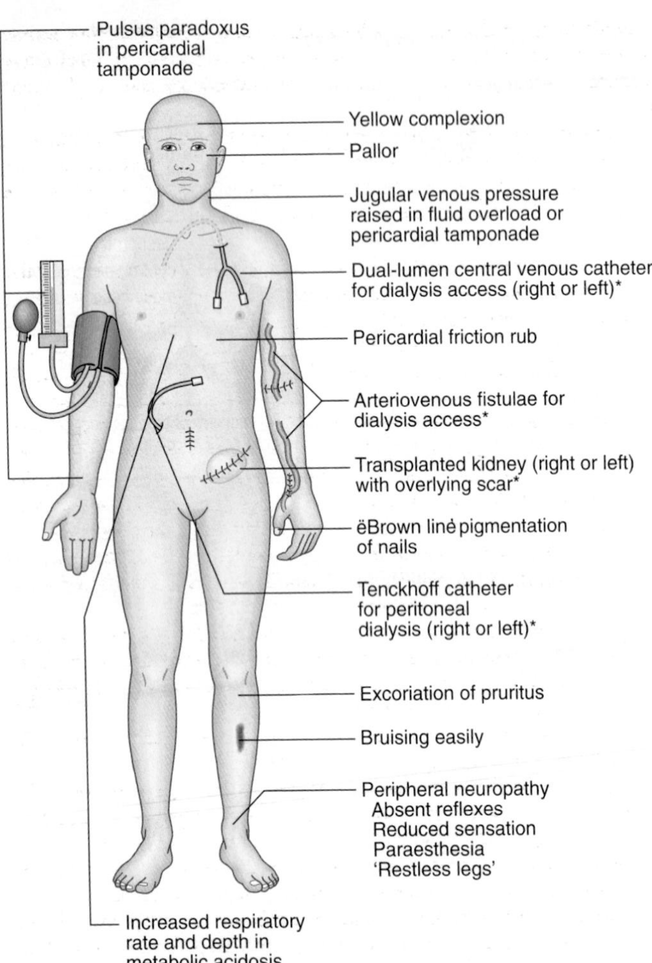

Fig. 7.4 Physical signs in CKD. (* Features of renal replacement therapy)

(Kussmaul's respiration), anorexia and nausea. Later, hiccoughs, pruritus, vomiting, muscular twitching, fits, drowsiness and coma ensue.

Investigations and management

Identify the underlying renal disease: Suggested screening tests in CKD are similar to those for ARF (Box 7.10).

Address reversible factors which are making renal function worse: These include hypertension, reduced renal perfusion (e.g. in renal artery stenosis), urinary tract obstruction or infection, and nephrotoxic medications.

Attempt to prevent further renal damage: Once the plasma creatinine exceeds about 300 μmol/l (3.4 mg/dl), there is usually progressive deterioration in renal function, irrespective of aetiology. The rate of deterioration is very variable between patients but is relatively constant for an individual patient.

- *Control BP.* In many types of renal disease, but particularly in glomerular disease, control of BP may retard deterioration of GFR. This has been proven for diabetic nephropathy, but is probably true for other diseases as well, particularly those associated with heavy proteinuria. No threshold for this effect has been found; reduction of any level of BP is beneficial. The very high incidence of left ventricular hypertrophy, heart failure and occlusive vascular disease in patients with long-standing renal disease also justifies vigorous BP control. ACE inhibitors have been shown to be more effective at retarding the progression of renal failure than other therapies which lower BP to a similar degree. This may be because they reduce glomerular perfusion pressure, although this causes an immediate reduction in GFR when therapy is initiated. Angiotensin II receptor antagonists also reduce glomerular perfusion pressure, and the same effect may be achieved by certain non-dihydropyridine calcium antagonists.
- *Diet.* Moderate protein restriction (to 60 g protein/day) should be accompanied by an adequate intake of calories to prevent malnutrition. Anorexia and muscle loss may indicate a need to commence dialysis treatment.

Limit the adverse effects of CKD:

- *Anaemia.* Anaemia is common and, in part, related to the relative deficiency of erythropoietin; it usually correlates with the severity of renal failure and contributes to many of the non-specific symptoms of CKD. Recombinant human erythropoietin is effective in correcting the anaemia of CKD. The target haemoglobin is between 100 and 120 g/l. Complications of treatment include hypertension, and adjustment of antihypertensive medication is often necessary. Erythropoietin is less effective in the presence of iron deficiency, active inflammation or malignancy. These factors should be sought and, if possible, corrected before treatment. Iron supplementation should be used to keep ferritin >100 μg/l and transferrin saturation >20%.
- *Fluid and electrolyte balance.* Due to the reduced concentrating ability of the failing kidney, a relatively high urine volume is needed to excrete products of metabolism and a fluid intake of around 3 litres/day is desirable. Limitation of potassium intake (e.g. 70 mmol/day) and sodium intake (e.g. 100 mmol/day) may be required in late CKD if there is evidence of accumulation. Disproportionate fluid retention in milder renal failure, sometimes leading to episodic pulmonary oedema, is particularly associated with renal artery stenosis.

- *Acidosis*. Declining renal function is associated with metabolic acidosis (p. 153). This is often asymptomatic but may also contribute to reduced renal function and increased tissue catabolism. Plasma bicarbonate should be maintained >22 mmol/l by giving sodium bicarbonate supplements (starting dose of 1 g 8-hourly, increasing as required).
- *Cardiovascular disease and lipids*. CKD is an independent risk factor for cardiovascular disease. Atherosclerosis is common and may be accelerated by hypertension. Vascular calcification, accelerated by a high calcium × phosphate product, may be sufficiently severe to cause limb ischaemia. Pericarditis is common in untreated or inadequately treated ESRF. It may lead to pericardial tamponade and, later, constrictive pericarditis. Hypercholesterolaemia is almost universal in patients with significant proteinuria, and increased triglyceride levels are also common in patients with CKD. It has been suggested that, as well as influencing the development of vascular disease, this may accelerate the progression of chronic renal disease. HMG-CoA reductase inhibitors are of benefit in CKD.
- *Infection*. Infections are the second most common cause of death in dialysis patients, after cardiovascular disease; they must be recognised and treated promptly.
- *Bleeding*. There is an increased bleeding tendency in renal failure, leading to cutaneous ecchymoses and mucosal bleeds in patients with advanced disease. Platelet function is impaired and bleeding time prolonged. Adequate dialysis partially corrects the bleeding tendency.
- *Renal osteodystrophy*. This metabolic bone disease, which accompanies CKD, consists of a mixture of osteomalacia, hyperparathyroid bone disease (osteitis fibrosa), osteoporosis and osteosclerosis (Fig. 7.5). To minimise the effects of CKD on bone, plasma calcium and phosphate should be kept as near to normal as possible. Hypocalcaemia is corrected by giving 1α-hydroxylated synthetic analogues of vitamin D, adjusting the dose to avoid hypercalcaemia. This will usually prevent or control osteomalacia. Hyperphosphataemia is controlled by dietary restriction of high-phosphate foods (milk, cheese, eggs) and the use of phosphate-binding drugs with food. These agents form insoluble complexes with dietary phosphate and prevent its absorption (e.g. calcium carbonate). Secondary hyperparathyroidism is usually controlled by these measures but, in severe bone disease with autonomous parathyroid function, parathyroidectomy may become necessary.
- *Myopathy*. Generalised myopathy is due to a combination of poor nutrition, hyperparathyroidism, vitamin D deficiency and disorders of electrolyte metabolism. Muscle cramps are common and quinine sulphate may be helpful. The 'restless leg syndrome', in which the patient's legs are jumpy during the night, may be troublesome and is often improved by clonazepam.

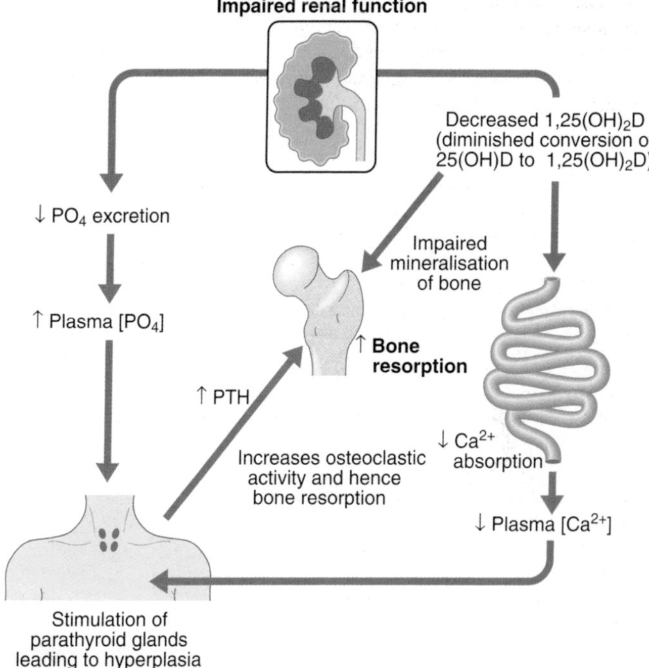

Fig. 7.5 Pathogenesis of renal osteodystrophy. The net result of decreased $1,25(OH)_2$ cholecalciferol levels and increased parathyroid hormone (PTH) levels in the presence of high $[PO_4]$ is bone which exhibits increased osteoclastic activity and increased osteoid as a consequence of decreased mineralisation.

- *Other adverse effects*. Sensory/motor/autonomic neuropathy appears late in the course of CKD but may improve or resolve on dialysis. Hyperprolactinaemia may cause loss of libido and sexual function. The half-life of insulin is prolonged and requirements go down in CKD. GI effects are common at low GFRs and include nausea, vomiting and anorexia. There is a high incidence of peptic ulcer disease and depression.

RENAL REPLACEMENT THERAPY (RRT)

Dialysis is now routine in patients with acute or chronic renal failure. It does not replace the endocrine and metabolic functions of the kidney, but aims to maintain the plasma biochemistry (uraemic toxins, electrolytes and acid–base status) at acceptable levels. Dialysis can also remove

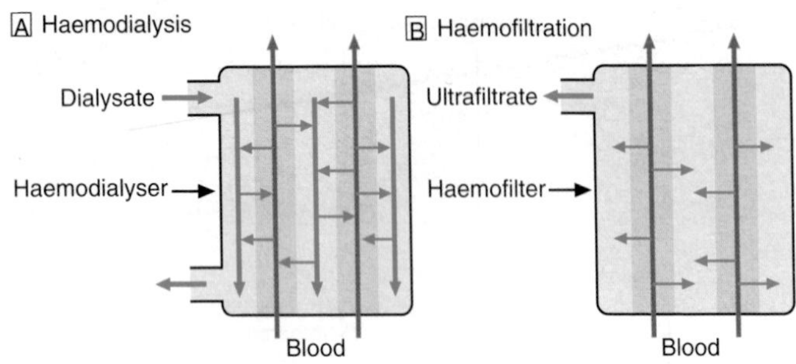

Fig. 7.6 Renal replacement therapy: haemodialysis and haemofiltration. A In haemodialysis solutes diffuse between plasma and dialysate across a semi-permeable membrane. Dialysate composition is chosen to achieve a suitable concentration gradient. Fluid is removed by applying negative pressure to the dialysate (ultrafiltration). B In haemofiltration water is filtered from plasma to ultrafiltrate by applying pressure across a more porous semi-permeable membrane, with removal of solutes by convection. 'Replacement' electrolyte solution is added to the circuit after the filter. For both haemodialysis and filtration, access to the circulation is required. Arteriovenous fistulae, temporary or semi-permanent tunnelled central venous lines or arteriovenous shunts (e.g. Scribner shunt) may be used. The extracorporeal circuit requires anticoagulation, typically with heparin.

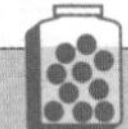

7.13 PROBLEMS WITH DIALYSIS	
Problems with haemodialysis	
• Hypotension during dialysis • Cardiac arrhythmias • Haemorrhage • Air embolism	• Dialyser hypersensitivity • Emergencies between treatments (pulmonary oedema, sepsis)
Problems with continuous ambulatory peritoneal dialysis	
• CAPD peritonitis • Catheter exit site infection	• Ultrafiltration failure • Peritoneal membrane failure

fluid from the circulation (ultrafiltration) to maintain euvolaemia. The major side-effects of dialysis relate to haemodynamic disturbance caused by fluid removal or the extracorporeal circulation of blood, and reactions between blood and components of the dialysis system (bioincompatibility) (Box 7.13). The different types of dialysis are shown in Figures 7.6–7.7.

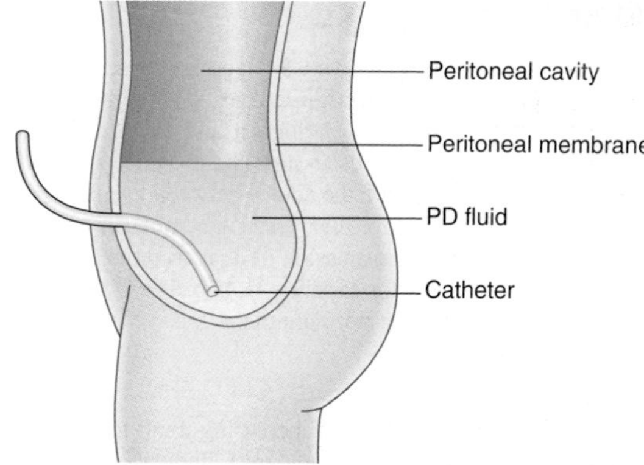

Fig. 7.7 Renal replacement therapy: peritoneal dialysis. Peritoneum is used as a semi-permeable dialysis membrane. Solutes move down a concentration gradient, and water down an osmotic gradient achieved by using an osmolar compound (typically glucose) in the dialysis fluid.

RENAL REPLACEMENT IN ARF

The decision to institute RRT is made on an individual basis, taking account of other aspects of the patient's care. Guideline indications are as follows:

- *Increased plasma urea and creatinine.* Plasma urea >30 mmol/l (180 mg/dl) and creatinine >600 μmol/l (6.8 mg/dl) are undesirable. At lower levels, if there is progressive biochemical deterioration and particularly if there is little or no urine output, it may be appropriate to commence dialysis.
- *Hyperkalaemia.* A plasma potassium >6 mmol/l is hazardous. Elevated plasma potassium can usually be reduced by medical measures in the short term (p. 151), but dialysis is often required for definitive control.
- *Metabolic acidosis.* This will often occur together with hyperkalaemia and raise the plasma potassium further.
- *Fluid overload and pulmonary oedema.* In patients with continued urine output, this may be controlled by careful fluid balance and use of diuretics, but in oligo-/anuric patients they may be an indication for RRT.
- *Uraemic pericarditis/uraemic encephalopathy.* These are features of severe untreated renal failure; they are uncommon in ARF but are strong indications for RRT.

RENAL REPLACEMENT IN CKD

When patients are known to have progressive CKD and are under regular clinic review, preparation for RRT should begin at least 12 months before the predicted start date. This involves psychological and social support, assessment of home circumstances and discussion about choice of treatment. The principal decisions required are the choice between haemodialysis and peritoneal dialysis, and referral for renal transplantation. In view of the historical high incidence of viral transmission in dialysis units, all such patients must be screened in advance for hepatitis B, hepatitis C and HIV, and have hepatitis B vaccine if they are not immune.

CONSERVATIVE TREATMENT OF STAGE V CKD

Partly as a result of survival data, there is an increasing trend to consider conservative non-dialytic treatment in patients in a high-risk category. Patients are offered full medical, psychological and social support to optimise and sustain their existing renal function for as long as possible, and appropriate palliative care in the terminal phase of their disease. Many of these patients enjoy a good quality of life for several years. It is also appropriate to discontinue dialysis treatment, with the consent of the patient, and to offer conservative therapy and palliative care when quality of life on dialysis is clearly inadequate.

RENAL TRANSPLANTATION

Renal transplantation offers the best chance of long-term survival in patients with ESRF. It can restore normal kidney function and correct all the metabolic abnormalities of CKD. All patients should be considered for transplantation unless there are active contraindications (Box 7.14).

Kidney grafts may be taken from a cadaver or from a living donor. The matching of a donor to a specific recipient is strongly influenced by immunological factors, since graft rejection is the major cause of failure of the transplant. ABO (blood group) compatibility between donor and recipient is essential, and the degree of matching for major histocompatibility (MHC) antigens—particularly HLA–DR—influences the incidence of rejection. T cells are the major cell involved in graft rejection; cytotoxic antibodies against HLA antigens, which may be present pre-transplant (sensitisation), are also important. A cytotoxicity test for these antibodies, along with T- and B-cell cross-match tests (donor lymphocytes mixed with patient serum), is performed pre-transplant. Positive tests predict early rejection.

In the transplant operation, the donor vessels are anastomosed to the recipient iliac artery and vein, and the donor ureter to the bladder (Fig. 7.8). Perioperative problems include:

- *Fluid balance.* Careful matching of input to output is required.
- *Primary graft non-function.* Causes include hypovolaemia, ATN or other pre-existing renal damage, hyperacute rejection, vascular occlusion and urinary tract obstruction.

7.14 CONTRAINDICATIONS TO RENAL TRANSPLANTATION

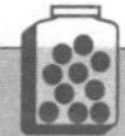

Absolute

- Active malignancy—a period of at least 2 yrs of complete remission is recommended for most tumours prior to transplantation
- Active vasculitis or anti-GBM disease, with positive serology—at least 1 yr of remission is recommended prior to transplantation
- Severe ischaemic heart disease
- Severe occlusive aorto-iliac vascular disease

Relative

- Age—while practice varies, transplants are not routinely offered to very young children (<1 yr) or older people (>75 yrs)
- High risk of disease recurrence in the transplant kidney
- Disease of the lower urinary tract—in patients with impaired bladder function, an ileal conduit may be considered
- Significant comorbidity

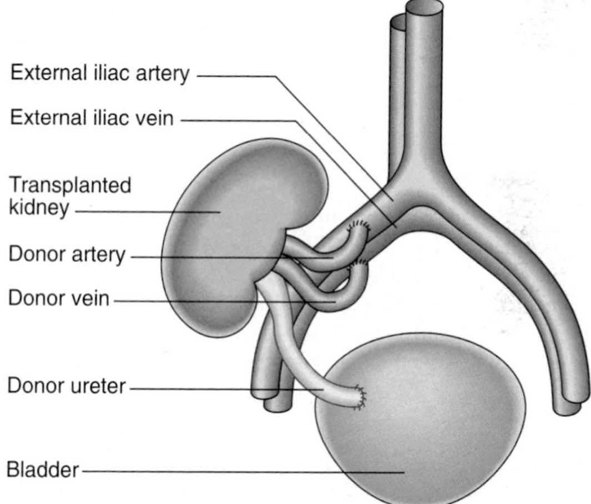

Fig. 7.8 Renal replacement therapy: transplantation. A functioning transplant replaces all of the functions of the failed kidneys. Successful transplantation extends the life expectancy of patients with end-stage CKD, but necessitates long-term use of immunosuppressant drugs.

- *Sepsis* (related to immunosuppression).

Once the graft begins to function, normal or near-normal biochemistry is usually achieved within a few days. All transplant patients require regular life-long clinic follow-up to monitor renal function and immunosuppression.

Management after transplantation

Immunosuppressive therapy is required throughout the life of the transplant to prevent rejection. This is associated with an increased incidence of infection, particularly opportunistic infections such as cytomegalovirus and *Pneumocystis jirovecii*. There is also an increased risk of malignancy, especially of the skin. Approximately 50% of white patients develop skin malignancy by 15 yrs post-transplant. Lymphomas are rare but may occur early and are often related to infection with herpes viruses, especially Epstein–Barr virus (p. 65).

In the UK, the prognosis for transplants from cadaver donors is 96% patient and 92% graft survival at 1 yr, and 84% patient and 76% graft survival at 5 yrs. Even better results follow living donor transplantation (92% patient and 86% graft survival at 5 yrs). Living donor operations are becoming more common in the UK and can even be performed successfully with genetically unrelated donors.

RENAL VASCULAR DISEASES

Diseases which affect renal blood vessels may cause renal ischaemia, leading to acute or chronic renal failure or secondary hypertension. The rising prevalence of atherosclerosis and diabetes in ageing populations has made renovascular disease an important cause of ESRF.

LARGE-VESSEL DISEASE: RENAL ARTERY STENOSIS

Presentations

Hypertension: This is driven by activation of the renin–angiotensin system in response to renal ischaemia. In atherosclerotic renal artery disease, there is usually evidence of vascular disease elsewhere, particularly in the legs. Factors which predict renovascular disease are shown in Box 7.15.

Deterioration of renal function on ACE inhibitors: When renal perfusion pressure drops, the renin–angiotensin–aldosterone system is activated and angiotensin-mediated glomerular efferent arteriolar vasoconstriction

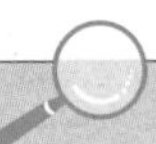

7.15 RENAL ARTERY STENOSIS

Renal artery stenosis is more likely if:
- Hypertension is severe, *or* of recent onset, *or* difficult to control
- Kidneys are asymmetrical in size
- Flash pulmonary oedema occurs repeatedly
- There is peripheral vascular disease of lower limbs
- Renal function has deteriorated on ACE inhibitors

maintains glomerular filtration pressure. ACE inhibitors or angiotensin II receptor antagonists block this physiological response. A drop in GFR (>20% rise in creatinine) on ACE inhibitors raises the possibility of renal artery stenosis.

Flash pulmonary oedema: Repeated episodes of acute pulmonary oedema associated with severe hypertension, occurring without other obvious cause (e.g. myocardial infarction) in patients with normal or only mildly impaired renal and cardiac function, can occur in renal artery stenosis.

Acute renal infarction: Sudden occlusion of the renal arteries causes acute loin pain, usually with dipstick haematuria. It may be caused by local atherosclerosis (atheroembolic) or by thromboemboli from a distant source, e.g. mural cardiac thrombus.

Atherosclerosis is the most common cause of renal artery stenosis, especially in older patients. There is usually vascular disease present elsewhere, e.g. in the aorta and iliac vessels.

In younger patients (<50 yrs), fibromuscular dysplasia is a more likely cause of renal artery stenosis. This is an uncommon congenital disorder of unknown cause affecting the media ('medial fibroplasia'), which narrows the artery but rarely leads to total occlusion. It most commonly presents with hypertension in patients aged 15–30 yrs, and in women more frequently than men.

Investigations

• USS may reveal renal asymmetry, with Doppler USS revealing significant renal artery stenosis. • Renal isotope scanning may show delayed uptake and reduced excretion by the affected kidney. • Renal arteriography is the definitive investigation, but carries the risk of contrast nephropathy. • Non-invasive tests, such as CT/MRI angiography, are increasingly used. • Invasive tests should be limited to those in whom intervention would be considered (e.g. those with uncontrollable hypertension, recurrent flash pulmonary oedema, deteriorating renal function).

Management

Left untreated, atheromatous renal artery stenosis will progress to complete arterial occlusion and loss of kidney function in about 15% of cases.

Treatment options are:

• Medical management with low-dose aspirin, antihypertensive and lipid-lowering drugs. This will usually have been attempted before angiography is performed. • Angioplasty, with stenting of atherosclerotic areas. • Surgical resection of the stenosed segment and reanastomosis.

Response to treatment remains hard to predict from investigations.

DISEASES OF SMALL INTRARENAL VESSELS

A number of conditions are associated with acute damage and occlusion of small blood vessels (arterioles and capillaries) in the kidney (Box 7.16). They may be associated with similar changes elsewhere in the body. A common feature of these syndromes is microangiopathic haemolytic

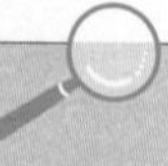

7.16 MICROVASCULAR DISORDERS ASSOCIATED WITH ACUTE RENAL DAMAGE

- Thrombotic microangiopathy (haemolytic uraemic syndrome and thrombotic thrombocytopenic purpura)
  - Associated with verotoxin-producing *E. coli*
  - Other (familial, drugs, cancer etc.)
- Disseminated intravascular coagulation
- Malignant hypertension
- Small-vessel vasculitis
- Systemic sclerosis (scleroderma)
- Atheroemboli ('cholesterol' emboli)

anaemia, in which fragmented red cells can be seen on a blood film as a consequence of damage during passage through the abnormal vessels.

GLOMERULAR DISEASES

Glomerular diseases may cause acute and chronic renal failure, and may follow a number of insults: immunological injury, inherited abnormality (e.g. Alport's syndrome), metabolic stress (e.g. diabetes mellitus), deposition of extraneous materials (e.g. amyloid), or other direct glomerular injury. The response of the glomerulus to injury varies according to the nature of the insult (Fig. 7.9). At one extreme, specific podocyte injury, or structural alteration of the glomerulus affecting podocyte function (e.g. by scarring or deposition of excess matrix or other material), causes proteinuria and nephrotic syndrome (p. 174). At the other end of the spectrum, inflammation leads to cell damage and proliferation, breaks form in the GBM and blood leaks into urine. In its extreme form, with acute sodium retention and hypertension, such disease is labelled nephritic syndrome.

GLOMERULONEPHRITIS

Glomerulonephritis literally means 'inflammation of glomeruli', although inflammation is not apparent in all varieties. Most types of glomerulonephritis seem to be immunologically mediated and several respond to immunosuppressive drugs. Classifications of glomerulonephritis are largely histopathological and may appear daunting, but the details are largely a specialist concern. Only clinically important types are described here.

MINIMAL CHANGE NEPHROPATHY AND PRIMARY FOCAL SEGMENTAL GLOMERULOSCLEROSIS (FSGS)

Patients with minimal change nephropathy and a subgroup of patients with FSGS can be seen as opposite ends of a spectrum of conditions causing idiopathic nephrotic syndrome. Minimal change disease occurs at all ages but accounts for nephrotic syndrome in most children and about one-quarter

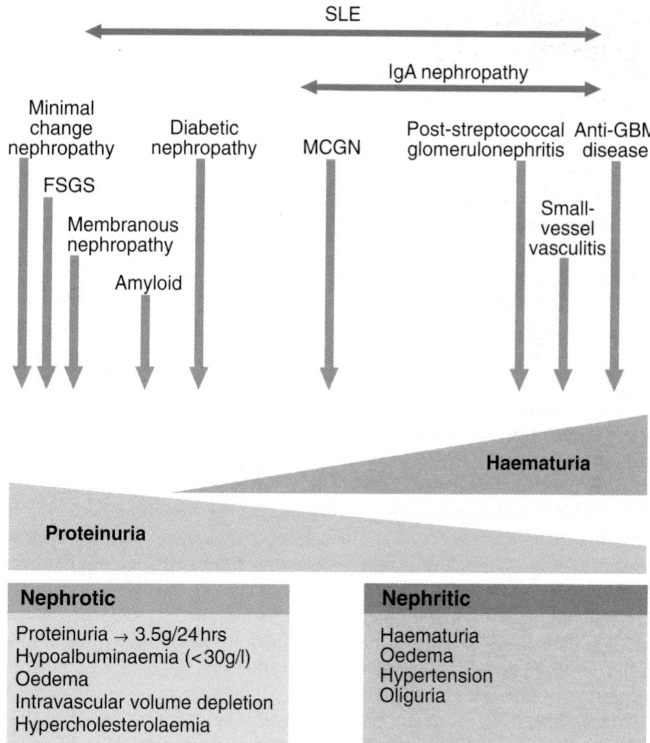

Fig. 7.9 Spectrum of glomerular diseases. (FSGS = focal and segmental glomerulosclerosis; MCGN = mesangiocapillary glomerulonephritis)

of adults. Proteinuria usually remits on high-dose corticosteroid therapy, although those who respond incompletely or relapse frequently need maintenance corticosteroids or cytotoxic treatments. Minimal change disease does not progress to CKD; the main problems are those of the nephrotic syndrome and complications of treatment.

FSGS is a histological description with many causes. The primary FSGS group that presents with idiopathic nephrotic syndrome and no other cause of renal disease typically shows little response to corticosteroid treatment and often progresses to renal failure; the disease frequently recurs after renal transplantation, and sometimes proteinuria recurs almost immediately. However, some patients with FSGS do respond to corticosteroids (a good prognostic sign). As FSGS is a focal process, abnormal glomeruli may not be seen on renal biopsy if only a few are sampled, leading to an initial diagnosis of minimal change nephropathy.

MEMBRANOUS NEPHROPATHY

This is the most common cause of nephrotic syndrome in adults. Some cases are associated with known causes (malignancy, hepatitis B virus) but most are idiopathic. Of this group, approximately one-third remit spontaneously, one-third remain in a nephrotic state, and one-third show progressive loss of renal function. Short-term immunosuppressive treatment may improve both the nephrotic syndrome and the long-term prognosis. However, because of the toxicity of these regimens, most nephrologists reserve such treatment for those with severe nephrotic syndrome or deteriorating renal function.

IgA NEPHROPATHY AND HENOCH–SCHÖNLEIN PURPURA

IgA nephropathy is the most common glomerulonephritis world-wide and a common cause of ESRF. Presentation is with haematuria (almost universal), proteinuria (usual) and hypertension (very common). There may be severe proteinuria and nephrotic syndrome, or in some cases progressive loss of renal function. Some individuals develop acute exacerbations, often with gross haematuria, a few days after minor respiratory infections. These episodes usually subside spontaneously.

In children and occasionally in adults a systemic vasculitis occurring in response to similar infections is called Henoch–Schönlein purpura. A characteristic petechial rash (cutaneous vasculitis, typically affecting buttocks and lower legs) and abdominal pain (GI vasculitis) usually dominate the clinical picture, with mild glomerulonephritis indicated by haematuria. The glomerulonephritis is usually more prominent in older children or adults. Renal biopsy shows mesangial IgA deposition and appearances indistinguishable from acute IgA nephropathy.

Management of IgA nephropathy is largely directed towards control of BP and proteinuria reduction in an attempt to prevent or retard progressive renal disease.

GLOMERULONEPHRITIS ASSOCIATED WITH INFECTION

Bacterial infections, usually subacute (typically subacute bacterial endocarditis), may cause a variety of histological patterns of glomerulonephritis, but usually with plentiful immunoglobulin deposition and often with evidence of complement consumption. In the developed world, hospital-acquired infections are now a common cause of these syndromes. World-wide, glomerulonephritis associated with malaria, HIV, hepatitis B, hepatitis C, schistosomiasis, leishmaniasis and other chronic infections is very common. The usual histological patterns are membranous and mesangiocapillary lesions, although many other types may be seen.

Acute post-infectious glomerulonephritis

This is most common following infection with certain strains of streptococcus (post-streptococcal nephritis), but can occur after other infections. It is much more common in children than adults but is now rare in the developed world. The latency is usually about 10 days after a throat infection or longer after skin infection, suggesting an immune mechanism rather than direct infection.

An acute nephritis of varying severity occurs. Sodium retention, hypertension and oedema are particularly pronounced. There is also reduction of GFR, proteinuria, haematuria and reduced urine volume. Characteristically, this gives the urine a red or smoky appearance. There are low serum concentrations of C3 and C4 and evidence of streptococcal infection. (Perform ASO titre, culture of throat swab, and other swab tests if skin infection is suspected.)

Renal function begins to improve spontaneously within 10–14 days, and management by fluid and sodium restriction and use of diuretic and hypotensive agents is usually followed by full recovery.

RAPIDLY PROGRESSIVE GLOMERULONEPHRITIS

This extreme inflammatory nephritis causes rapid loss of renal function over days to weeks. Renal biopsy shows crescentic lesions often associated with necrotising lesions within the glomerulus. It is typically seen in Goodpasture's disease, where there are specific anti-GBM antibodies, and in small-vessel vasculitides (p. 609), but can also be seen in SLE (p. 603) and occasionally IgA and other nephropathies.

INHERITED GLOMERULAR DISEASES

Alport's syndrome is an uncommon X-linked condition in which abnormal collagen deposition results in haematuria, progressive renal failure and sensorineural deafness. There is no effective treatment apart from renal replacement therapy.

TUBULO-INTERSTITIAL DISEASES

INTERSTITIAL NEPHRITIS

A group of inflammatory, inherited and other diseases affect renal tubules and the surrounding interstitium. The clinical presentation is often renal failure, but electrolyte abnormalities are common, especially hyperkalaemia and acidosis. Haematuria and pyuria are common, and proteinuria (and albuminuria) is rarely >1 g/24 hrs.

ACUTE INTERSTITIAL NEPHRITIS (AIN)

AIN may be caused by allergic reactions (e.g. penicillins, NSAIDs), autoimmune nephritis, infections (e.g. pyelonephritis, TB) or toxins (e.g. mushrooms or myeloma light chains). Renal biopsies show intense inflammation surrounding tubules and blood vessels and invading tubules (tubulitis), with occasional eosinophils (especially in drug-induced disease).

Diagnosis

• Urinalysis shows leucocytes and eosinophils in 70% of patients. • There is non-oliguric ARF with a rapid deterioration in renal function. Renal biopsy is usually required. • Only about 30% of patients with drug-induced AIN have a generalised drug hypersensitivity reaction (e.g. fever, rash, eosinophilia).

Management

• Remove/treat the cause. • Steroids may accelerate recovery and prevent long-term scarring. • Short-term dialysis is sometimes required.

7.17 CAUSES OF CHRONIC INTERSTITIAL NEPHRITIS

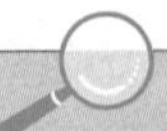

- Acute interstitial nephritis
- Glomerulonephritis
- Immune/inflammatory (sarcoid, SLE)
- Toxic (mushrooms, Balkan nephropathy)
- Drugs (ciclosporin, analgesic nephropathy)
- Infection
- Congenital/developmental (sickle cell nephropathy)
- Metabolic and systemic diseases (amyloid)

CHRONIC INTERSTITIAL NEPHRITIS (CIN)

Known causes of CIN are shown in Box 7.17; however, it is often diagnosed late and with no apparent aetiology.

Clinical and biochemical features

• Most patients present in adult life with moderate CKD (urea <25 mmol/l or 150 mg/dl), hypertension and small kidneys. • Due to tubular dysfunction electrolyte abnormalities (e.g. hyperkalaemia, acidosis) may be severe. • Urinalysis is non-specific.

SICKLE-CELL NEPHROPATHY

The longer survival of patients with sickle-cell disease (p. 545) means that a larger proportion live to develop chronic complications of microvascular occlusion.

Clinical features

• Damage to medullary vasa recta is most common. • There is early loss of urine concentrating ability with polyuria. • Distal renal tubular acidosis with hyperkalaemia is typical. • Papillary necrosis is common. • A minority of patients develop ESRF.

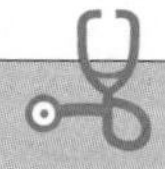

7.18 ADULT POLYCYSTIC KIDNEY DISEASE: COMMON CLINICAL FEATURES

- Asymptomatic until later life
- Vague discomfort in loin or abdomen due to increasing mass of renal tissue
- One or both kidneys palpable, with nodular surface
- Acute loin pain or renal colic due to haemorrhage into a cyst
- Hypertension gradually develops over age 20 yrs
- Haematuria (with little or no proteinuria)
- UTI
- Gradual-onset renal failure
- Associated features:
  - Hepatic cysts (30%)
  - Berry aneurysms of the cerebral vasculature
  - Mitral and aortic regurgitation (common but rarely severe)
  - Colonic diverticula
  - Abdominal wall hernias
  - Pulmonary cyst

CYSTIC KIDNEY DISEASES

POLYCYSTIC KIDNEY DISEASE (PKD)

Adult PKD is a common condition (prevalence ~1 : 1000) that is inherited as an autosomal dominant trait. Small cysts lined by tubular epithelium develop from infancy or childhood and enlarge slowly and irregularly. Surrounding normal kidney tissue is progressively attenuated. Renal failure is associated with grossly enlarged kidneys. PKD is not a pre-malignant condition. Mutations in *PKD1* account for 85% of cases and *PKD2* for about 15%. ESRF occurs in ~50% of patients with *PKD1* with a mean age of onset of 52 yrs, but in a minority of patients with *PKD2* with a mean age of onset of 69 yrs. Rarely, other genes are responsible.

Clinical features

See Box 7.18.

Investigations and screening

• These are based on family history, clinical examination and USS. • USS demonstrates cysts in ~95% of affected patients over 20 yrs but may not detect smaller cysts in younger patients. It is important to identify multiple cysts, not just two or three. • Genetic diagnosis is possible but difficult. • Screening for intracranial aneurysms is not generally indicated (low yield and unknown risk : benefit ratio of intervention in asymptomatic aneurysms).

Management

• Nothing has yet been found to alter the rate of progression of renal failure in PKD. • Good BP control is important because of cardiovascular morbidity and mortality, but there is no evidence that this retards the development of renal failure in PKD. • Patients with PKD are usually good candidates for dialysis and transplantation. Sometimes kidneys are so large that one or both have to be removed to make space for a renal transplant.

OTHER CYSTIC DISEASES

Medullary sponge kidney

Characterised by cysts confined to papillary collecting ducts, this disease is not inherited and its cause is unknown. Patients usually present as adults with renal stones. These are often recurrent, but the prognosis is generally good. The diagnosis is made by USS or IVU. Contrast medium is seen to fill dilated or cystic tubules, which are sometimes calcified.

Acquired cystic disease

Patients with a very long history of renal failure (usually on long-term dialysis) often develop multiple renal cysts in their shrunken kidneys: acquired cystic kidney disease. Kidneys are enlarged but not to the size seen in PKD. Acquired cystic disease is associated with increased erythropoietin production and an increased risk of renal cell carcinoma.

ISOLATED DEFECTS OF TUBULAR FUNCTION

An increasing number of disorders (e.g. renal glycosuria and cystinuria) are now known to be due to specific defects of transporter molecules in renal tubular cells.

The term 'Fanconi syndrome' is used to describe generalised proximal tubular dysfunction. It is not related to Fanconi anaemia. Notable abnormalities include low blood phosphate and uric acid, the finding of glucose and amino acids in urine, and proximal renal tubular acidosis. Renal tubular acidosis describes the common endpoint of a variety of diseases affecting distal (classical or type 1) or proximal (type 2) renal tubular function. They cause metabolic acidosis with a normal anion gap (p. 153).

DISEASES OF THE COLLECTING SYSTEM AND URETERS

RETROPERITONEAL FIBROSIS

Fibrosis of retroperitoneal connective tissue may compress and obstruct the ureters.

Causes are idiopathic (most commonly), drugs, aortic aneurysm or malignancy. Presentation is with symptoms of ureteric obstruction. Investigations show high ESR/CRP; IVU/CT shows obstruction and medial deviation of ureters. The idiopathic type responds to steroids; surgical relief of obstruction is necessary if there is no response.

REFLUX NEPHROPATHY (CHRONIC PYELONEPHRITIS)

This chronic interstitial nephritis (p. 196) is associated with vesico-ureteric reflux (VUR) in early life, and with the appearance of 'scars' in the kidney.

Clinical features

Usually the renal scarring and renal/ureteric dilatation are asymptomatic. Presentation may be at any age, with hypertension, proteinuria or features of CKD. Frequency, dysuria and lumbar back pain may be present; the history of UTIs may be absent. Urinalysis shows leucocytes and proteinuria (usually <1 g/24 hrs). There is an increased prevalence of urinary calculi.

Investigations

• USS: will exclude significant obstruction but is not helpful in identifying renal scarring. • Longitudinal CT/MRI: may be useful. • Radionuclide scans: sensitive but seldom required, as surgery for VUR is uncommon.

Management and prognosis

• Treat infection. If recurrent, use prophylactic measures (p. 167). • Nephrectomy may be indicated for pyelonephrosis, unilateral renal infection or persistent pain. • Hypertension is occasionally cured by the removal of a diseased kidney when disease is unilateral. • Otherwise, surgery is rarely indicated as most childhood reflux disappears spontaneously. Children and adults with small or unilateral renal scars have a good prognosis, provided renal growth is normal. • Deteriorating renal function, hypertension and proteinuria predict poor prognosis in more severe bilateral disease. If the serum creatinine is normal and hypertension and proteinuria are absent, long-term prognosis is good.

URINARY TRACT CALCULI AND NEPHROCALCINOSIS

While stones may be asymptomatic, more commonly patients present with pain (p. 168), recurrent urinary infection (p. 163) or clinical features of urinary tract obstruction (p. 168). Investigation and management are described on page 169.

DISEASES OF THE PROSTATE GLAND

BENIGN PROSTATIC HYPERPLASIA (BPH)

From 40 yrs of age the prostate increases in volume by 2.4 cm^3/yr on average. Associated symptoms are common from 60 yrs of age, and some 50% of men over 80 yrs will have lower urinary tract symptoms associated with BPH.

Clinical features

• There is hesitancy, urinary frequency and urgency, poor urine flow and a sensation of incomplete voiding. • Presentation may be with acute urinary retention, often precipitated by alcohol, constipation or prostatic infection. The painful distended bladder requires emergency catheter drainage. • Chronic urinary retention involves a painless distended bladder that may lead to dilatation of the ureters and kidneys, with eventual renal failure. These patients may develop acute on chronic retention.

Investigations

• Symptom scoring systems allow baseline values to be established and further deterioration/improvement to be assessed. • Urine flow meter readings. • Prostate volume assessment (PR and USS). • Urodynamic studies. • Renal function and renal USS.

Management

• Medical treatment (α-adrenoceptor blockers, 5α-reductase inhibitors): for mild symptoms. • Non-surgical intervention by thermotherapy: may help in those unfit for surgery. • Transurethral resection of prostate (TURP) or open prostatectomy is indicated for severe symptoms.

PROSTATE CANCER

Prostatic cancer is common in northern Europe and the USA but rare in China and Japan. In the UK it is the second most common malignancy in males. It rarely occurs before the age of 50 yrs and has a mean age at presentation of 70 yrs.

Almost all prostate cancers are carcinomas. Metastatic spread to pelvic lymph nodes occurs early and metastases to bone, mainly the lumbar spine and pelvis, are common. Prostate specific antigen (PSA) is a good tumour marker and 40% of patients with a serum PSA > 4.0 ng/ml will have prostate cancer on biopsy. This has led to the introduction of screening programmes, principally in the USA, despite a lack of consensus about their utility.

Clinical features

• Symptoms are usually indistinguishable from BPH. • Symptoms and signs due to metastases are much less common and include back pain, weight loss, anaemia and obstruction of the ureters. • Prostate often feels nodular and hard (although 10–15% of tumours are impalpable).

Investigations

• Needle biopsy: to confirm diagnosis. • USS of urinary tract and U&Es. • Plain XR of pelvis and lumbar spine may show osteosclerotic metastases. • Radioisotope bone scan: although high levels of serum PSA (>100 ng/ml) almost always indicate distant bone metastases. • PSA: most useful for monitoring response to treatment and disease progression.

Management and prognosis

Tumour confined to the prostate is potentially curable by either radical prostatectomy or radical radiotherapy, and these options should be considered in all patients with more than 10 yrs life expectancy. A small focus of tumour found incidentally at TURP does not significantly alter life expectancy and only requires follow-up.

Approximately half of men with prostate cancer will have metastatic disease at the time of diagnosis. Prostatic cancer is sensitive to hormonal influences; androgen depletion either by orchidectomy or more commonly by androgen-suppressing drugs leads to a high initial response rate in locally advanced or metastatic prostate cancer; however, the disease progresses after a year or two. A small proportion of patients fail to respond to endocrine treatment. Radiotherapy is useful for localised bone pain.

The life expectancy of a patient with an incidental finding of focal prostate carcinoma is normal. With more substantial tumours localised to the prostate, the 10-yr survival rate is 60–75%, but if metastases are present this falls to 10%.

TUMOURS OF THE KIDNEY AND URINARY TRACT

RENAL ADENOCARCINOMA

This is by far the most common malignant tumour of the kidney in adults, with a prevalence of 16 cases per 100 000 population. It is twice as common in males as in females. The peak incidence is between 65 and 75 yrs of age and it is uncommon before 40. Spread may be local, lymphatic or blood-borne.

Clinical features

• Presentation: haematuria (60%), loin pain (40%), abdominal mass (25%), PUO. • Systemic effects: fever, raised ESR, coagulopathy. • Tumour may secrete ectopic hormones, e.g. EPO, PTH, renin. The effects of these disappear when the tumour is removed.

Investigations

• USS: allows differentiation between solid tumour and simple renal cysts.
• CT abdomen/chest: for staging.

Management and prognosis

Radical nephrectomy should be performed whenever possible (even in the presence of metastases, which may regress after surgery). Renal adenocarcinoma is resistant to radiotherapy and chemotherapy but some benefit has been seen with immunotherapy. If the tumour is confined to the kidney, 5-yr survival is 75%. This falls to only 5% when there are distant metastases.

BLADDER CANCER

These are usually transitional cell in origin, and are three times more common in men than women. The appearance of a transitional cell tumour ranges from a delicate papillary structure to a solid ulcerating mass. Appearance correlates well with subsequent behaviour; papillary tumours are relatively benign cancers while those which ulcerate are much more aggressive.

Clinical features and investigations

• 80% of patients have painless, visible haematuria (see p. 173 for investigation of haematuria). • Obstructive symptoms may occur. • Examination is generally unhelpful. • CT chest/abdomen/pelvis allows invasive tumour staging.

Management and prognosis

• Superficial tumours are treated by transurethral surgery and/or intravesical chemotherapy; cystectomy is rarely required. • Regular cystoscopy is needed to detect recurrence. • Carcinoma in situ responds well to intravesical BCG treatment. • Invasive bladder tumours are generally treated with radical cystectomy and urinary diversion. • The 5-yr survival rate varies from 50–60% in those with superficial tumours to 20–30% for those with deep muscle invasion. Overall, ~33% of patients survive for 5 yrs.

RENAL INVOLVEMENT IN SYSTEMIC DISORDERS

DIABETES MELLITUS

Patients with diabetes show a steady advance from microalbuminuria to dipstick-positive proteinuria, the development of hypertension and the progression to frank nephrotic syndrome.

Few require renal biopsy for diagnosis, but atypical features should raise suspicion of an alternative condition.

Management with ACE inhibitors and other hypotensive agents to slow progression has been dramatically effective. In some patients, proteinuria may be eradicated and progression completely halted, even if renal function is abnormal.

MALIGNANT DISEASES

Cancer may affect the kidney in many ways (Box 7.19).

TUBERCULOSIS OF THE KIDNEY AND URINARY TRACT

TB may involve any part of the kidney and urinary tract, and results from haematogenous spread of infection from elsewhere in the body.

Clinical features

• Bladder symptoms, haematuria, malaise, fever, night sweats, loin pain, CKD as a result of urinary tract obstruction or destruction of renal tissue. • Renal calcification and ureteric strictures are typical.

7.19 RENAL EFFECTS OF MALIGNANCIES	
Direct involvement	e.g. Renal and urinary tract tumours
Immune reaction	e.g. Glomerulonephritis, especially membranous nephropathy
Metabolic consequences	e.g. Hypercalcaemia
Remote effects of tumour products	e.g. Amyloid, light chains in myeloma

Investigations and management

• Sterile pyuria is typical and early morning urine cultures should be sent to identify tubercle bacilli. • Perform cystoscopy if there is bladder involvement. • Radiology of urinary tract and CXR are mandatory. • Antituberculous chemotherapy (p. 300) is effective. • Surgical relief of obstruction and nephrectomy are sometimes necessary for severe infection.

SYSTEMIC VASCULITIS

Medium- to large-vessel vasculitis (e.g. polyarteritis nodosa)

This only causes renal disease when arterial involvement leads to hypertension or renal infarction.

Small-vessel vasculitis

This causes a focal inflammatory glomerulonephritis, often with crescentic changes. It may be a kidney-limited disorder with rapidly deteriorating renal function, or associated with a systemic illness with acute phase response, weight loss and arthralgia; in some patients it causes pulmonary haemorrhage, which can be life-threatening.

The most important causes of this syndrome, microscopic polyangiitis and Wegener's granulomatosis, are usually associated with ANCA (p. 611), but these antibodies are non-specific and cannot be relied upon to make the diagnosis, so biopsy is often required.

Vasculitis in other organs may give clues to the underlying systemic disorder and its subtype: e.g. ENT involvement and lung disease in Wegener's granulomatosis.

Treatment of small-vessel vasculitis is with immunosuppressive drugs. Death from extrarenal manifestations of the disease is prevented and renal function can be salvaged in acute disease, even if the glomerulonephritis is so severe as to cause oliguria. In these circumstances, plasma exchange offers additional benefit.

SYSTEMIC LUPUS ERYTHEMATOSUS (SLE)

Subclinical renal involvement, with low-level haematuria and proteinuria but minimally impaired or normal renal function, is common in SLE. Usually this is due to glomerular disease, although serologically and sometimes clinically overlapping syndromes (e.g. mixed connective tissue disorder, Sjögren's syndrome) may cause interstitial nephritis. SLE can produce almost any histological pattern of glomerular disease and an accordingly wide range of clinical features, ranging from florid rapidly progressive glomerulonephritis to nephrotic syndrome.

DRUGS AND THE KIDNEY

The kidney is susceptible to damage due to concentration of drugs and metabolites during excretion. Specific examples are shown in Box 7.20.

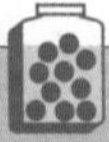

7.20 MECHANISMS AND EXAMPLES OF DRUG- AND TOXIN-INDUCED RENAL DISEASE/DYSFUNCTION

Mechanism	Drug or toxin	Comments
Haemodynamic	NSAIDs	Especially as a co-factor. Via inhibition of prostaglandin synthesis
	ACE inhibitors	Reduce efferent glomerular arteriolar tone. Toxic in the presence of renal artery stenosis and other conditions of renal hypoperfusion
	Radiographic contrast media	May cause intense vasoconstriction, as well as other toxic effects
Acute tubular necrosis	Aminoglycosides, amphotericin	Direct tubular toxicity, but haemodynamic factors probably contribute
	Paracetamol	May occur with or without serious hepatotoxicity
	Radiographic contrast media	May precipitate in tubules. Furosemide is a co-factor
Loss of tubular/ collecting duct function	Lithium	Loss of concentrating ability
	Cisplatin	
	Aminoglycosides, amphotericin	At lower exposures than cause acute tubular necrosis
Immune (glomerular)	Penicillamine, gold	Membranous nephropathy
	Mercury and heavy metals	Membranous nephropathy
	Penicillamine	Crescentic or focal necrotising glomerulonephritis in association with ANCA and systemic small-vessel vasculitis
	NSAIDs	Minimal change nephropathy
Immune (interstitial)	NSAIDs, penicillins and others	Acute interstitial nephritis

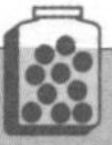

7.20 MECHANISMS AND EXAMPLES OF DRUG- AND TOXIN-INDUCED RENAL DISEASE/DYSFUNCTION (*Continued*)

Mechanism	Drug or toxin	Comments
Chronic interstitial nephritis (alone)	Lithium	As a consequence of acute toxicity
	Ciclosporin, tacrolimus	The major problem with these drugs
	Lead, cadmium	Consequence of chronic toxicity
	Bence Jones protein	Only some light chains are nephrotoxic
	Ochratoxin and other fungal toxins	From *Aspergillus* sp. Putative cause of Balkan nephropathy
	Aristolochic acid and other plant toxins	Found in *Aristolochia* clematis. Putative cause of 'Chinese herb' nephropathy
Chronic interstitial nephritis (with papillary necrosis)	Combination analgesics with caffeine and/or codeine	Incidence reduced since phenacetin withdraw
Obstruction (crystal formation)	Aciclovir, sulphonamides	Drug crystalises in tubules
	Chemotherapy	Uric acid crystals form as a consequence of tumour lysis
Retroperitoneal fibrosis	Methysergide, practolol	No longer used in UK. Idiopathic form is more common

8

Cardiovascular disease

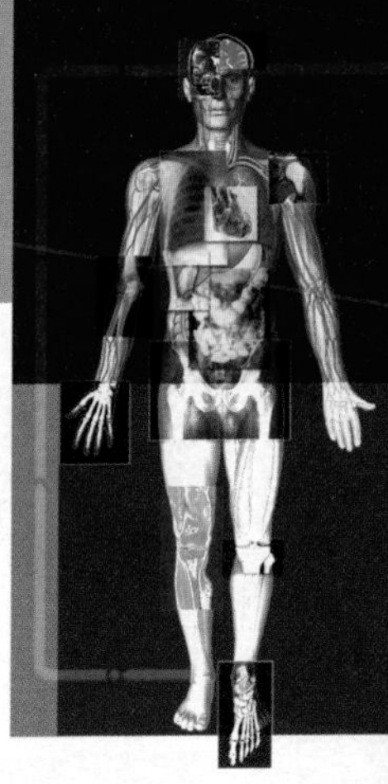

Cardiovascular disease is the leading cause of mortality in the Western world, with most deaths arising from ischaemic heart disease. Although the incidence of ischaemic heart disease is declining in many developed countries, it continues to rise in Eastern Europe and on the Indian subcontinent. Valvular heart disease is also common, but while rheumatic fever still predominates in the Indian subcontinent, degenerative disease of the aortic valve is now the leading aetiology in developed nations. The diversity of symptoms attributable to heart disease is limited and patients often remain asymptomatic despite the presence of advanced disease. However, prompt recognition of the development of heart disease is important, as many highly effective and evidence-based treatments are available.

PRESENTING PROBLEMS

A close relationship between symptoms and exercise is a hallmark of cardiovascular disease. The New York Heart Association (NYHA) functional classification is often used to grade disability (Box 8.1).

CHEST PAIN

Chest pain is a common presentation of cardiac disease, but may also arise from anxiety or disease of the lungs, musculoskeletal system or GI system.

CLINICAL EXAMINATION OF THE CARDIOVASCULAR SYSTEM

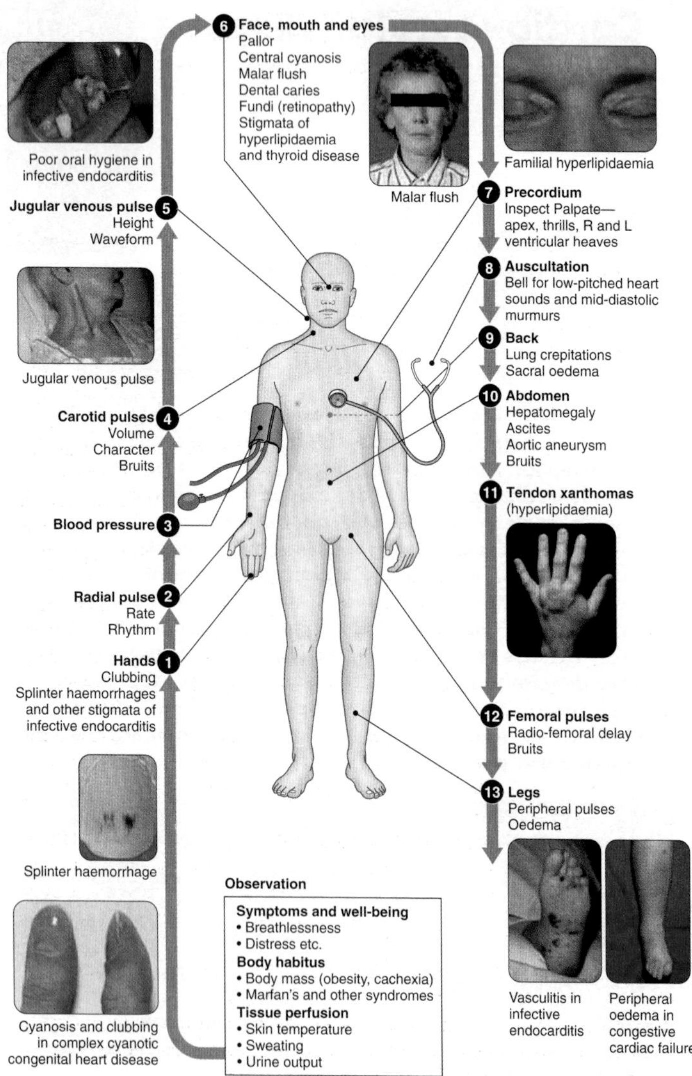

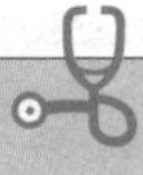

8.1 NEW YORK HEART ASSOCIATION (NYHA) FUNCTIONAL CLASSIFICATION

Class I	No limitation during ordinary activity
Class II	Slight limitation during ordinary activity
Class III	Marked limitation of normal activities without symptoms at rest
Class IV	Unable to undertake physical activity without symptoms; symptoms may be present at rest

CHRONIC EPISODIC CHEST PAIN

Angina pectoris: The pain of myocardial ischaemia is usually central and diffuse, and may radiate to the neck, jaw and arms. It is typically described as dull, heavy, squeezing or crushing but not sharp or stabbing. The sensation may be described as discomfort, breathlessness ('angina equivalent') or 'indigestion' rather than pain. It arises during (not after) exertion and may also be precipitated or exacerbated by emotion, a large meal or a cold wind. The pain builds up gradually in proportion to the intensity of exertion and is promptly relieved (<5 mins) by resting. In unstable angina (see below), similar pain may be precipitated by minimal exertion and may occur at rest. Physical examination is often unremarkable but may reveal xanthoma, gallop rhythm or evidence of arterial disease. A resting 12-lead ECG may be normal. Exercise ECG or stress radionuclide imaging helps to confirm the diagnosis and also identifies high-risk patients who require further investigation and treatment.

Oesophageal pain: Can mimic angina very closely, is sometimes precipitated by exercise and may be relieved by nitrates; however, it is usually possible to elicit a history relating chest pain to supine posture or to eating, drinking or oesophageal reflux. Upper GI endoscopy may reveal evidence of oesophagitis or hiatus hernia.

Bronchospasm: May be described by patients as exertional chest tightness and can be difficult to distinguish from ischaemic chest tightness. Persistent tightness after exercise, associated wheeze, cough or symptoms of atopy suggest the diagnosis.

Musculoskeletal chest pain: Common, with a very variable presentation. The pain may vary with posture or occur with specific movements (bending, stretching, turning). It is sometimes accompanied by local tenderness over a rib or costal cartilage. Causes include minor soft tissue injuries, arthritis, costochondritis and Coxsackie viral infection.

Anxiety-related chest pain: A very common cause of atypical chest pain that should be considered in patients with features of anxiety or neurosis, particularly when pain lacks a predictable relationship with exercise. Anxiety may also amplify the effects of organic disease or lead to exercise avoidance and secondary deconditioning.

ACUTE CHEST PAIN

Acute coronary syndromes: Prolonged and severe ischaemic chest pain may be due to unstable angina (which comprises recent-onset limiting angina, rapidly worsening or crescendo angina, and angina at rest) or acute myocardial infarction (MI); these are known collectively as the acute coronary syndromes. Although there may be a history of antecedent chronic stable angina, an episode of chest pain at rest is often the first presentation of coronary disease. The pain of MI typically takes several minutes to develop, is very severe and is often accompanied by autonomic disturbance including sweating, nausea and vomiting. Physical examination may reveal signs of important comorbidity (e.g. peripheral and/or cerebrovascular disease), autonomic disturbances, arrhythmia or heart failure. A 12-lead ECG may show features of ischaemia (ST elevation or depression, T-wave inversion) and helps guide initial treatment. An ECG obtained during the episode of pain is particularly useful. Plasma troponin concentrations should be measured and, if these are normal, the test should be repeated a minimum of 12 hrs after the onset of symptoms. If these tests are negative, an exercise test can help to confirm or refute a diagnosis of underlying coronary disease.

Arrhythmia: In patients with underlying coronary artery disease, the onset of a tachyarrhythmia may result in ischaemic chest pain at rest and can mimic an acute coronary syndrome.

Aortic dissection: An important differential diagnosis of acute coronary syndrome. The pain is severe, sharp and tearing, often felt in or penetrates through to the back, and is typically very sudden in onset. CXR may show a widened mediastinum but is normal in 10% of cases; transoesophageal echocardiography, CT or MRI can provide a definitive diagnosis.

Massive pulmonary embolism: May produce severe central chest pain with breathlessness and autonomic disturbance and can mimic MI. Sudden onset is typical. ECG may show right heart strain, and echocardiography right heart dilatation. CXR is frequently normal.

Myocarditis and pericarditis: Produce pain that is characteristically felt retrosternally, to the left of the sternum, or in the left or right shoulder. It varies in intensity with movement and with phase of respiration. It is usually described as 'sharp' and may 'catch' the patient during inspiration or coughing; there is occasionally a history of a prodromal viral illness.

BREATHLESSNESS (DYSPNOEA)

The differential diagnosis of dyspnoea is wide and includes many respiratory disorders (p. 271). However, both acute and chronic dyspnoea may have a cardiac aetiology. Acute left heart failure with pulmonary oedema is a common cause of the former. With pulmonary oedema:

• Patients are typically distressed, agitated and sweaty, and may produce frothy pink sputum. • There is often a history of chronic heart failure or

MI. • Extensive crepitations are audible in the chest and signs of right heart failure (e.g. elevated jugular venous pulse (JVP), peripheral oedema) may be evident. • CXR confirms the presence of pulmonary oedema. • Underlying causes may be revealed by ECG (e.g. MI, arrhythmia) and echocardiography (e.g. acute valvular regurgitation).

Arrhythmias can also cause acute breathlessness, but usually do so only if the heart is structurally abnormal (e.g. onset of atrial fibrillation in a patient with mitral stenosis).

Chronic exertional dyspnoea is the predominant symptom in chronic heart failure. Lying down increases venous return to the heart so patients may also complain of breathlessness on lying flat (orthopnoea) or of waking up during the night profoundly breathless (paroxysmal nocturnal dyspnoea). There may be a history of ischaemic heart disease, hypertension or valvular disorders.

• Relevant physical signs include an elevated JVP, displaced apex beat and cardiac murmurs. • Echocardiography permits assessment of left ventricular (LV) function and is the key investigation.

Breathlessness may also be the dominant or sole feature of myocardial ischaemia ('angina equivalent'). Patients sometimes describe chest tightness as 'breathlessness' but ischaemia may also cause dyspnoea by inducing transient LV dysfunction. Associated chest tightness, close correlation of symptoms with exercise, and objective evidence of myocardial ischaemia from stress testing may all help to establish the diagnosis.

SYNCOPE AND PRESYNCOPE

Cardiovascular disorders that cause an abrupt fall in cerebral perfusion may lead to recurrent or isolated episodes of syncope (sudden loss of consciousness) and presyncope (lightheadedness and near-collapse). Other causes of blackouts and 'funny turns' include seizure, hyperventilation and hypoglycaemia; dizziness, in the form of vertigo, may also result from labyrinthine or central vestibular dysfunction (p. 619). An accurate description of events from the patient and a witness is invaluable and helps to guide investigations. In cardiac syncope (i.e. secondary to arrhythmia or structural heart disease), onset is usually sudden and recovery rapid. In contrast, patients with vasovagal syncope often feel nauseated and unwell for several minutes before and after the episode. Patients with seizures may exhibit abnormal movements, usually take many minutes to recover and are confused on recovery.

Arrhythmias: May cause lightheadedness or blackouts, the latter with profound bradycardia or malignant ventricular tachyarrhythmias. Ambulatory ECG recordings may establish the diagnosis, although a close temporal relationship must be demonstrated between symptoms and a recorded arrhythmia. Patient-activated ECG recorders are useful for patients with recurrent dizziness but clearly unhelpful in sudden collapse. Where necessary, an implantable 'loop recorder' can be placed beneath the skin of the upper chest under local anaesthesia. This device continuously records an ECG, storing arrhythmic events in its digital memory for subsequent analysis.

Structural heart disease: Severe aortic stenosis, hypertrophic obstructive cardiomyopathy and severe coronary artery disease can cause lightheadedness or syncope on exertion. Profound hypotension occurs when cardiac output fails to rise normally as peripheral vascular resistance falls during exercise. Syncope may also result from an arrhythmia in these conditions. Echocardiography demonstrates the presence of structural heart disease. Exercise testing may reveal myocardial ischaemia, arrhythmia or an abnormal haemodynamic response during exertion.

Vasovagal syncope: Usually triggered by a reduction in venous return due to prolonged standing, excessive heat or a large meal. Initial sympathetic activation leads to vigorous contraction of the relatively underfilled ventricles. This stimulates ventricular mechanoreceptors, causing rebound parasympathetic activation and sympathetic withdrawal leading to bradycardia, vasodilatation or both. Often the diagnosis is clear from the history, but for repeated problematic episodes, head-up tilt testing (the patient lies on a table tilted to an angle of 70° for up to 45 mins with monitoring of ECG and BP) assists the diagnosis. In severe cases β-blockers or disopyramide may be helpful.

Carotid sinus hypersensitivity: May cause lightheadedness or syncope through inappropriate bradycardia and vasodilatation. Monitoring of the ECG and BP during carotid sinus massage can establish the diagnosis but should not be performed in patients with suspected carotid vascular disease (risk of a transient ischaemic attack).

Postural hypotension: May result from hypovolaemia (e.g. excessive diuretic therapy), sympathetic degeneration (e.g. diabetes mellitus, ageing) and drug therapy (e.g. vasodilators, antidepressants). Withdrawal of unnecessary medication, graduated elastic stockings and, in some cases, treatment with fludrocortisone may be helpful.

PALPITATION

The term 'palpitation' may be used to describe a variety of sensations, including an erratic, fast, slow or forceful heart beat. A detailed description is essential (Box 8.2) and patients should be asked to tap out the heart beat on the table.

• Recurrent but short-lived bouts of an irregular heart beat, such as dropped or missed beats, are usually due to atrial or ventricular extrasystoles. • Poorly defined attacks of a pounding, forceful, fast heart beat are a common manifestation of anxiety but may also occur in anaemia, pregnancy and thyrotoxicosis. • Discrete bouts of a very rapid (>120/min) heart beat suggest a paroxysmal arrhythmia. • Atrial fibrillation typically presents with a completely irregular tachycardia.

An ECG recording during an attack of palpitation (ambulatory monitoring or patient-activated recorder) may be necessary to establish a definitive

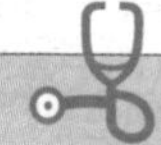

8.2 THE EVALUATION OF PALPITATION

- Is the palpitation continuous or intermittent?
- Is the heart beat regular or irregular?
- What is the approximate heart rate?
- Do symptoms occur in discrete attacks?
- Is the onset abrupt? How do attacks terminate?
- Are there any associated symptoms, e.g. chest pain, lightheadedness, polyuria (a feature of supraventricular tachycardia, p. 218)?
- Are there any precipitating factors, e.g. exercise, alcohol?
- Is there a history of structural heart disease, e.g. coronary artery disease, valvular heart disease?

diagnosis. Most cases are due to an awareness of the normal heart beat, sinus tachycardia or benign extrasystoles triggered by stress, intercurrent illness, caffeine or alcohol. In such cases, careful explanation and reassurance will often suffice but a low-dose β-blocker may be helpful in patients with distressing symptoms. Arrhythmia management is described on pages 215–225.

ANKLE SWELLING

Dependent peripheral oedema is a feature of both right and left heart failure (the latter due to salt and water retention) and, in ambulant patients, results in ankle swelling. Other important causes to consider include:
• Chronic venous insufficiency (e.g. elderly patients, previous DVT). • Hypoalbuminaemia (e.g. nephrotic syndrome, chronic liver disease). • Chronic lymphatic obstruction (e.g. malignancy). • Drugs, especially calcium channel blockers.

Patients should be asked about associated symptoms, such as exertional dyspnoea and orthopnoea, and examined carefully for evidence of cardiac disease (e.g. displaced apex beat, raised JVP, cardiac murmurs). Echocardiography may be helpful if the suspected aetiology is heart failure.

ABNORMAL HEART SOUNDS AND MURMURS

The first clinical manifestation of heart disease may be the incidental discovery of an abnormal sound on auscultation. Clinical evaluation is helpful (Box 8.3) but an echocardiogram is often necessary to confirm the nature of an abnormal heart sound or murmur. Some added sounds are physiological but may also occur in pathological conditions; for example, a third sound is common in young people and in pregnancy but is also a feature of heart failure. Similarly, an ejection systolic murmur may occur in hyperdynamic states (e.g. anaemia, pregnancy) but also in aortic stenosis. Benign murmurs do not occur in diastole and systolic murmurs that radiate or are

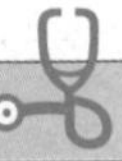

8.3 AUSCULTATORY FEATURES OF HEART MURMURS
When does it occur?
• Time the murmur using heart sounds, carotid pulse and apex beat. Is it systolic or diastolic? • Does the murmur extend throughout systole or diastole or is it confined to a shorter part of the cardiac cycle?
How loud is it? (intensity)
• Grade 1 Very soft (only audible in ideal conditions) • Grade 2 Soft • Grade 3 Moderate • Grade 4 Loud with associated thrill • Grade 5 Very loud • Grade 6 Heard without stethoscope **N.B.** Diastolic murmurs are sometimes graded 1–4.
Where is it heard best? (location)
• Listen over the apex and base of the heart, including the aortic and pulmonary areas
Where does it radiate?
• Evaluate radiation to the neck, axilla or back
What does it sound like? (pitch and quality)
• Pitch is determined by flow (high pitch indicates high-velocity flow) • Is the intensity constant or variable?

associated with a thrill are almost always pathological. Individual murmurs are dealt with below (pp. 254–260).

DISORDERS OF HEART RATE, RHYTHM AND CONDUCTION

Arrhythmias can cause palpitation, dizziness, syncope, chest pain or breathlessness, and trigger heart failure or even sudden death. They are generally classified as either tachycardias (heart rate >100/min) or bradycardias (heart rate <60/min).

• 'Supraventricular' (sinus, atrial or junctional) arrhythmias usually produce narrow QRS complexes because the ventricles are depolarised via normal pathways. • Ventricular arrhythmias give rise to broad QRS complexes because the ventricles are activated in an abnormal sequence.

SINUS RHYTHMS

Sinus arrhythmia: Refers to a physiological increase of the sinus rate during inspiration and slowing during expiration. It is mediated by the parasympathetic nervous system and may be pronounced in children.

Sinus bradycardia: May occur in healthy people at rest, especially athletes. Pathological causes include MI (sinus node ischaemia), raised intracranial pressure, hypothermia, hypothyroidism, cholestatic jaundice and drug therapy (e.g. β-blockers, verapamil, digoxin). Asymptomatic sinus bradycardia requires no treatment; symptomatic patients usually respond to i.v. atropine.

Sinus tachycardia: Usually due to an increase in sympathetic activity with exercise or emotion. Pathological causes include anaemia, fever, thyrotoxicosis, phaeochromocytoma, cardiac failure, shock and drug therapy (e.g. inhaled β-agonists).

TACHYARRHYTHMIAS

There are two main mechanisms of tachycardia:

Increased automaticity: The tachycardia is produced by repeated spontaneous depolarisation of an ectopic focus, often in response to catecholamines.

Re-entry: Occurs when there are two alternative pathways with different conducting properties (e.g. an area of normal tissue and an area of ischaemic tissue). In sinus rhythm each impulse passes down both pathways before entering a common distal pathway. However, owing to different refractory periods, a premature impulse may travel selectively down one pathway then retrogradely up the alternative pathway, establishing a closed loop or re-entry circuit and thus initiating a tachycardia.

ATRIAL TACHYARRHYTHMIAS

Atrial ectopic beats (extrasystoles): Usually cause no symptoms but can give the sensation of a missed beat or abnormally strong beat. The ECG shows a premature but otherwise normal QRS complex; the preceding P wave has a different morphology because the atria activate from an abnormal site. Treatment is rarely necessary.

Atrial tachycardia: Produces a narrow complex tachycardia with abnormal P-wave morphology caused by increased atrial automaticity, sinoatrial disease or digoxin toxicity. It may respond to β-blockers, which reduce automaticity, or class I or III anti-arrhythmic drugs (p. 760).

Atrial flutter: Results from a large re-entry circuit within the right atrium. The atrial rate is approximately 300/min, but associated 2 : 1, 3 : 1 or 4 : 1 atrioventricular (AV) block usually produces a ventricular heart rate of 150, 100 or 75/min. The ECG shows saw-toothed flutter waves. With regular 2 : 1 AV block these may be buried in the QRS complexes and T-waves but can be revealed by transiently increasing the degree of AV block through

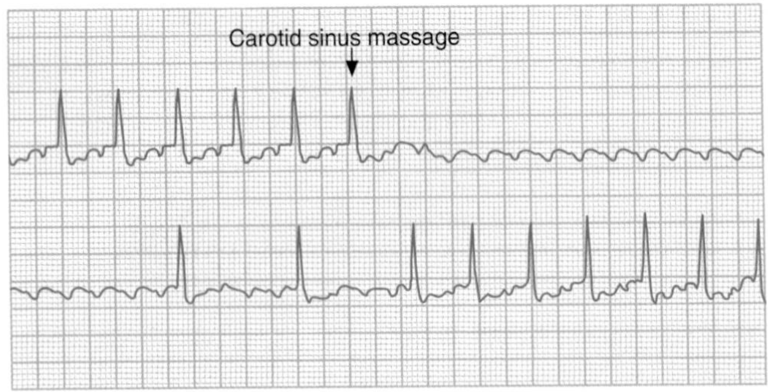

Fig. 8.1 Atrial flutter with 2:1 block; flutter waves revealed by carotid sinus massage.

carotid sinus massage (Fig. 8.1) or i.v. adenosine. Digoxin, β-blockers or verapamil can limit the ventricular rate but electrical or chemical cardioversion is often preferable. In addition to restoring sinus rhythm, flecainide, amiodarone or propafenone may prevent recurrent episodes of atrial flutter, though catheter ablation is now the treatment of choice for patients with persistent and troublesome symptoms.

ATRIAL FIBRILLATION (AF)

AF is the most common sustained cardiac arrhythmia, its prevalence rising with age. The atria beat rapidly, but in an uncoordinated and ineffective manner. The ventricles are activated irregularly at a rate determined by conduction through the AV node, giving rise to an 'irregularly irregular' pulse. The ECG (Fig. 8.2) shows normal but irregularly spaced QRS complexes with absent P waves.

AF can be classified as:

• Paroxysmal (intermittent, self-terminating episodes). • Persistent (prolonged episodes that can be terminated by electrical or chemical cardioversion). • Permanent.

Initially, classification may be difficult but paroxysmal AF often becomes permanent with progression of the underlying disease process. Common causes of AF are shown in Box 8.4; however, many patients have 'lone atrial fibrillation' where no underlying cause is identified.

AF is often asymptomatic but can cause palpitation, breathlessness and fatigue. It may provoke myocardial ischaemia in patients with underlying coronary disease or precipitate cardiac failure in those with poor ventricular function or valve disease. The risk of cerebral embolism is increased.

Management of an acute episode

Objectives are to optimise heart rate during AF, restore sinus rhythm as soon as possible, prevent thromboembolism and identify/treat precipitating factors.

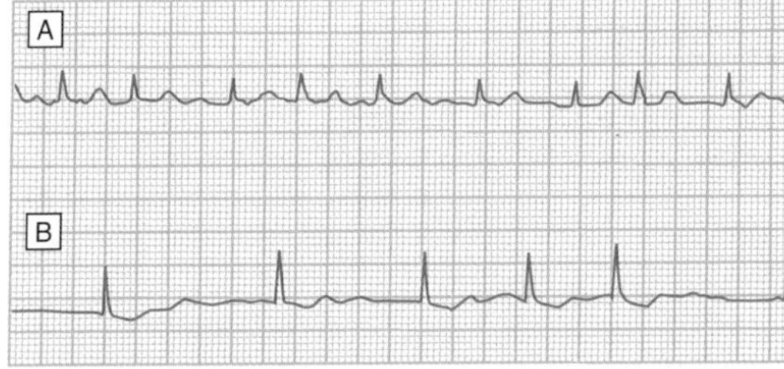

Fig. 8.2 Two examples of atrial fibrillation. The QRS complexes are irregular and there are no P waves. **A** There is usually a fast ventricular rate, often between 120 and 160/min, at the onset of AF. **B** In chronic AF the ventricular rate may be much slower due to the effects of medication and AV nodal fatigue.

8.4 COMMON CAUSES OF ATRIAL FIBRILLATION

- Coronary artery disease (including acute MI)
- Valvular heart disease, especially rheumatic mitral valve disease
- Hypertension
- Sinoatrial disease
- Hyperthyroidism
- Alcohol
- Cardiomyopathy
- Congenital heart disease
- Chest infection
- Pulmonary embolism
- Pericardial disease
- Idiopathic (lone AF)

Within 48 hrs of AF onset, heparinisation and cardioversion with a synchronised DC shock or drug therapy (flecainide or amiodarone) can be attempted. Beyond 48 hrs, the ventricular rate should be controlled and cardioversion deferred until anticoagulation with warfarin (INR 2–3) has been established for at least 3 wks. When AF complicates an acute illness (e.g. chest infection), treatment of the primary disorder usually restores sinus rhythm. All patients with haemodynamic compromise (e.g. hypotension) should receive immediate i.v. heparin and DC cardioversion.

Long-term management

In paroxysmal AF or after successful cardioversion of persistent AF, the aim is to maintain sinus rhythm. If sinus rhythm cannot be restored, treatment is aimed at achieving an appropriate heart rate.

Rhythm control—prevention of recurrent episodes: Treatment with amiodarone or β-blockers may reduce risk of recurrence following successful cardioversion; if relapse occurs, a repeat cardioversion may be appropriate. In paroxysmal AF, β-blockers are usual first-line therapy, especially in patients with associated ischaemic heart disease, hypertension or cardiac failure. Amiodarone is more effective in preventing AF but its use is limited

8.5 RISK FACTORS FOR THROMBOEMBOLISM IN AF

- Previous ischaemic stroke or TIA
- Mitral valve disease
- Age >65 yrs
- Hypertension
- Diabetes mellitus
- Heart failure
- Echocardiographic features of LV dysfunction, left atrial enlargement or mitral annular calcification

by side-effects. Class Ic drugs such as flecainide, though effective, should be avoided in patients with coronary disease or LV dysfunction. Digoxin and verapamil limit ventricular rate in AF but do not prevent episodes. Radiofrequency ablation is a promising treatment for lone paroxysmal AF.

Rate control: β-blockers and rate-limiting calcium antagonists (e.g. verapamil) are often more effective than digoxin at controlling the heart rate during exercise. In exceptional cases, AF can be treated by inducing complete heart block with transvenous catheter radiofrequency ablation after first implanting a permanent pacemaker.

Prevention of thromboembolism: Left atrial dilatation and loss of contraction cause stasis of blood and may lead to atrial thrombus formation, predisposing patients to stroke and other systemic embolic events. Warfarin (target INR 2.0–3.0) reduces the risk of stroke by two-thirds (with an annual risk of bleeding of 1–1.5%), while aspirin reduces it by only one-fifth. Warfarin is indicated for patients with AF and specific risk factors for stroke (Box 8.5). Patients <65 yrs with no evidence of structural heart disease have a very low risk of stroke and can receive aspirin. With intermittent AF, the risk of stroke depends on the frequency and duration of AF episodes; patients with frequent, prolonged (>24-hr) episodes should be considered for warfarin. Anticoagulation with warfarin should be maintained for at least 1 mth following successful cardioversion.

'SUPRAVENTRICULAR' TACHYCARDIAS

AV NODAL RE-ENTRY TACHYCARDIA (AVNRT)

This is due to re-entry in the right atrium and AV node, and tends to occur in hearts that are otherwise normal. It produces episodes of regular tachycardia with a rate of 140–220/min that last from a few seconds to many hours.

• The patient is usually aware of a fast heart beat and may feel faint or breathless. • Polyuria may occur, and also angina if there is underlying coronary disease. • The ECG (Fig. 8.3) usually shows a regular tachycardia with normal QRS complexes but occasionally there may be rate-dependent bundle branch block. • Attacks may be terminated by carotid sinus pressure or Valsalva manoeuvre, but if not, i.v. adenosine or verapamil will restore sinus rhythm in most cases. • When there is severe haemodynamic compromise, the tachycardia should be terminated by DC cardioversion

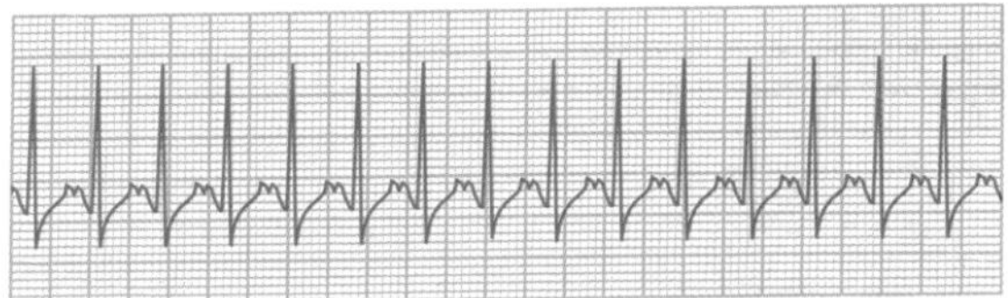

Fig. 8.3 Supraventricular tachycardia. The rate is 180/min and the QRS complexes are normal.

(p. 226). • If attacks are frequent or disabling, prophylactic oral therapy (e.g. β-blocker, verapamil) may be indicated but catheter ablation (p. 228) offers a very high chance of complete cure and is usually preferable to long-term drug treatment.

ATRIOVENTRICULAR RE-ENTRANT TACHYCARDIA (AVRT) AND WOLFF–PARKINSON–WHITE SYNDROME

An abnormal band of rapidly conducting tissue ('accessory pathway') connects the atria and ventricles. In around half of cases, premature activation of ventricular tissue via the pathway produces a short PR interval and a 'slurring' of the QRS complex, called a delta wave (Fig. 8.4). As the AV node and bypass tract have different conduction speeds and refractory periods, a re-entry circuit can develop, causing tachycardia; when associated with symptoms, the condition is known as Wolff–Parkinson–White syndrome.

• The ECG appearance of AVRT may be indistinguishable from that of AVNRT. • Carotid sinus pressure, Valsalva manoeuvre or i.v. adenosine can terminate the tachycardia. • If AF occurs, it may produce a dangerously rapid ventricular rate (since the accessory pathway lacks the rate-limiting properties of the AV node) and should be treated as an emergency, usually with DC cardioversion. • Digoxin and verapamil shorten the refractory period of the accessory pathway and must be avoided. • Prophylactic treatment is only indicated in symptomatic patients; catheter ablation (p. 228) of the accessory pathway is now preferred to drug therapy (flecainide or amiodarone).

VENTRICULAR TACHYARRHYTHMIAS

VENTRICULAR ECTOPIC BEATS (EXTRASYSTOLES, PREMATURE BEATS)

Ventricular ectopic beats (VEBs) produce a low stroke volume and premature broad, bizarre abnormal QRS complexes on ECG.

• Patients are usually asymptomatic but may complain of an irregular heart beat, missed beats or abnormally strong beats. • VEBs are frequently found in healthy people and treatment (β-blockers) is only necessary in highly symptomatic cases. • Frequent VEBs in patients with heart failure or those who have survived the acute phase of MI are associated with an adverse prognosis. • Treatment should be directed at the underlying cause.

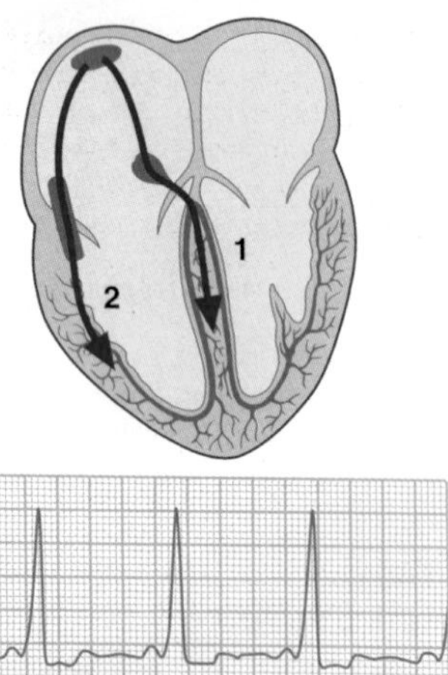

Fig. 8.4 **Wolff–Parkinson–White syndrome.** A strip of accessory conducting tissue allows electricity to bypass the AV node and spread from atria to ventricles without delay. When ventricular activation occurs through the AV node (1), the ECG is normal; however, when it occurs through the accessory pathway (2), a very short PR interval and a broad QRS complex are seen. In sinus rhythm, ventricular activation occurs by both paths, causing the characteristic short PR and slurring of the upstroke of the QRS complex (delta wave). The proportion of activation occurring via the accessory pathway may vary; therefore, at times, the ECG can look normal.

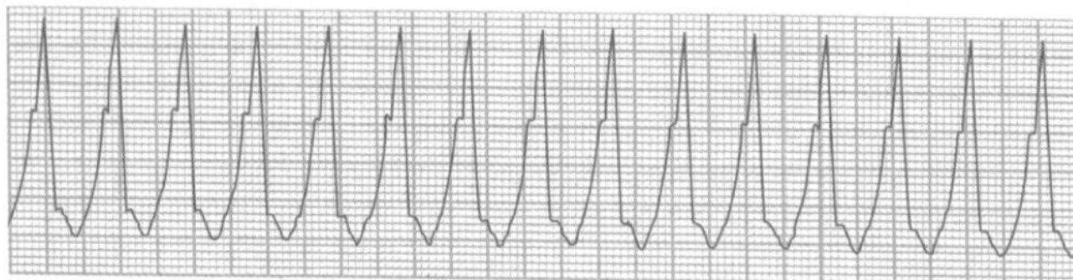

Fig. 8.5 **Ventricular tachycardia: rhythm strip.** Typical broad bizarre QRS complexes with a rate of 160/min.

VENTRICULAR TACHYCARDIA (VT)

VT usually occurs in patients with coronary heart disease or cardiomyopathies and may cause haemodynamic compromise or degenerate into ventricular fibrillation (p. 221). The ECG shows tachycardia with broad, abnormal QRS complexes and a rate >120/min (Fig. 8.5). VT is by far the most common cause of a broad-complex tachycardia but may be difficult to distinguish from supraventricular tachycardia with bundle branch block or Wolff–Parkinson–White syndrome. When there is doubt, it is safer to manage the problem as VT.

• Emergency DC cardioversion is required if systolic BP is <90 mmHg, but if VT is well tolerated then i.v. amiodarone or lidocaine may be tried.

• Hypokalaemia, hypomagnesaemia, acidosis and hypoxaemia must be corrected. • β-blockers and/or amiodarone may be effective for subsequent prophylaxis. • Long-term treatment with class I anti-arrhythmic drugs is dangerous in patients with ischaemic heart disease. • An implantable cardiac defibrillator may be indicated in patients with refractory VT or at high risk of arrhythmic death (e.g. poor LV function, associated haemodynamic compromise). • VT occasionally occurs in patients with otherwise healthy hearts; in such cases prognosis is good and catheter ablation can be curative.

TORSADES DE POINTES (TWISTING POINTS)

This form of VT complicates prolonged ventricular repolarisation (prolonged QT interval), which may be congenital or secondary to drugs (e.g. class Ia and class III anti-arrhythmics, macrolide antibiotics, tricyclic antidepressants, phenothiazines) or electrolyte disturbance (↓Ca^{2+}, ↓Mg^{2+}, ↓K^+). The ECG shows rapid irregular complexes that oscillate from an upright to an inverted position, seeming to twist around the baseline. It is typically non-sustained but may degenerate into ventricular fibrillation. The ECG in sinus rhythm shows a prolonged QT interval.

• I.v. magnesium should be given in all cases. • Atrial pacing or i.v. isoprenaline shortens the QT interval by increasing heart rate. • Otherwise, treatment is directed at the underlying cause. • Patients with congenital long QT syndrome often require an implantable cardiac defibrillator.

CARDIAC ARREST

Cardiac arrest describes the sudden, complete loss of cardiac output. The patient is unconscious, pulseless and apnoeic. Death is inevitable without prompt effective treatment.

VENTRICULAR FIBRILLATION (VF) AND PULSELESS VENTRICULAR TACHYCARDIA (VT)

These rhythms frequently arise in patients with MI or a history of previous MI.

• VF produces rapid, uncoordinated movement of the ventricles, which produces no pulse. The ECG (Fig. 8.6) shows chaotic, bizarre, irregular

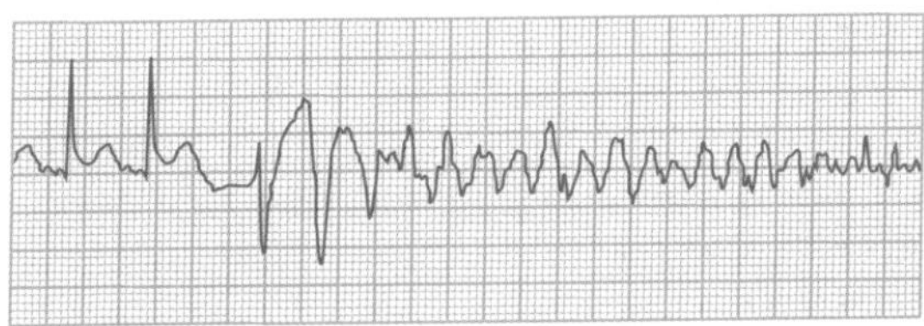

Fig. 8.6 Ventricular fibrillation. A bizarre chaotic rhythm initiated in this case by two ectopic beats in rapid succession.

ventricular complexes. • VT can cause cardiac arrest by preventing effective mechanical contraction and relaxation, and may degenerate into VF.

Defibrillation restores cardiac output in >80% of patients if delivered immediately.

ASYSTOLE AND PULSELESS ELECTRICAL ACTIVITY (PEA)

Asystole occurs when there is no electrical activity within the ventricles due to failure of the conducting tissue or massive ventricular damage. PEA refers to the absence of cardiac output despite the presence of organised electrical activity, often due to a catastrophic event such as cardiac rupture. These rhythms do not respond to defibrillation; treatment consists of cardiopulmonary resuscitation (CPR) with the additional support of atropine and adrenaline (epinephrine) whilst seeking potentially reversible causes; prognosis is poor.

MANAGEMENT OF CARDIAC ARREST

The management of cardiac arrest is shown in Figure 8.7.

• Basic life support (BLS) encompasses manoeuvres that attempt to maintain a low level of circulation pending more definitive treatment with advanced life support (ALS). • ALS aims to restore cardiac output by defibrillation or correction of other reversible causes of cardiac arrest.

In the absence of an identifiable, treatable cause (e.g. ischaemia, aortic stenosis), survivors of VT or VF arrest should be considered for anti-arrhythmic therapy or an implantable cardiac defibrillator (p. 226). • Patients who survive cardiac arrest in the context of acute MI require no specific additional treatment.

BRADYARRHYTHMIAS

SINOATRIAL DISEASE (SICK SINUS SYNDROME)

Sinoatrial disease results from degeneration of the sinus node and is common in the elderly. It may present with palpitation, dizzy spells or syncope, due to intermittent tachycardia, bradycardia, or pauses with no atrial or ventricular activity (sinus arrest or sinoatrial block). A permanent pacemaker may benefit patients with symptomatic bradycardias but is not indicated in asymptomatic patients.

ATRIOVENTRICULAR (AV) BLOCK

AV block may be congenital or result from:

• Idiopathic fibrosis. • Myocardial infarction/ischaemia. • Trauma (e.g. cardiac surgery). • Inflammation (e.g. sarcoidoisis). • Drugs (e.g. verapamil, digoxin or β-blockers).

First-degree AV block

AV conduction is delayed, producing a prolonged PR interval (>0.20 secs). It rarely causes symptoms.

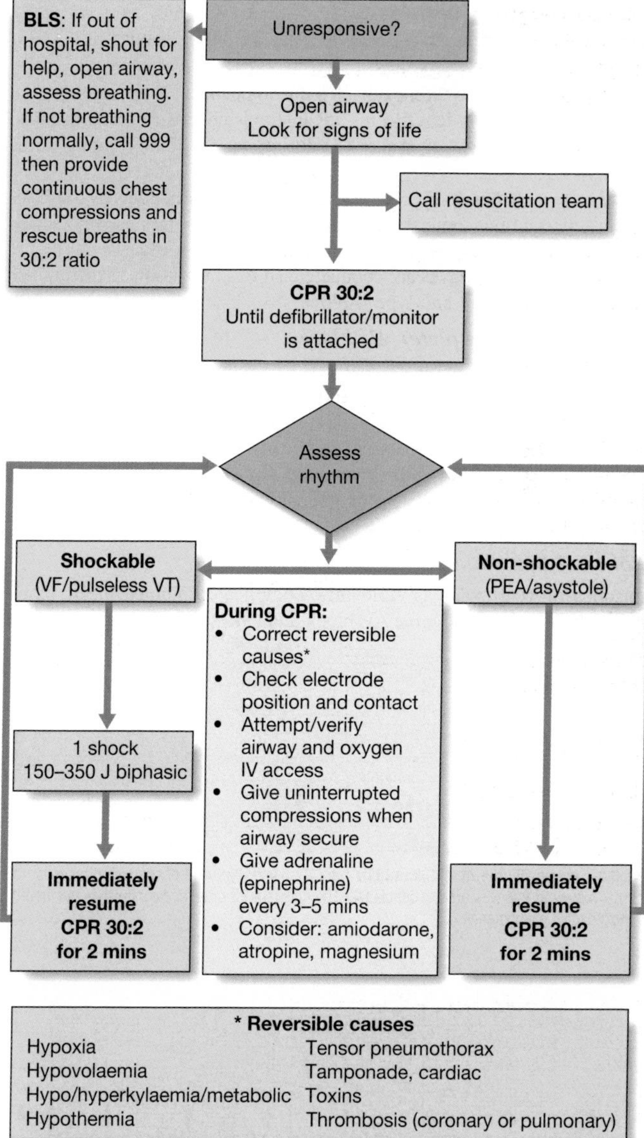

Fig. 8.7 Algorithm for basic and adult advanced life support. For further information see www.resus.org.uk. (BLS = basic life support; CPR = cardiopulmonary resuscitation; PEA = pulseless electrical activity; VF = ventricular fibrillation; VT = pulseless ventricular tachycardia)

Second-degree AV block

In second-degree AV block some atrial impulses fail to conduct to the ventricles resulting in dropped beats.

Mobitz type I block ('Wenckebach's phenomenon'): There are repeated cycles of progressively lengthening PR intervals culminating in a dropped beat. It is sometimes observed at rest or during sleep in athletic young adults with high vagal tone.

Mobitz type II block (Fig. 8.8): The PR interval of conducted impulses remains constant but some P waves are not conducted. It is usually caused by disease of the His–Purkinje system and carries a risk of asystole. In 2 : 1 AV block alternate P waves are conducted, so it is impossible to distinguish between Mobitz type I and type II block.

Third-degree (complete) AV block

AV conduction fails completely, the atria and ventricles beat independently (AV dissociation, Fig. 8.9), and ventricular activity is maintained by an escape rhythm arising in the AV node or bundle of His (narrow QRS complexes) or the distal Purkinje tissues (broad QRS complexes). Distal escape rhythms are completely regular but slower and less reliable. Cannon waves may be visible in the neck, and the intensity of the first heart sound varies due to the loss of AV synchrony.

Stokes–Adams attacks

Episodes of ventricular asystole may complicate complete heart block, Mobitz type II second-degree AV block and sinoatrial disease, resulting in

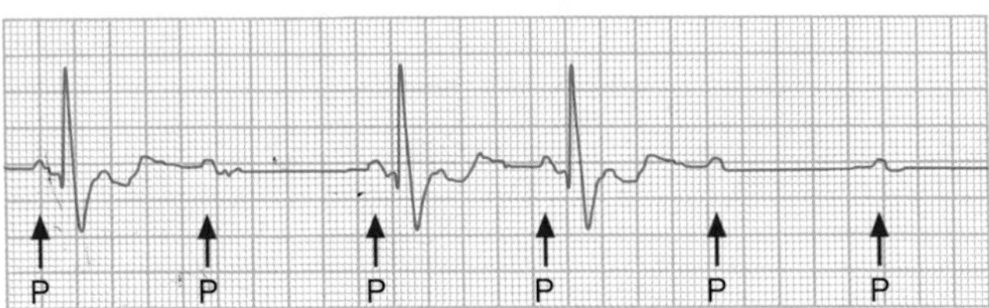

Fig. 8.8 Second-degree AV block (Mobitz type II). The PR interval of conducted beats is normal but some P waves are not conducted. The constant PR interval distinguishes this from Wenckebach's phenomenon.

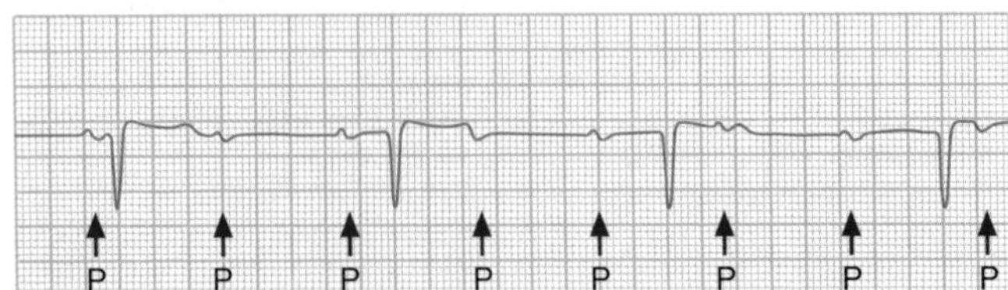

Fig. 8.9 Complete (third-degree) AV block. There is complete dissociation of atrial and ventricular complexes. The atrial rate is 80/min and the ventricular rate is 38/min.

recurrent syncope ('Stokes–Adams' attacks). Episodes are characterised by a sudden loss of consciousness, typically without warning, which may result in a fall. Convulsions (due to cerebral ischaemia) can occur if asystole is prolonged. There is pallor and a death-like appearance during the attack, but when the heart starts beating again there may be a characteristic flush. In contrast to epilepsy, recovery is rapid.

Management

AV block complicating acute MI: Acute *inferior* MI is often complicated by transient AV block because the right coronary artery supplies the AV junction. There is usually a reliable escape rhythm, and if the patient remains well, no treatment is required. Symptomatic second-degree or complete heart block may respond to i.v. atropine or, if this fails, a temporary pacemaker. In most cases the AV block will resolve within 7–10 days. Second-degree or complete heart block complicating acute *anterior* MI is usually a sign of extensive ventricular damage involving both bundle branches and carries a poor prognosis. Asystole may ensue and a temporary pacemaker should be inserted as soon as possible. If the patient presents with asystole, i.v. atropine (3 mg) or i.v. isoprenaline (2 mg in 500 ml 5% dextrose, infused at 10–60 ml/hr) may help to maintain the circulation until a temporary pacing electrode can be inserted.

Chronic AV block: Patients with symptomatic bradyarrhythmias associated with AV block should receive a permanent pacemaker. Asymptomatic first-degree or Mobitz type I second-degree AV block does not require treatment, but a permanent pacemaker is usually indicated in patients with asymptomatic Mobitz type II second-degree or complete heart block on prognostic grounds.

BUNDLE BRANCH BLOCK AND HEMIBLOCK

Interruption of the right or left branch of the bundle of His delays activation of the corresponding ventricle, broadens the QRS complex (≥0.12 secs) and produces characteristic alterations in QRS morphology (Figs 8.10 and 8.11). Right bundle branch block (RBBB) can be a normal variant but left bundle branch block (LBBB) usually signifies important underlying heart disease (Box 8.6).

8.6 COMMON CAUSES OF BUNDLE BRANCH BLOCK	
Right	
• Normal variant • Right ventricular hypertrophy or strain, e.g. pulmonary embolism	• Congenital heart disease, e.g. atrial septal defect • Coronary artery disease
Left	
• Coronary artery disease • Hypertension	• Aortic valve disease • Cardiomyopathy

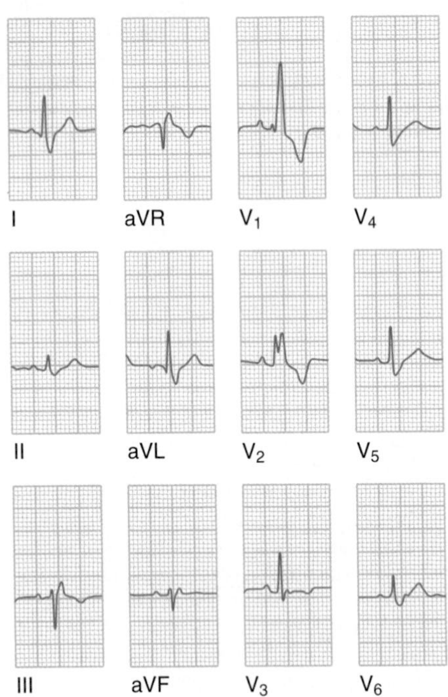

Fig. 8.10 Right bundle branch block. Note the wide QRS complexes with 'M'-shaped configuration in leads V_1 and V_2 and a wide S wave in lead I.

THERAPEUTIC PROCEDURES

EXTERNAL DEFIBRILLATION AND CARDIOVERSION

The heart can be depolarised by passing an electrical current through it from an external source. This will interrupt any arrhythmia and produce a brief period of asystole, usually followed by the resumption of normal sinus rhythm. Elective cardioversion requires a general anaesthetic. In this situation, a low-amplitude shock synchronised to occur 0.02 secs after the R wave peak is used. Patients with long-standing atrial arrhythmias are at risk of systemic embolism before and after cardioversion, so should be adequately anticoagulated for at least 4 wks either side of the procedure.

IMPLANTABLE CARDIAC DEFIBRILLATORS (ICDs)

These devices sense rhythm and deliver current through leads implanted in the heart via the subclavian or cephalic vein. They automatically sense and terminate life-threatening ventricular arrhythmias. ICDs have all of the

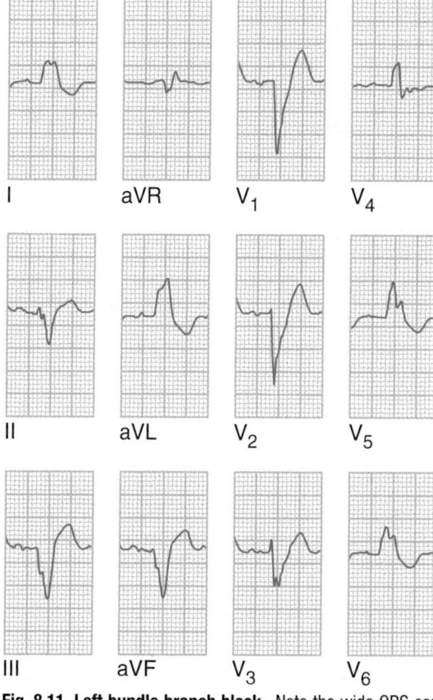

Fig. 8.11 Left bundle branch block. Note the wide QRS complexes with the loss of the Q wave or septal vector in lead I and 'M'-shaped QRS complexes in V_5 and V_6.

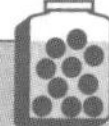

8.7 KEY INDICATIONS FOR ICD THERAPY
Primary prevention
• After MI, if LV ejection fraction <30% • Mild to moderate symptomatic heart failure, on optimal drug therapy, with LV ejection fraction <35%
Secondary prevention
• Survivors of VF or VT cardiac arrest not due to transient or reversible cause • VT with haemodynamic compromise or significant LV impairment (LV ejection fraction <35%)

functions of a pacemaker (to deal with bradycardias) but in addition can treat ventricular tachyarrhythmias using overdrive pacing, synchronised cardioversion, or defibrillation. ICD implantation is subject to similar complications as pacemaker implantation (see below). Indications for ICDs are shown in Box 8.7.

CATHETER ABLATION

Catheter ablation therapy has become the treatment of choice for many patients with recurrent arrhythmias (e.g. AV nodal and AV re-entry tachycardias), as it offers the prospect of a lifetime cure without the need for long-term drug therapy. A series of catheter electrodes are inserted into the heart via the venous system and used to record the activation sequence of the heart in sinus rhythm, during tachycardia and after pacing manoeuvres. Once the arrhythmia focus or circuit is identified, a catheter is placed into this critical zone and the culprit tissue is selectively ablated using radiofrequency current or cryoablation. Serious complications are rare (<1%) but include inadvertent complete heart block requiring pacemaker implantation, and cardiac tamponade.

TEMPORARY AND PERMANENT PACEMAKERS

Temporary pacemakers

Transcutaneous pacing: Administered by delivering an electrical stimulus sufficient to induce cardiac contraction through two adhesive gel pad electrodes placed externally over the apex and upper right sternal edge. It is easy and quick to set up, but causes significant discomfort.

Transvenous pacing: Delivered by positioning a pacing electrode at the apex of the right ventricle via the internal jugular, subclavian or femoral vein using fluoroscopic imaging. The electrode is then connected to an external pulse generator which can be adjusted to alter the energy output or pacing rate. Temporary pacing may be indicated in the management of transient heart block or of other causes of transient bradycardia (e.g. drug overdose), or as a prelude to permanent pacing. Complications include:

• Pneumothorax. • Brachial plexus or subclavian artery injury. • Infection (usually *Staphylococcus aureus*). • Pericarditis.

Permanent pacemakers

Permanent pacemakers utilise the same principles but the pulse generator is implanted under the skin. Electrodes can be placed in the right ventricular apex, the right atrial appendage or both (dual-chamber). Atrial pacing may be appropriate for patients with sinoatrial disease without AV block. In dual-chamber pacing the atrial electrode can be used to detect spontaneous atrial activity and trigger ventricular pacing, thereby preserving AV synchrony and allowing the ventricular rate to increase together with the atrial rate during exercise, leading to improved exercise tolerance. A code is used to signify the pacing mode (Box 8.8). Most dual-chamber pacemakers are programmed to a mode termed DDD. Rate-responsive pacemakers trigger a rise in heart rate in response to movement or increased respiratory rate and are used in patients unable to mount an increase in heart rate during exercise. Early complications of permanent pacing include:

8.8 INTERNATIONAL GENERIC PACEMAKER CODE		
Chamber paced	**Chamber sensed**	**Response to sensing**
0 = none	0 = none	0 = none
A = atrium	A = atrium	T = triggered
V = ventricle	V = ventricle	I = inhibited
D = both	D = both	D = both

• Pneumothorax. • Cardiac tamponade. • Infection. • Lead displacement.

Late complications include:

• Infection. • Erosion of the generator or lead. • Lead fracture due to mechanical fatigue.

CARDIAC RESYNCHRONISATION THERAPY (CRT)

CRT is a new treatment for selected patients with heart failure and LBBB. This conduction defect is associated with uncoordinated LV contraction, which may exacerbate heart failure. CRT devices carry an additional lead that is placed via the coronary sinus into one of the veins on the epicardial surface of the left ventricle. Simultaneous septal and LV epicardial pacing resynchronises LV contraction, improving exercise tolerance in selected patients.

CORONARY HEART DISEASE (CHD)

CHD, also known as ischaemic heart disease, is the leading cause of premature death in the developed world and is estimated to become, by 2020, the major cause of death world-wide. In the UK 1 in 3 men and 1 in 4 women die from CHD. Disease of the coronary arteries is almost always due to atherosclerosis and its complications, particularly thrombosis. Atherosclerosis is a progressive inflammatory disorder of the arterial wall, characterised by focal lipid-rich deposits of atheroma that remain clinically silent until they become large enough to impair arterial perfusion or until disruption of the lesion results in thrombotic occlusion or embolisation of the affected vessel. The pathogenesis of atherosclerosis is complex but several risk factors have been identified:

Age and sex: Age is the most powerful independent risk factor for atherosclerosis. Pre-menopausal women have much lower rates of disease than age- and risk-matched males but thereafter risk is similar.

Family history: A 'positive' family history is present when clinical problems occur in first-degree relatives aged <50 yrs (male) or <55 yrs (female). Increased risk reflects a combination of shared genetic and environmental (e.g. smoking, exercise, diet) factors.

Hypertension: The incidence of atherosclerosis increases as BP (systolic and diastolic) rises. Antihypertensive therapy reduces coronary mortality and stroke.

Hypercholesterolaemia: The risk of CHD and other atherosclerotic vascular disease rises with plasma cholesterol concentration, especially the ratio of total cholesterol to high-density lipoprotein (HDL) cholesterol. A weaker correlation exists with plasma triglyceride concentration. Lowering low-density lipoprotein (LDL) and total cholesterol concentrations reduces the risk of cardiovascular events.

Diabetes mellitus: A potent risk factor for all forms of atherosclerosis and is often associated with diffuse disease. Insulin resistance (normal glucose homeostasis with high levels of insulin) is also a risk factor for CHD.

Lifestyle factors: There is a strong, dose-linked relationship between cigarette smoking and CHD. Physical inactivity and obesity are associated with other risk factors (hypertension, diabetes) but are both independent risk factors for atherosclerosis. Diets deficient in fresh fruit, vegetables and polyunsaturated fatty acids are associated with an increased risk of vascular disease. Regular exercise appears to have a protective effect.

STABLE ANGINA

Stable angina occurs when coronary blood flow is impaired by fixed or stable atheroma of the coronary arteries. During exertion, an imbalance between myocardial oxygen supply and demand causes transient myocardial ischaemia. Coronary atheroma is by far the most common cause of angina; however, the symptom may also be a manifestation of other forms of heart disease such as aortic valve disease, hypertrophic cardiomyopathy or coronary vasopasm (Prinzmetal's angina). Occasionally, the coronary arteries are involved in other disorders such as polyarteritis and other connective tissue disorders.

Clinical features

The history is by far the most important factor in making the diagnosis of stable angina (p. 209). The condition is characterised by central chest pain, discomfort or breathlessness that is precipitated by exertion or other forms of stress, and is promptly relieved by rest. Physical examination is frequently negative but may reveal evidence of:

• Aortic stenosis (an occasional cause of angina). • CHD risk factors (e.g. hypertension, diabetes). • LV dysfunction (e.g. cardiomegaly). • Other arterial disease (e.g. carotid bruits, peripheral vascular disease). • Conditions that exacerbate angina (e.g. anaemia, thyrotoxicosis). • Retinopathy (diabetic or hypertensive).

Investigations

Resting ECG: May show evidence of previous MI but is often normal even in patients with left main or severe three-vessel coronary artery disease. The most convincing ECG evidence of myocardial ischaemia is obtained by demonstrating reversible ST segment depression or elevation, with or without T-wave inversion, during symptoms.

Exercise ECG: The patient's ECG and BP are monitored during exercise to a standard treadmill or bicycle ergometer protocol. Planar or down-sloping ST segment depression of ≥1 mm is indicative of ischaemia; up-sloping ST depression is less specific. Exercise testing can provide objective evidence of myocardial ischaemia and is also a useful means of assessing the severity of coronary disease and identifying high-risk individuals. However, false negatives and positives do occur and the predictive accuracy of exercise testing is lower in women than men.

Myocardial perfusion scanning: Has a higher predictive accuracy than exercise ECG and is particularly helpful in patients who are unable to exercise or who have an equivocal or uninterpretable exercise test. Scinti-scans of the myocardium are obtained at rest and during stress (exercise or pharmacological, e.g. dobutamine) after i.v. administration of a radioactive isotope that is taken up by viable perfused myocardium. A perfusion defect present during stress but not at rest indicates reversible myocardial ischaemia; a persistent defect suggests previous MI.

Stress echocardiography: An alternative to myocardial perfusion scanning with similar predictive accuracy (superior to exercise ECG). Ischaemic segments of myocardium exhibit reversible defects in contractility (visualised by echocardiography) during exercise or pharmacological stress; areas of infarction do not contract at rest or during stress. The technique is particularly useful for identifying areas of viable 'hibernating' myocardium in patients with heart failure and CHD being considered for revascularisation (p. 232).

Coronary arteriography: Provides detailed anatomical (as opposed to functional) information about the extent and nature of coronary artery disease. It may be indicated when non-invasive tests have failed to elucidate the cause of atypical chest pain but is usually performed with a view to revascularisation.

Management

Secondary prevention: In all forms of atheromatous vascular disease including angina, patients are at increased risk of major vascular events such as MI or stroke and can be offered a variety of treatments and measures to improve their outlook.

• The most important lifestyle modification is smoking cessation but other steps include regular exercise and aiming for ideal body weight. • Total cholesterol should be lowered to <5 mmol/l but all patients with CHD should receive statin therapy, irrespective of serum cholesterol concentration. • BP should be treated to a target of ≤130/80 mmHg, although ACE inhibitors (unless contraindicated) are of benefit in all patients with vascular disease. • Aspirin reduces the risk of adverse events such as MI and should be prescribed indefinitely for all patients with CHD; clopidogrel is an equally effective alternative in patients intolerant of aspirin.

Relief of symptoms: Patients should be advised to avoid vigorous exertion after a heavy meal or in cold weather. Sublingual glyceryl trinitrate (GTN) in spray or tablet form will usually relieve an attack of angina in

2–3 mins. Patients should be encouraged to use GTN prophylactically before engaging in exercise that is liable to provoke symptoms. Four groups of drugs are used to prevent the symptoms of angina:

• Nitrates. • β-blockers. • Calcium antagonists. • Potassium channel activators (nicorandil).

These drugs are discussed in detail on pages 757–759. There is little convincing evidence that one group is more effective than another, although it is conventional to start with a β-blocker, then add a calcium channel antagonist or a long-acting nitrate later, if necessary. The goal is control of angina with minimum side-effects and the simplest possible drug regimen. Revascularisation should be considered if symptoms persist despite the use of two drugs.

Percutaneous coronary intervention (PCI): This is performed by passing a fine guidewire across a coronary stenosis under radiographic control and using it to position a balloon which is then inflated to dilate the stenosis. A coronary stent is a piece of coated metallic 'scaffolding' that can be deployed on a balloon and used to maximise and maintain dilatation of a stenosed vessel. PCI is an effective symptomatic treatment but has not been shown to improve survival in patients with stable angina. It is mainly used in single or two-vessel disease; coronary artery bypass graft (CABG) surgery is usually the preferred option in patients with three-vessel or left main disease. The main acute complication is vessel occlusion by thrombus or dissection, which may lead to acute MI (2%) or the need for emergency CABG. The overall mortality risk is <0.5%. The main long-term complication is restenosis. The routine use of stents in appropriate vessels reduces both acute complications and the incidence of restenosis. Drug-eluting stents can reduce this risk even further but their use is currently controversial owing to a possible increased risk of stent thrombosis. In combination with aspirin and heparin, adjunctive therapy with potent platelet inhibitors, such as clopidogrel or glycoprotein IIb/IIIa receptor antagonists, improves the outcome of PCI, with lower short- and long-term rates of death and MI.

Coronary artery bypass grafting (CABG): The internal mammary arteries, radial arteries or reversed segments of saphenous vein can be used to bypass coronary artery stenoses, usually under cardiopulmonary bypass. The operative mortality is ~1.5%, but higher in elderly patients and those with poor LV function or significant comorbidity (e.g. renal failure). There is a 1–5% risk of perioperative stroke. CABG improves survival in patients with left main coronary stenosis and those with symptomatic three-vessel coronary disease; the benefit is greatest in those with impaired LV function or positive stress testing prior to surgery. Approximately 90% of patients are free of angina 1 yr after surgery, but <60% of patients are asymptomatic ≥5 yrs after CABG. Arterial grafts have much better long-term patency rates than vein grafts. Treatment with aspirin or clopidogrel improves graft patency, while intensive lipid-lowering therapy slows progression of disease in the native coronary arteries and grafts. Persistent smokers are twice as likely to die in the 10 yrs following surgery compared with those who give up at surgery.

UNSTABLE ANGINA

Unstable angina refers to new-onset or rapidly worsening angina (crescendo angina), angina on minimal exertion or angina at rest. It may present de novo or against a background of chronic stable angina. The underlying pathophysiology (fissured atheromatous plaque with adherent thrombus formation) is the same as in acute MI. The term 'acute coronary syndrome' is used to describe these disorders collectively and encompasses ischaemia with no myocardial damage, partial thickness (non-ST elevation) myocardial infarction (NSTEMI), and full-thickness (ST-elevation) myocardial infarction (STEMI).

Investigations

• ECG is the most important investigation in the assessment of acute chest pain and guides initial therapy (Fig. 8.12). In patients with unstable angina or NSTEMI, the ECG may show ST/T-wave changes including ST depression, transient ST elevation and T-wave inversion. • Serial measurements of biochemical markers of cardiac damage, such as troponins, also assist in diagnosis and risk stratification. • Unstable angina and NSTEMI carry a high risk of progression to STEMI or death, and risk stratification guides the use of more complex pharmacological and interventional treatment (Box 8.9). • Risk markers indicative of an adverse prognosis include recurrent ischaemia, extensive ECG changes, elevated troponin, arrhythmias and haemodynamic complications (e.g. hypotension) during ischaemic episodes.

Management

• Initial treatment includes combined antiplatelet therapy with aspirin and clopidogrel, low molecular weight heparin and a β-blocker. • I.v. nitrates

8.9 UNSTABLE ANGINA: RISK STRATIFICATION

	High risk	Low risk
Clinical	Post-infarct angina Recurrent pain at rest Heart failure	No history of MI Rapid resolution of symptoms
ECG	Arrhythmia ST depression Transient ST elevation Persistent deep T-wave inversion	Minor or no ECG changes
Biochemistry	Troponin T >0.1 μg/l	Troponin T <0.1 μg/l

N.B. There is a 5- to 10-fold difference in risk between the lowest and highest risk groups.

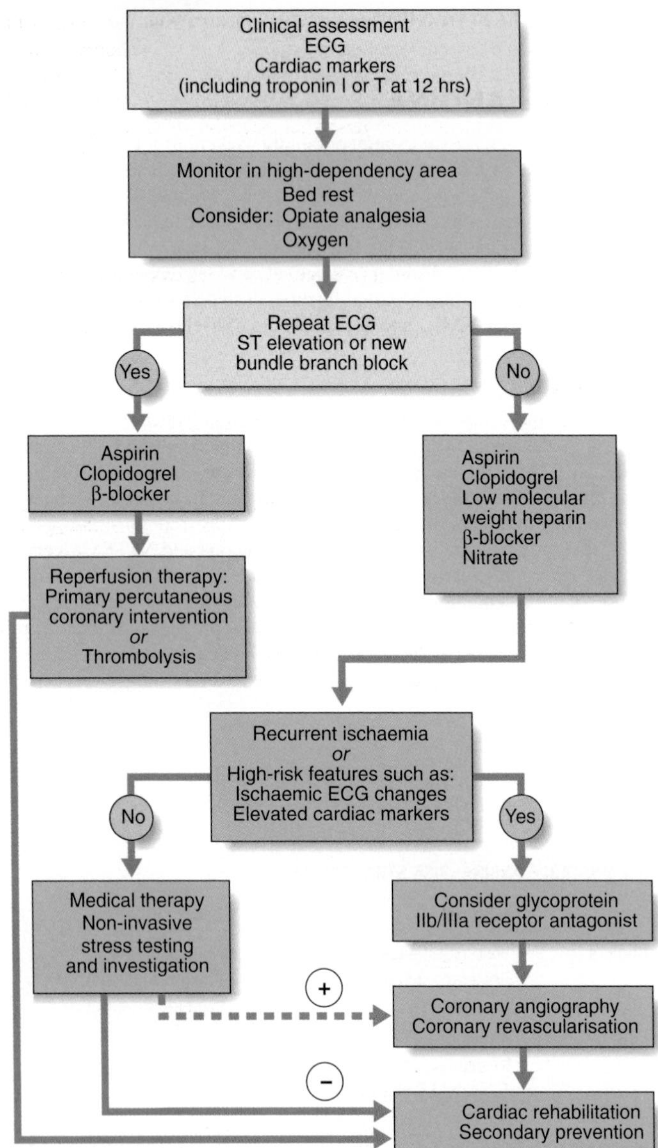

Fig. 8.12 Summary of treatment for unstable angina and non-ST elevation myocardial infarct. (BBB = bundle branch block; LMWH = low molecular weight heparin; PCI = percutaneous coronary intervention)

may help if pain persists or recurs. • Most low-risk patients stabilise with these measures and can undergo exercise testing prior to or shortly following discharge. • Coronary angiography, with a view to PCI or surgery, should be considered in all patients at moderate or high risk, those who fail to settle on medical therapy and those with extensive ECG changes or elevated plasma troponin. • The addition of a glycoprotein IIb/IIIa antagonist may be helpful in these patients.

MYOCARDIAL INFARCTION (MI)

MI is almost always due to the formation of occlusive thrombus at the site of rupture or erosion of an atheromatous plaque in a coronary artery. Most patients present when it is still possible to salvage myocardium and improve outcome.

Clinical features

The typical presentation of MI is described on page 210.

• In some patients breathlessness is the only symptom, while in others (particularly older or diabetic patients) the infarct may go unrecognised (silent MI). • Syncope may occur due to an arrhythmia or profound hypotension. • Vomiting and sinus bradycardia resulting from vagal stimulation are particularly common with inferior MI. • Sudden death, from VF or asystole, frequently occurs within the first hour.

Investigations

ECG: Shows a characteristic series of changes (Fig. 8.13):

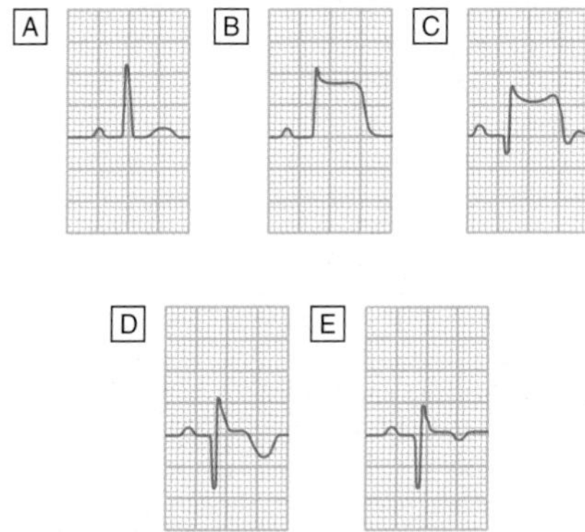

Fig. 8.13 The serial evolution of ECG changes in full-thickness MI. **A** Normal ECG complex. **B** (Minutes) Acute ST elevation. **C** (Hours) Progressive loss of the R wave, developing Q wave, resolution of the ST elevation and terminal T-wave inversion. **D** (Days) Deep Q wave and T-wave inversion. **E** (Weeks or months) Old or established infarct pattern; the Q wave tends to persist but the T-wave changes become less marked.

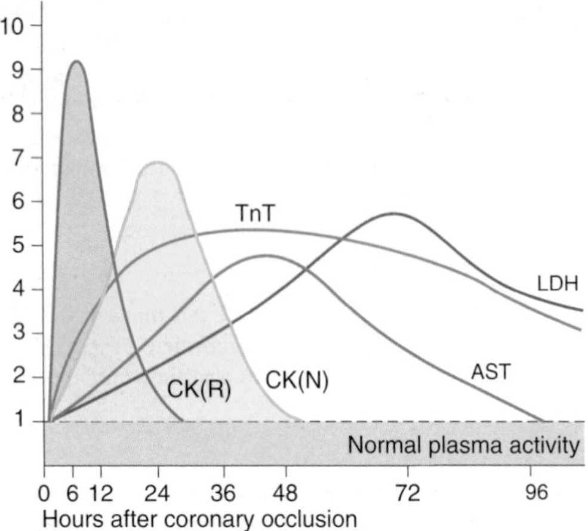

Fig. 8.14 Changes in plasma enzyme concentrations after MI. Creatine kinase (CK) and troponin T (TnT) are the first to rise, followed by aspartate aminotransferase (AST) and then lactate (hydroxybutyrate) dehydrogenase (LDH). In patients treated with a thrombolytic agent, reperfusion is usually accompanied by a rapid rise in plasma creatine kinase (curve CK(R)) due to a washout effect; if there is no reperfusion, the rise is less rapid but the area under the curve is often greater (curve CK(N)).

• The earliest change is usually ST elevation followed by diminution in the size of the R wave, and development of a Q wave (indicating full-thickness infarction). • Subsequently, the T wave becomes inverted and this change persists after the ST segment has returned to normal. • ECG changes are best seen in the leads that 'face' the infarcted area. • With anteroseptal infarction, abnormalities are found in one or more leads from V_1 to V_4. • Anterolateral infarction produces changes from V_4 to V_6, in aVL and lead I. • Inferior infarction is best shown in leads II, III and aVF. • Infarction of the posterior wall of the left ventricle does not cause ST elevation or Q waves in the standard leads, but can be diagnosed by the presence of reciprocal changes (ST depression and a tall R wave in leads V_1–V_4). • Occasionally, new onset LBBB is the only CCG change.

***Plasma biochemical markers* (Fig. 8.14):** The plasma concentration of enzymes and proteins normally concentrated within cardiac cells is increased in MI. Creatine kinase (CK) and CK-MB (a cardiospecific isoform) start to rise at 4–6 hrs, peak at about 12 hrs and fall to normal within 48–72 hrs. The most sensitive markers of myocardial cell damage are the cardiac troponins T and I, which are released within 4–6 hrs and remain elevated for up to 2 wks.

Echocardiography: Can be performed at the bedside. This is a very useful technique for assessing LV and RV function and for detecting important complications such as mural thrombus, cardiac rupture, ventricular septal defect, mitral regurgitation and pericardial effusion.

EARLY MANAGEMENT

Immediate measures include:

• High-flow oxygen. • Analgesia (i.v. opiates). • I.v. antiemetic (metoclopramide). • Oral aspirin (300 mg).

Analgesia is essential to relieve distress, and also to lower adrenergic drive and susceptibility to arrhythmias.

Acute reperfusion therapy

Thrombolysis: Helps to restore coronary patency, preserves LV function and reduces the mortality of MI by 25–50%. Successful thrombolysis leads to reperfusion with relief of pain and resolution of acute ST elevation. It is indicated only in patients presenting within 12 hrs of the onset of symptoms and with ECG changes of LBBB or ST segment elevation of >1 mm in the limb leads or 2 mm in the chest leads. The benefit is greatest when treatment is given within the first few hours.

• Streptokinase (1.5 million U in 100 ml normal saline i.v. over 1 hr) is widely used but may cause hypotension and, due to its antigenicity, serious allergic manifestations. Circulating neutralising antibodies are formed following treatment and this can render subsequent infusions of streptokinase ineffective. • Alteplase (human tissue plasminogen activator (tPA) 15 mg bolus then 0.75 mg/kg up to 50 mg over 30 mins, then 0.5 mg/kg up to 35 mg over 60 mins) is not antigenic, seldom causes hypotension and may produce better survival rates than streptokinase, particularly among high-risk patients (e.g. large anterior infarct), but with a slightly higher risk of intracerebral bleeding. • Newer-generation analogues of tPA such as tenecteplase and reteplase have equivalent efficacy to alteplase but have a longer plasma half-life and can be given by bolus administration. • The major hazard of thrombolytic therapy is bleeding, particularly cerebral haemorrhage. Serious risk of bleeding is one of several relative contraindications to thrombolytic therapy (Box 8.10).

PCI: Offers a 50% greater reduction in the risk of death, recurrent MI or stroke compared with thrombolytic therapy and, when available, is the reperfusion treatment of choice. PCI is especially useful in patients with contraindications to thrombolytic therapy.

8.10 RELATIVE CONTRAINDICATIONS TO THROMBOLYTIC THERAPY (POTENTIAL CANDIDATES FOR PRIMARY ANGIOPLASTY)

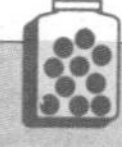

- Active internal bleeding
- Previous subarachnoid or intracerebral haemorrhage
- Uncontrolled hypertension
- Recent surgery (within 1 mth)
- Recent trauma (including traumatic resuscitation)
- High probability of active peptic ulcer
- Pregnancy

Maintaining vessel patency

Antiplatelet therapy: Oral administration of aspirin (300 mg initially then 75 mg daily) improves survival (30% reduction in mortality) on its own, and complements the effect of thrombolytic therapy. In combination with aspirin, the early (within 12 hrs) use of clopidogrel (75 mg daily) confers a further 10% reduction in mortality.

Unfractionated or low molecular weight heparin: May prevent reinfarction after successful thrombolysis and reduce the risk of thromboembolic complications.

Adjunctive therapy

• I.V. β-blockers relieve pain, reduce arrhythmias and improve short-term mortality in patients who present within 12 hrs of the onset of symptoms, but should be avoided if there is heart failure, AV block or bradycardia. • I.V. nitrates are useful for the treatment of LV failure and the relief of recurrent or persistent ischaemic pain.

COMPLICATIONS OF INFARCTION

Arrhythmias

Nearly all patients with acute MI have some form of arrhythmia; pain relief, rest and the correction of hypokalaemia are important preventative measures. • VF occurs in about 5–10% of patients who reach hospital. Prompt defibrillation usually restores sinus rhythm. Early VF (within the first 48 hrs) does not adversely alter long-term prognosis, provided patients are promptly resuscitated. • AV block complicating inferior infarction is usually temporary and often resolves following reperfusion. • AV block complicating anterior infarction carries a risk of asystole and a prophylactic temporary pacemaker should be inserted. • Other common peri-infarct arrhythmias include sinus tachycardia, sinus bradycardia, AF, VT and idioventricular rhythm.

Acute circulatory failure

Acute circulatory failure usually reflects extensive myocardial damage and indicates a bad prognosis.

Hypotension, oliguria, confusion and cold, clammy peripheries are the manifestations of a low cardiac output, whereas breathlessness, hypoxia, cyanosis and inspiratory crackles at the lung bases are typical features of pulmonary oedema. If necessary, a Swan–Ganz catheter can be used to measure the pulmonary artery wedge pressure: an indirect measure of left atrial pressure that guides fluid replacement. Inotropic agents may be required to augment cardiac output and insertion of an intra-aortic balloon pump can be very beneficial. Since viable myocardium surrounding a fresh infarct may contract poorly for a few days and then recover (myocardial stunning), it is often worth treating cardiogenic shock energetically in the hope that cardiac function will improve.

Pericarditis

This is particularly common on the second and third days. Opiate analgesics are preferred over non-steroidal and steroidal anti-inflammatory drugs as the latter may increase the risk of aneurysm formation and myocardial rupture. Dressler's syndrome is an autoimmune disorder that occurs weeks to months after the infarct and is characterised by persistent fever, pericarditis and pleurisy. Severe symptoms may require treatment with an NSAID or corticosteroids.

Mechanical complications

Papillary muscle damage may cause acute pulmonary oedema and shock with a pansystolic murmur due to the sudden onset of severe mitral regurgitation. Emergency mitral valve replacement may be necessary. Rupture of the interventricular septum usually presents with sudden haemodynamic deterioration accompanied by a new loud pansystolic murmur. It may be difficult to distinguish from acute mitral regurgitation but tends to cause right heart failure rather than pulmonary oedema. Doppler echocardiography will confirm the diagnosis. Without prompt surgery, the condition is usually fatal. Rupture of the ventricle leads to cardiac tamponade and is usually fatal.

Other recognised peri-infarct complications

These include:

• Recurrent ischaemia. • Systemic embolism from a cardiac thrombus. • Development of a ventricular aneurysm.

LATE MANAGEMENT

Risk stratification and further investigation

• Patients without spontaneous ischaemia should undergo an exercise tolerance test ~4 wks after the infarct. • Coronary angiography, with a view to revascularisation, should be considered in patients with spontaneous ischaemia, significant angina on effort, or a strongly positive exercise tolerance test. • The presence of ventricular arrhythmias in the weeks following MI may be a marker of poor ventricular function and risk of sudden death. • Empirical anti-arrhythmic treatment appears to be of no value, but selected patients may benefit from specific anti-arrhythmic therapy (e.g. ICDs).

Mobilisation and rehabilitation

When there are no complications, the patient can return home in 5 days and gradually increase activity with the aim of returning to work in 4–6 wks. The majority of patients may resume driving after 4–6 wks. Emotional problems, such as anxiety and depression, are common, and must be recognised and dealt with accordingly. Formal rehabilitation programmes based on graded exercise protocols with individual and group counselling are often very successful.

Secondary prevention

• Smoking cessation reduces 5-yr mortality of post-MI patients by 50% and is the single most effective contribution a patient can make to his or her own future. • Statins reduce the subsequent risk of death, reinfarction and stroke, and should be prescribed for all patients after MI. • Maintaining an ideal body weight, taking regular exercise, and achieving good control of hypertension and diabetes may all improve the long-term outlook. • Low-dose aspirin therapy reduces the risk of further infarction and other vascular events by ~25% and should be continued indefinitely. • Clopidogrel should be given in addition to aspirin for 4 wks and is a suitable alternative in aspirin-intolerant patients. • Long-term β-blocker therapy reduces mortality by ~25% in survivors of acute MI and should be prescribed unless there are specific contraindications (p. 763). • ACE inhibitors can prevent the onset of heart failure, improve survival and reduce hospitalisation, and should be considered in all post-infarct patients. • Patients with acute MI complicated by heart failure and LV dysfunction appear to benefit from additional aldosterone receptor antagonism (e.g. eplerenone 25–50 mg daily). • ICDs reduce the incidence of sudden cardiac death in patients with severe LV impairment (ejection fraction ≤30%) post-MI.

Prognosis

Of those who survive an acute attack, >80% live for a further year, ~75% for 5 yrs and 50% for 10 yrs. Early death is usually due to an arrhythmia but later on the outcome is determined by the extent of myocardial damage. Unfavourable features include poor LV function, AV block and persistent ventricular arrhythmias. The prognosis is worse for anterior than for inferior infarcts.

VASCULAR DISEASE

PERIPHERAL ARTERIAL DISEASE (PAD)

Almost all PAD is due to atherosclerosis and it shares the same risk factors as CHD. Around 20% of UK adults aged 55–75 yrs have PAD but only one-quarter have symptoms. PAD affects the leg eight times more often than the arm. The presence and severity of lower limb ischaemia can be determined by clinical examination (Box 8.11) and measurement of the ankle : brachial pressure index, the ratio between systolic ankle and brachial BPs (ABPI, normal >1.0). Chronic lower limb ischaemia presents as two distinct clinical entities: intermittent claudication (IC, ABPI 0.5–0.9) and critical limb ischaemia (CLI, ABPI <0.5).

INTERMITTENT CLAUDICATION (IC)

IC refers to ischaemic pain of the leg muscles precipitated by walking and relieved by rest. It is usually felt in the calf muscles (superficial femoral artery disease) but may occur in the thigh or buttock (iliac artery disease).

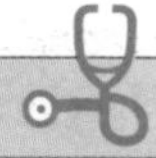

8.11 FEATURES OF CHRONIC LOWER LIMB ISCHAEMIA

- Pulses—diminished or absent
- Bruits—denote turbulent flow but bear no relationship to the severity of the underlying disease
- Reduced skin temperature
- Pallor on elevation and rubor on dependency (Buerger's sign)
- Superficial veins that fill sluggishly and empty ('gutter') upon minimal elevation
- Muscle-wasting
- Skin and nails—dry, thin and brittle
- Loss of hair

Typically, the pain comes on after a reasonably constant 'claudication distance' and rapidly resolves on stopping.

All patients with PAD should receive 'best medical therapy' (BMT), which comprises standard secondary prevention measures for atherosclerosis (smoking cessation, regular exercise, low-dose aspirin, identification and treatment of hypercholesterolaemia, hypertension and diabetes) and optimisation of exacerbating conditions (e.g. heart failure, anaemia). Peripheral vasodilators such as cilostazol can improve symptoms. Intervention (angioplasty, stenting, endarterectomy or bypass) is usually only considered after 6 mths of BMT, and then only in patients whose disability is severe or threatens their livelihood. Provided patients comply with BMT, only 1–2%/yr will require amputation and/or revascularisation, but the annual mortality rate exceeds 5%, reflecting a high incidence of MI and stroke.

CRITICAL LIMB ISCHAEMIA (CLI)

This is defined as rest (night) pain, requiring opiate analgesia, and/or tissue loss (ulceration or gangrene), present for >2 wks, in the presence of an ankle BP <50 mmHg. Whereas IC is usually due to single-segment plaque, CLI is always due to multi-level disease. Patients are at risk of losing their limb (or life) in a matter of weeks or months without surgical bypass or endovascular revascularisation, but treatment is difficult because they are often elderly with significant multisystem comorbidity and have severe multi-level disease.

• Imaging is performed using duplex ultrasonography. • More detailed non-invasive imaging can be provided by contrast MRI or CT. • Intra-arterial digital subtraction angiography is mainly used for patients considered suitable for endovascular revascularisation.

ACUTE LOWER LIMB ISCHAEMIA (ALI)

ALI is most frequently caused by acute thrombotic occlusion of a pre-existing arterial stenosis or thromboembolism (often secondary to AF). All

8.12 SYMPTOMS AND SIGNS OF ACUTE LIMB ISCHAEMIA	
Symptoms/signs	**Comment**
Pain Pallor Pulselessness	May be absent in complete acute ischaemia, and can be present in chronic ischaemia
Perishing cold	Unreliable, as the ischaemic limb takes on the ambient temperature
Paraesthesia Paralysis	Important features of impending irreversible ischaemia

suspected acutely ischaemic limbs (Box 8.12) must be discussed immediately with a vascular surgeon. If there are no contraindications, an i.v. bolus of heparin (3000–5000 U) should be given to limit thrombus propagation and protect the collateral circulation. Distinguishing thrombosis from embolism is frequently difficult. Evidence of chronic lower limb ischaemia (e.g. previous IC symptoms, bruits, diminished contralateral pulses) favours thrombosis, while the absence of such features and the presence of AF favour embolism.

• ALI due to thrombosis can often be treated medically with i.v. heparin (target APTT 2.0–3.0), antiplatelet agents, high-dose statins, i.v. fluids and oxygen. • ALI due to embolus (no collateral circulation) normally results in extensive tissue necrosis within 6 hrs unless the limb is revascularised. • Irreversible ischaemia mandates early amputation or palliative therapy.

DISEASES OF THE AORTA

ABDOMINAL AORTIC ANEURYSMS (AAAs)

An aortic aneurysm is an abnormal dilatation of the aortic wall. The most important risk factors for aneurysmal disease are male gender, family history, hypertension and smoking. Median age at presentation is 65 yrs for elective and 75 yrs for emergency cases.

• Many AAAs are asymptomatic and found incidentally, but they may cause central abdominal pain or lower limb embolic complications. • USS establishes the diagnosis and is used to follow up the size of asymptomatic AAAs; elective repair is considered if the diameter exceeds 5.5 cm. • All symptomatic AAAs should be considered for repair, not least because pain often predates rupture. Distal embolisation is a strong indication for repair. • Rupture of an AAA produces severe abdominal pain with hypovolaemic shock and is rapidly fatal. Operative mortality for ruptured AAA is ~50% but patients who survive to leave hospital have a good prognosis. • Some AAAs may be treated with a covered stent insertion under radiological guidance.

THORACIC AORTIC ANEURYSM

These may produce chest pain similar to cardiac pain, associated with expansion of the aneurysm, or aortic valve regurgitation if they extend proximally. Occasionally, they may erode into the adjacent structures, causing haemorrhage, tamponade and death. In Marfan's syndrome, an autosomal dominant connective tissue disorder caused by mutation in the fibrillin gene, weakening of the aortic media leads to progressive dilatation of the ascending aorta that may be complicated by aortic regurgitation and aortic dissection (see below). CXR, echocardiography, MRI or CT may detect aortic dilatation at an early stage and can be used to monitor the disease. Treatment with β-blockers reduces the rate of aortic dilatation and the risk of rupture.

AORTIC DISSECTION

A tear in the intima of the aortic wall allows arterial blood to burst into the media of the aorta, which is then split into two layers, creating a 'false lumen' alongside the existing or 'true lumen'. It is classified into type A and type B, involving or sparing the ascending aorta respectively. Aortic atherosclerosis and hypertension are common aetiological factors but other predisposing conditions include thoracic aortic aneurysm, aortic coarctation, previous aortic surgery, Marfan's syndrome and pregnancy.

• The patient typically presents with sudden-onset, severe 'tearing' chest pain often associated with collapse. • In type A dissection, the aortic valve may be damaged, causing acute regurgitation. • Occlusion of aortic branches may cause a variety of symptoms as well as asymmetry of the brachial, carotid or femoral pulses. • The CXR may show broadening of the upper mediastinum and distortion of the aortic 'knuckle', but these findings are absent in 10% of cases. • Transthoracic echocardiography can only image the first 3–4 cm of the ascending aorta but transoesophageal echocardiography, CT and MRI are all very useful. • Early mortality of acute dissection is ~1%/hr. • Initial management comprises pain control and i.v. labetalol (target systolic BP <120 mmHg). • Type A dissections require emergency surgical repair. • Type B dissections can usually be treated medically.

HYPERTENSION

High BP represents a quantitative rather than a qualitative deviation from the norm and any definition of hypertension is therefore arbitrary. The British Hypertension Society defines hypertension as a BP >140/90 mmHg. However, the incidence of cardiovascular disease (particularly stroke and CHD) is closely related to average BP at all ages, even when readings are within the 'normal range'.

In >95% of cases, no specific underlying cause of hypertension can be found and such patients are said to have essential hypertension. Important predisposing factors for essential hypertension include:

• Race (higher incidence in Black Americans and Japanese). • Genetic factors. • High salt intake. • Alcohol excess. • Obesity. • Lack of exercise. • Impaired intrauterine growth.

In ~5% of cases, hypertension results from a specific underlying disorder (secondary hypertension). Causes include:

• Renal disease (renal vascular disease, glomerulonephritis, polycystic kidney disease; see Ch. 7). • Endocrine disorders (phaeochromocytoma, Cushing's syndrome, Conn's syndrome, acromegaly, thyrotoxicosis, congenital adrenal hyperplasia; see Ch. 10). • Pregnancy. • Coarctation of the aorta. • Drugs (corticosteroids, oestrogen-containing oral contraceptive pill, anabolic steroids).

Target organ damage

Blood vessels: Widespread atheroma develops and may lead to coronary and/or cerebrovascular disease, particularly if other risk factors are present. Hypertension is also implicated in the pathogenesis of aortic aneurysm and aortic dissection. Structural changes in the vasculature often perpetuate and aggravate hypertension by increasing peripheral vascular resistance and reducing renal function.

CNS: Stroke, due to either cerebral haemorrhage or infarction, and TIAs are common complications. Subarachnoid haemorrhage is also associated with hypertension. Hypertensive encephalopathy is a rare condition characterised by high BP, neurological symptoms (e.g. speech and visual disturbance, disorientation, fits) and evidence of haemorrhage in and around the basal ganglia on CT scan. The neurological deficit is usually reversible with adequate control of hypertension.

Retina: The optic fundi reveal a gradation of changes linked to the severity of hypertension (Box 8.13). Hypertension is also associated with central retinal vein thrombosis.

Heart: The excess cardiac mortality and morbidity associated with hypertension are largely due to a higher incidence of CHD. High BP also places a pressure load on the heart and may lead to left ventricular hypertrophy (LVH) or, if severe, LV failure, even in the absence of coronary disease. ECG or echocardiographic evidence of LVH is highly predictive

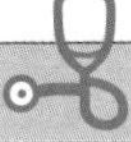

8.13 HYPERTENSIVE RETINOPATHY

Grade 1	Arteriolar thickening, tortuosity and increased reflectiveness ('silver wiring')
Grade 2	Grade 1 plus constriction of veins at arterial crossings ('arteriovenous nipping')
Grade 3	Grade 2 plus evidence of retinal ischaemia (flame-shaped or blot haemorrhages and 'cotton wool' exudates)
Grade 4	Grade 3 plus papilloedema

of cardiovascular complications and therefore particularly useful in risk assessment.

Kidneys: Long-standing hypertension may cause proteinuria and progressive renal failure (p. 180) by damaging the renal vasculature.

'Malignant' or 'accelerated' phase hypertension: This rare condition is characterised by accelerated microvascular damage and intravascular thrombosis. The diagnosis is based on evidence of high BP and rapidly progressive end organ damage such as retinopathy (grade 3 or 4), renal dysfunction (especially proteinuria) and/or hypertensive encephalopathy.

Clinical features

Hypertension occasionally causes headache but most patients remain asymptomatic. Accordingly, the diagnosis is usually made at routine examination or when a complication arises. Initial evaluation in hypertension includes:

• Accurate and representative measurements of BP. • Identification of underlying disorders (secondary hypertension). • Assessment of cardiovascular risk. • Detection of any target organ damage.

The history may reveal a family history, lifestyle factors (exercise, salt intake, smoking, alcohol intake) and potential drug causes. There may be symptoms suggesting a secondary cause such as phaeochromocytoma (paroxysmal headache, palpitation and sweating) or complications such as CHD (e.g. angina).

Examination may reveal radio-femoral delay (coarctation of the aorta), enlarged kidneys (polycystic kidney disease), abdominal bruits (renal artery stenosis) or features of endocrine disease. More commonly there may be signs attributable to the complications of hypertension, such as LVH (apical heave, fourth heart sound) or retinopathy (Box 8.13).

Investigations

Antihypertensive therapy is commonly life-long treatment, so it is vital that the BP readings on which the treatment decision is based are as accurate as possible. Sphygmomanometry, particularly when performed by a doctor, can cause an unrepresentative surge in BP ('white coat' hypertension). A series of automated ambulatory BP measurements, obtained over 24 hrs or longer, provides a better profile than a limited number of clinic readings. These may be particularly helpful in patients with unusually labile BP, those with refractory hypertension, those who may be experiencing symptomatic hypotension, and those in whom white coat hypertension is suspected.

• Routine investigations in all hypertensive patients should include urinalysis for blood, protein and glucose, U&Es, blood glucose, serum lipids and 12-lead ECG. • Additional investigations are appropriate in selected patients to identify target organ damage (e.g. echocardiography) or potential causes of secondary hypertension (e.g. renal USS, urinary catecholamines).

Management

The sole objective of antihypertensive therapy is to reduce the incidence of adverse cardiovascular events. The relative benefit of BP reduction (~30% reduction in risk of stroke and 20% reduction in risk of CHD) is similar in all patient groups, so the absolute benefit of treatment is greatest in those at highest risk. Decisions on treatment should therefore be guided by an overall assessment of cardiovascular risk. The British Hypertension Society guidelines for treatment thresholds are shown in Figure 8.15. The lower threshold for initiating antihypertensive therapy in patients with diabetes or cardiovascular disease reflects the high risk in these groups.

The following measures can not only lower BP but also directly reduce cardiovascular risk:

• Correcting obesity. • Reducing alcohol intake. • Restricting salt intake. • Taking regular physical exercise. • Increasing consumption of fruit and vegetables.

The major classes of hypertensive drug are:

• Thiazide diuretics. • β-blockers. • Calcium channel blockers. • ACE inhibitors. • Angiotensin receptor blockers. • Alpha-blockers.

A detailed description of these agents is provided in Chapter 18. Combination therapy is often required to achieve adequate control, and a recommended treatment algorithm is shown in Figure 8.16. However, comorbid conditions may have an important influence on initial drug selection (e.g. a β-blocker might be the most appropriate treatment for a patient with angina, but should be avoided in asthma). Adjuvant therapy with antiplatelet and lipid-lowering agents may be indicated in hypertensive patients with a high cardiovascular risk.

In accelerated phase hypertension, rapid lowering of BP may compromise tissue perfusion, leading to cerebral damage or to coronary or renal insufficiency. A controlled reduction, to a level of about 150/90 mmHg, over a period of 24–48 hrs, is ideal. In most patients it is possible to bring BP under control with oral agents. Where necessary, i.v. labetalol, GTN and sodium nitroprusside are all effective remedies but require careful supervision, preferably in a high-dependency unit.

HEART FAILURE

Heart failure describes the state that develops when the heart cannot maintain an adequate cardiac output or can do so only at the expense of elevated filling pressures. The prevalence rises from ~1% in the age group 50–59 yrs to between 5 and 10% of those aged 80–89 yrs. Overall, the prognosis is poor; ~50% of patients with severe heart failure due to LV dysfunction die within 2 yrs, many from ventricular arrhythmias or MI.

Almost all forms of heart disease can lead to heart failure (Box 8.14) but, irrespective of the original insult, the resulting decline in cardiac output may establish a downward spiral of events. Cardiac output is a function of

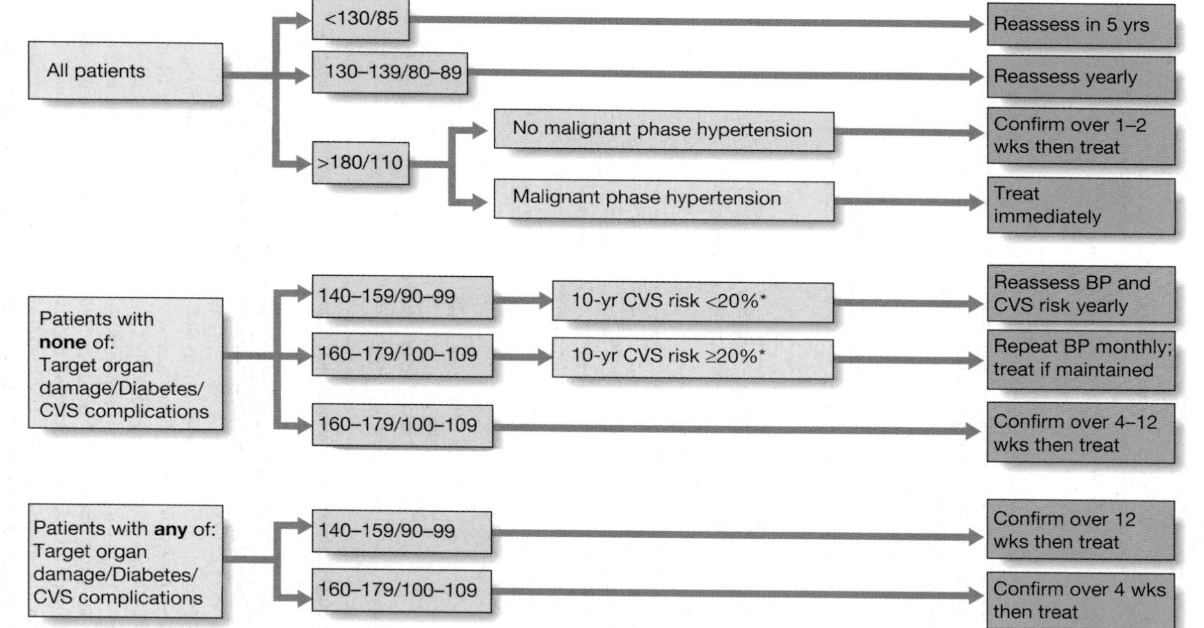

Fig. 8.15 Management of hypertension: British Hypertension Society guidelines. Initial blood pressure thresholds shown in mmHg. (* Assessed with risk chart for cardiovascular disease. See http://www.bhsoc.org/resources/prediction_chart.htm)

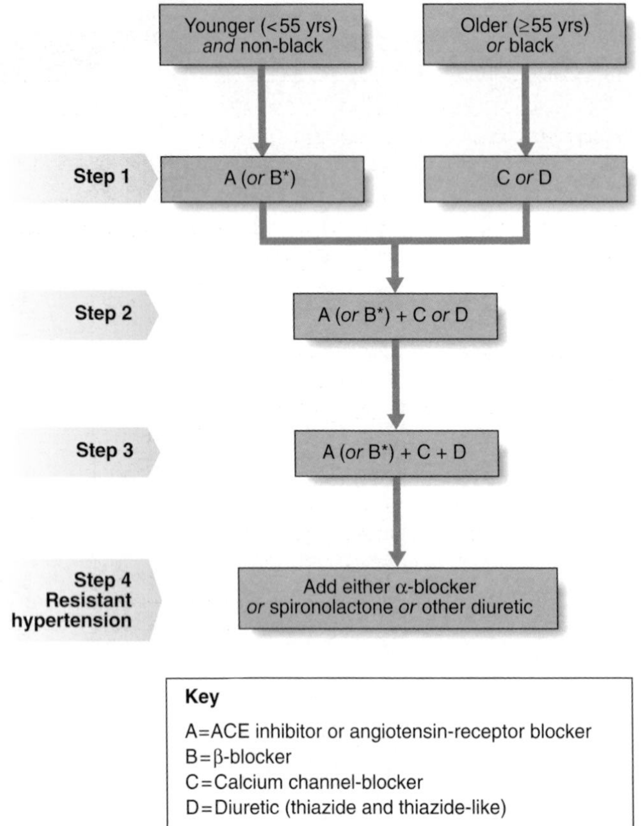

Fig. 8.16 Antihypertensive drug combinations. (* Combination therapy involving B and D may induce more new-onset diabetes compared with other combination therapies.)

the preload, the afterload and myocardial contractility (Figure 8.17). When cardiac output falls, impaired renal perfusion causes stimulation of the renin–angiotensin–aldosterone system (RAAS), leading to arteriolar vasoconstriction (↑afterload) and salt and water retention. Activation of the sympathetic nervous system also occurs and may initially maintain cardiac output through an increase in myocardial contractility, heart rate and venous return. However, prolonged stimulation leads to cardiac myocyte apoptosis, hypertrophy and focal myocardial necrosis (↓contractility), as well as peripheral vasoconstriction (↑afterload). These changes produce a further fall in cardiac output, which leads to even greater neurohormonal activation, thus establishing a vicious circle. The onset of pulmonary and/or

8.14 MECHANISMS OF HEART FAILURE

Cause	Examples
Reduced ventricular contractility	MI (segmental dysfunction) Myocarditis/cardiomyopathy (global dysfunction)
Ventricular outflow obstruction (pressure overload)	Hypertension, aortic stenosis (left heart failure) Pulmonary hypertension, pulmonary valve stenosis (right heart failure)
Ventricular inflow obstruction	Mitral stenosis, tricuspid stenosis
Ventricular volume overload	LV volume overload (e.g. mitral or aortic regurgitation) Ventricular septal defect RV volume overload (e.g. atrial septal defect)
Arrhythmia	Tachycardia-induced cardiomyopathy Complete heart block
Diastolic dysfunction	Constrictive pericarditis Restrictive cardiomyopathy LV hypertrophy and fibrosis Cardiac tamponade

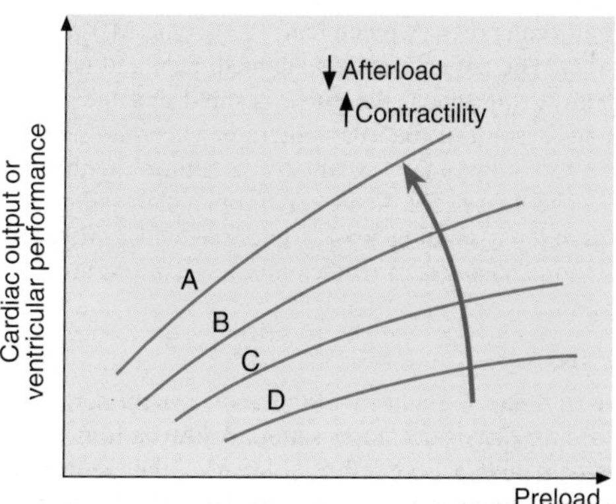

Fig. 8.17 Starling's Law. Normal (A), mild (B), moderate (C) and severe (D) heart failure. Ventricular performance is related to the degree of myocardial stretching. An increase in preload (end-diastolic volume, end-diastolic pressure, filling pressure or atrial pressure) will therefore enhance function; however, overstretching causes marked deterioration. In heart failure the curve moves to the right and becomes flatter. An increase in myocardial contractility or a reduction in afterload will shift the curve upwards and to the left.

peripheral oedema is due to high atrial pressures compounded by salt and water retention.

TYPES OF HEART FAILURE

• In left-sided heart failure, there is a reduction in LV output and/or an increase in the left atrial or pulmonary venous pressure. An acute increase in left atrial pressure may cause pulmonary oedema; a more gradual increase leads to reflex pulmonary vasoconstriction and pulmonary hypertension. • In right-sided heart failure (e.g. chronic lung disease, multiple pulmonary emboli) there is a reduction in RV output for any given right atrial pressure. • Biventricular heart failure may develop because the disease process (e.g. dilated cardiomyopathy) affects both ventricles, or because left heart failure leads to chronic elevation of left atrial pressure, pulmonary hypertension and right heart failure. Heart failure may develop suddenly (acute heart failure) or gradually (chronic heart failure). • The phrase 'compensated heart failure' is sometimes used to describe a patient with impaired cardiac function in whom adaptive changes have prevented the development of overt heart failure. • Acute left heart failure occurs either de novo or as an acute decompensated episode on a background of chronic heart failure (acute-on-chronic heart failure). • Heart failure may develop as a result of impaired myocardial contraction (systolic dysfunction) or poor ventricular filling caused by abnormal ventricular relaxation (diastolic dysfunction).

CLINICAL FEATURES

Acute de novo LV failure

This usually presents with sudden-onset dyspnoea at rest that rapidly progresses to acute respiratory distress. A precipitant (e.g. acute MI) may be apparent from the history. The patient appears agitated, pale and clammy. The peripheries are cool to the touch, the pulse is rapid and the JVP is usually elevated. The apex is not displaced, as there has been no time for ventricular dilatation. Auscultation may reveal a triple 'gallop' rhythm and crepitations are heard at the lung bases. Acute-on-chronic heart failure will have additional features of long-standing heart failure (see below). Potential precipitants (e.g. arrhythmia, changes in medication, intercurrent infective illness) should be identified.

Chronic heart failure

This commonly follows a relapsing and remitting course, with periods of stability interrupted by episodes of decompensation. A low cardiac output causes fatigue, listlessness and a poor effort tolerance; the peripheries are cold and BP is low. Pulmonary oedema due to left heart failure may present with breathlessness, orthopnoea, paroxysmal nocturnal dyspnoea and inspiratory crepitations over the lung bases. Right heart failure produces a high JVP, with hepatic congestion and dependent peripheral oedema. In ambulant patients the oedema affects the ankles, whereas in bed-bound patients it collects around the thighs and sacrum.

In advanced heart failure a number of non-specific complications may occur:

• Marked weight loss (cardiac cachexia) is caused by a combination of anorexia and impaired absorption due to GI congestion. • Renal failure arises from poor renal perfusion due to a low cardiac output and may be exacerbated by diuretic therapy, ACE inhibitors and angiotensin receptor blockers. • Hyperkalaemia may occur due to the effects of drug treatment (particularly the combination of ACE inhibitors and spironolactone) and renal dysfunction. • Hyponatraemia is caused by diuretic therapy or inappropriate water retention due to high ADH secretion and is a poor prognostic sign. • Atrial and ventricular arrhythmias are very common and may be related to electrolyte changes (e.g. hypokalaemia, hypomagnesaemia), underlying structural heart disease, and the pro-arrhythmic effects of increased circulating catecholamines. • Sudden death occurs in up to 50% of patients, often due to ventricular arrhythmias.

INVESTIGATIONS

• ECG may give clues to the aetiology of heart failure (e.g. LVH, evidence of previous MI). • CXR may reveal cardiomegaly and shows characteristic changes in pulmonary oedema, including distension of upper lobe pulmonary veins, Kerley B lines (horizontal lines in the costophrenic angles indicating interstitial oedema), hazy hilar opacification (alveolar oedema) and pleural effusions (Fig. 8.18). • U&Es, LFTs, TFTs and FBC may help

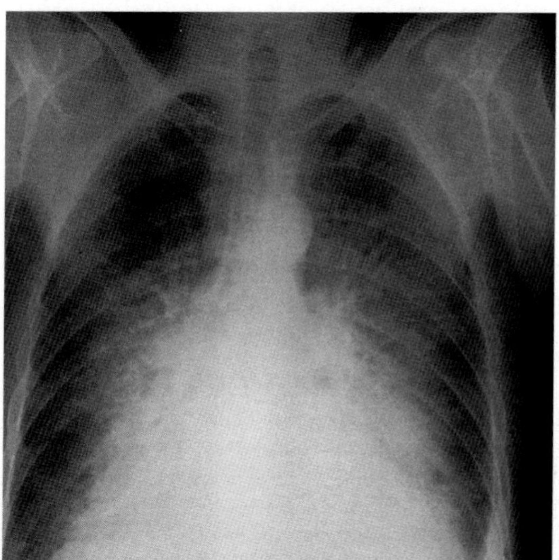

Fig. 8.18 Radiological features of heart failure. CXR of a patient with pulmonary oedema.

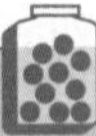

8.15 TREATMENT OF ACUTE PULMONARY OEDEMA
Immediate
• Sitting the patient up in order to reduce pulmonary congestion
• High-concentration oxygen (e.g. 60%)
• Continuous monitoring of cardiac rhythm, BP and oxygen saturation
• Nitrates (e.g. i.v. glyceryl trinitrate 10–200 μg/min or buccal glyceryl trinitrate 2–5 mg) titrated upwards every 10 mins, until clinical improvement occurs or systolic BP falls <110 mmHg
• A loop diuretic such as furosemide 50–100 mg i.v.
Consider
• Continuous positive airway pressure (CPAP) by mask
• I.V. opiates—with caution; can cause respiratory depression
If above measures are ineffective, consider
• Inotropic agents (particularly in hypotensive patients)
• Mechanical ventilation
• Insertion of an intra-aortic balloon pump (particularly in myocardial ischaemia)

to identify some of the complications above, as well as exacerbating factors such as anaemia. • Brain natriuretic peptide (BNP) is elevated in heart failure and can be used as a screening test in breathless patients and those with oedema. • Echocardiography should be considered in all patients with heart failure to determine the aetiology (e.g. valvular disease, regional wall motion defect in MI) and assess the severity of LV impairment.

MANAGEMENT OF ACUTE PULMONARY OEDEMA

This is summarised in Box 8.15.

MANAGEMENT OF CHRONIC HEART FAILURE

General measures

These include:

• Effective education about the condition. • Maintenance of nutritional status. • Smoking cessation. • Avoidance of excessive salt or alcohol intake. • Regular moderate exercise. • Vaccinations for influenza and pneumococcus.

In some cases (e.g. valvular disease, hypertension) it may be possible to remove the underlying cause. In patients with CHD, secondary preventative measures are required (p. 231).

Drug therapy

Diuretics: Reduce plasma volume and cause a small but significant degree of arterial and venous dilatation, thereby reducing preload and improving pulmonary and systemic venous congestion. In some patients with severe chronic heart failure i.v. loop diuretics or combination therapy with a loop and thiazide diuretic may be required. Aldosterone receptor antagonists such as spironolactone and eplerenone are potassium-sparing diuretics that improve long-term clinical outcome in patients with severe heart failure and those with heart failure following acute MI.

ACE inhibitors: Interrupt the vicious circle of neurohormonal activation in chronic heart failure, preventing salt and water retention, peripheral arterial and venous vasoconstriction, and sympathetic nervous system activation. The major haemodynamic benefit of ACE inhibitor therapy in heart failure is a reduction in afterload, possibly accompanied by a small reduction in preload. ACE inhibitors have been clearly shown to reduce mortality and morbidity in chronic heart failure and should be given to all patients. First-dose hypotension can occur and these drugs must be started cautiously.

Angiotensin receptor blockers: Produce beneficial haemodynamic changes similar to those produced by ACE inhibitors, have comparable effects on mortality and are a useful alternative for patients who cannot tolerate ACE inhibitors.

Other vasodilators: May also be useful in the treatment of chronic heart failure. The combination of nitrates (venodilator) and hydralazine (arterial dilator) is effective in patients unable to tolerate either ACE inhibitors or angiotensin receptor blockers.

β-blockers: Help to counteract the deleterious effects of enhanced sympathetic stimulation in chronic heart failure and reduce the risk of arrhythmias and sudden death. They must be introduced gradually to avoid precipitating acute-on-chronic failure but when used appropriately have been shown to increase ejection fraction, improve symptoms and reduce mortality.

Digoxin: Should be used as first-line therapy in patients with heart failure and AF. It may reduce the need for hospitalisation in patients with severe chronic heart failure who are in sinus rhythm, but has no effect on mortality.

Non-drug therapies

Cardiac resynchronisation therapy (p. 229): Restores the normal contraction pattern of the left ventricle, which may be dysynchronous in patients with impaired LV function and LBBB.

Implantable cardiac defibrillators (p. 226): Reduce the risk of sudden death in selected patients with chronic heart failure, particularly those with a history of ventricular arrhythmia.

Revascularisation with CABG or PCI: May improve function in areas of 'hibernating' myocardium with inadequate blood supply, and can be used to treat carefully selected patients with heart failure and coronary artery disease.

Cardiac transplantation: An established and very successful form of treatment for patients with intractable heart failure. Coronary artery disease and dilated cardiomyopathy are the most common indications. The use of transplantation is limited by the availability of donor hearts so it is generally reserved for young patients with severe symptoms. Serious complications include rejection, infection (due to immunosuppressive therapy) and accelerated atherosclerosis.

Ventricular assist devices: Have been employed as a bridge to cardiac transplantation, and more recently as potential long-term therapy. They assist cardiac output by using a roller, centrifugal or pulsatile pump. Their use currently carries a high rate of complication (e.g. haemorrhage, systemic embolism, infection).

DISEASES OF THE HEART VALVES

A diseased valve may be narrowed (stenosed) or it may fail to close adequately, and thus permit regurgitation (or reflux) of blood. Doppler echocardiography is the most useful technique for assessing patients with valvular heart disease, but often detects minor, unimportant abnormalities, such as trivial mitral regurgitation. Disease of the heart valves may progress with time and selected patients require regular review to ensure that deterioration is detected before complications such as heart failure ensue. Patients with valvular heart disease are susceptible to bacterial endocarditis, the risk of which can be reduced by good dental hygiene.

ACUTE RHEUMATIC FEVER (ARF)

ARF usually affects children or young adults. It has become very rare in Western Europe and North America but remains endemic in parts of Asia, Africa and South America. It is triggered by an immune-mediated delayed response to infection with specific strains of group A streptococci that possess antigens which cross-react with cardiac myosin and sarcolemmal membrane protein. Antibodies produced against the streptococcal antigens mediate inflammation in the endocardium, myocardium and pericardium, as well as the joints and skin.

Clinical features

• ARF typically follows an episode of streptococcal pharyngitis and usually presents with fever, anorexia, lethargy and joint pains. • The diagnosis is based on the revised Jones criteria (Box 8.16). • Carditis may involve the endocardium, myocardium and pericardium to varying degrees and manifest as breathlessness (heart failure or pericardial effusion), palpitations or chest pain (pericarditis). • Other features include tachycardia, cardiac enlargement, new murmurs of mitral regurgitation or aortic regurgitation, or a soft diastolic murmur due to mitral valvulitis (Carey Coombs murmur). • Arthritis is the most common major manifestation and is characterised by acute, painful, asymmetric and migratory inflammation of the large joints

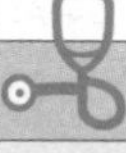

8.16 JONES CRITERIA FOR THE DIAGNOSIS OF RHEUMATIC FEVER	
Major manifestations	
• Carditis • Polyarthritis • Chorea	• Erythema marginatum • Subcutaneous nodules
Minor manifestations	
• Fever • Arthralgia • Previous rheumatic fever	• Raised ESR or CRP • Leucocytosis • First-degree AV block
Notes	
• Diagnosis depends on two or more major manifestations, or one major and two or more minor manifestations PLUS supporting evidence of preceding streptococcal infection: recent scarlet fever, raised antistreptolysin O or other streptococcal antibody titre, positive throat culture • Evidence of recent streptococcal infection is particularly important if there is only one major manifestation	

(knees, ankles, elbows, wrists). • Erythema marginatum appears as red macules which fade in the centre but remain red at the edges and occur mainly on the trunk and proximal extremities but not the face. • Subcutaneous nodules are small, firm, painless and best felt over extensor surfaces of bone or tendons. They usually appear >3 wks after the onset of other manifestations. • Sydenham's chorea (St Vitus dance) is a late (>3 mths) neurological manifestation characterised by emotional lability and purposeless involuntary choreiform movements of the hands, feet or face; spontaneous recovery usually occurs within a few months.

Investigations

• Evidence of preceding streptococcal infection is required (Box 8.17). • Raised WCC, ESR and CRP indicate systemic inflammation and are useful for monitoring progress of the disease. • ECG (AV block, pericarditis) and echocardiography (cardiac dilatation, valve abnormalities) may reveal evidence of carditis.

Management

• Penicillin is given to eliminate any residual streptococcal infection. • Bed rest lessens joint pain and reduces cardiac workload. • Cardiac failure should be treated as necessary. • High-dose aspirin (60–100 mg/kg up to 8 g per day) usually relieves the symptoms of arthritis rapidly and a prompt response helps to confirm the diagnosis. • Corticosteroids (prednisolone 1–2 mg/kg) produce more rapid symptomatic relief and are indicated in carditis or severe arthritis, until the ESR returns to normal. • Patients are

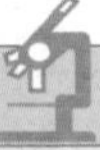

8.17 INVESTIGATIONS IN ACUTE RHEUMATIC FEVER
Evidence of a systemic illness (non-specific)
• Leucocytosis, raised ESR, raised CRP
Evidence of preceding streptococcal infection (specific)
• Throat swab culture: group A β-haemolytic streptococci (also from family members and contacts) • Antistreptolysin O antibodies (ASO titres): rising titres, or levels of >200 U (adults) or >300 U (children)
Evidence of carditis
• CXR: cardiomegaly; pulmonary congestion • ECG: first- and rarely second-degree heart block; features of pericarditis; T-wave inversion; reduction in QRS voltages • Echocardiography: cardiac dilatation and valve abnormalities

susceptible to further attacks of rheumatic fever if subsequent streptococcal infection occurs, and long-term prophylaxis with penicillin should be given, usually until the age of 21.

CHRONIC RHEUMATIC HEART DISEASE

This is characterised by progressive valve fibrosis and develops in at least half of those affected by rheumatic fever with carditis. Some episodes of rheumatic fever may pass unrecognised and it is only possible to elicit a positive history in about half of patients. The mitral valve is affected in >90% of cases, with the aortic valve the next most frequently involved.

MITRAL STENOSIS

Mitral stenosis is almost always rheumatic in origin. The valve orifice is slowly diminished by progressive fibrosis, leaflet calcification and fusion of the cusps and subvalvular apparatus. Restricted blood flow from left atrium to left ventricle causes a rise in left atrial pressure, leading to pulmonary venous congestion and breathlessness, while a low cardiac output may cause fatigue. Patients usually remain asymptomatic until the mitral valve area is approximately 2 cm^2 or less (normal = 5 cm^2). At first, symptoms occur only on exercise; however, in severe stenosis, left atrial pressure is permanently elevated and symptoms may occur at rest. AF due to progressive dilatation of the left atrium is very common. The onset of AF causes a rapid rise in left atrial pressure because ventricular filling depends on left atrial contraction and adequate diastolic filling time. Pulmonary hypertension may lead to RV hypertrophy and dilatation, tricuspid regurgitation and right heart failure. All patients with mitral stenosis, and particularly those with AF, are at risk from left atrial thrombosis and systemic thromboembolism.

Clinical features

• Effort-related dyspnoea is usually the dominant symptom and produces a gradual reduction in exercise tolerance over many years. • The onset of AF may precipitate acute pulmonary oedema. • Haemoptysis and systemic embolism may also occur. • On examination, the patient is usually in AF and a malar flush may be apparent. • The apex beat is characteristically tapping in nature. On auscultation there may be a loud first heart sound, an opening snap and a low-pitched mid-diastolic murmur. • An elevated JVP, RV heave, loud pulmonary component of the second heart sound and features of tricuspid regurgitation all signify the presence of pulmonary hypertension.

Investigations

• ECG may show bifid P waves (P mitrale) due to left atrial hypertrophy, or AF. • CXR may show an enlarged left atrium and features of pulmonary congestion. • Echocardiography provides the definitive evaluation of mitral stenosis, allowing estimation of valve area, pressure gradient across the valve and pulmonary artery pressure.

Management

• Medical management consists of diuretics for pulmonary congestion, and anticoagulants and rate-limiting agents in the presence of AF. • Valve replacement (or where possible, balloon valvuloplasty or valvotomy) should be considered if symptoms persist or if pulmonary hypertension develops.

MITRAL REGURGITATION

Causes of mitral regurgitation are shown in Box 8.18. Chronic mitral regurgitation causes gradual dilatation of the left atrium with little increase in pressure; progressive LV dilatation occurs due to chronic volume overload. Acute mitral regurgitation causes a rapid rise in left atrial pressure, resulting in pulmonary oedema.

Clinical features

• Chronic mitral regurgitation typically causes progressive exertional dyspnoea and fatigue, while sudden-onset mitral regurgitation usually presents

8.18 CAUSES OF MITRAL REGURGITATION

- Mitral valve prolapse
- Dilatation of the left ventricle and mitral valve ring (e.g. coronary artery disease, cardiomyopathy)
- Damage to papillary muscle
- Damage to valve cusps and chordae (e.g. rheumatic heart disease, endocarditis, valvotomy or valvuloplasty)
- MI

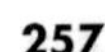

with acute pulmonary oedema. • The regurgitant jet causes an apical systolic murmur which radiates to the axilla. • The first heart sound is quiet and there may be a third heart sound. • The apex beat feels hyperdynamic and is usually displaced to the left, indicating LV dilatation. • Signs of AF, pulmonary venous congestion and pulmonary hypertension may be present.

Investigations

• CXR may show left atrial or ventricular enlargement or features of pulmonary venous congestion (pulmonary oedema if acute). • Echocardiography allows assessment of chamber dimensions, LV function and severity of regurgitation, as well as detection of structural abnormalities of the valve.

Management

• Medical treatment includes diuretics and afterload reduction with vasodilators (e.g. ACE inhibitors). • Regular review is important to detect worsening symptoms, progressive cardiac enlargement and LV impairment, as these are all indications for surgical intervention (mitral valve replacement or repair). • Acute severe mitral regurgitation necessitates emergency valve replacement or repair.

Mitral valve prolapse

This is a common cause of mild mitral regurgitation. It arises from congenital anomalies or degenerative myxomatous changes and is sometimes a feature of connective tissue disorders such as Marfan's syndrome. In mild mitral prolapse, the valve remains competent but bulges back into the atrium during systole, causing a mid-systolic click but no murmur. In the presence of a regurgitant valve, the click is followed by a late systolic murmur. The condition is associated with a variety of benign arrhythmias and atypical chest pain but the overall long-term prognosis is good. If regurgitation becomes severe, mitral valve repair can be used to treat most forms of mitral valve prolapse and is preferred to mitral valve replacement.

AORTIC STENOSIS

The three common causes of aortic stenosis are:

• Rheumatic fever (usually associated with mitral valve disease). • Calcification of a congenitally bicuspid valve. • In the elderly, calcification of a structurally normal valve.

Cardiac output is initially maintained but the left ventricle becomes increasingly hypertrophied. Eventually it can no longer overcome the outflow tract obstruction and heart failure supervenes. Patients with aortic stenosis typically remain asymptomatic for many years but deteriorate rapidly when symptoms develop.

Clinical features

Mild to moderate aortic stenosis is usually asymptomatic but may be detected incidentally on routine examination. The three cardinal symptoms are angina, syncope and breathlessness.

• Angina arises because of the increased oxygen demands of the hypertrophied left ventricle working against the high-pressure outflow tract obstruction (or coexisting coronary artery disease). • Syncope usually occurs on exertion when cardiac output fails to rise to meet demand because of severe outflow obstruction, causing a fall in BP. • Exertional breathlessness suggests cardiac decompensation as a consequence of chronic excessive pressure overload.

The characteristic clinical signs are:

• A slow rising carotid pulse. • A narrow pulse pressure. • A heaving but undisplaced apex beat. • A harsh ejection systolic murmur radiating to the neck (often with a thrill). • A soft second heart sound.

Investigations

• The ECG usually shows features of LVH, often with down-sloping ST segments and T inversion ('strain pattern'), but can be normal despite severe stenosis. • Doppler echocardiography may show a calcified valve with restricted opening and permits calculation of the gradient across the valve and identification of any associated valvular pathology. • Cardiac catheterisation is usually necessary to assess the coronary arteries before aortic valve replacement.

Management

• All patients with asymptomatic aortic stenosis should be kept under review, as the development of symptoms is an indication for prompt aortic valve replacement. • Surgery in the absence of symptoms is controversial. • Old age is not a contraindication to valve replacement and results are very good, even for those in their eighties.

AORTIC REGURGITATION

This condition may be due to disease of the aortic valve cusps (e.g. rheumatic fever, infective endocarditis) or dilatation of the aortic root (e.g. ankylosing spondylitis, Marfan's syndrome, aortic dissection). The left ventricle dilates and hypertrophies to compensate for the regurgitation, producing a large increase in stroke volume. As disease progresses, LV diastolic pressure rises and breathlessness develops.

Clinical features

• In mild to moderate aortic regurgitation, patients are frequently asymptomatic but may experience an awareness of the heart beat due to the increased stroke volume. • Exertional dyspnoea is the dominant symptom in more severe disease. • The pulse is typically of large volume and collapsing in nature, the pulse pressure is wide and the apex beat is heaving and displaced. • The characteristic soft early diastolic murmur is usually best heard to the left of the sternum with the patient leaning forward with the breath held in expiration. • A systolic murmur due to the increased stroke volume is common. • In acute severe regurgitation (e.g. perforation of aortic cusp in endocarditis) there may be no time for compensatory LVH and dilatation to develop and the features of heart failure may predominate.

Investigations

• CXR may show dilatation of the heart and possibly of the ascending aorta. • ECG typically shows evidence of LVH. • Echocardiography confirms the diagnosis, and may show a dilated, hyperdynamic left ventricle. • Cardiac catheterisation and aortography can also be helpful in assessing the severity of regurgitation, aortic dilatation and the presence of coexisting coronary artery disease.

Management

• Aortic valve replacement is indicated in symptomatic regurgitation. • Asymptomatic patients should also be followed up annually to detect the development of symptoms or increasing ventricular size on echocardiography; if the end-systolic dimension increases to ≥55 mm, then aortic valve replacement should be undertaken. • Systolic BP should be controlled with vasodilating drugs such as nifedipine or ACE inhibitors.

TRICUSPID VALVE DISEASE

Tricuspid stenosis: Uncommon, usually rheumatic in origin and almost always associated with mitral and aortic valve disease. It may cause signs and symptoms of right heart failure.

Tricuspid regurgitation: Common and most frequently 'functional' as a result of RV dilatation. It may also be caused by endocarditis (especially in i.v. drug-users), rheumatic fever or carcinoid syndrome. Symptoms result from reduced forward flow (tiredness) and venous congestion (oedema, hepatic enlargement). The most prominent sign is a large systolic wave in the JVP. Other features include a pansystolic murmur at the left sternal edge and pulsatile hepatomegaly. Tricuspid regurgitation due to RV dilatation often improves when the cause of RV overload is corrected, e.g. diuretic and vasodilator therapy in congestive cardiac failure.

PULMONARY VALVE DISEASE

Pulmonary stenosis: Can occur in the carcinoid syndrome but is usually congenital, when it may be isolated or associated with other abnormalities. The principal finding on examination is an ejection systolic murmur, loudest to the left of the upper sternum and radiating towards the left shoulder. Mild to moderate isolated pulmonary stenosis is relatively common, does not usually progress, does not require treatment and is a low-risk lesion for infective endocarditis. Severe pulmonary stenosis is treated by percutaneous pulmonary balloon valvuloplasty or, if this is not available, by surgical valvotomy.

Pulmonary regurgitation: Rarely an isolated phenomenon and usually associated with pulmonary artery dilatation due to pulmonary hypertension.

INFECTIVE ENDOCARDITIS

Infective endocarditis is due to microbial infection of a heart valve (native or prosthetic) or of the lining of a cardiac chamber or blood vessel, or to a congenital anomaly (e.g. ventricular septal defect (VSD)). It typically occurs at sites of pre-existing endocardial damage, although infection with particularly virulent organisms (e.g. *Staph. aureus*) can cause endocarditis in a previously normal heart. Areas of endocardial damage caused by a high-pressure jet of blood (e.g. VSD, mitral regurgitation, aortic regurgitation) are particularly vulnerable. When the infection is established, vegetations composed of organisms, fibrin and platelets grow and may break away as emboli. Adjacent tissues are destroyed, abscesses may form and valve regurgitation may develop through cusp perforation, distortion or rupture of chordae. Extracardiac manifestations such as vasculitis and skin lesions are due to emboli or immune complex deposition.

• The *viridans* group of streptococci (from the upper respiratory tract or gums) and enterococci (from the gut or urinary tract) may enter the blood stream and are common causes of subacute endocarditis, while *Staph. aureus* is often responsible for acute endocarditis. • *Staph. epidermidis*, a normal skin commensal, is the most common organism in post-operative endocarditis after cardiac surgery. • Other offending organisms include the Gram-negative HACEK group (*Haemophilus* spp.; *Actinobacillus actinomycetem-comitans; Cardiobacterium hominis; Eikenella* spp. and *Kingella kingae*). • *Coxiella burnetii* (Q fever) and *Brucella* cause occasional cases in patients exposed to farm animals. • Yeasts and fungi may be responsible in immunocompromised patients.

Clinical features

Subacute endocarditis: Should be suspected when a patient with congenital or valvular heart disease develops a persistent fever, unusual tiredness, night sweats, weight loss or new signs of valve dysfunction. Other features include a petechial rash, splinter haemorrhages and splenomegaly. Osler's nodes (painful swellings at the fingertips) are rare and finger clubbing is a late sign.

Acute endocarditis: Usually presents as a severe febrile illness with prominent and changing heart murmurs and petechiae. Clinical stigmata of chronic endocarditis are usually absent but embolic events (e.g. cerebral) are common, and cardiac or renal failure may develop rapidly.

Post-operative endocarditis: Should be considered in any patient who develops an unexplained fever after heart valve surgery. The pattern may resemble subacute or acute endocarditis, depending on the virulence of the organism. Morbidity and mortality are high and redo surgery is often required.

Investigations

• Diagnosis of endocarditis is based on the modified Duke criteria (Box 8.19). • Blood culture is the crucial investigation because it may identify the infection and guide antibiotic therapy; three sets should be taken prior

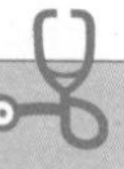

8.19 DIAGNOSIS OF INFECTIVE ENDOCARDITIS (MODIFIED DUKE CRITERIA)
Major criteria
• Positive blood culture Typical organism from two cultures Persistent positive blood cultures taken >12 hrs apart Three or more positive cultures taken over >1 hr • Endocardial involvement Positive echocardiographic findings of vegetations New valvular regurgitation
Minor criteria
• Predisposing valvular or cardiac abnormality • I.v. drug misuse • Pyrexia ≥38°C • Embolic phenomenon • Vasculitic phenomenon • Blood cultures suggestive—organism grown but not achieving major criteria • Suggestive echocardiographic findings
• **Definite endocarditis**: two major, or one major and three minor, or five minor • **Possible endocarditis**: one major and one minor, or three minor

to commencing therapy using scrupulous aseptic technique. • Echocardiography allows detection of vegetations and abscess formation, as well as assessment of valve damage. Transoesophageal echo has a higher sensitivity than transthoracic echo for detecting vegetations (90% vs 65%) and is particularly valuable for investigating patients with prosthetic heart valves. Failure to detect vegetations does not exclude the diagnosis. • A normochromic, normocytic anaemia and elevated WCC, ESR and CRP are common; CRP is particularly useful for monitoring progress. • Microscopic haematuria is usually present. • The ECG may show the development of AV block (due to abscess formation). • CXR may show evidence of cardiac failure.

Management

• Any source of infection (e.g. dental abscess) should be removed as soon as possible. • Empirical antibiotic therapy is with vancomycin and gentamicin if the presentation is acute, or with benzyl penicillin and gentamicin if it is subacute or indolent. Subsequent antibiotic treatment is guided by culture results and is usually continued for at least 4 wks. • Indications for surgery (débridement of infected material; valve replacement) include development of heart failure, abscess formation, failure of antibiotic therapy and large vegetations on left-sided heart valves (high risk of systemic emboli).

Prevention

Patients with valvular or congenital heart disease should be made aware of the risk of endocarditis, and the importance of maintaining good dental health. Recent U.K. advice states that routine antibiotic prophylaxis to cover invasive or dental procedures is no longer recommended.

CONGENITAL HEART DISEASE

ATRIAL SEPTAL DEFECT

This common congenital defect results in shunting of blood from the left to the right atrium, and then to the right ventricle and pulmonary arteries. As a result there is gradual enlargement of the right side of the heart and of the pulmonary arteries.

• The condition is frequently asymptomatic. • Characteristic physical signs include wide fixed splitting of the second heart sound and a systolic flow murmur over the pulmonary valve. • The CXR typically shows enlargement of the heart and the pulmonary artery, as well as pulmonary plethora. • The ECG usually shows incomplete RBBB. The defect is often first detected when a CXR or ECG is carried out for incidental reasons. • Echocardiography can directly demonstrate the defect and may show RV dilatation or hypertrophy. • Atrial septal defects in which pulmonary flow is increased by 50% above systemic flow should be closed either surgically or by percutaneous catheter implantation of a closure device.

VENTRICULAR SEPTAL DEFECT

This is the most common congenital cardiac defect; it may be isolated or form part of complex congenital heart disease.

• Flow from the high-pressure left ventricle to the low-pressure right ventricle produces a pansystolic murmur usually heard best at the left sternal edge but radiating all over the precordium. • Ventricular septal defect may present as cardiac failure in infants, as a murmur with only minor haemodynamic disturbance in older children or adults, or rarely as Eisenmenger's syndrome (see below). • The CXR shows pulmonary plethora and the ECG shows bilateral ventricular hypertrophy. • Small ventricular septal defects require no specific treatment, apart from endocarditis prophylaxis. • Eisenmenger's syndrome is avoided by monitoring for signs of rising pulmonary resistance (serial ECG and echocardiography) and carrying out surgical repair when appropriate. • Long-term prognosis is very good, except in the case of Eisenmenger's syndrome.

PERSISTENT DUCTUS ARTERIOSUS

During fetal life, before the lungs begin to function, most of the blood from the pulmonary artery passes through the ductus arteriosus into the aorta.

Normally the ductus closes soon after birth but sometimes it fails to do so. Since the pressure in the aorta is higher than that in the pulmonary artery, there will be a continuous left to right shunt.

• Usually there is no disability in infancy but cardiac failure may eventually ensue, dyspnoea being the first symptom. • A continuous 'machinery' murmur is heard, maximal in the second left intercostal space below the clavicle. • It is now usual practice to close a patent ductus at cardiac catheterisation with an implantable occlusive device.

COARCTATION OF THE AORTA

This condition is associated with other abnormalities, including bicuspid aortic valve and 'berry' aneurysms of the cerebral circulation. It is an important cause to consider in younger patients with hypertension.

• BP is raised in the upper body but normal or low in the legs. • The femoral pulses are weak, and delayed in comparison with the radial pulse. • A systolic murmur is usually heard posteriorly, over the coarctation. • CXR may show changes in the contour of the aorta and notching of the under-surfaces of the ribs from collateral vessel development. • MRI is ideal for demonstrating the lesion. • Surgical correction is advisable in all but the mildest cases. If this is done sufficiently early in childhood, persistent hypertension can be avoided but patients repaired in late childhood or adult life often remain hypertensive. • Recurrence of stenosis may be managed by balloon dilatation, which can also be used as the primary treatment in some cases.

EISENMENGER'S SYNDROME

Congenital lesions that produce a left-to-right shunt (e.g. ventricular septal defect, patent ductus arteriosus) cause an increase in pulmonary blood flow leading to increased pulmonary resistance. If severe pulmonary hypertension develops, a left-to-right shunt may reverse, resulting in right-to-left shunting and marked cyanosis (Eisenmenger's syndrome). Patients with Eisenmenger's syndrome are at particular risk from changes in afterload that exacerbate right-to-left shunting, e.g. vasodilatation, anaesthesia, pregnancy.

TETRALOGY OF FALLOT

This is the most common cause of cyanotic disease in childhood and comprises:

• Ventricular septal defect (VSD). • Right ventricular outflow obstruction (usually subvalvular). • Aorta overriding the septum and • Right ventricular hypertrophy.

The subvalvular obstruction may increase suddenly after feeding or crying, causing apnoea and unconsciousness ('Fallot's spells'). In older children, Fallot's spells are uncommon but cyanosis increases as rising right ventricular pressure causes increasing right-to-left shunt across the VSD, together with stunted growth, clubbing and polycythaemia. A loud ejection systolic murmur is heard in the pulmonary area. Cyanosis may be absent in the newborn or in patients with only mild right ventricular outflow obstruction. Investigation is by ECG (right ventricular hypertrophy), CXR (a 'boot-shaped' heart) and echocardiography, which is diagnostic. Definitive management is by surgical relief of the outflow obstruction and closure of the VSD, and the prognosis is good following surgery in childhood.

ADULT CONGENITAL HEART DISEASE

Many patients who would not previously have survived childhood now do so following corrective surgery; in Western countries there are now more adults than children with congenital heart disease. These patients may develop problems in adult life. For example, following correction of coarctation of the aorta, adults may develop hypertension. Adults with repaired tetralogy of Fallot may develop ventricular arrhythmias secondary to hypertrophy and post-operative ventricular scarring, or right ventricular dilatation from chronic pulmonary regurgitation. Such patients require careful follow-up from the teenage years through adult life in specialist clinics.

DISEASES OF THE MYOCARDIUM

ACUTE MYOCARDITIS

This is an acute inflammatory condition of the myocardium. Viral infection is the most common cause, particularly Coxsackie and influenza viruses A and B. Other causes include Lyme disease (p. 85), Chagas disease (p. 112) and acute rheumatic fever.

The clinical picture ranges from a symptomless disorder, sometimes recognised by the presence of an inappropriate tachycardia or abnormal ECG, to fulminant heart failure. ECG changes are common but non-specific. Biochemical markers of myocardial injury (e.g. troponins, creatine kinase) are elevated in proportion to the extent of damage. Echocardiography may reveal LV dysfunction which is sometimes regional (due to focal myocarditis).

In most patients the disease is self-limiting and the immediate prognosis is excellent; however, death may occur due to ventricular arrhythmia or rapidly progressive heart failure. Some forms of myocarditis (e.g. Chagas disease) may lead to chronic low-grade myocarditis or dilated cardiomyopathy. Treatment for cardiac failure or arrhythmias may be required and intense physical exertion should be avoided.

DILATED CARDIOMYOPATHY

This condition is characterised by dilatation and impaired contraction of the left (and sometimes the right) ventricle. The differential diagnosis includes coronary artery disease and some specific disorders of heart muscle (Box 8.20); a diagnosis of dilated cardiomyopathy should only be offered when these conditions have been excluded. At least 25% of cases are

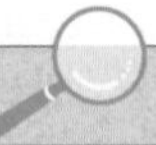

8.20 SPECIFIC DISEASES OF HEART MUSCLE
Infections
• Viral, e.g. Coxsackie A and B, influenza, HIV • Bacterial, e.g. diphtheria, *Borrelia burgdorferi* • Protozoal, e.g. trypanosomiasis
Endocrine and metabolic disorders
• e.g. Diabetes, hypo- and hyperthyroidism, acromegaly, carcinoid syndrome, phaeochromocytoma, inherited storage diseases
Connective tissue diseases
• e.g. Systemic sclerosis, SLE, polyarteritis nodosa
Infiltrative disorders
• e.g. Haemochromatosis, haemosiderosis, sarcoidosis, amyloidosis
Toxins
• e.g. Doxorubicin, alcohol, cocaine, irradiation
Neuromuscular disorders
• e.g. Dystrophia myotonica, Friedreich's ataxia

inherited as an autosomal dominant trait and a variety of single gene mutations (mostly affecting cytoskeletal proteins) have been identified. Alcohol and a late autoimmune reaction to viral myocarditis are important aetiological factors in some patients.

• Most patients present with heart failure. • Arrhythmia, thromboembolism and sudden death are common and may occur at any stage. • Echocardiography is useful in establishing the diagnosis. • Treatment is aimed at controlling the resulting heart failure and preventing arrhythmias. • The prognosis is variable and cardiac transplantation may be required.

HYPERTROPHIC CARDIOMYOPATHY

This is the most common form of cardiomyopathy and is characterised by elaborate LV hypertrophy with malalignment of the myocardial fibres. The hypertrophy may be generalised or confined largely to the interventricular septum. Heart failure develops because the stiff non-compliant ventricles impede diastolic filling. Septal hypertrophy may also cause dynamic LV outflow tract obstruction (hypertrophic obstructive cardiomyopathy). The condition is a genetic disorder with autosomal dominant transmission, a high degree of penetrance and variable expression.

• Effort-related symptoms (angina and breathlessness), arrhythmia and sudden death (mainly from ventricular arrhythmias) are the dominant clinical problems. • Signs are similar to those of aortic stenosis, except that in hypertrophic cardiomyopathy the character of the arterial pulse is jerky.

8.21 RISK FACTORS FOR SUDDEN DEATH IN HYPERTROPHIC CARDIOMYOPATHY

- A history of previous cardiac arrest or sustained VT
- Recurrent syncope
- An adverse genotype and/or family history
- Exercise-induced hypotension
- Multiple episodes of non-sustained VT on ambulatory ECG
- Marked increase in LV wall thickness

• The ECG is usually abnormal and may show features of LVH or deep T-wave inversion. • Echocardiography is usually diagnostic. • β-blockers and rate-limiting calcium antagonists can help to relieve angina and sometimes prevent syncopal attacks but no pharmacological treatment is definitely known to improve prognosis. • Outflow tract obstruction can be improved by partial surgical resection or by iatrogenic infarction of the basal septum using a catheter-delivered alcohol solution. • An ICD should be considered in patients with clinical risk factors for sudden death (Box 8.21).

RESTRICTIVE CARDIOMYOPATHY

In this rare condition, ventricular filling is impaired because the ventricles are 'stiff'. This leads to high atrial pressures with atrial hypertrophy, dilatation and later AF. Amyloidosis is the most common cause of restrictive cardiomyopathy in the UK.

• Diagnosis can be very difficult and may require complex Doppler echocardiography, CT or MRI, and endomyocardial biopsy. • Treatment is symptomatic but the prognosis is poor and transplantation may be indicated.

DISEASES OF THE PERICARDIUM

ACUTE PERICARDITIS

Pericardial inflammation may be due to infection (viral, bacterial, TB), immunological reaction (e.g. post-MI, connective tissue disorder), trauma, uraemia or neoplasm. Pericarditis and myocarditis often coexist, and all forms of pericarditis may produce a pericardial effusion (see below).

Clinical features

• The characteristic pain of pericarditis is retrosternal, radiates to the shoulders and neck, and is aggravated by deep breathing and movement. • A low-grade fever is common. • A pericardial friction rub is a high-pitched superficial scratching or crunching noise produced by movement of the inflamed pericardium, and is diagnostic of pericarditis.

Investigations

The ECG shows ST elevation with upward concavity over the affected area, which may be widespread. PR interval depression is a very sensitive indicator of acute pericarditis.

Management

• The pain is usually relieved by aspirin but a more potent anti-inflammatory agent such as indometacin may be required. • Corticosteroids may suppress symptoms but there is no evidence that they accelerate cure.

PERICARDIAL EFFUSION

This refers to accumulation of fluid within the pericardial sac. Cardiac tamponade describes acute heart failure due to compression of the heart by a large or rapidly developing effusion.

• Typical physical findings include hypotension, tachycardia, a markedly raised JVP which rises paradoxically with inspiration (Kussmaul's sign), pulsus paradoxus (dramatic fall in BP during inspiration) and muffled heart sounds. • The QRS voltages on the ECG are often reduced in the presence of a large effusion. • CXR may show an increase in the size of the cardiac shadow, which may have a globular appearance if the effusion is large. • Echocardiography confirms the diagnosis and helps identify the optimum site for aspiration of fluid. • The patient usually responds promptly to percutaneous pericardiocentesis or (particularly in cases of cardiac rupture or aortic dissection) surgical drainage.

CHRONIC CONSTRICTIVE PERICARDITIS

Constrictive pericarditis is due to progressive thickening, fibrosis and calcification of the pericardium. In effect, the heart is encased in a solid shell and cannot fill properly. The condition often follows an attack of tuberculous pericarditis but can also complicate haemopericardium, viral pericarditis, rheumatoid arthritis and purulent pericarditis.

Clinical features

• The symptoms and signs of systemic venous congestion are the hallmarks of constrictive pericarditis; AF is common and there is often dramatic ascites and hepatomegaly. • Breathlessness is not a prominent symptom because the lungs are seldom congested. • The condition should be suspected in any patient with unexplained right heart failure and a small heart. • CXR (pericardial calcification) and echocardiography often help to establish the diagnosis, though it is may be difficult to distinguish from restrictive cardiomyopathy.

Management

Surgical resection of the diseased pericardium can lead to a dramatic improvement but carries a high morbidity and produces disappointing results in up to 50% of patients.

9

Respiratory disease

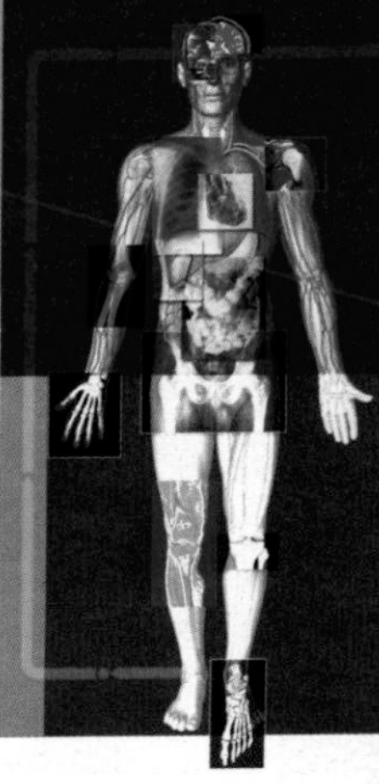

Respiratory symptoms are the most common cause of presentation to the family practitioner. Asthma occurs in more than 10% of British adults, and bronchial carcinoma is the most common fatal malignancy in the developed world. The lung is the major site of opportunistic infection in immunocompromised patients, and TB (including multiple drug-resistant strains) continues to increase, infecting one-third of the world's population.

PRESENTING PROBLEMS

COUGH

Cough is the most common respiratory symptom and the underlying cause is often clear from other clinical features, particularly in more serious disease. Common causes of acute or transient cough are:

• Viral lower respiratory tract infection. • Post-nasal drip (rhinitis/sinusitis). • Foreign body aspiration. • Laryngitis or pharyngitis. • Pneumonia. • Congestive heart failure. • Pulmonary embolism.

Chronic cough presents more of a diagnostic challenge, especially if physical examination, CXR and lung function are normal. In this context, consider:

• Post-nasal drip. • Cough-variant asthma. • Gastro-oesophageal reflux with aspiration. • Drug-induced cough (ACE inhibitors). • *Bordetella pertussis* infection.

While most patients with bronchogenic carcinoma have an abnormal CXR on presentation, fibreoptic bronchoscopy or spiral CT of the airways is advisable for an unexplained cough in adults (particularly smokers), as

CLINICAL EXAMINATION OF THE RESPIRATORY SYSTEM

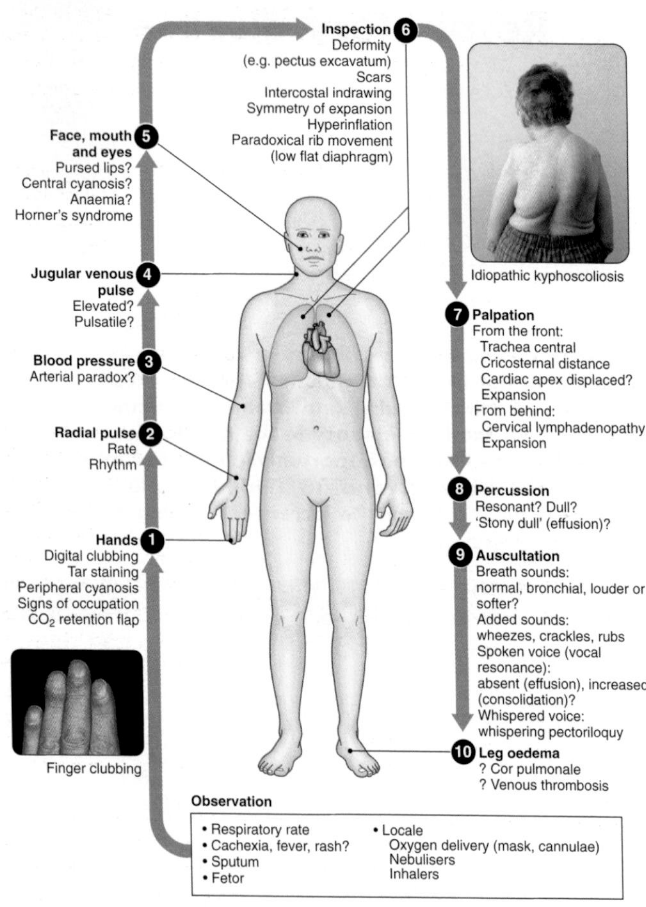

Observation

- Respiratory rate
- Cachexia, fever, rash?
- Sputum
- Fetor
- Locale
  Oxygen delivery (mask, cannulae)
  Nebulisers
  Inhalers

this may reveal a small endobronchial tumour or unexpected foreign body.

BREATHLESSNESS (DYSPNOEA)

Breathlessness or dyspnoea can be defined as the feeling of an uncomfortable need to breathe. It is unusual among sensations in having no defined receptors, no localised representation in the brain, and multiple causes both in health (e.g. exercise) and in diseases of the lungs, heart or muscles.

CHRONIC EXERTIONAL DYSPNOEA

Chronic obstructive pulmonary disease (COPD): Dyspnoea typically varies little day to day, but exercise capacity falls steadily over months or years. Patients usually report relief of dyspnoea at rest and overnight, a useful distinction from asthma. Orthopnoea may be present due to cranial displacement of the diaphragm on lying flat. Chronic cough and sputum (particularly in the morning) indicate bronchitis, but sputum may be absent when emphysema predominates. Recurrent acute exacerbations of breathlessness occur, usually in winter. Most but not all patients have a significant smoking history. In advanced disease, ankle swelling may develop as a result of cor pulmonale.

Asthma: Dyspnoea in asthma is associated with episodes of wheeze or chest tightness, varying in severity over time, but usually worse in the morning and often waking the patient overnight. There may be a history of childhood wheeze, or of wheeze or rhinitis provoked by pollens, dusts, household pets or occupational allergens. In exercise-induced asthma, wheeze and chest tightness typically come on immediately after exercise.

Heart disease: Impaired left ventricular function can cause exertional dyspnoea. Orthopnoea, cough and wheeze may also be present, as in lung disease. A history of angina or hypertension, or examination findings of displaced apex beat, raised JVP or cardiac murmurs may be useful in implicating a cardiac cause.

Interstitial or alveolar disease of the lung: Dyspnoea in these conditions is usually relentless and progressive. A detailed history should be obtained, including lifetime occupation and exposure to birds, dusts and other sources of organic agents which may provoke lung disease.

Diseases of the chest wall or respiratory muscles: May be obvious on history, examination and chest radiography. Other rarer causes of alveolar hypoventilation, e.g. brain-stem defects, and alveolar hypoventilation in gross obesity, may cause disordered breathing and cyanosis, but are not usually associated with breathlessness. Diaphragmatic weakness or palsy characteristically causes orthopnoea, with an abnormally large drop in the vital capacity on lying down. Respiratory failure tends to occur initially during sleep, with nocturnal hypoxaemia and hypercapnia, which resolve during the day.

Pulmonary thromboembolism: Often presents with acute breathlessness with or without chest pain. However, chronic thromboembolic disease should be suspected in patients who present with more gradual onset of breathlessness, particularly if there is a previous history of thromboembolic events or marked exertional breathlessness but a relatively normal examination and CXR. Leg swelling and an elevated JVP may be present, but are non-specific.

Psychogenic breathlessness and hyperventilation syndrome: Breathlessness not caused by organic disease of the heart or lungs is relatively common. It is particularly difficult to diagnose in patients with coexisting disease, such as asthma or heart disease. Suggestive features include an 'inability to take a deep enough breath', leading to extra deep sighs being taken, digital and perioral paraesthesiae, light-headedness, central chest discomfort or even carpopedal spasm due to acute respiratory alkalosis. Psychogenic breathlessness rarely disturbs sleep, frequently occurs at rest, may be provoked by stressful situations and may even be relieved by exercise. Arterial blood gases show normal PO_2, low PCO_2 and an alkalosis.

ACUTE SEVERE DYSPNOEA

This is one of the most common and dramatic medical emergencies.

It is important to ascertain the rate of onset and severity of the breathlessness, and whether associated cardiovascular symptoms (chest pain, palpitations, sweating and nausea) or respiratory symptoms (cough, wheeze, haemoptysis and stridor) are present. A previous history of repeated episodes of left ventricular failure, asthma or exacerbations of COPD is valuable. In children, the possibility of inhalation of a foreign body or acute epiglottitis should always be considered.

Common causes of acute breathlessness and their clinical features are in listed in Box 9.1.

Investigations and management

• Arterial blood gases (ABG), CXR and an ECG should be obtained to confirm the clinical diagnosis, and oxygen given pending results. • Urgent endotracheal intubation may become necessary if the conscious level declines or severe respiratory acidosis is present.

CHEST PAIN

• Pleural or chest wall involvement by lung disease gives rise to peripheral chest pain which is exacerbated by deep breathing or coughing ('pleuritic' pain). • Central chest pain suggests heart disease but can occur with tumours affecting the mediastinum or massive pulmonary embolism. • Tracheitis produces raw upper retrosternal pain which is worse on coughing. • Musculoskeletal chest wall pain is usually exacerbated by movement and associated with local tenderness.

HAEMOPTYSIS

Coughing up blood, irrespective of the amount, is an alarming symptom and nearly always brings the patient to the doctor.

9.1 DIFFERENTIAL DIAGNOSIS OF ACUTE SEVERE DYSPNOEA

Condition	History	Signs	CXR	ABG	ECG
Pulmonary oedema	Chest pain, orthopnoea, palpitations, cardiac history*	Central cyanosis, ↑JVP, sweating, cool extremities, basal crepitations*	Cardiomegaly, oedema/pleural effusions*	↓PaO_2 ↓$PaCO_2$	Sinus tachycardia, ischaemia*, arrhythmia
Massive pulmonary embolus	Risk factors (Box 9.16), chest pain, pleurisy, syncope*, dizziness*	Severe central cyanosis, ↑JVP*, absence of signs in the lung*, shock (tachycardia, reduced BP)	Often normal; prominent hilar vessels, oligaemic lung fields*	↓PaO_2 ↓$PaCO_2$	Sinus tachycardia, RBBB, $S_1Q_3T_3$ pattern, ↓T (V_1–V_4)
Acute severe asthma	History of asthma, wheeze*	Tachycardia, pulsus paradoxus, cyanosis (late), JVP→*, ↓peak flow, rhonchi*	Hyperinflation only (unless complicated by pneumothorax)*	↓PaO_2 ↓$PaCO_2$ (↑$PaCO_2$ in extremis)	Sinus tachycardia (bradycardia in extremis)
Acute exacerbation of COPD	Previous episodes*. If in type II resp[y] failure may be drowsy	Cyanosis, hyperinflation*, signs of CO_2 retention (flapping tremor, bounding pulses)*	Hyperinflation*, bullae, complicating pneumothorax	↓ or ⇓ PaO_2; $PaCO_2$↑ in type II failure ± ↑H^+, ↑HCO_3^-	Nil, or signs of R ventricular strain
Pneumonia	Prodromal illness*, fever*, rigors*, pleurisy*	Fever, confusion, pleural rub*, consolidation*, cyanosis (if severe)	Pneumonic consolidation*	↓PaO_2 ↓or →$PaCO_2$	Tachycardia
Metabolic acidosis	Diabetes/renal disease, aspirin or ethylene glycol overdose	Fetor (ketones), hyperventilation without heart or lung signs*, dehydration*, air hunger	Normal	PaO_2 normal ↓$PaCO_2$, ↑H^+	
Psychogenic	Previous episodes	Not cyanosed, no heart or lung signs; carpopedal spasm	Normal	PaO_2 normal* ↓$PaCO_2$, H^+↓*	

*Denotes a valuable discriminatory feature. (RBBB = right bundle branch block)

A clear history should be taken to establish that it is true haemoptysis and not haematemesis, gum bleeding or nosebleed. Haemoptysis must always be assumed to have a serious cause until proven otherwise. A history of repeated small haemoptyses, or blood-streaking of sputum, is highly suggestive of bronchial carcinoma. Fever, night sweats and weight loss suggest TB. Pneumococcal pneumonia is often the cause of 'rusty'-coloured sputum but can cause frank haemoptysis, as can all the pneumonic infections which lead to suppuration or abscess formation. Bronchiectasis and intracavitary mycetoma can cause catastrophic bronchial haemorrhage and in these patients there may be a history of previous TB or pneumonia in early life. Pulmonary thromboembolism is a common cause of haemoptysis and should always be considered. Many episodes of haemoptysis are unexplained, even after full investigation, and are likely to be caused by simple bronchial infection.

Investigations and management

In severe acute haemoptysis, the patient should be nursed upright (or on the side of the bleeding if this is known), given oxygen and haemodynamically resuscitated. In the vast majority of cases, however, haemoptysis itself is not life-threatening and it is possible to follow a logical sequence of investigations which include: CXR, FBC, clotting screen, bronchoscopy and CT pulmonary angiography (CTPA).

THE SOLITARY RADIOGRAPHIC PULMONARY LESION

The incidental finding of a solitary pulmonary nodule (SPN) on a plain CXR in an adult patient is a common dilemma and the differential diagnosis is broad (Box 9.2). Between 20 and 30% of all cancers present in this way; the incidence increases with age and accounts for >50% of nodules in patients aged >50 yrs.

9.2 THE SOLITARY PULMONARY NODULE	
Common causes	
• Bronchial carcinoma	• Lung abscess
• Single metastasis	• Tuberculoma
• Localised pneumonia	• Pulmonary infarct
Uncommon causes	
• Benign tumours	• Bronchogenic cyst
• Lymphoma	• Rheumatoid nodule
• Arteriovenous malformation	• Pulmonary sequestration
• Hydatid cyst	• Wegener's granuloma
• Pulmonary haematoma	• Aspergilloma ('halo' sign)

Radiology

• A nodule that has been present for >2 yrs and has not changed can be assumed to be benign (previous radiology is therefore invaluable). • Any new nodule requires a CT scan to define the lesion more precisely. • Benign disease is favoured by the presence of calcification or fat. • Features suggestive of malignancy include size >3 cm or a spiculated appearance, particularly in a smoker. • CT with i.v. contrast provides information regarding the vascularity of the lesion, with malignant tumours tending to show greatest contrast enhancement. • CT may also demonstrate additional unsuspected nodules, or hilar and mediastinal lymphadenopathy, important in the staging of a primary bronchial carcinoma.

Management

Percutaneous needle biopsy under CT guidance has proved to be the most effective procedure for the diagnosis of SPNs, which are usually beyond the reach of the bronchoscope. However, if the lesion has a high probability of malignancy and the patient is fit for surgery, the best option may be to proceed to resection. If bacterial infection is included in the differential diagnosis, an antibiotic should be given during the period in which the investigations are being performed. In elderly patients in whom a primary malignant lesion is suspected but who are considered unfit for any form of curative treatment, an interval CXR may be the most appropriate management.

PLEURAL EFFUSION

The accumulation of fluid within the pleural space is termed pleural effusion. Accumulations of frank pus (empyema) or blood (haemothorax) represent separate conditions. Pleural fluid accumulates due either to increased hydrostatic pressure or decreased osmotic pressure ('transudative effusion' as seen in cardiac, liver or renal failure), or to increased microvascular permeability caused by disease of the pleural surface itself, or injury in the adjacent lung ('exudative effusion'). Some causes of pleural effusion are shown in Box 9.3. Particular attention should be paid to a recent history of

9.3 CAUSES OF PLEURAL EFFUSION

- Pneumonia ('para-pneumonic effusion')
- TB
- Pulmonary infarction
- Malignant disease
- Cardiac failure
- Subdiaphragmatic disease (subphrenic abscess, pancreatitis)
- Asbestos-related benign pleural effusion
- Hypoproteinaemia (nephrotic syndrome, liver failure)
- Connective tissue diseases (SLE, rheumatoid arthritis)
- Acute rheumatic fever
- Post-MI syndrome
- Meigs' syndrome (ovarian tumour plus pleural effusion)
- Myxoedema
- Uraemia

respiratory infection, the presence of heart, liver or renal disease, occupation (e.g. exposure to asbestos), contact with TB, and risk factors for thromboembolism.

Symptoms and signs of pleurisy often precede the development of an effusion, especially in patients with underlying pneumonia, pulmonary infarction or connective tissue disease. However, the onset may be insidious. Breathlessness is often the only symptom related to the effusion and its severity depends on the size and rate of accumulation.

Radiology

The classical appearance of pleural fluid on CXR is of a curved shadow at the lung base, blunting the costophrenic angle and ascending towards the axilla. Fluid appears to track up the lateral chest wall. In fact, fluid surrounds the whole lung at this level, but casts a radiological shadow only where the X-ray beam passes tangentially through the fluid against the lateral chest wall. Around 200 ml of fluid is required to be detectable on a PA CXR, but smaller effusions can be identified by USS or CT. Previous scarring or adhesions in the pleural space can cause localised effusions. USS is more accurate than plain CXR for determining the volume of pleural fluid and frequently provides additional helpful information. The presence of loculation suggests an evolving empyema or resolving haemothorax. CT displays pleural abnormalities more readily than either plain radiography or USS, and may distinguish benign from malignant pleural disease.

Pleural aspiration and biopsy

Pleural aspiration reveals the colour and texture of fluid and on appearance alone may immediately suggest an empyema or chylothorax. The presence of blood is consistent with pulmonary infarction or malignancy, but may represent a traumatic tap. Biochemical analysis allows classification into transudate and exudate. An exudate usually has a protein concentration of >30 g/l or can be distinguished using Light's criteria (Box 9.4). The predominant cell type provides useful information and cytological examination is essential. A low pH suggests infection but may also be seen in rheumatoid arthritis, ruptured oesophagus or advanced malignancy. In some clinical settings (e.g. left ventricular failure) it should not be necessary to sample fluid unless atypical features are present. Combining pleural aspiration with biopsy (using an Abrams needle) increases the diagnostic yield, but the best results are obtained from CT-guided biopsy or video-assisted thoracoscopy,

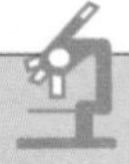

9.4 LIGHT'S CRITERIA FOR DISTINGUISHING PLEURAL TRANSUDATE FROM EXUDATE

Pleural fluid is an exudate if one or more of the following criteria are met:

- Pleural fluid protein : serum protein ratio >0.5
- Pleural fluid LDH : serum LDH ratio >0.6
- Pleural fluid LDH > two-thirds of the upper limit of normal serum LDH

allowing the operator to visualise the pleura and guide the biopsy directly.

Management

Therapeutic aspiration may be required to palliate breathlessness, but removing >1.5 litres in one episode is inadvisable as this can cause re-expansion pulmonary oedema. An effusion should never be drained to dryness before establishing a diagnosis as further biopsy may be precluded until further fluid accumulates. Treatment of the underlying cause—e.g. heart failure, pneumonia, pulmonary embolism or subphrenic abscess—will often be followed by resolution of the effusion. The management of pleural effusion in association with pneumonia, TB and malignancy is dealt with later in this chapter.

SLEEP-DISORDERED BREATHING

A variety of respiratory disorders manifest themselves during sleep, e.g. nocturnal cough and wheeze in asthma. Nocturnal hypoventilation may exacerbate respiratory failure in patients with restrictive lung disease such as kyphoscoliosis, diaphragmatic palsy, muscle weakness (e.g. muscular dystrophy) or intrinsic lung disease (e.g. COPD, pulmonary fibrosis). In contrast, a small but important group of disorders cause problems only during sleep due to upper airway obstruction (obstructive sleep apnoea) or abnormalities of ventilatory drive (central sleep apnoea).

THE SLEEP APNOEA/HYPOPNOEA SYNDROME (SAHS)

It is now recognised that 2–4% of the middle-aged population suffers from recurrent upper airway obstruction during sleep, which causes sleep fragmentation leading to daytime sleepiness. This results in a threefold increased risk of road traffic accidents.

A reduction in upper airway muscle tone during sleep results in pharyngeal narrowing, which often manifests as snoring. Negative pharyngeal pressure during inspiration can then cause complete upper airway occlusion, usually at the level of the soft palate. This leads to transient wakefulness and recovery of upper airway muscle tone. The subject rapidly returns to sleep, snores and becomes apnoeic once more. This cycle repeats itself many times, causing severe sleep fragmentation. Predisposing factors include:

• Obesity. • Male sex. • Nasal obstruction. • Acromegaly. • Hypothyroidism. • Familial causes (back-set mandible and maxilla). • Alcohol and sedatives (relaxation of the upper airway dilating muscles).

Clinical assessment

• Excessive daytime sleepiness is the principal symptom. • Snoring is virtually universal; bed partners report loud snoring in all body positions and often notice multiple breathing pauses (apnoeas). • Sleep is unrefreshing. •

Patients have difficulty with concentration, impaired cognitive function and work performance, depression, irritability and nocturia.

Investigations

• A quantitative assessment of daytime sleepiness can be obtained by questionnaire (Epworth Sleepiness Scale). • Overnight studies of breathing, oxygenation and sleep quality are diagnostic (SAHS defined as >15 apnoeas/hypopnoeas per hr of sleep).

Differential diagnosis

Narcolepsy is a rare cause of sleepiness, occurring in 0.05% of the population and is associated with cataplexy (when muscle tone is lost in fully conscious people in response to emotional triggers), hypnagogic hallucinations (hallucinations at sleep onset) and sleep paralysis.

Idiopathic hypersomnolence occurs in younger individuals and is characterised by long nocturnal sleeps.

Management

• Weight reduction and avoiding alcohol and sedatives can lead to an improvement in symptoms. • Most patients need overnight continuous positive airway pressure (CPAP) by nasal/face mask, which prevents upper airway collapse during sleep. CPAP often leads to dramatic improvements in symptoms, daytime performance and quality of life. Unfortunately, 30–50% of patients are poorly compliant or do not tolerate CPAP. • Mandibular advancement devices are an alternative approach. • There is no evidence that palatal surgery has any role in management.

RESPIRATORY FAILURE

The term respiratory failure is used when pulmonary gas exchange fails to maintain normal arterial oxygen and carbon dioxide levels. Its classification into type I and type II relates to the absence or presence of hypercapnia (raised $PaCO_2$). The main causes are shown in Box 9.5.

Management

• Treat the underlying cause. Occasionally, rapid reversal of the precipitating event will restore good gas exchange, e.g. tracheostomy for laryngeal obstruction, reversal of narcotic poisons. • In acute left ventricular failure, in massive pulmonary embolism and when pulmonary infarction or pneumonia is the cause of pleural pain, treatment with opiates is entirely appropriate, but these drugs depress respiratory drive and should never be used in asthma or COPD, except during assisted mechanical ventilation. • Common to all cases is the need to restore adequate arterial oxygen levels, for which oxygen therapy with or without mechanically assisted ventilation is important.

The consequences of untreated severe hypoxaemia include:

• Systemic hypotension. • Pulmonary hypertension. • Polycythaemia. • Tachycardia. • Cerebral dysfunction ranging from confusion to coma.

9.5 RESPIRATORY FAILURE: UNDERLYING CAUSES AND BLOOD GAS ABNORMALITIES

	Type I Hypoxia (PaO_2 <8.0 kPa (60 mmHg)) Normal or low $PaCO_2$ (<6.6 kPa (50 mmHg))		Type II Hypoxia (PaO_2 <8.0 kPa (60 mmHg)) Raised $PaCO_2$ (>6.6 kPa (50 mmHg))	
	Acute	**Chronic**	**Acute**	**Chronic**
H^+	→ or ↑	→	↑	→ or ↑
Bicarbonate	→	→	→	↑
Causes	Acute asthma Pulmonary oedema Pneumonia Lobar collapse Pneumothorax Pulmonary embolus ARDS	Emphysema Lung fibrosis Lymphangitis carcinomatosa Right-to-left shunts	Acute severe asthma Acute exacerbation COPD Upper airway obstruction Acute neuropathies/paralysis Narcotic drugs Primary alveolar hypoventilation Flail chest injury	COPD Sleep apnoea Kyphoscoliosis Myopathies/muscular dystrophy Ankylosing spondylitis

Oxygen therapy

Oxygen delivery depends on many factors:

• Inspired oxygen concentration. • Alveolar ventilation. • Ventilation–perfusion distribution within the lung. • Haemoglobin and the oxygen–haemoglobin dissociation curve. • Cardiac output. • Distribution of capillary blood flow within the tissues.

Normally, high-flow oxygen (35–60%) is appropriate treatment in respiratory failure (e.g. severe asthma, pulmonary oedema or pneumonia) because respiratory drive is high. A small percentage of patients with severe chronic COPD and type II respiratory failure develop abnormal tolerance of raised CO_2 and may become dependent on hypoxic drive to breathe. In these patients only, lower concentrations of oxygen (24–28% via a Venturi mask) may be needed to avoid precipitating worsening respiratory depression.

Close monitoring of ABGs is essential to ensure acceptable PaO_2 levels. If there is persistent hypoxia, progressive respiratory acidosis, or the patient becomes exhausted, an early decision should be made about whether it is appropriate to commence non-invasive ventilation or formal intubation and mechanical ventilation. Very ill patients may require immediate ventilatory support on presentation.

CHRONIC AND 'ACUTE ON CHRONIC' TYPE II RESPIRATORY FAILURE

The most common cause of chronic type II respiratory failure is COPD. When CO_2 retention is chronic, the acidaemia is corrected by renal retention of bicarbonate, which results in a plasma pH within the normal range. This 'compensated' pattern, which is also seen in some patients with chronic neuromuscular disease or kyphoscoliosis, is maintained until there is a further pulmonary insult, such as an exacerbation of COPD which precipitates an episode of 'acute on chronic' respiratory failure. The further acute increase in $PaCO_2$ results in acidaemia and worsening hypercapnia, and may lead to drowsiness and eventually to coma.

The principal aim of treatment in acute on chronic type II respiratory failure is to achieve a safe PaO_2 (>7.0 kPa (52 mmHg)) without increasing $PaCO_2$ and acidosis, while identifying and treating the precipitating condition. These patients usually have severe pre-existing lung disease, and only a small insult may be required to tip the balance towards severe respiratory failure. Moreover, in contrast to acute severe asthma, a patient with 'acute on chronic' type II respiratory failure due to COPD may not feel overtly distressed despite being critically ill with severe hypoxaemia, hypercapnia and acidaemia.

If controlled oxygen treatment causes a further increase in the $PaCO_2$ associated with a reduction in pH, non-invasive or invasive ventilatory support is usually indicated. In these patients the decision regarding invasive ventilation can be particularly complex and difficult. Ideally, an early decision should be made, based on whether there is a potentially remediable precipitating condition and whether the patient is likely to regain an acceptable quality of life.

LUNG TRANSPLANTATION

Lung transplantation is now an established treatment for carefully selected patients with advanced lung disease unresponsive to medical treatment. Single-lung transplantation may be used for older patients with emphysema and patients with intrapulmonary restrictive disorders such as lung fibrosis. It is contraindicated in patients with chronic bilateral pulmonary infection, such as cystic fibrosis and bronchiectasis, where bilateral lung transplantation is the favoured option. Heart–lung transplantation remains necessary for the treatment of patients with advanced congenital heart disease such as Eisenmenger's syndrome and is preferred by some surgeons for the treatment of primary pulmonary hypertension unresponsive to medical therapy. Although prognosis is good with modern immunosuppressive drugs, the availability of lung transplants remains limited due to shortage of donor lungs.

OBSTRUCTIVE PULMONARY DISEASES

ASTHMA

Asthma is characterised by chronic airway inflammation and increased airway hyper-responsiveness leading to wheeze, cough, chest tightness and dyspnoea. Airflow obstruction in asthma is variable over time and reversible with treatment. Around 300 million people world-wide suffer from asthma and the prevalence is increasing, particularly in countries with a Western lifestyle. In childhood, asthma is more common in boys, but following puberty females are more frequently affected. Multiple environmental and genetic determinants are implicated in the aetiology of asthma. The 'hygiene hypothesis' proposes that decreased infections in early life bias the immune system towards an allergic phenotype. There is a strong association between atopy—a propensity to produce IgE—and asthma.

Clinical features

Asthma is not a uniform disease but a dynamic clinical syndrome characterised by episodes of wheezing, chest tightness, breathlessness and cough. There is diurnal variation in symptoms (worse in early morning); sleep is often disturbed by cough and wheeze. In mild intermittent asthma, patients may be asymptomatic between exacerbations. In persistent asthma the pattern is one of chronic wheeze and breathlessness.

Symptoms may be precipitated by:

• Exercise. • Cold weather. • Allergen exposure (may be occupational). • Viral respiratory tract infections. • Drugs (β-blockers, aspirin and NSAIDs).

Investigations

Pulmonary function tests: Diagnosis is based on a compatible history and an increase in FEV_1 of ≥15% and at least 200 ml following bronchodilator/trial of corticosteroids; or >20% diurnal variation on ≥3 days in a week for 2 wks on PEF (peak expiratory flow) diary; or a decrease in FEV_1 of ≥15% after 6 mins of exercise.

Radiological examination: Often normal. There is lobar collapse if mucus has occluded a large bronchus. Hyperinflation is present in acute asthma. Flitting infiltrates may be seen in allergic bronchopulmonary aspergillosis (ABPA).

Measurement of allergic status: Total IgE ± allergen-specific IgE and/or skin prick tests are carried out. There may be a peripheral blood eosinophilia or sputum eosinophilia (the latter also used to measure airway inflammation).

Management

The goals of asthma therapy are to:

• Control symptoms. • Prevent exacerbations. • Maintain pulmonary function as close to normal as possible. • Avoid adverse effects from medications. • Prevent irreversible airflow limitation. • Prevent mortality.

Patient education: Patients should be taught the relationship between symptoms and inflammation, the importance of key symptoms (e.g. nocturnal waking), about different types of medication and the use of PEF to guide management decisions. Written action plans may be helpful.

Avoidance of aggravating factors: Asthma control may be improved by reducing exposure to trigger antigens, e.g. household pets. In occupational asthma, removal from the offending agent may lead to cure. Many patients are sensitised to several antigens, making avoidance almost impossible. Patients should be advised not to smoke.

Pharmacological treatment

Step 1—Occasional use of inhaled short-acting β_2-adrenoreceptor agonist bronchodilators: This is used for patients with mild intermittent asthma (symptoms < once/wk for 3 mths and <2 nocturnal episodes/mth). Patients often underestimate the severity of asthma.

Step 2—Regular anti-inflammatory therapy (preferably inhaled corticosteroids (ICS)): This is used for any patient who has experienced an exacerbation in the last 2 yrs, uses inhaled β_2-agonists >3 times/wk, reports symptoms >3 times/wk, or is awakened by asthma 1 night/wk.

Step 3—Add-on therapy: If poor control remains, despite regular ICS up to a dose of 800 μg/day BDP or equivalent, add-on therapy should be considered with either long-acting β_2-agonists (LABAs), such as salmeterol and formeterol, or leukotriene receptor antagonists (e.g. montelukast 10 mg daily). LABAs have consistently been demonstrated to improve asthma control and reduce exacerbations compared to increasing the dose of ICS alone. Fixed-combination inhalers of ICS and LABAs are convenient and help compliance.

Step 4—Poor control on a moderate dose of inhaled steroid and add-on therapy: The ICS dose may be increased to 2000 μg BDP or equivalent daily. A nasal corticosteroid should be used if upper airway symptoms are prominent. Consider trials of leukotriene receptor antagonists or theophyllines. Further studies on new therapies, such as monoclonal antibodies directed against IgE, are awaited.

Step 5—Continuous or frequent use of oral steroids: Prednisolone therapy should be prescribed in the lowest amount necessary to control symptoms. Long-term corticosteroid tablets (>3 mths) or receiving more than three or four courses per year put patients at risk of systemic side-effects. Osteoporosis may be prevented using bisphosphonates.

Step-down therapy: Once asthma control is established, inhaled (or oral) corticosteroid dose should be titrated to the lowest dose at which effective control of asthma is maintained.

Exacerbations of asthma

Asthma exacerbations are characterised by increased symptoms, deterioration in PEF and an increase in airway inflammation. They may be precipitated by infections (most commonly viral), moulds (*Alternaria* and *Cladosporium*) and, on occasion, pollen (particularly following thunderstorms). Most attacks are characterised by a gradual deterioration over several hours to days, but some appear to occur with little or no warning: so-called brittle asthma.

Management of mild–moderate exacerbations

• It is widely believed that an impending exacerbation may be avoided by doubling the dose of ICS; however, recent studies have failed to confirm this. • Short courses of 'rescue' oral corticosteroids (prednisolone 30–60 mg daily) are often required where there are worsening symptoms (morning symptoms persisting until midday, nocturnal wakening or diminishing response to bronchodilator) and a fall of PEF to <60% of best recording. • Tapering of the dose is not necessary unless given for >3 wks.

Management of acute severe asthma (Box 9.6 and Fig. 9.1)

9.6 IMMEDIATE ASSESSMENT OF ACUTE SEVERE ASTHMA	
Acute severe asthma	
• PEF 33–50% predicted (<200 l/min) • Inability to complete sentences in 1 breath	• Heart rate ≥110/min • Respiratory rate ≥25/min
Life-threatening features	
• PEF 33–50% predicted (<100 l/min) • SpO_2 <92% or PaO_2 <8 kPa (60 mmHg) • Normal $PaCO_2$ • Silent chest/feeble respiratory effort • Cyanosis	• Hypotension • Exhaustion • Confusion • Coma • Bradycardia or arrhythmias
Near-fatal asthma	
• ↑$PaCO_2$ and/or requiring mechanical ventilation with raised inflation pressures	

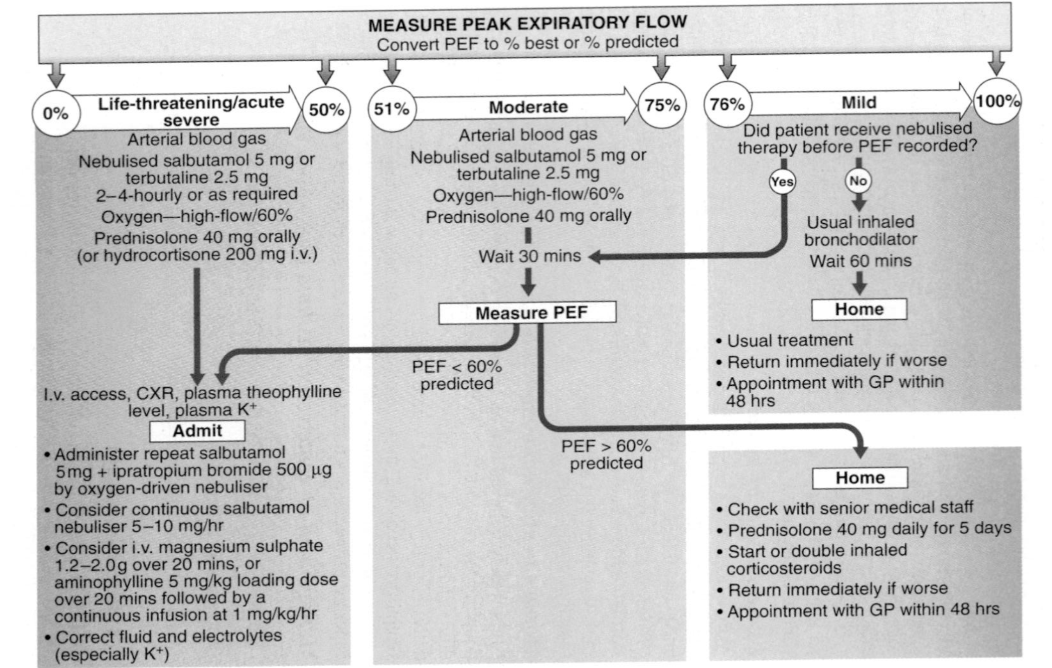

Fig. 9.1 Immediate treatment of patients with acute severe asthma.

CHRONIC OBSTRUCTIVE PULMONARY DISEASE (COPD)

COPD is a heterogeneous condition embracing several overlapping pathological processes including chronic bronchitis, chronic bronchiolitis (small airway disease) and emphysema. Many patients also exhibit a systemic component characterised by impaired nutrition, weight loss and skeletal muscle dysfunction. COPD is defined by the presence of airways obstruction, which does not change markedly over several months and, unlike asthma, is not fully reversible. The prevalence of COPD in the UK is estimated at 1–2%, but is probably greater. Exacerbations of COPD account for 10% of hospital admissions in the UK, and with ~30 000 deaths/yr it represents the sixth most common cause of death in the UK. Following the marked increase in tobacco consumption in developing countries, COPD is gaining in global importance. Cigarette smoking is the most important risk factor. Susceptibility to cigarette smoke varies but both the dose and duration of smoking appear to be important. Other risk factors are solid fuel fires, air pollution, occupation (coal miners) and low socio-economic class. Rarely, an inherited deficiency of α_1 antitrypsin predisposes to premature emphysema.

Clinical features

COPD should be suspected in any patient over the age of 40 yrs who has persistent cough and sputum production and/or breathlessness.

• Chronic bronchitis is defined as cough and sputum on most days for >3 consecutive mths for >2 successive yrs. • The level of breathlessness should be quantified for future reference (e.g. MRC dyspnoea scale, Box 9.7). • In advanced disease there may be oedema or morning headaches (hypercapnia). • Physical signs (Fig. 9.2) are non-specific, but may help to indicate the severity of disease.

Two classical phenotypes have been described:

• 'Pink puffers' are thin and breathless, and maintain a normal $PaCO_2$. • 'Blue bloaters' develop hypercapnia, oedema and secondary polycythaemia.

In practice, these phenotypes often overlap.

Investigations

• CXR reveals hyperinflation and occasionally demonstrates large bullae or other complications of smoking (lung cancer). • FBC may demonstrate polycythaemia. • α_1 antitrypsin level should be checked in younger patients with a basal distribution of emphysema. • Spirometry reveals FEV_1 <80% predicted value and FEV_1/FVC (forced vital capacity) <70%. Severity of disease is defined according to percentage predicted FEV_1: mild disease 50–80%, moderate 30–49%, severe <30%. • Lung volumes using helium dilution or body plethysmography quantify any hyperinflation. • Carbon monoxide transfer factor is low in emphysema. • Exercise tests provide an objective assessment of exercise tolerance. • Pulse oximetry may prompt

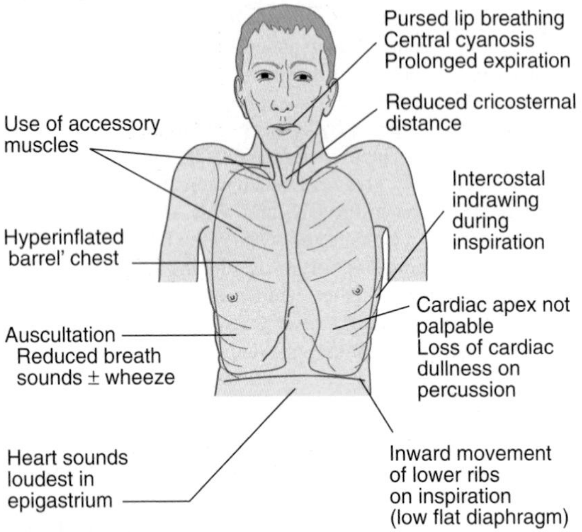

Fig. 9.2 Key features on examination in COPD.

9.7 MODIFIED MRC DYSPNOEA SCALE

Grade	Degree of breathlessness related to activities
0	No breathlessness except with strenuous exercise
1	Breathlessness when hurrying on the level or walking up a slight hill
2	Walks slower than contemporaries on level ground because of breathlessness or has to stop for breath when walking at own pace
3	Stops for breath after walking about 100 m or after a few mins on level ground
4	Too breathless to leave the house, or breathless when dressing or undressing

referral for a domiciliary oxygen assessment if <93%. • CT is likely to play an increasing role in the assessment of COPD as it allows the detection, characterisation and quantification of emphysema.

Management and prognosis

Pessimism is unjustified, as it is usually possible to improve breathlessness, reduce the frequency and severity of exacerbations, and improve health status and prognosis.

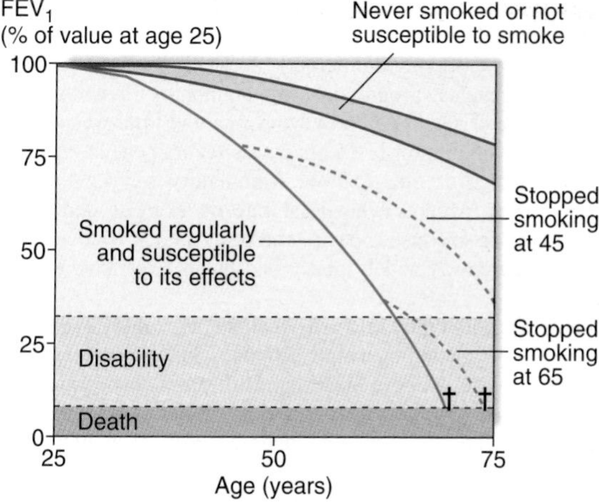

Fig. 9.3 Model of annual decline in FEV_1 with accelerated decline in susceptible smokers. When smoking is stopped, subsequent loss is similar to that in healthy non-smokers.

Smoking cessation: Offer help to stop smoking at every opportunity. Combine pharmacotherapy with appropriate support as part of a programme. It is the only intervention proven to decelerate the decline in FEV_1 (Fig. 9.3).

Bronchodilators: Short-acting bronchodilators for mild disease (β_2-agonist or anticholinergic). Longer-acting bronchodilators are more appropriate for patients with moderate to severe disease. From the wide range available, select a device which the patient can use effectively. Significant improvements in breathlessness may be reported despite minimal changes in FEV_1, probably reflecting reduced hyperinflation. Theophylline preparations improve breathlessness, but use is limited by side-effects. Oral bronchodilators may be contemplated in patients who cannot use inhaled devices efficiently.

Inhaled corticosteroids: Reduce the frequency and severity of exacerbations; they are recommended in patients with moderate to severe disease (FEV_1 <50%) who report >2 exacerbations requiring antibiotics or oral steroids/yr. Regular use leads to a small improvement in FEV_1 but no change in the rate of decline of lung function. ICS/LABA combinations produce further improvements in breathlessness and exacerbation rate. Oral corticosteroids are useful during exacerbations, but maintenance therapy contributes to osteoporosis and impaired muscle function and should be avoided.

Pulmonary rehabilitation: Encourage exercise. Multidisciplinary programmes (usually 6–12 wks' duration) incorporating physical training, education and nutritional counselling reduce symptoms, improve health status and enhance confidence.

Oxygen therapy: Long-term domiciliary oxygen therapy (LTOT) improves survival, prevents progression of pulmonary hypertension, decreases the incidence of secondary polycythaemia and improves neuropsychological health. A minimum of 15 hrs/day is recommended, to keep PaO_2 >8 kPa (60 mmHg) or SaO_2 >90%. Ambulatory oxygen therapy should be considered in patients who desaturate on exercise and show objective improvement in exercise capacity and/or dyspnoea with oxygen. Short-burst oxygen therapy is widely prescribed but is expensive and of unproven benefit.

Surgical intervention: In highly selected patients, lung volume reduction surgery (removing non-functioning emphysematous lung tissue) reduces hyperinflation and decreases work of breathing. Bullectomy is occasionally performed to remove large bullae that compress surrounding lung tissue.

Other measures: Influenza vaccination; pneumococcal vaccination; trial of mucolytic therapy.

COPD has a variable natural history. Prognosis is inversely related to age and directly related to FEV_1. Poor prognostic indicators include weight loss and pulmonary hypertension.

Acute exacerbations of COPD

These are characterised by an increase in symptoms and deterioration in lung function. They are more common in severe disease and may be caused by bacteria, viruses or a change in air quality. Respiratory failure and/or fluid retention may be present. Many patients can be managed at home with the use of increased bronchodilator therapy, a short course of oral corticosteroids and, if appropriate, antibiotics. Cyanosis, peripheral oedema or altered conscious level should prompt hospital referral.

Oxygen therapy: High concentrations of oxygen may cause respiratory depression and worsening acidosis (p. 280). Controlled oxygen at 24% or 28% should be used, aiming for PaO_2 >8 kPa (60 mmHg) (or an SaO_2 >90%) without worsening acidosis.

Bronchodilators: Nebulised short-acting β_2-agonists and anticholinergics are used. If concern exists regarding oxygen sensitivity, nebulisers may be driven by compressed air.

Corticosteroids: Oral prednisolone (usually 30 mg for 5–10 days) reduces symptoms and improves lung function. Prophylaxis against osteoporosis should be considered if frequent courses are needed.

Antibiotic therapy: Recommended for an increase in sputum purulence, sputum volume or breathlessness. An aminopenicillin or a macrolide should be used. Co-amoxiclav is only required in regions where β-lactamase-producing organisms are known to be common.

Non-invasive ventilation (NIV): If patients have persistent tachypnoea and a respiratory acidosis ($H^+ \geq 45$/pH < 7.35), NIV is associated with reduced requirements for mechanical ventilation and reductions in mortality. Consider mechanical ventilation where there is a reversible cause for deterioration (e.g. pneumonia), or if there is no prior history of respiratory failure.

Additional therapy: Evidence for i.v. aminophylline is limited and there is a risk of arrhythmias and drug interactions. The respiratory stimulant doxapram has been largely superseded by NIV. Diuretics should be administered if peripheral oedema has developed.

BRONCHIECTASIS

Bronchiectasis is defined as abnormal dilatation of the bronchi due to chronic airway inflammation and infection. It is usually acquired, but may result from an underlying genetic or congenital defect of airway defences (Box 9.8).

Clinical features

• Chronic productive cough. • Malaise. • Haemoptysis. • Weight loss. • Exacerbations may cause fever, increased cough and sputum volume, and pleurisy. • Coarse crackles caused by sputum in bronchiectatic spaces may be unilateral or bilateral. • Diminished breath sounds may indicate lobar collapse. • Bronchial breathing due to scarring may be heard in advanced disease.

Investigations

Sputum: May reveal common respiratory pathogens. As disease progresses, *Pseudomonas aeruginosa* or fungi such as *Aspergillus* and various mycobacteria may be seen. Frequent cultures assist appropriate antibiotic selection.

Radiology: CXR may be normal in mild disease. In advanced disease, thickened airway walls, cystic bronchiectatic spaces, and associated areas

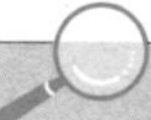

9.8 CAUSES OF BRONCHIECTASIS
Congenital
• Cystic fibrosis • Primary ciliary dyskinesia • Kartagener's syndrome (sinusitis and transposition of the viscera) • Primary hypogammaglobulinaemia
Acquired
• Pneumonia (complicating whooping cough or measles) • Inhaled foreign body • Suppurative pneumonia • Pulmonary TB • Allergic bronchopulmonary aspergillosis complicating asthma • Bronchial tumours

of pneumonic consolidation or collapse may be seen. CT is much more sensitive, and shows thickened dilated airways.

Assessment of ciliary function: Saccharin test or nasal biopsy may be used.

Management and prognosis

In patients with airflow obstruction, inhaled bronchodilators and corticosteroids may enhance airway patency.

Physiotherapy: Patients should perform regular daily physiotherapy to keep the dilated bronchi empty of secretions. Commonly used methods are postural drainage, 'active cycle of breathing' technique, chest percussion or mechanical oscillatory devices.

Antibiotic therapy: In most patients with bronchiectasis, the same antibiotics are used as in COPD, although higher doses are needed. Some patients are colonised with staphylococci and Gram-negative bacilli, especially *Pseudomonas* spp; in these, antibiotic therapy should be guided by microbiology results. Regular macrolides help reduce exacerbations in some patients with bronchiectasis, but their use is not yet supported by large trials (except in cystic fibrosis).

Surgical treatment: Only indicated in a few cases where bronchiectasis is unilateral and confined to a single lobe/segment on CT.

The disease is progressive when associated with ciliary dysfunction and cystic fibrosis, and eventually causes respiratory failure. In other patients the prognosis can be good with regular physiotherapy and judicious use of antibiotics. Bronchiectasis may be prevented by prophylaxis or treatment of common causes, e.g. measles, whooping cough, TB.

CYSTIC FIBROSIS (CF)

This is the most common fatal autosomal recessive disease in Caucasians, affecting 1 in 2500 births. It is caused by mutations of a gene (on chromosome 7) coding for a chloride channel known as cystic fibrosis transmembrane conductance regulator (*CFTR*). The carrier rate of CF mutations is 1 in 25. The most common mutation is *ΔF508,* but >800 mutations have been identified. The genetic defect causes increased sodium and chloride content in sweat and secretions, which predisposes indirectly to chronic bacterial infection in the lungs. The gut epithelium, pancreas, liver and reproductive tract are also affected. Neonatal screening for CF is now routine in the UK. The diagnosis is confirmed by genetic testing and sweat electrolyte measurements.

Clinical features

• The lungs are normal at birth, but bronchiectasis develops in childhood. • *Staph. aureus* is the most common childhood organism; *Ps. aeruginosa* infection affects the majority of patients by adolescence. • Recurrent exacerbations of bronchiectasis cause progressive lung damage, resulting ultimately in death from respiratory failure. • Other clinical manifestations of the gene defect include intestinal obstruction, exocrine pancreatic insufficiency with malabsorption, diabetes and hepatic cirrhosis. • Men with CF are infertile due to failure of development of the vas deferens.

Management and prognosis

• Regular chest physiotherapy is needed. • For exacerbations, *Staph. aureus* is often managed with oral antibiotics; i.v. treatment is usually needed for *Pseudomonas* spp. • Resistant strains of *Ps. aeruginosa, Stenotrophomonas maltophilia* and *Burkholderia cepacia* are a major problem. • *Aspergillus* and 'atypical mycobacteria' are also frequently found (may be benign 'colonisers'). • Nebulised antibiotic therapy (colomycin or tobramycin) is used to suppress chronic *Pseudomonas* infection. • Nebulised recombinant human deoxyribonuclease (DNase) to liquefy sputum can reduce exacerbations and improve pulmonary function in some patients. • Regular macrolides (e.g. azithromycin) reduce exacerbations and improve lung function in patients with *Pseudomonas* colonisation. • In advanced disease, home oxygen and non-invasive ventilation may be necessary to treat respiratory failure. • Ultimately, lung transplantation can produce dramatic improvements but is limited by donor organ availability.

Treatment of non-respiratory manifestations of CF: Malabsorption is treated with vitamins and pancreatic enzyme supplements. • Increased calorie requirements of CF patients are met by supplemental feeding, including nasogastric or gastrostomy tube feeding if required. • Diabetes eventually appears in ~25% of patients and often requires insulin. • Osteoporosis should be sought and treated.

The prognosis of CF has improved greatly in recent decades, mainly because of better nutrition and control of bronchial sepsis. The median survival of patients with CF born in the 21st century is now predicted to be at least 40 yrs.

INFECTIONS OF THE RESPIRATORY SYSTEM

UPPER RESPIRATORY TRACT INFECTIONS

Acute coryza (common cold): Sore throat and blocked nose with watery discharge. There is usually a viral cause, but disease may be complicated by lower respiratory tract infection, sinusitis or otitis media. Antibiotics are not necessary in uncomplicated coryza.

Acute laryngitis: Dry, sore throat and hoarse voice. Symptoms can be relieved with paracetamol; antibiotics are not usually required.

Acute laryngo-tracheobronchitis (croup): Coryzal symptoms and paroxysms of cough accompanied by stridor and breathlessness. Treat with steam inhalation or humidified oxygen. Intravenous co-amoxiclav or erythromycin is given for seriously ill patients. Croup can cause cyanosis and asphyxia in small children if appropriate treatment is not given. Intubation may be needed to relieve laryngeal obstruction.

Acute epiglottitis: Fever and sore throat, leading rapidly to stridor due to swollen epiglottis. Disease is usually caused by infection with *Haemophilus influenzae*. Asphyxia may be precipitated by attempts to examine the throat (ensure that resuscitation facilities are available). I.V. antibiotics (e.g. co-amoxiclav) are essential.

Acute bronchitis and tracheitis: Often follows acute coryza. Cough is productive of mucoid/mucopurulent sputum. Patients have pyrexia, and chest tightness, wheeze and breathlessness are present when the bronchi are involved. Tracheitis causes pain on coughing. Disease is usually self-limiting, but may lead to bronchopneumonia or an exacerbation of COPD/asthma.

Influenza: A specific viral infection caused by influenza A or B. Epidemics or pandemics occur due to mutations in virus surface proteins. Patients develop pyrexia, generalised aches and pains, anorexia, nausea and vomiting. During epidemics the diagnosis is usually easy; in sporadic cases, acute and convalescent serology samples aid diagnosis. Usually symptoms resolve in 3–5 days, although influenza may be complicated by secondary bacterial invasion. Treatment is usually symptomatic, although antibiotics are required if pneumonia develops.

PNEUMONIA

Pneumonia is defined as an acute respiratory illness associated with recently developed segmental, lobar or multilobar radiological shadowing. It is classified as community-acquired, hospital-acquired (nosocomial), or occurring in immunocompromised hosts. 'Lobar pneumonia' is a radiological and pathological term referring to homogeneous consolidation of one or more lung lobes, often with pleural inflammation; bronchopneumonia refers to more patchy alveolar consolidation with bronchial and bronchiolar inflammation often affecting both lower lobes.

COMMUNITY-ACQUIRED PNEUMONIA (CAP)

In the UK 5–11/1000 adults have CAP each year. The incidence is higher in the very young and the elderly. 20% of childhood deaths world-wide are due to pneumonia. Most patients may be safely managed at home, but hospital admission is necessary in 20–40%. In hospital, death rates are typically 5–10%, rising to 50% in severe illness. The most common organism is *Streptococcus pneumoniae. H. influenzae* should be considered in elderly patients, and *Mycoplasma* and *Chlamydia pneumoniae* are more often seen in the young. Recent influenza may predispose to *Staph. aureus* (although most cases of post-influenza pneumonia are caused by *Strep. pneumoniae*). Rarer causes of severe pneumonia include legionella (from infected warm water – ask about foreign travel) and psittacosis (from birds infected with chlamydia psittaci).

Clinical features

• Fever, rigors, shivering and vomiting often predominate. • Patients have poor appetite and headache. • Cough is followed by mucopurulent sputum

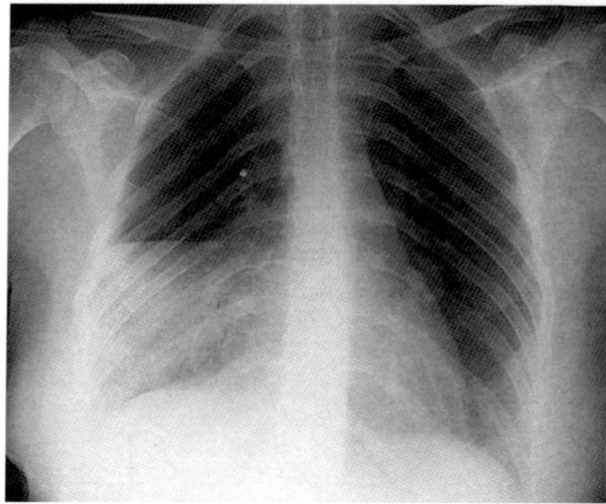

Fig. 9.4 Pneumonia of the right middle lobe.

(rust-coloured sputum may be seen in patients with *Strep. pneumoniae*). • Pleuritic chest pain is common and may be the presenting feature. • Haemoptysis occasionally occurs. • Examination may reveal crepitations or bronchial breathing, suggesting underlying consolidation.

Investigations

• ***CXR:*** In lobar pneumonia, CXR reveals a homogenous opacity localised to the affected lobe or segment (Fig. 9.4). • CXR may also identify complications such as a parapneumonic effusion, intrapulmonary abscess formation, or empyema.

• ***Microbiological investigations:*** Sputum in sent for microscopy (Gram and Ziehl–Neelsen stains), culture and sensitivity testing. • Blood culture is frequently positive in pneumococcal pneumonia. • Acute and convalescent samples for *Mycoplasma*, *Chlamydia*, *Legionella* and viral serology should be sent. • *Legionella* antigen can be detected in urine and pneumococcal antigen can be detected in blood or sputum. • Throat/nasopharyngeal swabs may be helpful in children or during an influenza epidemic. • Many cases of CAP are managed successfully without identification of the organism.

• ***Blood investigations:*** ABG if SaO_2 is <92% or if clinical features suggest severe pneumonia. • WCC is often marginally raised or even normal in patients with pneumonia caused by atypical organisms. Very high ($>20 \times 10^9$/l) or low ($<4 \times 10^9$/l) WCC may be seen in severe pneumonia. • U&Es and LFTs should be checked. • CRP is typically elevated.

Management

A scoring system to assess disease severity helps to guide antibiotic and admission policies (Fig. 9.5).

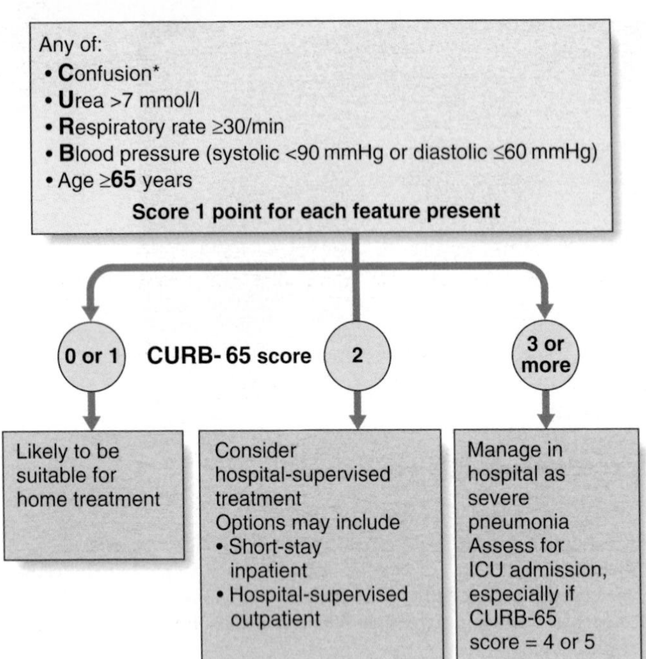

Fig. 9.5 Hospital CURB-65. * Defined as a Mental Test Score of 8 or less, or new disorientation in person, place or time. (A urea of 7 mmol/l ≅ 20 mg/dl.)

• High concentrations (>35%) of oxygen (preferably humidified) should be administered to all patients with tachypnoea, hypoxaemia, hypotension or acidosis, aiming to keep PaO_2 ≥8 kPa (60 mmHg) or SaO_2 ≥92% (except in hypercapnia associated with COPD). • I.V. fluids are given in severe disease, and in elderly or vomiting patients. • If possible, take blood cultures prior to starting antibiotics (Box 9.9) but do not delay treatment in severe pneumonia. • Consider analgesia for pleural pain, and physiotherapy if cough is suppressed, e.g. due to pain. • Refer to ITU if: CURB score 4–5 and failing to respond to treatment; persistent hypoxia despite high inspired O_2; progressive hypercapnia; severe acidosis; shock; or depressed conscious level.

Complications

• Parapneumonic effusion. • Empyema. • Lobar collapse. • Thromboembolic disease. • Pneumothorax. • Lung abscess (*Staph. aureus*). • Renal failure, the acute respiratory distress syndrome (ARDS), multi-organ failure. • Ectopic abscess formation (*Staph. aureus*). • Hepatitis, peri-

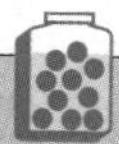

9.9 ANTIBIOTIC TREATMENT FOR COMMUNITY-ACQUIRED PNEUMONIA
Uncomplicated CAP
• Amoxicillin 500 mg 8-hourly orally for 7–10 days • If penicillin allergy, clarithromycin 500 mg 12-hourly/erythromycin 500 mg 6-hourly
If *Staphylococcus* is cultured or suspected
• Flucloxacillin 1–2 g i.v. 6-hourly *plus* clarithromycin 500 mg i.v. 12-hourly
If *Mycoplasma* or *Legionella* is suspected
• Clarithromycin 500 mg 12-hourly *or* erythromycin 500 mg–1 g 6-hourly *plus* • Rifampicin 600 mg i.v. 12-hourly in severe cases
Severe CAP
• Clarithromycin 500 mg i.v. 12-hourly *or* erythromycin 500 mg–1 g i.v. 6-hourly *plus* • Co-amoxiclav 1.2 g i.v. 8-hourly *or* ceftriaxone 1–2 g daily *or* cefuroxime 1.5 g 8-hourly

carditis, myocarditis, meningoencephalitis. • Pyrexia due to drug hypersensitivity.

Follow-up and prevention

Improvement in the CXR typically lags behind clinical recovery. Review should be arranged at around 6 wks and a CXR obtained if there are persistent symptoms, physical signs or reasons to suspect underlying malignancy.

Influenza vaccination is recommended for those at high risk of mortality from influenza or pneumonia. Pneumococcal vaccination is followed by a good antibody response but the efficacy in preventing pneumonia in high-risk groups remains uncertain.

HOSPITAL-ACQUIRED PNEUMONIA (HAP)

HAP is defined as a new episode of pneumonia occurring at least 2 days after admission to hospital. The most important distinction between HAP and CAP is the difference in the spectrum of organisms, with the majority of hospital-acquired infections caused by Gram-negative bacteria, including *Escherichia, Pseudomonas* and *Klebsiella* spp. *Staph. aureus*/MRSA are also common. The clinical features and investigation of patients with HAP are very similar to CAP.

Management and prognosis

• Adequate Gram-negative coverage is usually obtained with a third-generation cephalosporin (e.g. cefotaxime) + an aminoglycoside (e.g. gentamicin), or meropenem, or a monocyclic β-lactam (e.g. aztreonam) + flucloxacillin. • Aspiration pneumonia can be treated with co-amoxiclav 1.2 g 8-hourly + metronidazole 500 mg 8-hourly. • The nature and severity of most HAPs dictate that these antibiotics are all given intravenously, at least initially. • Physiotherapy is of particular importance in the immobile and elderly, and adequate oxygen therapy, fluid support and monitoring are essential.

The mortality from HAP is high (~30%).

SUPPURATIVE AND ASPIRATION PNEUMONIA (INCLUDING PULMONARY ABSCESS)

In suppurative pneumonia there is destruction of the lung parenchyma by the inflammatory process. Although microabscess formation is a characteristic histological feature of suppurative pneumonia, it is usual to restrict the term 'pulmonary abscess' to large localised collections of pus. Organisms include *Staph. aureus* or *Klebsiella pneumoniae.* Suppurative pneumonia may be produced by primary infection, inhalation of septic material from the oropharynx or haematogenous spread (e.g. in i.v. drug abusers). Bacterial infection of a pulmonary infarct or of a collapsed lobe may also produce suppurative pneumonia or lung abscess.

• CXR characteristically demonstrates a dense opacity with cavitation and/or a fluid level. • Treatment with oral amoxicillin may be effective. • If anaerobes are suspected, oral metronidazole should be added. • Prolonged treatment for 4–6 wks may be required.

PNEUMONIA IN THE IMMUNOCOMPROMISED PATIENT

Pulmonary infection is common in patients receiving immunosuppressive drugs and in diseases causing defects of cellular or humoral immune mechanisms. Most infections are caused by the same common pathogens that cause CAP. However, Gram-negative bacteria, especially *Ps. aeruginosa*, are more of a problem than Gram-positive organisms, and unusual organisms or those normally considered to be non-pathogenic may become 'opportunistic' pathogens. More than one organism may be present.

Clinical features and investigations

• Patients may have non-specific symptoms and the onset tends to be less rapid in patients with opportunistic organisms such as *Pneumocystis jirovecii* and mycobacterial infections. • In *P. jirovecii* pneumonia, cough and breathlessness can precede the appearance of CXR abnormality by several days. At presentation the patient is usually pyrexial and hypoxic with normal breath sounds. • Induced sputum or bronchoscopy with bronchoalveolar lavage or bronchial brushings may help to establish a diagnosis.

Management

• Whenever possible, treatment should be based on an established aetiological diagnosis. • Frequently the cause is not known and broad-spectrum antibiotic therapy is required (e.g. a third-generation cephalosporin, or a quinolone, + an antistaphylococcal antibiotic, or an antipseudomonal penicillin + an aminoglycoside); treatment is thereafter tailored according to the results of investigations and the clinical response. • The investigation and management of *P. jirovecii* infection is detailed on page 137.

SEVERE ACUTE RESPIRATORY DISTRESS SYNDROME (SARS)

SARS rose to prominence in late 2002 when a series of cases in the Guangdong Province, China, was followed by an international outbreak. The illness is characterised by fever, malaise and muscle aches, and later a dry cough with shortness of breath. Travel to an area affected by SARS or close contact with a person known to be a suspect SARS case is typical. SARS has recently been attributed to the Corona virus (Urbani SARS-associated coronavirus).

TUBERCULOSIS

TB is caused by infection with *Mycobacterium tuberculosis* (MTB), which is part of a complex of organisms that also includes *M. bovis* (reservoir cattle) and *M. africanum* (reservoir human). One-third of the world's population has latent TB. Current estimates suggest that, between 2002 and 2020, 1000 million people will become newly infected, the majority in the world's poorest nations. *M. bovis* infection arises from drinking non-sterilised milk from infected cows; otherwise, *M. tuberculosis* is spread by the inhalation of aerosolised droplet nuclei from other infected patients.

The formation of a mass of granulomas surrounding an area of caseation leads to the appearance of the primary lesion in the lung, referred to as the 'Ghon focus'. The combination of a primary lesion and regional lymph node involvement is termed the 'Ghon complex'. If the bacilli spread (either by lymph or blood) before immunity is established, secondary foci may be established in other organs including lymph nodes, serous membranes, meninges, bones, liver, kidneys and lungs. These foci resolve once an immune response is mounted and the organisms gradually lose viability. However, 'latent bacilli' may persist for many years. The estimated lifetime risk of developing disease after primary infection is 10%, with roughly half of this risk occurring in the first 2 yrs after infection. Factors predisposing to TB are summarised in Box 9.10.

Clinical features

Primary pulmonary TB: Refers to infection of a previously uninfected (tuberculin-negative) individual. In most cases, infection of a healthy individual is subclinical and indicated only by the appearance of a cell-mediated, delayed-type hypersensitivity reaction to tuberculin (demonstrated by tuberculin skin testing). If the organism cannot be contained, primary progressive disease ensues.

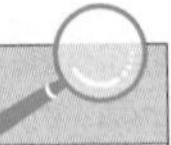

9.10 FACTORS INCREASING THE RISK OF TB

- Age (children > young adults < elderly)
- First-generation immigrants from high-prevalence countries
- Close contacts of patients with smear-positive pulmonary TB
- Overcrowding: prisons, collective dormitories
- CXR evidence of self-healed TB
- Primary infection <1 yr previously
- Immunosuppression: HIV, infliximab, high-dose corticosteroids, cytotoxic agents
- Malignancy (especially lymphoma and leukaemia)
- Type 1 diabetes mellitus
- Chronic renal failure
- Silicosis
- GI disease associated with malnutrition (gastrectomy, jejuno-ileal bypass, cancer of the pancreas, malabsorption)
- Deficiency of vitamin D or A

Miliary TB: Blood-borne dissemination gives rise to miliary TB which may present acutely but is often characterised by 2–3 wks of fever, night sweats, anorexia, weight loss and a dry cough. Hepatosplenomegaly may be present and the presence of a headache may indicate co-existent tuberculous meningitis. Auscultation of the chest is frequently normal, although with more advanced disease widespread crackles are evident. Fundoscopy may show choroidal tubercles. CXR demonstrates fine 1–2 mm lesions ('millet seed') distributed throughout the lung fields. Anaemia and leucopenia may be present.

Post-primary pulmonary TB: The most frequent form of post-primary disease. Onset occurs insidiously over several weeks. Systemic symptoms include fever, night sweats, malaise, and loss of appetite and weight, and are accompanied by cough, often with haemoptysis. CXR typically shows an ill-defined opacity situated in one of the upper lobes. As disease progresses, consolidation, collapse and cavitation may develop (a miliary pattern or cavitation suggest active disease).

Extrapulmonary disease (Fig. 9.6): Accounts for ~20% of cases in HIV-negative individuals and is more common in HIV-positive individuals. Cervical or mediastinal lymphadenitis is the most common extrapulmonary presentation. Meningeal disease represents the most important form of CNS TB, as it is rapidly fatal if unrecognised and untreated.

Investigations

• Mycobacterial infection is usually confirmed by direct microscopy (Ziehl–Neelsen or auramine staining) and culture of sputum or other samples from the respiratory tract or other infected site. • An estimated 5000–10 000

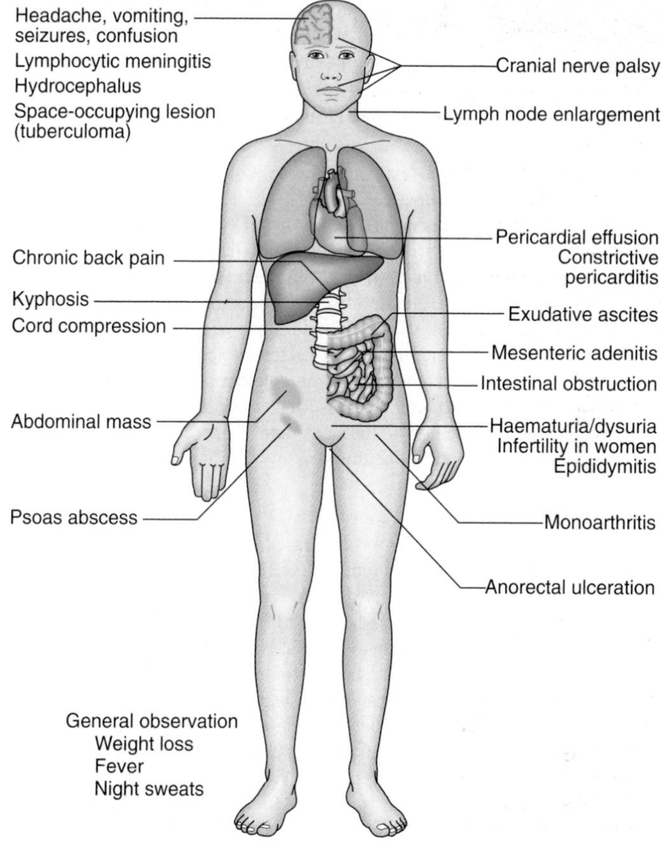

Fig. 9.6 Systemic presentations of extrapulmonary TB.

acid-fast bacilli must be present for sputum to be smear-positive, whereas only 10–100 viable organisms are required for sputum to be culture-positive. • Standard culture takes up to 8 wks. Liquid culture media can expedite growth and drug sensitivity testing (7–21 days). • Where multiple drug-resistant TB (MDRTB) is suspected, molecular tools may be employed to test for the presence of the *rpo* (rifampicin resistance) gene.

Control and prevention

BCG (the Calmette–Guérin bacillus) is a live attenuated vaccine used to stimulate protective immunity and prevent the dissemination of MTB (efficacy 20–60%). Vaccination policies vary world-wide according to incidence and health-care resources. In the UK vaccination is recommended for the following tuberculin skin test-negative groups:

• Contacts <2 yrs old. • Immigrants from countries where TB is endemic. • Infants in high-prevalence ethnic groups. • Health-care workers at high risk.

Grade 3–4 tuberculin skin test responders should be referred for clinical and radiological examination.

The identification of latent TB is an integral component of control. An asymptomatic contact with a positive tuberculin test but a normal CXR may be treated with chemoprophylaxis (e.g. rifampicin and isoniazid for 3 mths) to prevent progression to clinical disease. Tuberculin skin testing may be associated with false-positive reactions in those who have had a BCG and in areas where non-tuberculous mycobacteria exposure is high. Contact screening is a legal requirement in many countries. The aim is to identify the probable index case, other cases infected by the same index patient (with or without evidence of disease), and close contacts who should receive BCG vaccination or chemotherapy.

Chemotherapy

• Chemotherapy regimens for TB are based on the principle of an initial intensive phase (which rapidly reduces the bacterial population), followed by a continuation phase to destroy any remaining bacteria. • An initial 2 mths' therapy with four drugs (isoniazid, rifampicin, pyrazinamide and ethambutol), followed by 4 mths of two drugs (isoniazid and rifampicin), has become standard in the UK. Ethambutol may be omitted in non-cavitary smear-negative cases unless resistance is suspected. • Streptomycin is rarely prescribed in the UK, but is widely used in developing nations. • Six mths of therapy is appropriate in most cases; however, 9–12 mths of therapy should be considered if the patient is HIV-positive, or if drug intolerance occurs and a second-line agent is substituted. Meningitis should be treated for a minimum of 12 mths. • Pyridoxine should be prescribed in pregnant women and malnourished patients. • Regular monitoring of LFTs is important, as several antituberculous drugs are potentially hepatotoxic. • Corticosteroids reduce inflammation and limit tissue damage and are currently recommended when treating pericardial or meningeal disease, and in children with endobronchial disease. They may also be of benefit in pleural effusion, ureteric TB and severe pulmonary TB. • Poor adherence is a major factor in prolonged infectious illness, risk of relapse and the emergence of resistance. Directly observed therapy, in which supervised therapy is administered 2–3 times/wk, has been advocated as a method of improving adherence and control of TB in resource-poor nations.

TB and HIV/AIDS

Globally, ~9% of all new TB cases in adults are attributable to HIV infection. The clinical features vary according to the CD4 count, with low counts favouring atypical presentations. Chemotherapy regimens may be complicated by an increased potential for drug interactions between antituberculous agents and antiretroviral therapy.

Multidrug-resistant TB

The re-emergence of TB has been accompanied by a marked increase in drug-resistant strains, particularly in the poorest countries, and is closely linked to inadequate treatment. Cure is possible but prolonged treatment with less effective, more toxic and more expensive therapies is often necessary.

Prognosis

Cure should be anticipated in the majority of patients. There is a small (<5%) risk of relapse and most recurrences occur within 5 mths. Without treatment a patient with smear-positive TB will remain infectious for around 2 yrs; in 1 yr, 25% of untreated cases will die.

Opportunistic mycobacterial infection

Other species of environmental mycobacteria (often termed 'atypical') may cause human disease. These mycobacteria are low-grade pathogens (with the exception of *M. malmoense* and *M. ulcerans*), tending to cause disease in the setting of immunocompromised or scarred lungs. *M. kansasii, M. avium* complex (MAC), *M. malmoense* and *M. xenopi* are the species that most often cause lung disease. These organisms are not communicable but prolonged treatment is needed.

RESPIRATORY DISEASES CAUSED BY FUNGI

ASPERGILLOSIS

Aspergillus fumigatus may be an allergen in atopic asthma, and may cause allergic bronchopulmonary aspergillosis, an intracavitary aspergilloma or invasive pulmonary aspergillosis.

ALLERGIC BRONCHOPULMONARY ASPERGILLOSIS (ABPA)

This is a hypersensitivity reaction to *A. fumigatus.* The diagnosis may be suggested by pulmonary infiltrates on routine CXRs of patients with asthma. A persistent vigorous inflammatory response leads to bronchiectasis.

Investigations

• Proximal bronchiectasis on CT. • High serum IgE. • Elevated IgE-*A. fumigatus.* • Elevated *A. fumigatus* precipitins in serum. • Blood eosinophilia. • *A. fumigatus* in sputum.

Management

• Exacerbations are treated with prednisolone 40–60 mg daily and physiotherapy. • Maintenance therapy with low-dose oral corticosteroids may be needed to prevent disease progression.

INTRACAVITARY MYCETOMA

Inhaled air-borne spores may lodge and germinate in areas of damaged lung tissue, forming a fungal ball (mycetoma), usually in the upper lobes. As *A. fumigatus* is the most common organism, the term 'aspergilloma' is frequently used. Mycetomas are often asymptomatic, although in some patients they cause recurrent haemoptysis, which can be severe and life-threatening.

Investigations

• CXR classically demonstrates a dense rounded shadow in the upper lobe, with the 'crescent sign' (thin rim of air between the fungal ball and the upper wall of the cavity). • High-resolution CT (HRCT) provides greater sensitivity. • Serum precipitins (IgG) to *A. fumigatus* are usually positive.

Management

• Treatment is often disappointing. • Selected patients may benefit from surgery. • Bronchial artery embolisation provides a palliative approach to haemoptysis.

INVASIVE PULMONARY ASPERGILLOSIS

This is a serious and often fatal condition, which usually occurs in patients immunocompromised by either drugs or disease. It should be suspected in any patient with a severe suppurative pneumonia that has not responded to antibiotics. Demonstration of abundant fungal elements in sputum helps diagnosis. Mortality is high, but treatment with antifungal agents such as amphotericin and flucytosine may be successful.

TUMOURS OF THE BRONCHUS AND LUNG

Lung cancer is the most common cancer world-wide, accounting for 1.2 million new cases annually in 2000 and causing 18% of all cancer deaths. The prognosis of primary lung carcinoma is poor, with fewer than 30% surviving at 1 yr and 6–8% at 5 yrs. Smoking is thought to be directly responsible for at least 90% of lung carcinomas, the risk being directly proportional to the amount smoked and to the tar content of cigarettes. Risk falls slowly after smoking cessation, but remains above the risk in non-smokers for many years. Exposure to naturally occurring radon is another known risk. The incidence of lung cancer is slightly higher in urban than in rural dwellers; this may reflect differences in atmospheric pollution (including tobacco smoke) or occupation, since a number of industrial products (e.g. asbestos, beryllium, cadmium and chromium) are associated with lung cancer. The incidence of bronchial carcinoma increased dramatically during the 20th century. In women, smoking prevalence and deaths from lung cancer continue to increase.

BRONCHIAL CARCINOMA

These tumours arise from the bronchial epithelium or mucous glands. The common cell types are squamous (35%), adenocarcinoma (30%), small-cell (20%) and large-cell (15%). Lung cancer presents in many different ways. If the tumour arises in a large bronchus, symptoms arise early, but tumours originating in a peripheral bronchus can grow large without producing symptoms. Peripheral squamous tumours may cavitate. Local spread may occur into the mediastinum and invade or compress the pericardium, oesophagus, superior vena cava, trachea, or phrenic or left recurrent laryngeal nerves. Lymphatic spread to supraclavicular and mediastinal lymph nodes is also frequently observed. Blood-borne metastases most commonly affect liver, bone, brain, adrenals and skin. Even a small primary tumour may cause widespread metastatic deposits and this is a particular characteristic of small-cell-type lung cancers.

Clinical features

• Cough is the most common early symptom. • Haemoptysis occurs especially in central tumours. • Bronchial obstruction may cause breathlessness, stridor, lung collapse, pneumonia or distal abscess formation. • Breathlessness may also reflect development of a large pleural effusion. • Pleural pain usually indicates invasion of the pleura. • Pancoast's syndrome (pain in the shoulder and arm) is caused by involvement of the lower part of the brachial plexus by an apical tumour. • Horner's syndrome (ipsilateral ptosis, enophthalmos, a small pupil and hypohidrosis of the face) is due to involvement of the sympathetic chain. • Dysphagia may result from mediastinal spread. • Symptoms may be due to blood-borne metastases, such as focal neurological defects, epileptic seizures, personality change, jaundice, bone pain or skin nodules. • Lassitude, anorexia and weight loss usually indicate the presence of metastatic spread. • There are also several non-metastatic extra-pulmonary manifestations of lung cancer (Box 9.11).

Physical signs

• A large obstructing tumour produces the physical signs of lung collapse. • A monophonic or unilateral wheeze which fails to clear with coughing, or the presence of stridor, indicates incomplete large airway obstruction. • A hoarse voice with a 'bovine' cough usually indicates left recurrent laryngeal nerve palsy. • Phrenic nerve paralysis causes unilateral diaphragmatic palsy with dullness to percussion and absent breath sounds at a lung base. • There may be a pleural rub or signs of pleural effusion (stony dull percussion with absent breath sounds). • Superior vena cava obstruction leads to bilateral engorgement of the jugular veins and oedema affecting

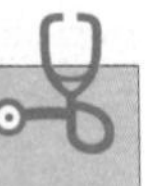

9.11 NON-METASTATIC EXTRAPULMONARY MANIFESTATIONS OF BRONCHIAL CARCINOMA

- Hyponatraemia (inappropriate ADH secretion)
- Ectopic ACTH secretion
- Hypercalcaemia (PTH-related peptide secretion)
- Myasthenia (Lambert–Eaton syndrome)
- Digital clubbing
- Hypertrophic pulmonary osteoarthropathy
- Polymyositis and dermatomyositis
- Carcinoid syndrome
- Gynaecomastia
- Polyneuropathy
- Myelopathy
- Cerebellar degeneration
- Nephrotic syndrome
- Eosinophilia

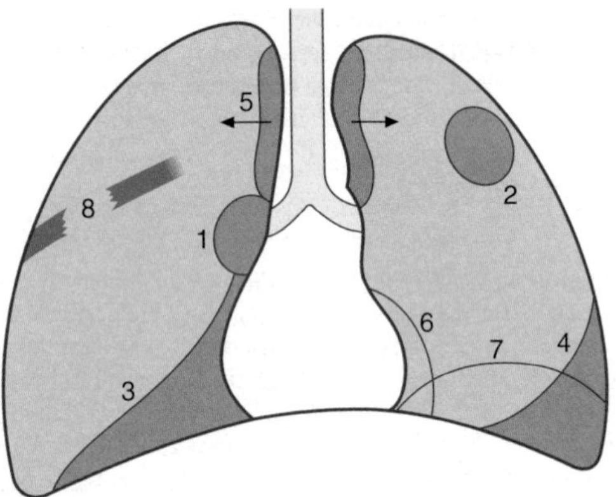

Fig. 9.7 Common radiological presentations of bronchial carcinoma. (1) Hilar mass. (2) Peripheral opacity. (3) Lung, lobe or segmental collapse. (4) Pleural effusion. (5) Broadening of mediastinum. (6) Enlarged cardiac shadow. (7) Elevation of hemidiaphragm. (8) Rib destruction.

the face, neck, arms and conjunctivae. • Finger clubbing is common and may be associated with a syndrome called hypertrophic pulmonary osteoarthropathy (HPOA).

Investigations

The main aims of investigation are to confirm the diagnosis, establish the histological cell type and define the extent of the disease.

• Common CXR features of bronchial carcinoma are illustrated in Figure 9.7. • CT thorax and abdomen is mandatory for disease staging. • Samples for pathology can be obtained in a variety of ways (Box 9.12).

After establishing a histological diagnosis, investigations should focus on determining whether the tumour is operable (Box 9.13).

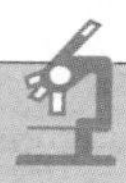

9.12 INVESTIGATIONS USED TO OBTAIN A HISTOLOGICAL DIAGNOSIS IN LUNG CANCER	
Bronchoscopy	~75% of primary lung tumours can be visualised; biopsies, mucosal brushings and bronchial washings should be taken
CT-guided biopsy	For peripheral lung tumours; small risk of pneumothorax
Needle aspiration/biopsy	Used to sample lymph nodes, skin lesions, liver or bone marrow
Sputum cytology	Not routine due to low yield; sometimes used if patient is unfit for bronchoscopy
Mediastinoscopy	Surgical procedure under general anaesthetic; required for staging prior to lung resection; can also be used in difficult cases where other investigations have not led to a diagnosis
Endoscopic USS	Used to sample abnormal mediastinal nodes through the oesophagus or bronchial wall using ultrasound guidance
Pleural aspiration ± biopsy	Indicated in all patients with a pleural effusion; 'blind' (Abrams needle) or radiologically guided pleural biopsy is performed
Thoracoscopy	May be required if pleural aspiration and biopsy are negative; allows direct visualisation of the pleura

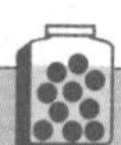

9.13 CONTRAINDICATIONS TO SURGICAL RESECTION IN BRONCHIAL CARCINOMA

- Distant metastasis (M1)
- Malignant pleural effusion (T4)
- Severe/unstable cardiac or other medical condition
- Invasion of mediastinal structures (T4)
- Contralateral mediastinal nodes (N3)
- FEV_1 <0.8 litres

• A PET scan detects elevated radiolabelled glucose metabolism in areas affected by tumour and can be used prior to surgery (or radical radiotherapy) to detect unsuspected metastatic disease. • Small-cell lung cancer tends to metastasise early; therefore patients with this tumour are not suitable for surgical intervention. • Head CT, radionuclide bone scanning, liver USS and bone marrow biopsy are reserved for patients with clinical, haematological or biochemical evidence of tumour spread to such sites.

Management and prognosis

Surgical resection carries the best hope of long-term survival; however, some patients treated with radical radiotherapy also achieve prolonged remission or cure. Following resection, 5-yr survival rates are >75% in stage I disease (N0, tumour confined within visceral pleura) and 55% in stage II disease (includes resection in patients with ipsilateral peribronchial or hilar node involvement). Unfortunately the majority of cases (>85%) have unresectable disease.

Radiotherapy can palliate distressing symptoms such as large airway obstruction, SVC obstruction, recurrent haemoptysis, and pain caused by chest wall invasion or by skeletal metastatic deposits. The treatment of small-cell carcinoma with chemotherapy, sometimes in combination with radiotherapy, can increase the median survival of patients with this highly malignant tumour from 3 mths to well over a year. Chemotherapy is generally less effective in non-small-cell bronchial cancers, although platinum-based regimens show some benefit. Malignant pleural effusions should be drained if the patient is symptomatic and pleurodesis should be considered.

The best outcomes are obtained when lung cancer is managed in specialist centres by multidisciplinary teams including oncologists, thoracic surgeons, respiratory physicians and specialist nurses. As in other forms of carcinoma, effective communication, pain relief and attention to diet are important.

Overall the prognosis in bronchial carcinoma is very poor, with ~70% of patients dying within 1 yr of diagnosis and <8% of patients surviving 5 yrs after diagnosis.

CARCINOID TUMOUR

This is a low-grade malignant neuroendocrine tumour. It typically presents with bronchial obstruction or cough. Unlike other primary lung tumours it carries a good prognosis (95% 5-yr survival with resection).

SECONDARY TUMOURS OF THE LUNG

The most common tumours that metastasise to the lung are those of the breast, kidney, uterus, ovary, testes, thyroid and bone, often with multiple deposits. Lymphatic infiltration (lymphangitis) may develop in patients with carcinoma of the breast, stomach, bowel, pancreas or bronchus. This grave condition causes severe and rapidly progressive breathlessness associated with marked hypoxaemia.

TUMOURS OF THE MEDIASTINUM

A variety of conditions can present radiologically as a mediastinal mass (Fig. 9.8). Benign tumours and cysts in the mediastinum are often an incidental finding. Malignant mediastinal tumours are distinguished by their power to invade as well as compress structures such as bronchi and lungs. CT (or MRI) is the investigation of choice for mediastinal tumours.

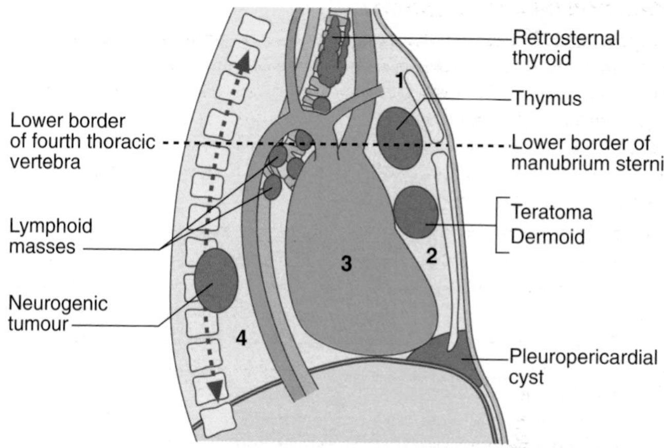

Fig. 9.8 The divisions of the mediastinum described in the diagnosis of mediastinal masses. (1) Superior mediastinum. (2) Anterior mediastinum. (3) Middle mediastinum. (4) Posterior mediastinum. Sites of the more common mediastinal tumours are also illustrated.

INTERSTITIAL AND INFILTRATIVE PULMONARY DISEASES

DIFFUSE PARENCHYMAL LUNG DISEASE

The diffuse parenchymal lung diseases (DPLDs) are a heterogeneous group of conditions associated with diffuse thickening of the alveolar walls with inflammatory cells and exudates (e.g. ARDS), granulomas (e.g. sarcoidosis), alveolar haemorrhage (e.g. Goodpasture's syndrome, p. 195) and/or fibrosis (e.g. idiopathic pulmonary fibrosis—IPF). Lung disease may occur in isolation or as part of a systemic connective tissue disorder. The classification of DPLD is shown in Figure 9.9. Establishing a diagnosis is important to determine prognosis, predict response to treatment and avoid inappropriate treatment. A lung biopsy taken when the patient is already established on empirical immunosuppressive therapy is associated with a higher morbidity and mortality and is more difficult to interpret. Particular attention should be paid to occupational history, drug history and any exposure to organic and inorganic dusts. Rashes, joint pains or renal disease may suggest an underlying connective tissue disorder or vasculitis.

Investigations

• FBC may show lymphopenia (sarcoid), eosinophilia (pulmonary eosinophilias, drug reactions) or neutrophilia (hypersensitivity pneumonitis). •

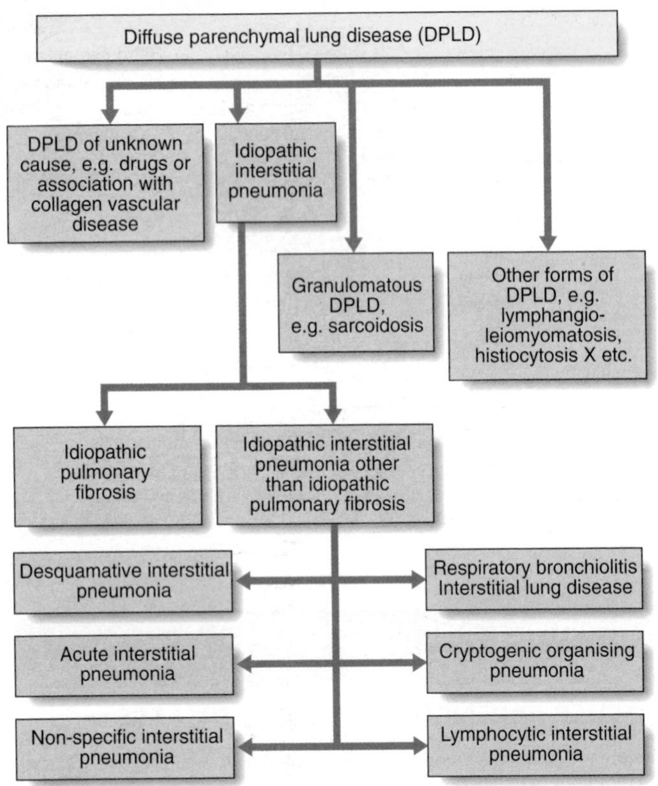

Fig. 9.9 Classification of diffuse parenchymal lung disease.

Ca^{2+} and serum ACE may be elevated in sarcoid. • Autoimmune screen or rheumatoid factor may help diagnose connective tissue disease. • CXR shows a reticulonodular pattern of infiltration, with honeycombing at the lung bases in advanced disease. • HRCT has become extremely valuable in detecting early interstitial lung disease, assessing the disease pattern and guiding further investigations and management. • Pulmonary function tests typically show a restrictive pattern with diminished lung volumes and a reduced gas transfer (although gas transfer may be elevated in alveolar haemorrhage). • Bronchoscopy with bronchoalveolar lavage (BAL) shows increased lymphocytes in sarcoid or hypersensitivity pneumonitis, while neutrophilia is more suggestive of IPF. Transbronchial biopsies are often diagnostic in sarcoidosis, but are less specific in heterogeneous disorders such as IPF, where video-assisted thoracoscopy (VATS) can obtain a more representative sample.

SARCOIDOSIS

Sarcoidosis is a multisystem granulomatous disorder, which is more common in colder parts of Northern Europe. In North America it is more common and more aggressive in Afro-Caribbean populations. The aetiology is unknown, although atypical mycobacteria, viruses and genetic factors have been proposed. Sarcoidosis is less common in smokers. The characteristic histological feature is a non-caseating epithelioid granuloma.

Clinical features

• Any organ may be affected, but 90% of cases affect the lungs. • Otherwise, lymph glands, liver, spleen, skin, eyes, parotid glands and phalangeal bones are the most frequently involved sites. • Löfgren's syndrome—erythema nodosum, peripheral arthropathy, uveitis, bilateral hilar lymphadenopathy (BHL), lethargy and occasionally fever—commonly presents in the third or fourth decade. • BHL may be detected in an otherwise asymptomatic individual undergoing CXR. • Pulmonary disease may present insidiously with cough, exertional breathlessness and radiographic infiltrates. • Fibrosis occurs uncommonly but may cause a silent loss of lung function.

Investigations

• FBC demonstrates lymphopenia. • LFTs may be mildly deranged. • Ca^{2+} may be elevated. • Serum ACE can sometimes provide a non-specific marker of disease activity. • CXR is used to stage sarcoid (Box 9.14). • Characteristic HRCT appearances include reticulonodular opacities that follow a perilymphatic distribution centred on bronchovascular bundles and the subpleural areas. • Bronchoscopy may demonstrate a 'cobblestone' appearance of the mucosa, and bronchial and transbronchial biopsies usually show non-caseating granulomas. • The occurrence of erythema nodosum in patients in the second to third decades with BHL on CXR is often sufficient for a confident diagnosis.

9.14 CXR CHANGES IN SARCOIDOSIS	
Stage I: BHL (usually symmetrical); paratracheal nodes often enlarged	Often asymptomatic but may be associated with erythema nodosum and arthralgia; majority of cases resolve in <1 yr
Stage II: BHL and parenchymal infiltrates	Patients may present with breathlessness or cough; majority of cases resolve spontaneously
Stage III: parenchymal infiltrates without BHL	Disease less likely to resolve spontaneously
Stage IV: pulmonary fibrosis	Can cause progression to ventilatory failure, pulmonary hypertension and cor pulmonale

Management

The majority of patients enjoy spontaneous remission and, if there is no evidence of organ damage, it is appropriate to withhold therapy for 4–6 mths. Patients who present with acute illness and erythema nodosum may require NSAIDs and on occasion a short course of corticosteroids. Systemic corticosteroids are also indicated in the presence of hypercalcaemia, pulmonary function impairment and renal impairment. In patients with severe disease both methotrexate and azathioprine have been used successfully and selected patients may be referred for consideration of single lung transplantation.

IDIOPATHIC PULMONARY FIBROSIS (IPF)

The term IPF has replaced cryptogenic fibrosing alveolitis and refers to a specific form of DPLD characterised by pathological (or radiological) evidence of usual interstitial pneumonia (UIP). The aetiology remains unknown; speculation has included exposure to infectious agents such as Epstein–Barr virus or to occupational dusts such as metal or wood dusts, prior use of antidepressants, and a possible role for chronic gastro-oesophageal reflux. A strong association with smoking exists.

Clinical features

• Uncommon before the age of 50 yrs. • Usually presents with progressive disabling breathlessness and a non-productive cough, reduced expansion, tachypnoea and central cyanosis. • Finger clubbing: present in 25–50% of cases. • Late inspiratory crackles likened to the parting of Velcro, classically heard at the lung bases.

Investigations

• Blood tests are of little value. • Pulmonary function tests show a restrictive defect with reduced lung volumes and gas transfer. • Exercise tests are useful to demonstrate arterial hypoxaemia on exercise, but as IPF advances, hypoxia is present at rest. • CXR demonstrates lower zone bi-basal reticular and reticulonodular opacities. A 'honeycomb' appearance may be seen in advanced disease. • HRCT may be diagnostic, demonstrating a patchy, predominantly peripheral, subpleural and basal reticular pattern with subpleural cysts (honeycombing) and/or traction bronchiectasis. • Patients with typical clinical features and HRCT appearances consistent with UIP do not require lung biopsy, particularly if other known causes of interstitial lung disease have been excluded.

Management

A median survival of 3 yrs is typical. However, the rate of progression varies from death within a few months to survival for many years. Serial lung function may be helpful in predicting survival; relative preservation of lung function is a predictor of longer survival but desaturation on exercise heralds a poor prognosis. Treatment options remain limited. Prednisolone therapy (0.5 mg/kg) combined with azathioprine (2–3 mg/kg) is currently recommended to patients who are highly symptomatic or have rapidly progressive disease, have a predominantly 'ground-glass' appearance on CT or have a sustained fall of >15% in their FVC or gas transfer over a 3–6-mth period. However, response rates are notoriously poor and side-effects guaranteed. Oxygen may be provided for palliation of breathlessness but opiates may be required for relief of severe dyspnoea.

HYPERSENSITIVITY PNEUMONITIS (HP)

HP (also called extrinsic allergic alveolitis) results from the inhalation of certain types of organic dust which give rise to a diffuse immune complex reaction in the walls of the alveoli and bronchioles. In the UK, 50% of reported cases of HP occur in farm workers; bird fanciers represent another important group.

Clinical features

• The acute form of the disease should be suspected when anyone exposed to organic dust complains of 'flu'-like symptoms (headache, malaise, myalgia, fever, dry cough, breathlessness) within a few hours of re-exposure to the same dust. • Chest auscultation reveals widespread end-inspiratory crackles and squeaks. • Onset of disease is more insidious with chronic low-level exposure (as may be the case with an indoor pet bird). • If unchecked, the disease may progress to cause fibrosis, severe respiratory disability, hypoxaemia, pulmonary hypertension, cor pulmonale and eventually death.

Investigations

• CXR demonstrates diffuse micronodular shadowing that is classically more pronounced in the upper zones. • In acute disease, HRCT shows bilateral areas of consolidation superimposed on small centrilobar nodular opacities and air-trapping on expiration. • In chronic disease, fibrosis may predominate. • Pulmonary function tests show a restrictive ventilatory defect with reduced lung volumes and impaired gas transfer. • ABG reveals reduced PaO_2, and in the presence of over-ventilation the $PaCO_2$ is often low. • Serology can be used to identify positive precipitating antibodies to the offending antigen, e.g. *Micropolyspora faeni* (farmer's lung) or avian serum proteins (bird fancier's lung). However, precipitating antibodies may also be present without evidence of HP. • Open lung biopsy may be necessary to establish the diagnosis.

Management

Whenever possible, the patient should cease exposure to the inciting agent. This may be difficult to achieve, either because of implications for livelihood (e.g. farmers) or addiction to hobbies (e.g. pigeon breeders). Dust masks with appropriate filters may minimise exposure and may be combined with methods of reducing levels of antigen (e.g. drying hay before storage). In acute cases prednisolone 40 mg/day should be given for 3–4 wks. Most patients recover completely, but the development of interstitial fibrosis causes permanent disability when there has been prolonged exposure to antigen.

LUNG DISEASES DUE TO INORGANIC DUSTS

Prolonged exposure to certain inorganic dusts may lead to diffuse pulmonary fibrosis (the pneumoconioses), although berylliosis causes an interstitial granulomatous disease similar to sarcoidosis. The dusts themselves cause little direct damage to the lung parenchyma and the pathological result depends largely on the inflammatory and fibrotic responses to the dust. The most important types of pneumoconiosis are coal worker's pneumoconiosis, silicosis and asbestosis.

COAL WORKER'S PNEUMOCONIOSIS

Prolonged inhalation of coal dust overwhelms alveolar macrophages, leading to a fibrotic reaction. Scattered discrete fibrotic lesions constitute simple coal worker's pneumoconiosis (SCWP), which is usually asymptomatic. Complicated pneumoconiosis is characterised by large dense masses appearing mainly in the upper lobes (also known as progressive massive fibrosis, PMF). Cavitation may occur, raising important differential diagnoses such as lung cancer, TB and Wegener's granulomatosis (p. 611). PMF is usually associated with cough, production of sputum that may be black (melanoptysis), and breathlessness. It may progress to respiratory failure even after cessation of exposure.

SILICOSIS

Silicosis occurs in stonemasons who inhale crystalline or free silica, usually in the form of quartz dust. The clinical and radiological features are similar to those of coal worker's pneumoconiosis. Enlargement of the hilar glands with an 'egg-shell' pattern of calcification is said to be characteristic but is uncommon and non-specific. Silica is highly fibrogenic and the disease is usually progressive (even when exposure ceases). The patient should, therefore, be removed from the offending environment as soon as possible.

ASBESTOSIS

The main types of the fibrous mineral asbestos are chrysotile (white asbestos), which accounts for 90% of the world's production, crocidolite (blue asbestos) and amosite (brown asbestos). Exposure occurs in a variety of occupations (e.g. demolition, ship breaking, pipe and boiler lagging) and is a recognised risk factor for several respiratory diseases (Fig. 9.10). The law in many countries now enforces improved industrial hygiene and provides compensation for asbestos-related disease.

Asbestosis is a diffuse interstitial fibrosis of the lungs. The condition seldom develops <20 yrs after the start of exposure and usually follows substantial and prolonged asbestos exposure over many years. The risk increases with the amount inhaled.

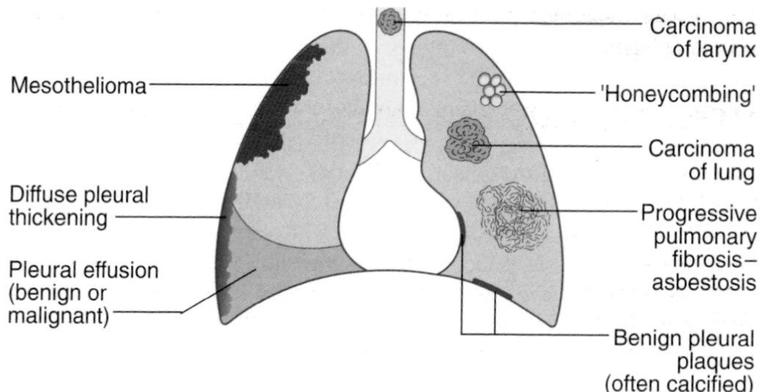

Fig. 9.10 Asbestosis: the range of possible effects on the respiratory tract.

• Patients usually present with exertional breathlessness and fine, late inspiratory crackles over the lower zones. • Digital clubbing (reported in 40% of patients) is an adverse prognostic feature. • CXR shows bi-basal reticulonodular shadowing, and asbestos-related pleural plaques are usually present. • HRCT typically shows basal, subpleural, curvilinear opacities, band-like opacities and occasionally 'honeycombing'. • Pulmonary function tests typically show a restrictive defect with decreased lung volumes and reduced gas transfer factor. • No specific treatment is available. • Asbestosis usually progresses very slowly. In advanced cases respiratory failure and cor pulmonale may develop. About 40% of patients (usually those who smoke) develop carcinoma of the lung and 10% may develop mesothelioma.

LUNG DISEASES DUE TO SYSTEMIC INFLAMMATORY DISEASE

ACUTE RESPIRATORY DISTRESS SYNDROME

See page 23.

RESPIRATORY INVOLVEMENT IN CONNECTIVE TISSUE DISORDERS

Pulmonary fibrosis is a recognised complication of most connective tissue diseases. The clinical features are usually indistinguishable from IPF (p. 310) and the response to immunosuppressive drugs is similarly unpredictable. Connective tissue disorders may also cause disease of the pleura, diaphragm and chest wall muscles. Pulmonary hypertension and cor pulmonale may result from advanced pulmonary fibrosis associated with connective tissue disorders and is particularly common in patients with systemic sclerosis.

Indirect associations between connective tissue diseases and respiratory disorders include:

• Those due to disease in other organs, e.g. thrombocytopenia causing haemoptysis. • Pulmonary toxic effects of drugs used to treat the connective tissue disorder (e.g. gold and methotrexate). • Secondary infection due to the disease itself, neutropenia or immunosuppressive drug regimens.

Rheumatoid disease: Pulmonary fibrosis is the most common pulmonary manifestation (rheumatoid lung). The clinical features, investigations, treatment and prognosis are usually similar to those of IPF. Pleural effusion is common, especially in men with seropositive disease. Most resolve spontaneously. Biochemical testing shows an exudative effusion with markedly reduced glucose levels and raised LDH. Effusions that fail to resolve spontaneously may respond to prednisolone (30–40 mg daily) but some become chronic. Rheumatoid pulmonary nodules are usually asymptomatic and detected incidentally on CXR. They are usually multiple and subpleural in site, but can mimic lung cancer. The combination of rheumatoid nodules and pneumoconiosis is known as Caplan's syndrome. Treatments given for rheumatoid arthritis may also be relevant; corticosteroid therapy predisposes to infections, methotrexate may cause pulmonary fibrosis, and anti-TNF therapy has been associated with the reactivation of TB. Obliterative bronchiolitis and bronchiectasis are also recognised pulmonary complications of rheumatoid arthritis.

Systemic lupus erythematosus (SLE): Pulmonary fibrosis is a relatively uncommon manifestation of SLE. Recurrent pleurisy is common in SLE, with or without effusions. An acute alveolitis may rarely be associated with diffuse alveolar haemorrhage. This condition is life-threatening and requires immunosuppression. Some patients with SLE present with exertional dyspnoea and orthopnoea but without pulmonary fibrosis. The CXR reveals elevated diaphragms, and pulmonary function testing shows reduced lung volumes. This condition has been described as 'shrinking lungs' and has been attributed to diaphragmatic myopathy. Antiphospholipid syndrome is associated with an increased risk of venous and pulmonary thromboembolism and these patients require life-long anticoagulation.

Systemic sclerosis: Most patients with systemic sclerosis eventually develop diffuse pulmonary fibrosis (up to 90% at autopsy). In some patients it is indolent, but when progressive, as in IPF, the median survival time is around 4 yrs. Pulmonary fibrosis is rare in the CREST variant of progressive systemic sclerosis but isolated pulmonary hypertension may develop. Other pulmonary complications include recurrent aspiration pneumonias secondary to oesophageal disease. Rarely, sclerosis of the skin of the chest wall may be so extensive and cicatrising as to restrict chest wall movement—the so-called 'hidebound chest'.

PULMONARY EOSINOPHILIA AND VASCULITIDES

This term is applied to a group of disorders of different aetiology in which lesions in the lungs produce a CXR abnormality associated with pulmonary eosinophilia with or without peripheral blood eosinophilia (Box 9.15).

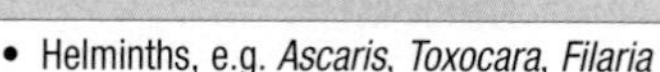

9.15 PULMONARY EOSINOPHILIA

- Helminths, e.g. *Ascaris, Toxocara, Filaria*
- Drugs, e.g. nitrofurantoin, para-aminosalicylic acid (PAS), sulfasalazine, imipramine, chlorpropamide, phenylbutazone
- Fungi, e.g. *Aspergillus fumigatus* causing ABPA (p. 301)
- Cryptogenic eosinophilic pneumonia
- Churg–Strauss syndrome (asthma, blood eosinophilia, neuropathy, pulmonary infiltrates, eosinophilic vasculitis)
- Hypereosinophilic syndrome

LUNG DISEASES DUE TO DRUGS AND IRRADIATION

Drugs may cause a number of parenchymal reactions:

ARDS: Hydrochlorothiazide, streptokinase, aspirin and opiates (in overdose).

Pulmonary eosinophilia: See Box 9.15.

Non-eosinophilic alveolitis: Amiodarone, gold, nitrofurantoin, bleomycin, methotrexate.

Pleural disease: Bromocriptine, amiodarone, methotrexate, methysergide, or others via induction of SLE (phenytoin, hydralazine, isoniazid).

Asthma: β-blockers, cholinergic antagonists, aspirin, NSAIDs.

Acute radiation pneumonitis is typically seen within 6–12 wks of lung irradiation, and causes cough and dyspnoea. This may resolve spontaneously but responds to corticosteroid treatment. Chronic interstitial fibrosis may present several months later.

PULMONARY VASCULAR DISEASE

VENOUS THROMBOEMBOLISM

Deep venous thrombosis (DVT) and pulmonary embolism (PE) can be considered under the heading of venous thromboembolism (VTE). The majority (75%) of PEs arise from the propagation of lower limb DVT. PE is common, occurring in ~1% of all patients admitted to hospital and accounting for ~5% of in-hospital deaths. Amniotic fluid, placenta, air, fat, tumour (especially choriocarcinoma) and septic emboli (from endocarditis affecting the tricuspid/pulmonary valves) are rare.

Clinical features

The varied clinical presentation, non-specific nature of the physical signs and the lack of sensitive and specific diagnostic tests can make the diagnosis of PE difficult. It is helpful to consider three questions:

9.16 RISK FACTORS FOR VENOUS THROMBOEMBOLISM	
Surgery	Major abdominal/pelvic surgery; hip/knee surgery; post-operative intensive care
Pregnancy/puerperium	
Cardiorespiratory disease	COPD, congestive cardiac failure or other disabling disease
Lower limb problems	Fracture; varicose veins; stroke/spinal cord injury
Malignant disease	Abdominal/pelvic; advanced/metastatic; concurrent chemotherapy
Increasing age	
Previous proven VTE	
Immobility	
Thrombotic disorders	Antiphospholipid syndrome; protein C, protein S deficiency
Trauma	

- Is the clinical presentation consistent with PE?
- Does the patient have risk factors for PE?
- Is there any alternative diagnosis that can explain the patient's presentation?

A recognised risk factor for PE (Box 9.16) is present in 80–90% of patients. The clinical features (Box 9.17) depend largely upon the size of embolism and comorbidity.

Investigations

CXR: PE may give rise to a variety of non-specific appearances but may be normal. A normal CXR in an acutely breathless and hypoxaemic patient should raise the suspicion of PE, as should bilateral changes in a patient with unilateral pleuritic chest pain. CXR can also exclude alternatives such as heart failure, pneumonia or pneumothorax.

ECG: ECG changes in PE are common but usually non-specific. The most common findings are a sinus tachycardia and anterior T-wave inversion; larger emboli may cause right heart strain revealed by an $S_1Q_3T_3$ pattern, ST-segment and T-wave changes, or right bundle branch block. The ECG may also suggest an alternative diagnosis such as myocardial infarction and pericarditis.

ABG: Typically show a reduced PaO_2 and a normal or low $PaCO_2$, but are occasionally normal. Metabolic acidosis may occur in acute massive PE with cardiovascular collapse.

D-dimer: This is a specific degradation product released into the circulation when cross-linked fibrin undergoes endogenous fibrinolysis. A low D-dimer level has a high negative predictive value and is a useful screening test (Fig. 9.11). However, a suggestive clinical picture in a high-risk patient must be investigated further even when the D-dimer level is normal. Non-

9.17 CATEGORISATION OF PULMONARY THROMBOEMBOLI

	Acute massive PE	Acute small/medium PE	Chronic PE
Symptoms	Faintness or collapse, central chest pain, apprehension, severe dyspnoea	Pleuritic chest pain, restricted breathing, haemoptysis	Exertional dyspnoea; late symptoms of pulmonary hypertension or right heart failure
Signs	Major circulatory collapse: tachycardia, hypotension, ↑JVP, right ventricular gallop rhythm, split P_2; severe cyanosis; ↓urinary output	Tachycardia; pleural rub, raised hemidiaphragm, crackles, effusion (often blood-stained); low-grade fever	May be minimal early in disease; later—RV heave, loud, split P_2; extensive right heart failure
CXR	Usually normal; may be subtle oligaemia	Pleuropulmonary opacities, pleural effusion, linear shadows, raised hemidiaphragm	Enlarged pulmonary artery trunk, enlarged heart, prominent RV
ECG	$S_1Q_3T_3$ anterior T-wave inversion; RBBB	Sinus tachycardia	RV hypertrophy and strain
ABG	Markedly abnormal with ↓PaO_2 and ↓$PaCO_2$; metabolic acidosis	May be normal or ↓PaO_2	Exertional ↓PaO_2 or desaturation on exercise testing
Alternative diagnoses	MI; pericardial tamponade; aortic dissection	Pneumonia, pneumothorax, musculoskeletal chest pain	Other causes of pulmonary hypertension

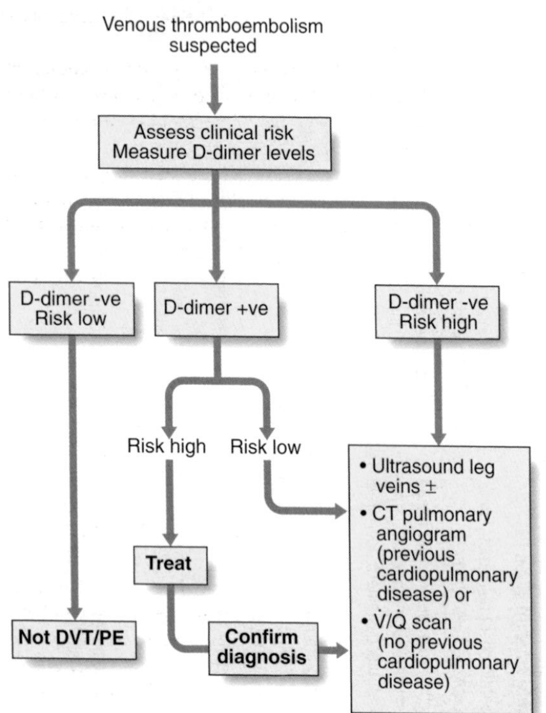

Fig. 9.11 Algorithm for the investigation of patients with suspected pulmonary thromboembolism. Clinical risk is based on the presence of risk factors for VTE and the probability of another diagnosis.

specific elevation of the D-dimer is observed in a number of conditions other than PE, including myocardial infarction, pneumonia and sepsis.

CT pulmonary angiography (CTPA): The development of rapid acquisition helical CT scanners has popularised the use of CTPA (Fig. 9.12). It not only may exclude PE but may also reveal an alternative diagnosis. Limited resolution may hinder the detection of small peripheral emboli but further advances in CT are likely to improve this.

Ventilation–perfusion scanning: The sensitivity and specificity of $\dot{V}/\dot{Q}$ scanning are enhanced by a clinical probability assessment. A normal $\dot{V}/\dot{Q}$ scan virtually excludes PE, and a low-probability scan in the presence of a low clinical probability makes PE unlikely. Similarly, the presence of a high-probability scan in a patient with a high clinical probability almost certainly establishes the diagnosis of PE. However, $\dot{V}/\dot{Q}$ scanning is of limited value when PE is suspected in patients with pre-existing cardiopulmonary pathology (e.g. COPD or cardiac failure) because in these cases 70% of scans are indeterminate.

Doppler USS of the leg veins: This is the investigation of choice in patients with clinical DVT, but may also be applied to patients in whom PE is suspected, particularly if there are clinical signs in a limb, as many will have identifiable proximal thrombus in the leg veins.

Echocardiography: This is helpful in the differential diagnosis and assessment of acute circulatory collapse. Acute dilatation of the right heart is usually present in massive PE, and thrombus (embolism in transit) may be visible. Alternative diagnoses, including left ventricular failure, aortic dissection and pericardial tamponade, can usually be established with confidence.

Pulmonary angiography: This has largely been superseded by CTPA.

Management

• Oxygen should be given to all hypoxaemic patients in a concentration necessary to restore SpO_2 to >90%. • Hypotension should be treated by giving i.v. fluid or plasma expander; diuretics and vasodilators should be avoided. • Opiates may be necessary to relieve pain and distress but should be used with caution. • Resuscitation by external cardiac massage may be successful in the moribund patient by dislodging and breaking up a large central embolus.

Anticoagulation: Should be commenced immediately in patients with a high or intermediate probability of PE, but can usually be safely withheld from patients with a low clinical probability pending further investigation. Low molecular weight heparin administered subcutaneously is as effective as i.v. unfractionated heparin and easier to administer. The dose is standardised for the weight of the patient and does not require monitoring by tests of coagulation. Heparin is effective in reducing mortality in PE by reducing the propagation of clot and the risk of further emboli. It should be administered for at least 5 days and anticoagulation continued using oral warfarin. Heparin should not be discontinued until the international normalised ratio (INR) is >2. The optimum duration of warfarin therapy is not clear. Current guidelines suggest that patients with an underlying prothrombotic risk or a history of previous emboli should be anticoagulated for life. Those with a reversible risk factor require 3 mths of therapy, although 6 wks may be sufficient for some. Six mths of therapy is currently recommended for idiopathic VTE.

Thrombolytic therapy: Thrombolysis appears to improve outcome when acute massive PE is accompanied by shock, but it is not clear whether there is any advantage of thrombolysis over heparin in patients with a normal BP. Patients with PE appear to have a high risk of intracranial haemorrhage and must be screened carefully for haemorrhagic risk.

Caval filters: Selected patients with recurrent PE despite adequate anticoagulation, or those in whom anticoagulation is contraindicated, may benefit from insertion of a filter in the inferior vena cava below the origin of the renal vessels.

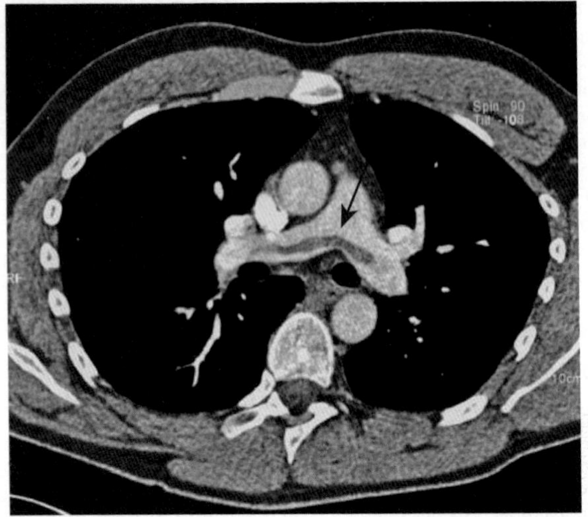

Fig. 9.12 CT pulmonary angiogram. The arrow points to a saddle embolism in the bifurcation of the pulmonary artery.

Prognosis

Patients who develop PE after an operation have the lowest recurrence rate; in other groups, recurrence rates may be as high as 9%/yr. Echocardiographic evidence of right ventricular dysfunction identifies patients at risk of developing cardiogenic shock and an increased risk of death. Persistent pulmonary hypertension and right ventricular dysfunction 6 wks after PE identify high-risk patients with an increased likelihood of developing overt right ventricular failure over the next 5 yrs.

PULMONARY HYPERTENSION

Pulmonary hypertension is defined as a mean pulmonary artery pressure >25 mmHg at rest or 30 mmHg with exercise. The causes of pulmonary hypertension are listed in Box 9.18. Further classification is based on the degree of functional disturbance using the New York Heart Association (NYHA) grades I–IV. Respiratory failure due to intrinsic pulmonary disease is the most common cause of pulmonary hypertension.

Primary pulmonary hypertension (PPH) is a rare but important disease that affects young people, predominantly women, aged between 20 and 30 yrs. It is usually sporadic or associated with an underlying cause, but may also be familial, caused by an inherited gene mutation. The median survival from time of diagnosis (without heart–lung transplantation) is 2–3 yrs.

9.18 CLASSIFICATION OF PULMONARY HYPERTENSION	
Pulmonary arterial hypertension	Primary pulmonary hypertension: sporadic and familial Related to: collagen vascular disease (limited cutaneous systemic sclerosis), congenital systemic to pulmonary shunts, portal hypertension, HIV infection, exposure to various drugs or toxins, persistent pulmonary hypertension of the newborn
Pulmonary venous hypertension	Left-sided valvular or ventricular disease, pulmonary veno-occlusive disease
Pulmonary hypertension associated with parenchymal lung disease and/or hypoxaemia	COPD; DPLD; sleep-disordered breathing; chronic high-altitude exposure
Chronic thromboembolic disease	

All patients should be anticoagulated with warfarin, as this has been demonstrated to improve prognosis in severe pulmonary hypertension. Treatment with the oral endothelin receptor antagonist bosentan, nebulised iloprost or infused epoprostamol has dramatically improved exercise performance, symptoms and prognosis in selected cases. Pulmonary thromboendarterectomy should be contemplated in patients with chronic proximal pulmonary thromboembolic disease and heart–lung transplantation may be considered in selected patients.

DISEASES OF THE NASOPHARYNX, LARYNX AND TRACHEA

DISEASES OF THE NASOPHARYNX

ALLERGIC RHINITIS

In this disorder there are episodes of nasal congestion, watery nasal discharge and sneezing. It may be seasonal or perennial (continuous symptoms). It is due to an immediate hypersensitivity reaction to seasonal antigens including pollens from grasses (hay fever), flowers, weeds or trees. Perennial allergic rhinitis may be a specific reaction to antigens derived from house dust, fungal spores or animal dander but similar symptoms can be caused by physical or chemical irritants. Skin hypersensitivity tests with the relevant antigen are usually positive in seasonal allergic rhinitis but are less useful in perennial rhinitis.

Management

• Exposure to trigger antigens (e.g. pollen) should be minimised. • The following medications may be used singly or in combination: an oral antihistamine, a topical steroid nasal spray and/or sodium cromoglicate nasal spray. • When severe symptoms interfere with school, business or social activities, oral corticosteroids are occasionally indicated.

LARYNGEAL DISORDERS

The most common symptom of laryngeal disorders is hoarseness. The differential diagnosis of hoarseness that persists beyond a few days is:

• Laryngeal tumour. • Vocal cord paralysis. • Inhaled corticosteroid treatment. • Chronic laryngitis due to excessive use of the voice (particularly in dusty atmospheres). • Heavy tobacco smoking. • Chronic infection of nasal sinuses.

LARYNGEAL PARALYSIS

Disease affecting the motor nerve supply of the larynx is nearly always unilateral and, because of the intrathoracic course of the left recurrent laryngeal nerve, usually left-sided. One or both recurrent laryngeal nerves may be damaged at thyroidectomy or by thyroid carcinoma. Symptoms are hoarseness, a 'bovine cough' and stridor, which may be severe if both vocal cords are affected. In some patients a CXR may bring to light an unsuspected bronchial carcinoma or pulmonary TB. If no such abnormality is found, laryngoscopy should be performed. In unilateral paralysis the voice may be improved by injection of Teflon into the affected cord. In bilateral paralysis, tracheal intubation, tracheostomy or laryngeal surgery may be necessary.

LARYNGEAL OBSTRUCTION

Laryngeal obstruction is more liable to occur in children than in adults because of the smaller size of the glottis. Sudden complete laryngeal obstruction by a foreign body causes acute asphyxia—violent but ineffective inspiratory efforts with indrawing of the intercostal spaces and the unsupported lower ribs, accompanied by cyanosis. Unrelieved, the condition is rapidly fatal. When, as in most cases, the obstruction is incomplete at first, the clinical features are progressive breathlessness accompanied by stridor and cyanosis.

Management

Urgent treatment to relieve obstruction is needed.

• When a foreign body causes laryngeal obstruction in children it can often be dislodged by turning the patient head downwards and squeezing the chest vigorously. • In adults this is often impossible, but a sudden forceful compression of the upper abdomen (Heimlich manoeuvre) may be effective. • In other circumstances the cause should be investigated by direct laryngoscopy, which may also permit the removal of an unsuspected foreign body or the insertion of a tube past the obstruction into the trachea. • Tracheostomy must be performed without delay if these procedures fail to relieve obstruction, but except in dire emergencies this operation should be performed in an operating theatre by a surgeon. • In angioedema complete laryngeal occlusion can usually be prevented by treatment with adrenaline (epinephrine) 0.5–1 mg (0.5–1 ml of 1 : 1000) i.m., chlorphenamine maleate 10–20 mg by slow i.v. injection and i.v. hydrocortisone sodium succinate 200 mg.

TRACHEAL DISORDERS

TRACHEAL OBSTRUCTION

External compression by enlarged mediastinal lymph nodes containing metastatic deposits, usually from a bronchial carcinoma, is a more frequent cause of tracheal obstruction than the uncommon primary benign or malignant tumours. Rarely, the trachea may be compressed by an aneurysm of the aortic arch, by a retrosternal goitre or in children by tuberculous mediastinal lymph nodes. Tracheal stenosis is an occasional complication of tracheostomy, prolonged intubation, Wegener's granulomatosis or trauma.

Clinical features

• Stridor can be detected in every patient with severe tracheal narrowing. • Bronchoscopy should be undertaken without delay to determine the site, degree and nature of the obstruction.

Management

• Localised tumours of the trachea can be resected, but reconstruction after resection may be technically difficult. • Endobronchial laser therapy, bronchoscopically placed tracheal stents, chemotherapy and radiotherapy are alternatives to surgery.

TRACHEO-OESOPHAGEAL FISTULA

This may be a congenital abnormality in newborn infants. In adults it is usually due to malignant lesions in the mediastinum, such as carcinoma or lymphoma, eroding both the trachea and oesophagus to produce a communication between them. Swallowed liquids enter the trachea and bronchi through the fistula and provoke coughing.

Management

• Surgical closure of a congenital fistula, if undertaken promptly, is usually successful. • There is usually no curative treatment for malignant fistulae, and death from overwhelming pulmonary infection rapidly supervenes.

DISEASES OF THE PLEURA, DIAPHRAGM AND CHEST WALL

DISEASES OF THE PLEURA

PLEURISY

Pleurisy is a term used when disease involving the pleura gives rise to pain on breathing or evidence of pleural friction. It commonly results from pulmonary infection, inflammation and infarction, but may also occur in malignancy. On examination rib movement is restricted and a pleural rub may be present. This may only be heard in deep inspiration or near the pericardium (pleuro-pericardial rub). Every patient should have a CXR but a normal CXR does not exclude a pulmonary cause of pleurisy. A history of cough, purulent sputum and pyrexia suggests pulmonary infection which may not have been severe enough to produce a radiographic abnormality or which may have resolved before the CXR was taken.

PLEURAL EFFUSION

See page 275.

EMPYEMA

Empyema means pus in the pleural space. The pus may be as thin as serous fluid or so thick that it is impossible to aspirate, even through a wide-bore needle. Microscopically, neutrophils are present in large numbers. The causative organism may or may not be isolated from the pus. An empyema may involve the whole pleural space or only part of it ('loculated' or 'encysted' empyema) and is almost invariably unilateral. Empyema is always secondary to infection in a neighbouring structure, usually the lung (bacterial pneumonias and TB). Over 40% of patients with community-acquired pneumonia develop an associated pleural effusion ('parapneumonic' effusion) and ~15% of these become secondarily infected, often where there is a delay in diagnosis or treatment.

Clinical features

• Persistence or recurrence of pyrexia in pulmonary infections, despite the administration of a suitable antibiotic. • Rigors, sweating, malaise and weight loss. • Pleural pain, breathlessness, cough, sputum (copious amounts if empyema ruptures into a bronchus—bronchopleural fistula). • Clinical signs of a pleural effusion.

Investigations

• Blood tests reveal a polymorphonuclear leucocytosis and high CRP. • CXR demonstrates a pleural effusion, which often appears loculated ('D-shaped opacity'). When air is present in addition to pus (pyopneumothorax), a horizontal 'fluid level' marks the air/liquid interface. • USS shows the position of the fluid, the extent of pleural thickening and whether fluid is in a single collection or multiloculated by fibrin and debris. • CT can be useful in assessing the underlying lung parenchyma and patency of the major bronchi. • Aspiration of pus confirms the presence of an empyema; the pus is frequently sterile when antibiotics have already been given. • The distinction between tuberculous and non-tuberculous disease can be difficult and often requires pleural histology and culture.

Management

• When the patient is acutely ill and the pus is thin, a large intercostal tube should be inserted for drainage of the pleural space. • If the initial aspirate reveals turbid fluid or frank pus, or if loculations are seen on USS, the tube should be put on suction (5–10 cmH_2O) and flushed regularly with 20 ml normal saline. • Although intrapleural fibrinolytic therapy is widely used in such situations, trial evidence of its benefit is conflicting. • An antibiotic directed against the organism causing the empyema should be given for 2–4 wks. • If the pleural fluid is difficult to drain, which can happen when the pus is thick or loculated, surgery is required to clear the empyema cavity. Surgical 'decortication' of the lung may also be required if thickening of the visceral pleura is preventing re-expansion of the lung.

Tuberculous empyema: Anti-TB chemotherapy must be started immediately and the pus in the pleural space drained until it ceases to reaccumulate. In many patients no other treatment is necessary but surgery is occasionally required to ablate a residual empyema space.

SPONTANEOUS PNEUMOTHORAX

Pneumothorax is the presence of air in the pleural space, which can either occur spontaneously, or result from iatrogenic injury or trauma to the lung or chest wall. Primary spontaneous pneumothorax occurs in patients with no history of lung disease. It principally affects males aged 15–30 in whom smoking, tall stature and the presence of apical subpleural blebs are additional risk factors. Secondary pneumothorax affects patients with pre-existing lung disease, especially COPD, bullous emphysema and asthma. It is most common in older patients and is associated with the highest mortality rates.

Clinical features

• There is sudden-onset unilateral pleuritic chest pain or breathlessness (those with underlying chest disease may have severe breathlessness). • With a small pneumothorax the physical examination may be normal; a larger pneumothorax (>15% of the hemithorax) results in decreased or absent breath sounds and a resonant percussion note. • A tension pneumothorax occurs when a small communication acts as a one-way valve allowing air to enter the pleural space from the lung during inspiration but not to escape on expiration; this causes raised intrapleural pressure which leads to mediastinal displacement, compression of the opposite lung and impaired systemic venous return and cardiovascular compromise.

Investigations

CXR shows the sharply defined edge of the deflated lung with complete lack of lung markings between this and the chest wall. CXR also shows any mediastinal displacement and gives information regarding the presence or absence of pleural fluid and underlying pulmonary disease. Care must be taken to differentiate between a large pre-existing emphysematous bulla and a pneumothorax to avoid misdirected attempts at aspiration; where doubt exists, CT is useful in distinguishing bullae from pleural air.

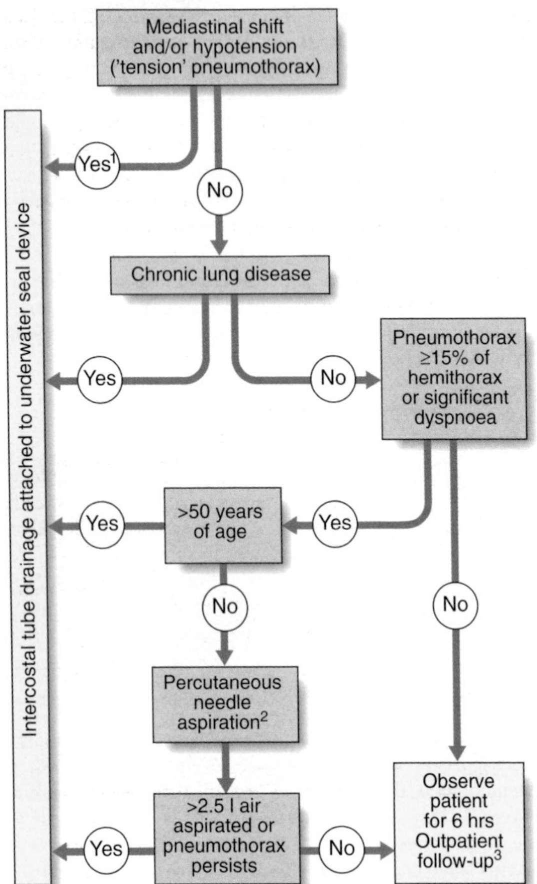

Fig. 9.13 Management of spontaneous pneumothorax. (1) Immediate decompression is required prior to insertion of intercostal drain. (2) Aspirate in the 2nd intercostal space anteriorly in the mid-clavicular line; discontinue if resistance is felt, the patient coughs excessively, or >2.5 litres are aspirated. (3) All patients should be told to attend again immediately in the event of noticeable deterioration.

Management (Fig. 9.13)

• Primary pneumothorax, where the lung edge is <2 cm from the chest wall and the patient is not breathless, normally resolves without intervention. • In young patients presenting with a moderate or large spontaneous primary pneumothorax an attempt at percutaneous needle aspiration of air should be made in the first instance, with a 60–80% chance of avoiding the need for a chest drain. • Patients with chronic lung disease always require a chest tube and inpatient observation, as even a small pneumothorax may cause respiratory failure.

Intercostal drains should be inserted in the 4th, 5th or 6th intercostal space in the mid-axillary line, following blunt dissection through to the parietal pleura, or by using a guidewire and dilator ('Seldinger' technique). The tube should be advanced in an apical direction, connected to an underwater seal or one-way Heimlich valve, and secured firmly to the chest wall. Clamping of the drain is potentially dangerous and never indicated. The drain should be removed 24 hrs after the lung has fully reinflated and bubbling stopped. Continued bubbling after 5–7 days is an indication for surgery.

Supplemental oxygen is given, as this accelerates the rate at which air is reabsorbed by the pleura. Patients with a closed pneumothorax should not fly until the pneumothorax has resolved, as the trapped gas expands at altitude. Patients should be advised to stop smoking and be informed about the risks of a recurrent pneumothorax (25% after primary spontaneous pneumothorax).

Recurrent spontaneous pneumothorax: Surgical pleurodesis, with thoracoscopic pleural abrasion or pleurectomy, is recommended in all patients following a second pneumothorax (even if ipsilateral), and should be considered following the first episode of secondary pneumothorax if low respiratory reserve makes recurrence hazardous. Patients who plan to continue activities where pneumothorax would be particularly dangerous (e.g. diving) should also undergo definitive treatment after the first episode of a primary spontaneous pneumothorax.

ASBESTOS-RELATED PLEURAL DISEASE (Fig. 9.10)

Benign pleural plaques: Areas of calcified pleural thickening that do not produce clinical symptoms and are usually identified on routine CXR.

Benign pleural effusion: May be associated with pleural pain, fever and leucocytosis. The pleural liquid may be blood-stained, and differentiation of this benign condition from a malignant effusion caused by mesothelioma can be difficult. The disease is self-limiting but may cause diffuse pleural fibrosis, which sometimes leads to breathlessness.

Diffuse pleural thickening: Diffuse pleural thickening is an important pleural manifestation of asbestos fibre inhalation and can restrict chest expansion and cause breathlessness. The restrictive defect caused by diffuse pleural thickening tends to progress and, like asbestosis and mesothelioma, qualifies a patient for industrial injury benefit in many countries.

Mesothelioma: A malignant tumour affecting the pleura or, less commonly, the peritoneum. Although all fibre types are implicated, crocidolite appears to be the most potent cause of mesothelioma. A time lag of ≥20 yrs between asbestos exposure and the development of mesothelioma is typical. The incidence of this tumour has increased markedly over the past 20 yrs and this trend is predicted to continue until 2010. Asbestos exposure is also a recognised risk factor for the development of bronchogenic carcinoma.

Clinical features: Chest pain is common. • A pleural effusion, often blood-stained, may develop and cause breathlessness. • Histological diagnosis is difficult and generous (often surgical) pleural biopsies are needed.

Treatment: Surgical resection is rarely successful and most tumours are resistant to chemotherapy. • Radiotherapy can prevent tumour growth through previous chest drain or biopsy sites. • There is no curative treatment and chest wall pain is often difficult to control, requiring expert palliative care.

DISEASES OF THE DIAPHRAGM

Congenital disorders: Congenital defects of the diaphragm (foramina of Bochdalek and Morgagni) can allow herniation of abdominal viscera. Abnormal elevation or bulging of one hemidiaphragm (eventration of the diaphragm), more often the left, may result from total or partial absence of muscular development of the septum transversum.

Acquired disorders: Phrenic nerve damage leading to diaphragmatic paralysis may be idiopathic, but is most often due to bronchial carcinoma. Other causes include disease of cervical vertebrae, tumours of the cervical cord, shingles, trauma including road traffic and birth injuries, surgery, and stretching of the nerve by mediastinal masses and aortic aneurysms. CXR demonstrates elevation of the hemidiaphragm. Screening USS can demonstrate paradoxical upward movement of the paralysed hemidiaphragm on sniffing. Bilateral diaphragmatic weakness occurs in neuromuscular disease of any type including Guillain–Barré syndrome, poliomyelitis, muscular dystrophies, motor neuron disease and connective tissue disorders such as SLE and polymyositis.

DEFORMITIES OF THE CHEST WALL

Thoracic kyphoscoliosis: Abnormalities of alignment of the dorsal spine and their consequent effects on thoracic shape may be congenital or caused by: vertebral disease, including TB; osteoporosis; ankylosing spondylitis; trauma; previous lung surgery and neuromuscular disease such as poliomyelitis. Kyphoscoliosis, if severe, restricts and distorts expansion of the chest wall. Patients with severe deformity may develop type II respiratory failure.

Pectus excavatum: In pectus excavatum (funnel chest) the body of the sternum, usually only the lower end, is curved backwards. This is rarely of any clinical consequence. Operative correction is usually only indicated for cosmetic reasons.

Pectus carinatum: Pectus carinatum (pigeon chest) is frequently caused by severe asthma during childhood.

10 Endocrine disease

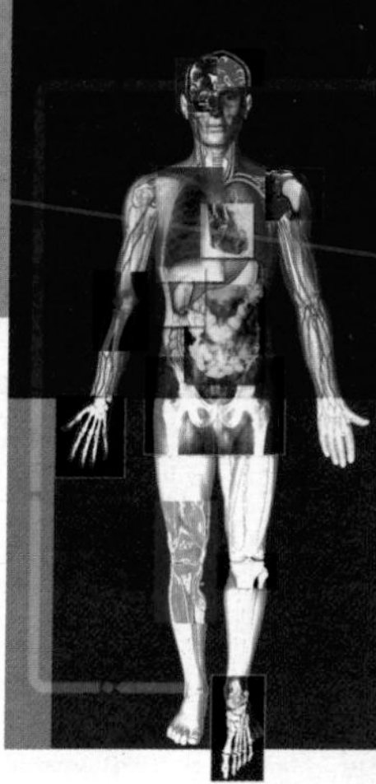

Endocrinology concerns the synthesis, secretion and action of hormones. These are chemical messengers released from endocrine glands that coordinate the activities of many different cells. Endocrine disease, therefore, has a wide range of manifestations in many organs.

MAJOR ENDOCRINE FUNCTIONS AND ANATOMY

Although some endocrine glands (e.g. the parathyroids and pancreas) respond directly to metabolic signals, most are controlled by hormones released from the pituitary gland. Anterior pituitary hormone secretion is controlled in turn by substances produced in the hypothalamus and released into portal blood which flows down the pituitary stalk. Posterior pituitary hormones are synthesised in the hypothalamus and transported down nerve axons to be released from the posterior pituitary. Hormone release in the hypothalamus and pituitary is regulated by numerous nervous, metabolic, physical or hormonal stimuli, in particular feedback control by hormones produced by target glands (thyroid, adrenal cortex and gonads). These integrated endocrine systems are called 'axes' (Figs 10.1, 10.2).

The classical model of endocrine function involves hormones which are synthesised in endocrine glands and are released into the circulation, acting at sites distant from those of secretion. However, most major organs also secrete hormones or contribute to the metabolism and activation of prohormones; many hormones act on adjacent cells (paracrine system, e.g. neurotransmitters) or even back on the cell of origin (autocrine system); and the sensitivity of target tissues is regulated in a tissue-specific

CLINICAL EXAMINATION IN ENDOCRINE DISEASE

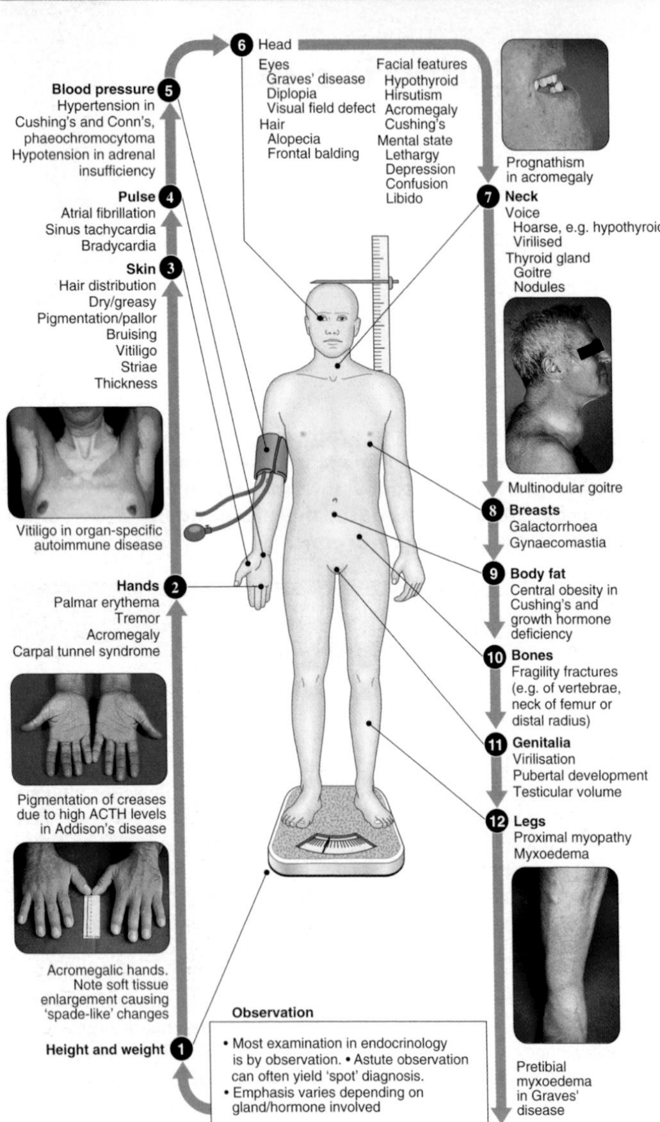

Prognathism in acromegaly

Vitiligo in organ-specific autoimmune disease

Multinodular goitre

Pigmentation of creases due to high ACTH levels in Addison's disease

Acromegalic hands. Note soft tissue enlargement causing 'spade-like' changes

Pretibial myxoedema in Graves' disease

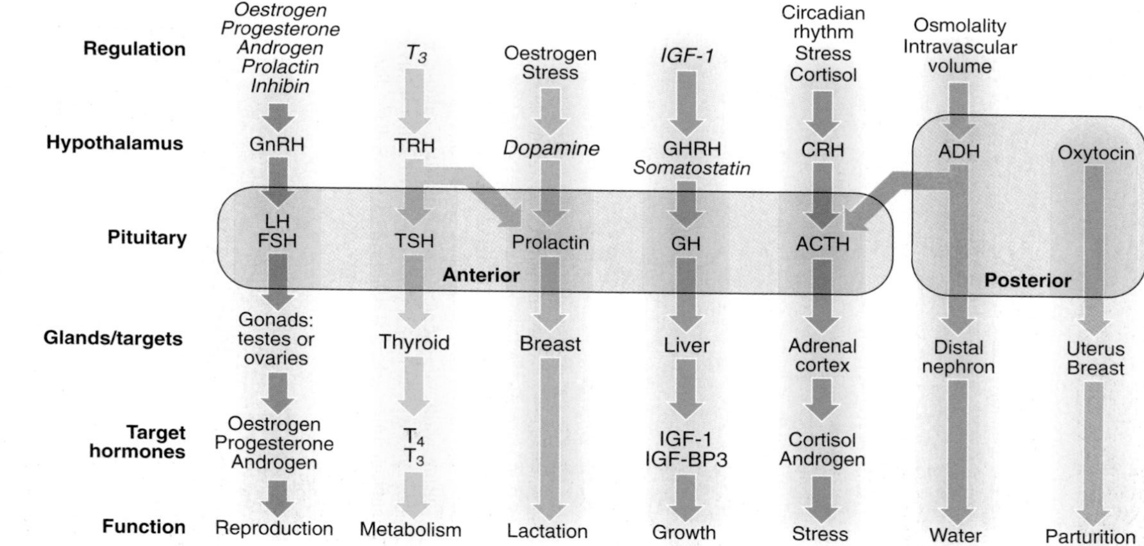

Fig. 10.1 The principal endocrine 'axes' and glands. Parathyroid glands, adrenal zona glomerulosa and endocrine pancreas are not controlled by the pituitary. Italics show negative regulation. (GnRH = gonadotrophin-releasing hormone. For other abbreviations see text.)

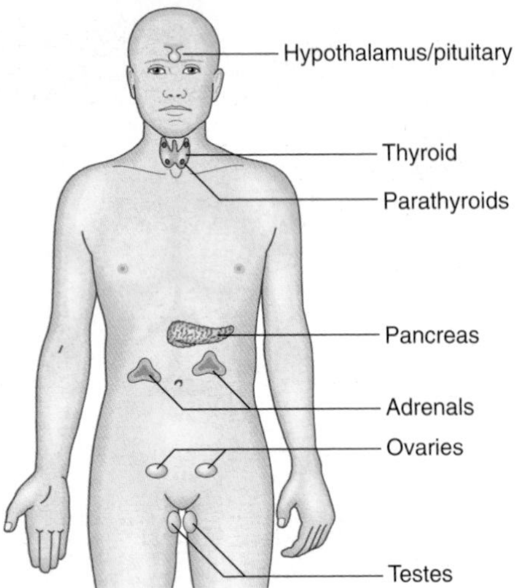

Fig. 10.2 The principal endocrine glands.

fashion. Some hormones (e.g. insulin, adrenaline (epinephrine)) act on specific cell surface receptors. Other hormones (e.g. steroids, triiodothyronine, vitamin D) bind to specific intracellular receptors, which in turn bind to response elements on DNA to regulate gene transcription.

Pathology arising within an endocrine gland is often called 'primary' disease (e.g. primary hypothyroidism in Hashimoto's thyroiditis), while abnormal stimulation of the gland is often called 'secondary' disease (e.g. secondary hypothyroidism in patients with thyroid-stimulating hormone (TSH) deficiency).

PRESENTING PROBLEMS IN ENDOCRINE DISEASE

Patients with endocrine disease present in many ways, to many different specialists, reflecting the diverse effects of hormone deficiency and excess. Presenting symptoms are often non-specific and long-standing (Box 10.1). In many patients, endocrine disease is asymptomatic and detected by routine biochemical testing. The most common classical presentations are of thyroid disease, reproductive disorders and hypercalcaemia. In addition, endocrine diseases are often part of the differential diagnosis of other disorders, including electrolyte abnormalities, hypertension, obesity and osteoporosis. Although diseases of the adrenal glands, hypothalamus and pituitary are relatively rare, their diagnosis often relies on astute clinical

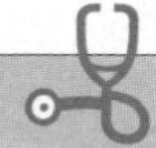

10.1 MOST COMMON PRESENTING SYMPTOMS OF ENDOCRINE DISEASE	
Symptom	**Most likely disorder(s)**
Lethargy/depression	Hypothyroidism, DM, Cushing's syndrome, hyperparathyroidism, hypogonadism, adrenal insufficiency
Weight gain	Hypothyroidism, Cushing's
Weight loss	Thyrotoxicosis, adrenal insufficiency, DM
Proptosis	Graves' disease
Thyroid nodule	Solitary thyroid nodule, dominant nodule in multinodular goitre
Polyuria/polydipsia	DM, diabetes insipidus, hyperparathyroidism, Conn's syndrome
Coarse features	Acromegaly, hypothyroidism
Galactorrhoea	Hyperprolactinaemia
Ureteric colic	Hyperparathyroidism
Paraesthesiae/tetany	Hypoparathyroidism
Muscle weakness (usually proximal)	Thyrotoxicosis, Cushing's, hypokalaemia (e.g. Conn's), hyperparathyroidism, hypogonadism
Heat intolerance	Thyrotoxicosis, menopause
Thyroid swelling	Simple goitre, Graves' disease, Hashimoto's thyroiditis
Palpitations	Thyrotoxicosis, phaeochromocytoma
Hirsutism	Idiopathic, PCOS, congenital adrenal hyperplasia, Cushing's
Amenorrhoea/ oligomenorrhoea	Menopause, PCOS, hyperprolactinaemia, thyrotoxicosis, premature ovarian failure, Cushing's
Pain over thyroid	Haemorrhage into nodule, de Quervain's thyroiditis
Loss of libido	Male hypogonadism
Headache	Acromegaly, pituitary tumour, phaeochromocytoma
Visual dysfunction	Pituitary tumour
(DM = diabetes mellitus; PCOS = polycystic ovarian syndrome)	

observation in a patient with non-specific complaints, so it is important that clinicians are familiar with their key features.

THE THYROID GLAND

Diseases of the thyroid affect 5% of the population, predominantly females. The thyroid axis is involved in the regulation of cellular differentiation and metabolism in virtually all nucleated cells, so that disorders of thyroid function have diverse manifestations. Follicular epithelial cells synthesise thyroid hormones by incorporating iodine into the amino acid, tyrosine. The thyroid secretes predominantly thyroxine (T_4) and only a small amount of triiodothyronine (T_3), the more active hormone; ~85% of T_3 in blood is produced from peripheral conversion of T_4. They both circulate in plasma almost entirely (>99%) bound to transport proteins, mainly thyroxine-binding globulin (TBG). The unbound hormones diffuse into tissues and exert diverse metabolic actions. The advantage of measuring free over total hormone is that the former is not influenced by changes in TBG concentrations; in pregnancy, for example, TBG levels are increased and total T_3/T_4 may be raised, but free thyroid hormone levels are normal.

Production of T_3 and T_4 in the thyroid is stimulated by thyroid-stimulating hormone (TSH), a glycoprotein released from the thyrotroph cells of the anterior pituitary in response to the hypothalamic tripeptide, thyrotrophin-releasing hormone (TRH). There is a negative feedback of thyroid hormones on the hypothalamus and pituitary such that in thyrotoxicosis, when plasma concentrations of T_3 and T_4 are raised, TSH secretion is suppressed. Conversely, in primary hypothyroidism low T_3 and T_4 are associated with high circulating TSH levels. TSH is, therefore, regarded as the most useful investigation of thyroid function. However, TSH may take several weeks to 'catch up' with T_4/T_3 levels, e.g. after prolonged suppression of TSH in thyrotoxicosis is relieved by antithyroid therapy. Common patterns of abnormal thyroid function tests (TFTs) are shown in Box 10.2.

PRESENTING PROBLEMS

THYROTOXICOSIS

• Approximately 75% of cases are due to Graves' disease, 15% to multinodular goitre and 5% to toxic adenoma. • Less common causes include transient thyroiditis (de Quervain's, post-partum), iodide-induced (drugs, supplementation), factitious and TSH-secreting pituitary tumour.

Clinical assessment

Manifestations of thyrotoxicosis are shown in Box 10.3. The most common symptoms are:

• Weight loss with a normal appetite. • Heat intolerance. • Palpitations. • Tremor. • Irritability.

10.2 PATTERNS OF THYROID FUNCTION TEST (TFT) RESULTS			
	TSH	**T_4**	**T_3**
Primary thyrotoxicosis	Undetectable	Raised	Raised
Primary T_3-toxicosis	Undetectable	Normal	Raised
Subclinical thyrotoxicosis	Undetectable	Normal	Normal
Sick euthyroidism/ non-thyroidal illness	Undetectable	Raised	Low, normal or raised
Secondary hypothyroidism	Undetectable	Low	Low
Primary hypothyroidism	Elevated >20 mU/l	Low	Low
Subclinical hypothyroidism	Mildly elevated 5–20 mU/l	Normal	Normal
Non-compliance with T_4 replacement and recent 'loading' dose	Elevated	High	High
Secondary thyrotoxicosis—TSH-secreting pituitary tumour			

All causes of thyrotoxicosis can cause lid retraction and lid lag, but only Graves' disease causes other ocular features (see Box 10.3).

Investigations

Figure 10.3 summarises the approach to establishing the diagnosis.

TFTs: T_3 and T_4 are elevated in most patients, but T_4 is normal and T_3 raised (T_3 toxicosis) in 5%. In primary thyrotoxicosis, serum TSH is undetectable (<0.05 mU/l).

Antibodies: TSH receptor antibodies (TRAb) are elevated in 80–95% of patients with Graves' disease. Other thyroid antibodies are unhelpful, as they are present in the healthy population.

Imaging: ^{99m}Technetium scintigraphy scans indicate trapping of isotope in the gland (see Fig. 10.3). Iodine can also be used but yields lower resolution images.

• In Graves' disease there is diffuse uptake. • In multinodular goitre, there is low, patchy uptake within the nodules. • A hot spot is seen in toxic adenoma, with no uptake in the dormant gland tissue. • In low-uptake thyrotoxicosis, the cause is usually a transient thyroiditis, although rarely patients may induce 'factitious thyrotoxicosis' by consuming thyroxine.

Management

Definitive treatment of thyrotoxicosis depends on the underlying cause (see pp. 343–346) and may include antithyroid drugs, radioactive iodine or surgery. A non-selective β-blocker (propranolol 160 mg daily) will alleviate symptoms within 24–48 hrs.

10.3 CLINICAL FEATURES OF THYROTOXICOSIS		
	Symptoms	**Signs**
General	*Weight loss (normal appetite), heat intolerance, fatigue,* apathy[1], osteoporosis	*Weight loss*, goitre with bruit[2], lymphadenopathy[3]
GI	*Hyperdefecation*, diarrhoea, steatorrhoea, anorexia[1], vomiting[3]	
Cardio-respiratory	*Palpitations, dyspnoea on exertion*, angina, ankle swelling, asthma exacerbation[3]	*Sinus tachycardia*, atrial fibrillation, systolic hypertension, cardiac failure
Neuromuscular	Anxiety, *irritability, emotional lability*, psychosis, tremor, weakness	*Tremor*, hyper-reflexia, ill-sustained clonus, proximal/bulbar[1] myopathy
Dermatological	*Sweating*, pruritus, alopecia	*Palmar erythema*, pretibial myxoedema[2], thyroid acropachy[2], onycholysis[3], pigmentation[3], vitiligo[2]
Reproductive	Oligo-/amenorrhoea, infertility, ↓libido, impotence	Gynaecomastia
Ocular	*Grittiness, red eyes*, excessive lacrimation, diplopia[2], loss of acuity[2]	*Lid retraction, lid lag*, chemosis[2], exophthalmos[2], periorbital oedema[2], corneal ulceration[2], ophthalmoplegia[2], papilloedema[2]

Italics indicate common features. [1] Particularly in elderly patients. [2] Graves' disease only. [3] Rare.

Atrial fibrillation (AF) in thyrotoxicosis: AF is present in ~10% of all patients with thyrotoxicosis (more in the elderly). Subclinical thyrotoxicosis is also a risk factor for AF. Ventricular rate responds better to β-blockade than digoxin. Thromboembolic complications are particularly common so anticoagulation with warfarin is indicated. Once the patient is biochemically euthyroid, AF reverts to sinus rhythm spontaneously in ~50% of patients.

Thyrotoxic crisis ('thyroid storm'): This is a medical emergency with a mortality of 10%. The most prominent signs are fever, agitation, confusion, tachycardia or AF, and cardiac failure. It is precipitated by infection in patients with unrecognised thyrotoxicosis and may develop after subtotal thyroidectomy or ^{131}I therapy.

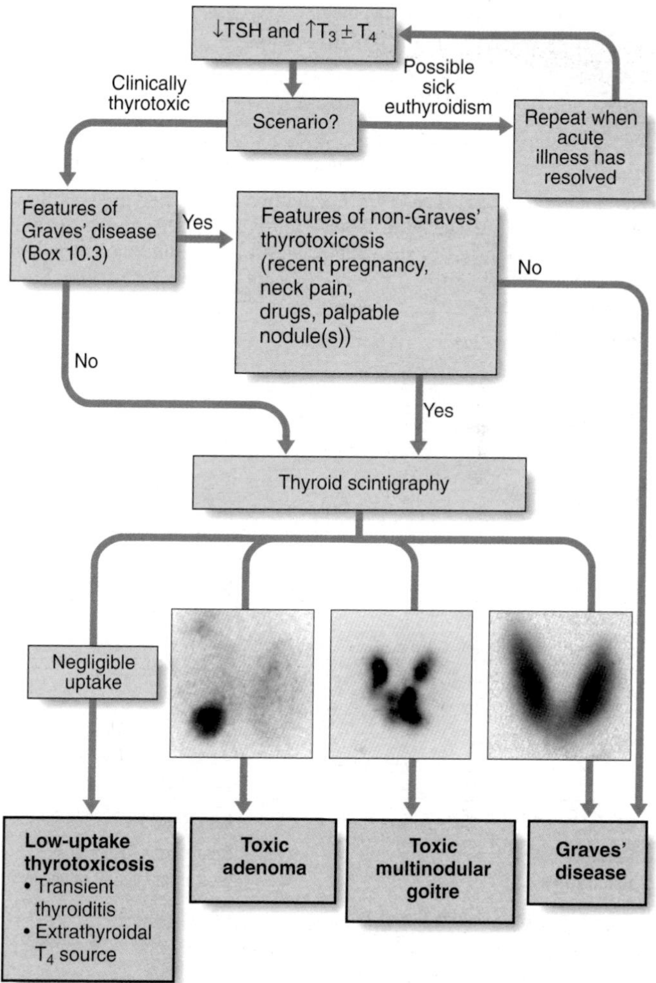

Fig. 10.3 Establishing the differential diagnosis in thyrotoxicosis. Scintigraphy is not necessary in most cases of drug-induced thyrotoxicosis.

Patients should be rehydrated and given broad-spectrum antibiotics. • Propranolol is rapidly effective orally (80 mg 6-hourly) or intravenously (1–5 mg 6-hourly). • Sodium ipodate (500 mg daily orally) restores serum T_3 levels to normal in 48–72 hrs by inhibiting release of hormones and conversion of T_4 to T_3. • Oral carbimazole 40–60 mg daily inhibits the synthesis of new hormones. In the unconscious patient, carbimazole can be administered rectally. After 10–14 days, maintenance with carbimazole alone is possible.

HYPOTHYROIDISM

The prevalence of primary hypothyroidism is 1 in 100, with a female : male ratio of 6 : 1.

• Autoimmune disease (Hashimoto's thyroiditis) and thyroid failure following ^{131}I or surgical treatment of thyrotoxicosis account for >90% of cases where the population is not iodine-deficient. • Less common causes include secondary hypothyroidism, transient thyroiditis, amiodarone-induced and dyshormonogenesis.

Clinical assessment

Clinical features depend on the duration and severity of the hypothyroidism. The classical clinical features listed in Box 10.4 occur when deficiency develops insidiously over months/years.

Investigations

• In primary hypothyroidism, T_4 is low and TSH elevated (>20 mU/l) (Fig. 10.4). T_3 is not a sensitive indicator of hypothyroidism and should not be

10.4 CLINICAL FEATURES OF HYPOTHYROIDISM

	Symptoms	Signs
General	*Weight gain*, *cold intolerance*, *fatigue*, *somnolence*, hoarseness	*Weight gain*, hoarseness, goitre, macrocytosis, anaemia
GI	Constipation	Ileus*, ascites*
Cardio-respiratory		Bradycardia, hypertension, pericardial/pleural effusions*
Neuromuscular	*Carpal tunnel syndrome*, muscle stiffness, deafness, depression, psychosis*	Delayed relaxation of reflexes, cerebellar ataxia*, myotonia*
Dermatological	*Dry skin*, *dry hair*, alopecia	Myxoedema, purplish lips, malar flush, vitiligo, erythema ab igne
Reproductive	*Menorrhagia*, infertility, galactorrhoea*, impotence*	
Ocular		Periorbital oedema, loss of lateral eyebrows

Italics indicate common features. *Rare.

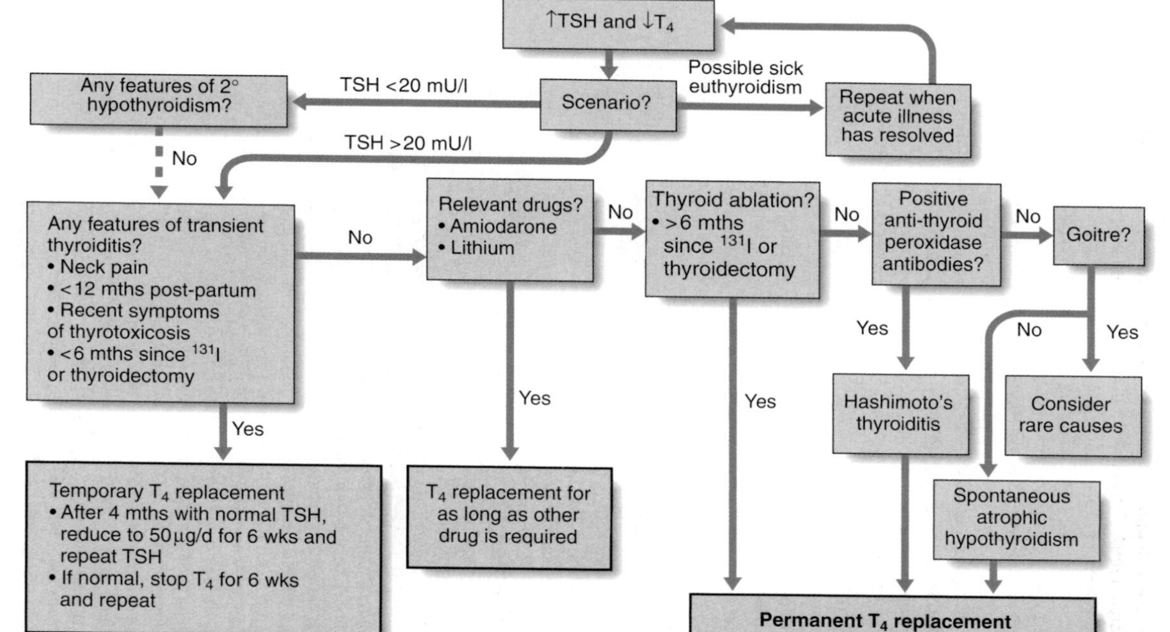

Fig. 10.4 Diagnostic approach to adults with suspected hypothyroidism. This scheme ignores congenital causes of hypothyroidism such as thyroid aplasia and dyshormonogenesis. Rare causes of hypothyroidism with goitre include amyloidosis and sarcoidosis.

measured. • In the rare secondary hypothyroidism there is thyroid atrophy caused by failure of TSH secretion due to hypothalamic or anterior pituitary disease, e.g. pituitary macroadenoma. T_4 is low and TSH is usually low but sometimes paradoxically detectable. • Other biochemical abnormalities associated with hypothyroidism include ↑CK, ↑LDH, ↑AST, ↑cholesterol, ↓Na^+ and anaemia (macrocytic or normocytic). • ECG may show sinus bradycardia with small complexes and ST–T abnormalities. • Thyroid peroxidase antibodies are usually elevated in autoimmune causes but are also common in the healthy population.

Management

Most patients require life-long thyroxine therapy. A replacement regimen is:

• Thyroxine 50 μg daily for 3 wks. • Then 100 μg daily for 3 wks. • Then maintenance 100–150 μg daily.

Thyroxine has a half-life of 7 days, and so 6 wks should pass before repeating TFTs following a dose change. Patients feel better within 2–3 wks; resolution of skin and hair texture and effusions may take 3–6 mths.

The long-term correct dose of thyroxine restores TSH to within the reference range. This usually requires a T_4 level in the upper normal range because the more active T_3 is derived exclusively from peripheral conversion of T_4 without the usual contribution from thyroid secretion. Some physicians advocate combined T_4/T_3 replacement but this approach remains controversial. TFTs should be checked every 1–2 yrs once the dose of thyroxine is stabilised.

Thyroxine requirements may increase with co-administration of other drugs (e.g. phenytoin, ferrous sulphate, rifampicin) and during pregnancy. In non-compliance, if thyroxine is taken just prior to clinic, the anomalous combination of a high T_4 and high TSH may result. Around 40% of patients with angina cannot tolerate full replacement thyroxine despite the use of β-blockers. Exacerbation of myocardial ischaemia, infarction and sudden death are well-recognised complications. In known ischaemic heart disease, thyroxine should be introduced at low dose and increased under specialist supervision. Coronary intervention may be required to allow full replacement dosage. Most pregnant women with primary hypothyroidism require a ~50 μg increase in thyroxine dose. This is due to increased TBG. Inadequate maternal T_4 therapy may be associated with impaired cognitive development in offspring.

Myxoedema coma: This is a rare presentation of hypothyroidism in which there is depressed consciousness, usually in an elderly patient who appears myxoedematous. Body temperature may be low, convulsions are not uncommon, and CSF pressure and protein content are raised. The mortality rate is 50% and survival depends upon early recognition and treatment.

Myxoedema coma is a medical emergency and treatment must begin before biochemical confirmation of the diagnosis. Triiodothyronine is given as an i.v. bolus of 20 μg followed by 20 μg 8-hourly until there is sustained clinical improvement. After 48–72 hrs, oral thyroxine (50 μg daily) may be substituted. Unless the patient has primary hypothyroidism, the thyroid failure should be assumed to be secondary to hypothalamic or pituitary disease and treatment given with hydrocortisone 100 mg 8-hourly, pending TFT and cortisol results. Other measures include slow rewarming, cautious i.v. fluids, broad-spectrum antibiotics and high-flow oxygen with or without assisted ventilation.

ASYMPTOMATIC ABNORMAL THYROID FUNCTION TEST RESULTS

Subclinical thyrotoxicosis: TSH is undetectable, while T_3/T_4 is in the upper normal range. This condition is usually found in older patients with multinodular goitre. There is an increased risk of AF and osteoporosis; hence the consensus view is that such patients require therapy (usually ^{131}I). Otherwise, annual follow-up is required, as overt thyrotoxicosis occurs in 5% annually.

Subclinical hypothyroidism: TSH is raised, while T_3/T_4 is in the lower normal range. Progression to overt thyroid failure is highest in those with antithyroid peroxidase antibodies or TSH >10 mU/l. This group should be treated with thyroxine to normalise TSH.

Non-thyroidal illness ('sick euthyroidism'): TSH is low, T_4 raised and T_3 normal or low. Other patterns are also seen. During illness, there is decreased conversion of T_4 to T_3 and alterations in affinity to binding proteins. TSH may be low as a result of the illness itself or drug treatments (e.g. corticosteroids). During convalescence, TSH may increase to levels found in primary hypothyroidism. TFTs should therefore not be checked during an acute illness in the absence of clear signs of thyroid disease. If an abnormal result is found, tests should be repeated after recovery.

THYROID ENLARGEMENT

Palpable thyroid enlargement affects 5% of the population but a minority seek medical attention. Multinodular goitres and solitary nodules sometimes present with acute painful enlargement due to haemorrhage into a nodule. There are several causes of thyroid enlargement (Box 10.5). Whereas diffuse and multinodular goitre are invariably benign, there is a 1 : 20 chance of malignancy in a solitary lesion. TFTs should always be performed.

Diffuse goitre: In the absence of thyrotoxicosis or hypothyroidism, a diffuse goitre rarely needs further investigation unless it is very large, causing cosmetic symptoms or compression. Absence of autoantibodies in a younger patient suggests a simple goitre. Thyroxine therapy may help to shrink the goitre.

Solitary thyroid nodule: It is important to determine whether the nodule is benign or malignant. Cervical lymphadenopathy increases the likelihood of malignancy, as does a solitary nodule presenting in the elderly. Rarely,

10.5 CAUSES OF THYROID ENLARGEMENT	
Diffuse goitre	
• Simple goitre[1] • Hashimoto's thyroiditis[1] • Graves' disease • Drugs: iodine, amiodarone	• Transient thyroiditis[2] • Riedel's thyroiditis[2] • Iodine deficiency (endemic goitre)[1]
Solitary nodule	
• Simple cyst • Colloid nodule • Primary thyroid cancer (see Box 10.7 below)	• Follicular adenoma • Metastasis
Multinodular goitre	
[1] May shrink with thyroxine therapy. [2] Usually tender.	

a metastasis from renal, breast or lung carcinoma presents as a painful, rapidly growing solitary nodule.

TFTs should be measured in all patients with a solitary nodule. Undetectable TSH is suggestive of an autonomously functioning benign follicular adenoma, which can only be confirmed by thyroid isotope scanning. For euthyroid patients, fine needle aspiration (FNA) of the nodule is undertaken. Aspiration may be therapeutic if the swelling is a cyst. Cytological examination will differentiate benign (80%) from suspicious nodules (20%), of which 25–50% are confirmed as cancer at surgery. The advantage of FNA over isotope scanning is that a higher proportion of patients avoid surgery. However, FNA cannot differentiate between follicular adenoma and carcinoma, and 10–20% of specimens are inadequate.

Solitary nodules with either inconclusive or malignant cytology are treated by surgical excision. Benign lesions are sometimes excised but the majority of patients can be reassured.

Multinodular goitre: The clinical diagnosis is confirmed using ^{99m}Tc scintigraphy or USS. Sometimes one nodule is larger than others (dominant); if 'cold' on isotope scanning, it is investigated as a solitary nodule since there is a risk of malignancy.

AUTOIMMUNE THYROID DISEASE

GRAVES' DISEASE

The most common manifestation is thyrotoxicosis with or without a diffuse goitre. Clinical features are described in Box 10.3. Graves' disease also causes ophthalmopathy and rarely pretibial myxoedema. These features can occur in the absence of thyroid dysfunction. Graves' disease most commonly affects women aged 30–50 yrs.

Graves' thyrotoxicosis

IgG antibodies are directed against the TSH receptors on follicular cells, stimulating hormone production and goitre formation. These TSH receptor antibodies (TRAb) can be detected in 80–95% of patients. The natural history of the disease follows one of three patterns:

• A prolonged period of hyperthyroidism of fluctuating severity. • Alternating relapse and remission. • A single, short-lived episode of hyperthyroidism, followed by prolonged remission and eventually hypothyroidism.

There is an association of Graves' disease with HLA-B8, DR3 and DR2. Smoking is weakly associated with Graves' thyrotoxicosis, but strongly linked with the development of ophthalmopathy.

Management

Symptoms respond to β-blockade but definitive treatment requires control of thyroid hormone secretion. The different options are compared in Box 10.6. For patients <40 yrs old many centres prescribe a course of carbima-

10.6 COMPARISON OF TREATMENTS FOR THE THYROTOXICOSIS OF GRAVES' DISEASE

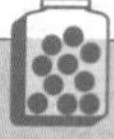

Management	Common indications	Contraindications	Disadvantages/ complications
Antithyroid drugs	First episode in patients <40 yrs	Breastfeeding (propylthiouracil suitable)	Hypersensitivity rash 2% Agranulocytosis 0.2% Recurrent thyrotoxicosis
Subtotal thyroidectomy	Large goitre	Previous thyroid surgery Dependence upon voice, e.g. opera singer	Hypothyroidism ~25% Transient hypocalcaemia 10% Hypoparathyroidism 1% Recurrent laryngeal nerve palsy 1%
Radio-iodine	Patients >40 yrs Recurrence following surgery	Pregnancy Active Graves' eye disease	Hypothyroidism: 40% in 1st yr, 80% by 15 yrs Worsens ophthalmopathy

zole and recommend surgery if relapse occurs, while ^{131}I is employed as first- or second-line treatment in older patients. It is unclear whether ^{131}I increases the incidence of some malignancies; the association may be with Graves' disease rather than its therapy. In many centres, however, ^{131}I is used more extensively, even in young patients.

Antithyroid drugs: The most commonly used are carbimazole and propylthiouracil. These drugs reduce thyroid hormone synthesis by inhibiting tyrosine iodination. Antithyroid drugs are introduced at high doses (carbimazole 40–60 mg daily, propylthiouracil 400–600 mg daily). There is subjective improvement within 2 wks and the patient is biochemically euthyroid at 4 wks, when the dose can be reduced. The maintenance dose is determined by measurement of T_4 and TSH. Carbimazole is continued for 12–18 mths in the hope that permanent remission will occur. Unfortunately, thyrotoxicosis recurs in at least 50% within 2 yrs of stopping treatment. Adverse effects of antithyroid drugs include rash and idiosyncratic but reversible agranulocytosis.

Subtotal thyroidectomy: Patients must be rendered euthyroid before operation. Potassium iodide, 60 mg 8-hourly orally, is given for 2 wks before surgery to inhibit thyroid hormone release and reduce the size and vascularity of the gland, making surgery technically easier. Complications are uncommon (see Box 10.6). One year post-surgery, 80% of patients are euthyroid, 15% are hypothyroid and 5% remain thyrotoxic. Hypothyroidism within 6 mths of operation may be temporary. Long-term follow-up is necessary, as the late development of hypothyroidism and recurrence of thyrotoxicosis are well recognised.

Radioactive iodine: ^{131}I is administered as a single dose (185–370 MBq, 5–10 mCi) and is trapped and organified in the thyroid. It is effective in 75% of patients within 4–12 wks. Symptoms can initially be controlled by β-blockade or with carbimazole. However, carbimazole reduces the efficacy of ^{131}I therapy and should be avoided until 48 hrs after radioiodine administration. If thyrotoxicosis persists after 12–24 wks, a further dose of ^{131}I should be employed. The majority of patients eventually develop hypothyroidism, necessitating long-term follow-up.

Thyrotoxicosis in pregnancy

TFTs must be interpreted with caution in pregnancy. Thyroid-binding globulin, and hence total T_4/T_3 levels, are increased and TSH normal ranges are lower; a fully suppressed TSH with elevated free hormone levels indicates thyrotoxicosis. The thyrotoxicosis is almost always caused by Graves' disease. Maternal thyroid hormones, TRAb and antithyroid drugs can all cross the placenta.

Treatment with propylthiouracil is preferred, as carbimazole is rarely associated with the childhood skin defect, aplasia cutis. The smallest dose of propylthiouracil (<150 mg/day) is used that maintains maternal TFTs within their normal ranges, thereby minimising fetal hypothyroidism and goitre. TRAb levels in the third trimester predict the likelihood of neonatal thyrotoxicosis; if they are not elevated, antithyroid drugs can be discontinued 4 wks before delivery to avoid fetal hypothyroidism at the time of maximum brain development. • During breastfeeding, propylthiouracil is used, as it is minimally excreted in the milk.

Graves' ophthalmopathy

Within the orbit, there is immune-mediated fibroblast proliferation, increased interstitial fluid and a chronic inflammatory cell infiltrate. This causes swelling and ultimately fibrosis of the extraocular muscles and a rise in retrobulbar pressure. The eye is displaced forwards (proptosis, exophthalmos) with optic nerve compression in severe cases.

Ophthalmopathy is typically episodic. It is detectable in ~50% of thyrotoxic patients at presentation, more commonly smokers, but may occur long before or after thyrotoxic episodes (exophthalmic Graves' disease). Presenting symptoms are related to increased corneal exposure due to proptosis and lid retraction:

• Excessive lacrimation worsened by wind and sun. • 'Gritty' sensations. • Pain due to corneal ulceration. • Reduced visual acuity/fields or colour vision due to optic nerve compression. • Diplopia resulting from extraocular muscle involvement.

Most patients require no treatment. Methylcellulose eye drops are used for dry eyes and sunglasses reduce the excessive lacrimation. Severe inflammatory episodes are treated with glucocorticoids (prednisolone 60 mg daily) and sometimes orbital irradiation. Loss of visual acuity requires urgent surgical decompression of the orbit. Surgery to ocular muscles may improve diplopia.

Pretibial myxoedema

This infiltrative dermopathy occurs in <10% of patients with Graves' disease.

• Pink-purple plaques on the anterior leg and foot are seen. • Lesions are itchy and the skin may have a 'peau d'orange' appearance with coarse hair. • In severe cases topical glucocorticoids may be helpful.

HASHIMOTO'S THYROIDITIS

Hashimoto's thyroiditis increases in incidence with age. It is characterised by destructive lymphoid infiltration leading to a varying degree of fibrosis and thus a varying degree of thyroid enlargement. There is a slightly increased risk of thyroid lymphoma. The term 'Hashimoto's thyroiditis' has been reserved for patients with thyroid peroxidase autoantibodies and a goitre (with or without hypothyroidism), whilst 'spontaneous atrophic hypothyroidism' has been used in hypothyroid patients without a goitre with TSH receptor-blocking antibodies. However, these syndromes are both variants of Hashimoto's.

• At presentation, a small or moderately sized firm diffuse goitre may be palpable. • 25% of patients are hypothyroid and the remainder are at risk of developing overt hypothyroidism in future years. • Thyroid peroxidase antibodies are present in >90%. • Thyroxine therapy is given.

TRANSIENT THYROIDITIS

SUBACUTE (DE QUERVAIN'S) THYROIDITIS

Subacute thyroiditis is a virus-induced (e.g. Coxsackie, mumps) transient inflammation of the thyroid usually affecting 20–40-yr-old females.

• There is classically pain around the thyroid radiating to the jaw and ears, which is worsened by swallowing and coughing. The thyroid is enlarged and tender. Painless transient thyroiditis also occurs. • Systemic upset is common. • Inflammation in the thyroid causes release of colloid and stored hormones, and damages follicular cells. As a result, T_4/T_3 levels are raised for 4–6 wks until depletion of colloid. A period of hypothyroidism follows, during which follicular cells recover, restoring thyroid function within 4–6 mths. In the thyrotoxic phase, iodine uptake and technetium trapping are low due to follicular cell damage and TSH suppression. • Pain and systemic upset respond to NSAIDs. Occasionally, prednisolone 40 mg daily for 3–4 wks is required. Mild thyrotoxicosis is treated with propranolol. • Monitoring of thyroid function is required so that thyroxine can be prescribed temporarily in the hypothyroid phase.

POST-PARTUM THYROIDITIS

The maternal immune response is enhanced after delivery and may unmask subclinical autoimmune thyroid disease. Transient asymptomatic disturbances of thyroid function occur in 5–10% of women post-partum. However, symptomatic thyrotoxicosis presenting within 6 mths of childbirth is likely to be due to post-partum thyroiditis and the diagnosis is confirmed by negligible radioisotope uptake. The clinical course is similar to painless subacute thyroiditis. Post-partum thyroiditis can recur after subsequent pregnancies and may progress to hypothyroidism.

IODINE-ASSOCIATED THYROID DISEASE

IODINE DEFICIENCY

In mountainous areas (e.g. Andes, Himalayas), dietary iodine deficiency causes thyroid enlargement (endemic goitre) affecting >10% of the population. Most patients are euthyroid and have normal or raised TSH levels.

IODINE-INDUCED DYSFUNCTION

Chronic excess of iodine inhibits thyroid hormone release; this is the basis for its utility in treatment of thyroid storm and prior to subtotal thyroidectomy. Transient thyrotoxicosis may be precipitated in iodine deficiency following prophylactic iodinisation programmes. In individuals who have underlying thyroid disease predisposing to thyrotoxicosis (e.g. multinodular goitre or Graves' disease), thyrotoxicosis can be induced by iodine administration (e.g. radiocontrast media).

AMIODARONE

The anti-arrhythmic agent amiodarone contains large amounts of iodine. Amiodarone also has a cytotoxic effect on thyroid follicular cells and inhibits T_4 to T_3 conversion. Around 20% of patients develop hypothyroidism or thyrotoxicosis. TSH provides the best indicator of thyroid function.

Thyrotoxicosis has been classified as:

- Type I (stimulatory effect of iodine in underlying thyroid disease).
- Type II (transient thyrotoxicosis due to cytotoxic thyroiditis).

In hypothyroid patients, thyroxine can be given while amiodarone is continued. Treatment of thyrotoxicosis, however, is difficult. Excess iodine renders the gland resistant to radio-iodine. Antithyroid drugs may be effective in patients with type I thyrotoxicosis, but not in type II. If the cardiac state allows, amiodarone should be discontinued. Prior to amiodarone therapy, thyroid function should be measured and avoided if TSH is suppressed. Thyroid function should be monitored regularly.

SIMPLE AND MULTINODULAR GOITRE

SIMPLE DIFFUSE GOITRE

This presents in 15–25-yr-olds, often during pregnancy. The goitre is visible, soft and symmetrical and the thyroid is 2–3 times its normal size. There is no tenderness, lymphadenopathy or bruit, and TFTs are normal. The goitre may may regress without treatment or may progress to multinodular goitre.

MULTINODULAR GOITRE

Occasionally, simple goitres become multinodular over 10–20 yrs. These nodules grow at varying rates and secrete thyroid hormone 'autonomously', thereby suppressing TSH-dependent growth and function in the remaining gland. Ultimately, complete TSH suppression occurs in ~25% of cases, with T_4/T_3 levels often within the normal range (subclinical thyrotoxicosis) but sometimes elevated (toxic multinodular goitre). The nodules may represent multiple adenomas or focal hyperplasia.

Clinical features and investigations

• Patients present with thyrotoxicosis, a large goitre or sudden painful swelling caused by haemorrhage into a nodule. The goitre is nodular or lobulated on palpation and may extend retrosternally. • Very large goitres may cause stridor, dysphagia and superior vena cava obstruction. Hoarseness due to recurrent laryngeal nerve palsy is more suggestive of thyroid carcinoma. • The diagnosis is confirmed by a radioisotope thyroid scan and USS. • A flow-volume loop is a good screening test for tracheal compression. • CT/MRI of the thoracic inlet can quantify the degree of tracheal compression and retrosternal extension. • In those with a dominant, cold nodule, FNA is indicated to exclude thyroid cancer.

Management

Small goitre: Annual review is required, as progression to toxic multinodular goitre can occur.

Large goitre: Partial thyroidectomy is indicated in cases of mediastinal compression or for cosmesis. ^{131}I is used in the elderly to reduce thyroid size but recurrence is common after 10–20 yrs.

Toxic multinodular goitre: ^{131}I is used; hypothyroidism is less common than in Graves' disease. Partial thyroidectomy may be required for a large goitre. Antithyroid drugs are not usually used, as drug withdrawal invariably leads to relapse.

Subclinical thyrotoxicosis: This is increasingly being treated with ^{131}I, as a suppressed TSH is a risk factor for AF and osteoporosis.

THYROID NEOPLASIA

Patients with thyroid tumours usually present with a solitary nodule (p. 341). Most are benign and a few (toxic adenomas) secrete excess thyroid hormones. Primary thyroid malignancy is rare (<1% of all carcinomas). As shown in Box 10.7, it can be classified according to the cell type of origin. With the exception of medullary carcinoma, thyroid cancer is more common in females.

TOXIC ADENOMA

The presence of a toxic solitary nodule is the cause of <5% of cases of thyrotoxicosis. The nodule is a follicular adenoma, usually >3 cm, which secretes excess thyroid hormones. The remaining gland atrophies following TSH suppression. Most patients are female and >40 yrs old.

- The diagnosis is made by isotope scanning. Thyrotoxicosis is mild, and in 50% of patients T_3 alone is elevated (T_3 thyrotoxicosis).
- ^{131}I is highly effective and is an ideal treatment since the atrophic cells surrounding the nodule do not take up iodine, making permanent hypothyroidism unusual.
- Hemi-thyroidectomy is an alternative.

10.7 MALIGNANT THYROID TUMOURS

Origin of tumour	Type of tumour	Frequency (%)	Age at presentation (yrs)	20-yr survival (%)
Follicular cells	Papillary	70	20–40	95
	Follicular	10	40–60	60
	Anaplastic	5	>60	<1
Parafollicular C cells	Medullary carcinoma	5–10	Childhood or >40	50
Lymphocytes	Lymphoma	5–10	>60	10

DIFFERENTIATED CARCINOMA

Papillary carcinoma: The most common thyroid malignancy. It may be multifocal and spread is to regional lymph nodes.

Follicular carcinoma: A single encapsulated lesion. Cervical lymph nodes spread is rare. Metastases are blood-borne and are found in bone, lungs and brain.

Management

• Total thyroidectomy is undertaken, followed by a large dose of ^{131}I in order to ablate remaining thyroid tissue. • Thereafter, long-term treatment with thyroxine in a dose sufficient to suppress TSH (150–200 μg daily) is important, as differentiated thyroid carcinomas are TSH-dependent. • Follow-up is by measurement of serum thyroglobulin, which should be undetectable in patients whose thyroid has been ablated. Detectable thyroglobulin suggests tumour recurrence or metastases which may respond to further radio-iodine therapy. • Most patients have an excellent prognosis. Those <50 yrs with papillary carcinoma have near-normal life expectancy if the tumour is <2 cm in diameter, confined to cervical nodes and of low grade; 10-yr survival is ~40% with distant metastases.

ANAPLASTIC CARCINOMA AND LYMPHOMA

These two conditions are difficult to distinguish clinically. Patients are usually elderly women with rapidly enlarging, hard and symmetrical goitre over 2–3 mths.

• There is stridor (tracheal compression) and hoarseness (recurrent laryngeal nerve palsy). • There is no effective treatment of anaplastic carcinoma, although radiotherapy may relieve mediastinal compression. • The prognosis for lymphoma, which may arise from Hashimoto's thyroiditis, is better. External irradiation dramatically shrinks the goitre and, with chemotherapy, may result in a >5-yr survival.

MEDULLARY CARCINOMA

This tumour arises from the parafollicular C cells of the thyroid. The tumour may secrete calcitonin, 5-HT (serotonin) and adrenocorticotrophic hormone (ACTH). As a consequence, carcinoid syndrome and Cushing's syndrome may occur.

• Patients present with a firm thyroid mass and cervical lymphadenopathy. • Distant metastases are rare. • Serum calcitonin is raised and useful in monitoring response to treatment. • Hypocalcaemia is rare. • Treatment is by total thyroidectomy with removal of cervical nodes. • Medullary carcinoma may occur in childhood in families as part of the multiple endocrine neoplasia (MEN) type 2 syndrome (p. 382).

RIEDEL'S THYROIDITIS

• This rare, non-malignant condition has a similar presentation to thyroid cancer, with a slow-growing goitre which is irregular and stony-hard.

• Diagnosis is by biopsy. The thyroid and surrounding structures are infiltrated with fibrous tissue. There may be mediastinal and retroperitoneal fibrosis. • Tracheal and oesophageal compression necessitate thyroidectomy. • Complications include recurrent laryngeal nerve palsy, hypoparathyroidism and hypothyroidism.

THE REPRODUCTIVE SYSTEM

In the male, the testis has two principal functions:

• Synthesis of testosterone by the interstitial Leydig cells controlled by luteinising hormone (LH). • Spermatogenesis by Sertoli cells under the control of follicle-stimulating hormone (FSH).

Negative feedback suppression of LH is mediated principally by testosterone, while inhibin suppresses FSH.

In the female, sex hormones vary during the menstrual cycle. FSH produces growth and development of ovarian follicles during the first 14 days. This leads to a gradual increase in oestradiol production which initially suppresses FSH secretion (negative feedback) but then, above a certain level, stimulates an increase in the frequency and amplitude of gonadotrophin-releasing hormone (GnRH) pulses, resulting in a marked increase in LH secretion (positive feedback). This LH surge induces ovulation. The follicle then differentiates into a corpus luteum which secretes progesterone. Withdrawal of progesterone results in menstrual bleeding.

The cessation of menstruation (the menopause) occurs in developed countries at a median age of 50.8 yrs. In the 5 yrs before there is an increase in the number of anovulatory cycles, referred to as the climacteric. Oestrogen and inhibin secretion falls, resulting in increased pituitary secretion of LH and FSH.

PRESENTING PROBLEMS

DELAYED PUBERTY

Genetic factors influence the timing of the onset of puberty, although body weight acts as a trigger. Puberty may be considered delayed if it has not begun by a chronological age >2.5 standard deviations (SD) above the national average (>14 in boys, >13 in girls in the UK).

The differential diagnosis is considered in Box 10.8. The key issue is to determine whether the delay in puberty is because the 'clock is running slow' (constitutional delay) or because of pathology in the hypothalamus/pituitary (hypogonadotrophic hypogonadism) or the gonads (hypergonadotrophic hypogonadism).

Constitutional delay of puberty: This should be considered a normal variant and is the most common cause of delayed puberty. Affected children are typically shorter than their peers throughout childhood. There is often a family history and bone age is lower than chronological age. Puberty will

10.8 CAUSES OF DELAYED PUBERTY AND HYPOGONADISM	
Constitutional delay	
Hypogonadotrophic hypogonadism	Structural hypothalamic/pituitary disease—see Box 10.16 Functional gonadotrophin deficiency Chronic systemic illness (e.g. asthma, coeliac disease, cystic fibrosis) Psychological stress, anorexia nervosa, excessive exercise Endocrine disease: hyperprolactinaemia, Cushing's, hypothyroidism Isolated gonadotrophin deficiency (Kallmann's)
Hypergonadotrophic hypogonadism	Chemotherapy/radiotherapy to gonads Gonadal trauma/surgery, cryptorchidism Autoimmune gonadal failure Mumps, TB, haemochromatosis Klinefelter's/Turner's syndrome

start spontaneously, but prolonged delay can have significant psychological consequences.

Hypogonadotrophic hypogonadism: This may be due to structural, inflammatory or infiltrative disorders of the pituitary/hypothalamus (p. 373). Other pituitary hormones are likely to be deficient. 'Functional' gonadotrophin deficiency is caused by a variety of factors (see Box 10.8). Isolated gonadotrophin deficiency is due to a genetic abnormality affecting GnRH or gonadotrophin synthesis. The most common form is Kallmann's syndrome which is also associated with olfactory bulb agenesis, resulting in anosmia. If left untreated, the epiphyses fail to fuse, resulting in tall stature with disproportionately long arms and legs (eunuchoid habitus). Cryptorchidism (undescended testes) and gynaecomastia are seen in all forms of hypogonadotrophic hypogonadism.

Hypergonadotrophic hypogonadism: Hypergonadotrophic hypogonadism associated with delayed puberty is usually due to sex chromosome abnormalities (Klinefelter's/Turner's syndromes, p. 356). Other causes of primary gonadal failure are shown in Box 10.8.

Investigations

• Height should be plotted on centile charts. • Key measurements are LH/FSH, testosterone, oestradiol, FBC, renal, liver and thyroid function, and coeliac disease autoantibodies. • Chromosome analysis is performed if gonadotrophin concentrations are elevated. • If gonadotrophin concentrations are low, the differential diagnosis lies between constitutional delay and hypogonadotrophic hypogonadism. • A wrist X-ray allows estimation of bone age. • Neuroimaging is required in hypogonadotrophic hypogonadism.

Management

• Puberty can be induced using low doses of oestrogen or testosterone. • Higher doses carry a risk of early fusion of epiphyses and therefore therapy should be administered and monitored by a specialist. • In constitutional delay, therapy is withdrawn once puberty is established. In other cases, hormone doses are gradually increased during puberty and full adult replacement doses given when development is complete.

SECONDARY AMENORRHOEA

Primary amenorrhoea describes a patient who has never menstruated. This is usually due to delayed puberty but may be a consequence of anatomical defects, e.g. endometrial hypoplasia, vaginal agenesis.

Secondary amenorrhoea describes the cessation of menstruation. The causes of this are:

• Physiological (pregnancy, menopause). • Hypogonadotrophic hypogonadism (see Box 10.8). • Ovarian dysfunction (hypergonadotrophic hypogonadism; see Box 10.8). • Polycystic ovarian syndrome (PCOS), androgen-secreting tumours. • Uterine dysfunction (Asherman's syndrome).

Premature ovarian failure (premature menopause) is defined as occurring before 40 yrs of age.

Clinical assessment

Hypothalamic/pituitary disease and premature ovarian failure result in oestrogen deficiency, which causes menopausal symptoms: hot flushes, sweating, anxiety, irritability, dyspareunia, vaginal infections. Weight loss may indicate anorexia nervosa or underlying disease, e.g. malabsorption. Weight gain may suggest hypothyroidism or Cushing's syndrome. Breast examination should be performed for galactorrhoea (suggesting hyperprolactinaemia).

Investigations

• Measurement of urinary human chorionic gonadotrophin (hCG) will exclude pregnancy. • LH, FSH, oestradiol, prolactin, testosterone, T_4 and TSH should be measured. • ↑LH, ↑FSH, ↓oestradiol suggest primary ovarian failure. Ovarian autoantibodies may be positive. • ↑LH, ↑prolactin, ↑testosterone with normal or ↑oestradiol are common in PCOS. • ↓LH, ↓FSH, ↓oestradiol suggest hypothalamic/pituitary disease. • ↑↑prolactin suggests prolactinoma or 'disconnection' (see p. 379). • Assessment of bone mineral density is appropriate in patients with low androgen and oestrogen levels.

Management

Where possible, the underlying cause should be treated. The management of structural pituitary/hypothalamic disease and PCOS is described below. In oestrogen deficiency, oestrogen replacement therapy is necessary to treat symptoms and to prevent osteoporosis. Oestrogen should not be given without progesterone to a woman with a uterus due to the risk of endometrial cancer. This is administered most conveniently as an oral contraceptive pill. In post-menopausal females, HRT relieves menopausal symptoms and prevents osteoporotic fractures, but is associated with adverse effects (e.g. stroke, breast cancer, pulmonary embolism). Many authorities recommend that women should take replacement therapy until the age of 50 and only continue if there are unacceptable menopausal symptoms.

Women with hypogonadotrophic hypogonadism who wish fertility are given injections of gonadotrophins (FSH for follicular development, followed by hCG to induce follicular rupture). Monitoring is mandatory because of the risk of multiple ovulation and the hyperstimulation syndrome (capillary leak with circulatory shock, pleural effusions and ascites).

MALE HYPOGONADISM

The clinical features of both hypo- and hypergonadotrophic hypogonadism in men include:

• Loss of libido. • Lethargy. • Muscle weakness. • Decreased frequency of shaving.

Patients may also present with:

• Gynaecomastia. • Infertility. • Delayed puberty. • Erectile dysfunction.

The causes of hypogonadism are listed in Box 10.8.

Investigations

• Male hypogonadism is confirmed by demonstrating a low serum testosterone level. • Hypo- and hypergonadotrophic hypogonadism are distinguished by measurement of random LH and FSH. • Patients with hypogonadotrophic hypogonadism should be investigated for pituitary disease (p. 375). • Patients with hypergonadotrophic hypogonadism should have the testes examined for cryptorchidism or atrophy and a karyotype should be performed (Klinefelter's syndrome).

Management

• Testosterone replacement is indicated to prevent osteoporosis and to restore muscle power and libido. • Testosterone administration should be avoided in prostatic carcinoma. In men over 50, prostate-specific antigen (PSA) should be monitored. • Men with hypogonadotrophic hypogonadism who wish fertility are usually given injections of hCG. Extraction of sperm from the epididymis, in vitro fertilisation and intracytoplasmic sperm injection (ICSI) are used in primary testicular disease.

GYNAECOMASTIA

Gynaecomastia is the presence of glandular breast tissue in males, resulting from an imbalance between androgen and oestrogen activity (androgen deficiency or oestrogen excess). Causes are listed in Box 10.9. The most common are physiological, i.e. in the newborn baby (maternal oestrogens),

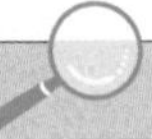

10.9 CAUSES OF GYNAECOMASTIA

- Idiopathic
- Physiological
- Drug-induced: cimetidine, digoxin, anti-androgens (cyproterone acetate, spironolactone)
- Hypogonadism (see Box 10.8)
- Androgen resistance syndromes
- Oestrogen excess: liver failure (impaired steroid metabolism), oestrogen-secreting tumour (e.g. testis), hCG-secreting tumour (e.g. testis, lung)

in pubertal boys (oestradiol concentrations reach adult levels before testosterone) and in elderly men (↓testosterone concentrations). Gynaecomastia is often asymmetrical.

• Palpation may allow breast tissue to be distinguished from adipose tissue observed in obesity. If a clinical distinction between gynaecomastia and adipose tissue cannot be made, then USS or mammography is required. • The testes should be examined for cryptorchidism, atrophy or a tumour. • Testosterone, LH, FSH, oestradiol, prolactin and hCG should be measured. Elevated oestrogen concentrations are found in testicular tumours and hCG-producing neoplasms. • The underlying cause should be addressed, e.g. changing drug treatments, excision of tumour. • In physiological gynaecomastia, reassurance is usually sufficient but if the condition is associated with significant psychological distress, surgical excision may be justified. • Androgen replacement improves gynaecomastia in hypogonadal males.

HIRSUTISM

Hirsutism refers to the excessive growth of thick terminal hair in an androgen-dependent distribution in women (upper lip, chin, chest, back, lower abdomen, thigh, forearm). It should be distinguished from hypertrichosis, which is generalised excessive growth of vellus hair. The aetiology of hirsutism is shown in Box 10.10.

• Important observations are a drug and menstrual history, BMI, BP, examination for virilisation (clitoromegaly, deep voice, male-pattern balding, breast atrophy) and associated features, e.g. Cushing's syndrome. • Recent hirsutism associated with virilisation is suggestive of an androgen-secreting tumour. • Testosterone, prolactin, LH and FSH should be measured. If testosterone levels are over twice the upper limit of the normal female range, especially with ↓LH and ↓FSH, then causes other than idiopathic hirsutism and PCOS are more likely. • See Box 10.10 for specific investigations and management.

POLYCYSTIC OVARIAN SYNDROME (PCOS)

The aetiology of PCOS remains poorly understood. It is characterised by loss of coordinate control of the menstrual cycle. PCOS often affects

10.10 CAUSES OF HIRSUTISM

Cause	Investigation findings	Treatment
Idiopathic	Normal	Cosmetic measures Anti-androgens
PCOS	LH : FSH ratio >2.5 : 1 Mild ↑androgens Mild hyperprolactinaemia	See below
Congenital adrenal hyperplasia (95% 21-hydroxylase deficiency)	↑Androgens suppress with dexamethasone ACTH test causes ↑17OH-progesterone	Glucocorticoid replacement administered in reverse rhythm to suppress early morning ACTH
Exogenous androgen administration	↓LH/FSH Urinalysis detects drug of misuse	Stop steroid misuse
Androgen-secreting tumour of ovary or adrenal cortex	↑Androgens do not suppress with dexamethasone/ oestrogen; ↓LH/FSH CT/MRI demonstrates tumour	Surgical excision
Cushing's syndrome	Normal or mild ↑adrenal androgens	Treat cause

several family members and is aggravated by obesity. Clinical and biochemical features include:

• Pituitary dysfunction: ↑LH, ↑prolactin. • Anovulatory menstrual cycles: oligomenorrhoea, secondary amenorrhoea, cystic ovaries, infertility. • Androgen excess: hirsutism, acne. • Obesity: hyperglycaemia, ↑oestrogens, dyslipidaemia, hypertension.

Management

Infertility: Treated under specialist supervision with clomifene or exogenous gonadotrophins.

Menses: High oestrogen concentrations can cause endometrial hyperplasia. Inducing a regular withdrawal bleed with cyclical progestogens can reduce the risk of endometrial neoplasia.

Hirsutism: Many patients use shaving, bleaching and waxing. Electrolysis and laser treatment are effective but expensive. Eflornithine cream inhibits ornithine decarboxylase in hair follicles and may reduce hair growth. Weight loss is important as it enhances insulin sensitivity, reduces the peripheral conversion of androgens to oestrogens by the aromatase enzyme in adipose, and reduces metabolic clearance of cortisol, thereby reducing ACTH-dependent adrenal androgen secretion.

Anti-androgen therapy: May be employed if other measures have failed. Treatments include:

• Androgen receptor antagonists (e.g. cyproterone acetate). • 5α-reductase inhibitors which prevent activation of testosterone (e.g. finasteride). • Exogenous oestrogen which suppresses ovarian hormone production. • In addition, insulin-sensitising drugs (metformin) may have a role.

Without weight loss, hirsutism will return if therapy is discontinued. Prolonged exposure to some of these agents is not desirable; they should be discontinued in advance of pregnancy and the prescription should be reviewed at least every 6 mths.

TURNER'S SYNDROME

Turner's syndrome affects approximately 1 in 2500 females. The syndrome is classically associated with a 45XO karyotype. Individuals with Turner's syndrome have short stature. The genitals are female in character, although gonadal dysgenesis results in 'streak ovaries'. The lack of oestrogen causes loss of negative feedback and elevation of FSH and LH concentrations. There is a wide variation in the spectrum of associated somatic abnormalities. These include:

• Webbing of the neck (25–40%). • Widely spaced nipples. • Shield chest. • Horse-shoe kidney. • Lymphoedema of hands and feet (30%). • Coarctation of the aorta. • Aortic root dilatation.

Short stature may be helped by high doses of growth hormone. Pubertal development is induced with oestrogen therapy and long-term oestrogen replacement is required.

KLINEFELTER'S SYNDROME

Klinefelter's syndrome affects approximately 1 in 1000 males and is usually associated with a 47XXY karyotype. Leydig cell function is impaired, resulting in hypergonadotrophic hypogonadism. The diagnosis is often made in adolescents with gynaecomastia and delayed puberty. Affected individuals usually have small, firm testes and may have learning difficulties. Tall stature is apparent from early childhood, with a long leg length exacerbated by lack of epiphyseal closure in puberty. Individuals with androgen deficiency require androgen replacement.

TESTICULAR TUMOURS

Tumours of the testes are uncommon (5/100 000 population) and occur mainly in young men aged 20–40 yrs. They often secrete tumour markers which are useful for diagnosis and prognosis. Seminoma and teratoma account for 85% of all tumours of the testis; Leydig cell tumours are less common.

• Seminomas arise from seminiferous tubules. Metastases occur via the lymphatics, often involving the lungs. • Teratomas arise from primitive germinal cells. They may contain cartilage, bone, muscle or fat. Well-differentiated tumours are the least aggressive; at the other extreme, trophoblastic teratoma is highly malignant. • Leydig cell tumours are usually small and benign, but secrete oestrogens leading to presentation with gynaecomastia.

Clinical features and investigations

• The common presentation is incidental discovery of a painless testicular lump, although some complain of testicular ache. • Suspicious scrotal lumps are imaged by USS. • Serum levels of the 'tumour markers' α-fetoprotein (AFP) and β-hCG are increased in extensive disease. • Oestradiol may be elevated, suppressing the levels of LH, FSH and testosterone. • Accurate staging is based on CT or MRI.

Management and prognosis

• The primary treatment is surgical orchidectomy. • Radiotherapy is the treatment of choice for early-stage seminoma. • Teratoma confined to the testes may be managed conservatively, but more advanced cancers are treated with chemotherapy. • Follow-up is by imaging and assessment of AFP and β-hCG. • 5-yr survival rates are 90–95% for seminomas and 60–95% for teratomas.

THE PARATHYROID GLANDS

The four parathyroid glands lie behind the lobes of the thyroid. Parathyroid hormone (PTH) interacts with vitamin D to control calcium metabolism. Calcium exists in serum as 50% ionised, and 50% complexed with organic ions and proteins. The parathyroid chief cells respond directly to changes in calcium concentrations, secreting PTH in response to a fall in ionised calcium. PTH promotes reabsorption of calcium from renal tubules and bone, stimulating alkaline phosphatase and lowering plasma phosphate. PTH also promotes renal conversion of 25-hydroxycholecalciferol to the more potent 1,25-dihydroxycholecalciferol, which results in increased calcium absorption from food.

To investigate disorders of calcium metabolism, measurement of calcium, phosphate, alkaline phosphatase and PTH should be undertaken. Most laboratories measure total calcium in serum. This needs to be corrected if serum albumin is low, by adjusting the value for calcium upwards by 0.1 mmol/l (0.4 mg/dl) for each 5 g/l reduction in albumin below 40 g/l.

PRESENTING PROBLEMS

HYPERCALCAEMIA

Causes of hypercalcaemia are listed in Box 10.11. Primary hyperparathyroidism and malignant hypercalcaemia are the most common causes. Famil-

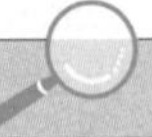

10.11 CAUSES OF HYPERCALCAEMIA
With normal/elevated (inappropriate) PTH levels
• Primary or tertiary hyperparathyroidism • Lithium-induced hyperparathyroidism • Familial hypocalciuric hypercalcaemia
With low (suppressed) PTH levels
• Malignancy (e.g. lung, breast, renal, colonic and thyroid carcinoma, lymphoma, multiple myeloma) • Elevated 1,25$(OH)_2$ vitamin D (vitamin D intoxication, sarcoidosis, HIV) • Thyrotoxicosis • Paget's disease with immobilisation • Milk-alkali syndrome • Thiazide diuretics • Glucocorticoid deficiency

ial hypocalciuric hypercalcaemia (FHH) is a rare autosomal dominant disorder in which a mutation in the calcium-sensing receptor results in increased PTH secretion with consequent calcium retention in the renal tubules. FHH is almost always asymptomatic and without complication. Unnecessary parathyroidectomy may be undertaken if FHH is misdiagnosed as primary hyperparathyroidism.

Clinical assessment

• Symptoms and signs of hypercalcaemia include polyuria, polydipsia, renal colic, lethargy, anorexia, nausea, dyspepsia, peptic ulceration, constipation, depression and impaired cognition ('bones, stones and abdominal groans'). • Patients with malignant hypercalcaemia can have a rapid onset of symptoms. • Hypertension is common in hyperparathyroidism. • Parathyroid tumours are almost never palpable. • A family history of hypercalcaemia raises the possibility of FHH or MEN.

Investigations

• ↓Plasma phosphate and ↑alkaline phosphatase support a diagnosis of primary hyperparathyroidism or malignancy. • ↑Plasma phosphate and ↑alkaline phosphatase accompanied by renal impairment suggest tertiary hyperparathyroidism (p. 360). • If PTH is normal or elevated and urinary calcium is elevated, then hyperparathyroidism is confirmed. • Low urine calcium excretion indicates likely FHH, confirmed by genetic analysis of the calcium-sensing receptor. • If PTH is low and no other cause is apparent, then malignancy with or without bony metastases is likely. The patient should be screened with a CXR, isotope bone scan, myeloma screen and serum ACE (elevated in sarcoidosis). PTH-related peptide, which causes hypercalcaemia associated with malignancy, can be measured by a specific assay.

Management

• Treatment of severe hypercalcaemia involves rehydration with normal saline. • Bisphosphonates (e.g. pamidronate 90 mg i.v. over 4 hrs) reduce serum calcium for a few weeks, working maximally at 2–3 days. If the underlying cause cannot be removed, oral bisphosphonates should be continued. • In very ill patients, forced diuresis with furosemide, glucocorticoids, calcitonin or haemodialysis may need to be employed. • For management of hyperparathyroidism, see page 361. • FHH does not require therapy.

HYPOCALCAEMIA

The differential diagnosis of hypocalcaemia is shown in Box 10.12. It is the ionised rather than total concentration which is biologically important. The most common cause of hypocalcaemia is a low serum albumin with normal ionised calcium concentration. Ionised calcium may be low with a normal total serum calcium in alkalosis, e.g. hyperventilation (respiratory) or Conn's syndrome (metabolic).

Causes of hypoparathyroidism include:

• Parathyroid gland damage during thyroid surgery (transient hypocalcaemia in 10%, permanent in 1%). • Infiltration of the glands, e.g. haemochromatosis, Wilson's disease. • Congenital/inherited, e.g. autoimmune polyendocrine syndrome (APS) type I, autosomal dominant hypoparathyroidism.

In pseudohypoparathyroidism there is tissue resistance to PTH. Clinical features include:

• Short stature. • Short 4th metacarpals and metatarsals. • Rounded face. • Obesity. • Calcification of the basal ganglia.

10.12 DIFFERENTIAL DIAGNOSIS OF HYPOCALCAEMIA

	Total serum calcium	Ionised serum calcium	Serum phosphate	Serum PTH concentration
Hypoalbuminaemia	↓	→	→	→
Alkalosis	→	↓	→	→ or ↑
Vitamin D deficiency	↓	↓	↓	↑
Chronic renal failure	↓	↓	↑	↑
Hypoparathyroidism	↓	↓	↑	↓
Pseudohypoparathyroidism	↓	↓	↑	↑
Acute pancreatitis	↓	↓	→ or ↓	↑
Hypomagnesaemia	↓	↓	Variable	↓ or →

The term 'pseudo-pseudohypoparathyroidism' describes those with these clinical features in whom serum calcium and PTH concentrations are normal. Due to genomic imprinting, pseudohypoparathyroidism results from inheritance of the gene defect from the mother, but inheritance from the father results in pseudo-pseudohypoparathyroidism.

Clinical assessment

• Low ionised calcium increases excitability of peripheral nerves. • Tetany can occur if total serum calcium is <2.0 mmol/l (8 mg/dl). • In children a characteristic triad of carpopedal spasm, stridor and convulsions occurs. Adults complain of tingling in the hands and feet and around the mouth. • When overt signs are lacking, latent tetany may be revealed by Trousseau's sign (inflation of a sphygmomanometer cuff to more than the systolic BP causes carpal spasm) or Chvostek's sign (tapping over the facial nerve produces twitching of the facial muscles). • Hypocalcaemia causes papilloedema and QT interval prolongation, predisposing to ventricular arrhythmias. • Prolonged hypocalcaemia with hyperphosphataemia may cause calcification of the basal ganglia, epilepsy, psychosis and cataracts. • Hypocalcaemia with hypophosphataemia (vitamin D deficiency) causes rickets in children and osteomalacia in adults.

Management

• To control tetany, alkalosis can be reversed by rebreathing expired air in a bag (↑$PaCO_2$). • Injection of 20 ml of 10% calcium gluconate slowly into a vein will raise the serum calcium concentration immediately. • I.V. magnesium is required to correct hypocalcaemia associated with hypomagnesaemia. • Vitamin D deficiency, persistent hypoparathyroidism and pseudohypoparathyroidism are treated with oral calcium salts and vitamin D analogues (alfacalcidol, calcitriol). • Monitoring of therapy is required because of the risks of iatrogenic hypercalcaemia, hypercalciuria and nephrocalcinosis.

PRIMARY HYPERPARATHYROIDISM

The three categories of hyperparathyroidism are shown in Box 10.13. • In primary hyperparathyroidism there is autonomous secretion of PTH, usually by a single parathyroid adenoma. • In secondary hyperparathyroidism there is increased PTH secretion to compensate for prolonged hypocalcaemia, thus increasing serum calcium levels by bone resorption. It is associated with hyperplasia of all parathyroid tissue. • In a small proportion of secondary hyperparathyroidism cases, continuous stimulation of the parathyroids results in adenoma formation and autonomous PTH secretion. This is known as tertiary hyperparathyroidism.

Primary hyperparathyroidism has a prevalence of 1 in 800 and is 2–3 times more common in women; 90% of patients are over 50. It also occurs in MEN syndromes. Clinical presentation is described under hypercalcaemia (p. 358).

10.13 HYPERPARATHYROIDISM		
Type	**Serum calcium**	**PTH**
Primary Single adenoma (90%), multiple adenomas (4%), nodular hyperplasia (5%), carcinoma (1%)	Raised	Not suppressed
Secondary Chronic renal failure, malabsorption, osteomalacia and rickets	Low	Raised
Tertiary	Raised	Not suppressed

Skeletal and radiological changes include:
• Osteoporosis-reduced bone mineral density on DEXA scanning. • Osteitis fibrosa results from increased bone resorption by osteoclasts with fibrous replacement. It presents as bone pain, fracture and deformity. • Chondrocalcinosis is due to deposition of calcium pyrophosphate crystals within articular cartilage, typically the knee, leading to osteoarthritis or acute pseudogout. • X-ray changes include subperiosteal erosions, terminal resorption in the phalanges, 'pepper-pot' skull and renal calcification.

Imaging to locate the adenoma or differentiate hyperplasia has traditionally not been necessary, but its increasing use allows more targeted resection through a smaller incision. Localisation of parathyroid tumours may be carried out using ^{99m}Tc-sestamibi scanning, USS, CT or selective neck vein catheterisation with PTH measurements. Without imaging, >90% of adenomas can be located at surgery.

Management

Treatment of severe hypercalcaemia is described above (p. 359). Hypercalcaemia in primary hyperparathyroidism responds less well to glucocorticoids and bisphosphonates. Most patients do not require urgent surgical treatment. However, the only long-term therapy is surgery, with excision of an adenoma or debulking of hyperplastic glands. Part of the hyperplastic gland can be transplanted to the forearm to allow further debulking at a later date. Post-operative hypocalcaemia can occur while residual suppressed parathyroid tissue recovers.

Surgery is indicated for patients under 50 and for those with symptoms or complications, e.g. peptic ulceration, renal stones, renal impairment or osteopenia. The remainder can be reviewed annually, with assessment of symptoms, renal function, serum calcium and bone mineral density.

THE ADRENAL GLANDS

The adrenals function as several separate endocrine glands within one anatomical structure.

• The adrenal medulla is an extension of the sympathetic nervous system which secretes catecholamines. • Most of the adrenal cortex is made up of cells which secrete cortisol and adrenal androgens, and form part of the hypothalamic–pituitary–adrenal axis. • The small outer glomerulosa of the cortex secretes aldosterone under the control of the renin–angiotensin system.

Adrenal anatomy and function are shown in Figure 10.5.

Glucocorticoids: Cortisol is the major glucocorticoid in humans. Levels are highest in the morning and lowest in the middle of the night. Cortisol rises dramatically during stress, including any illness. This elevation protects key metabolic functions and cortisol deficiency is, therefore, most obvious at times of stress.

Mineralocorticoids: Aldosterone is the body's most important sodium-retaining hormone, acting via mineralocorticoid receptors. Sodium is retained at the expense of increased excretion of potassium. Increased potassium in the lumen of the distal nephron also results in increased exchange with protons and metabolic alkalosis. The principal stimulus to aldosterone secretion is angiotensin II, a peptide produced by activation of the renin–angiotensin system (see Fig. 10.5). Renin secretion from the juxtaglomerular apparatus in the kidney is stimulated by low perfusion pressure in the afferent arteriole, low sodium filtration or increased sympathetic nerve activity.

Catecholamines: In humans, most circulating noradrenaline (norepinephrine) is derived from sympathetic nerve endings. However, noradrenaline is converted to adrenaline (epinephrine) in the adrenal medulla. The medulla is thus the major source of circulating adrenaline.

Adrenal androgens: Adrenal androgens are secreted in response to ACTH. They are probably important in the initiation of puberty (the adrenarche), are the major source of androgens in females and may be important in female libido.

PRESENTING PROBLEMS

CUSHING'S SYNDROME

Cushing's syndrome is caused by excessive activation of glucocorticoid receptors. Causes are shown in Box 10.14. By far the most common cause is iatrogenic, due to prolonged administration of synthetic glucocorticoids such as prednisolone. Pituitary-dependent cortisol excess (Cushing's disease) accounts for ~80% of endogenous cases.

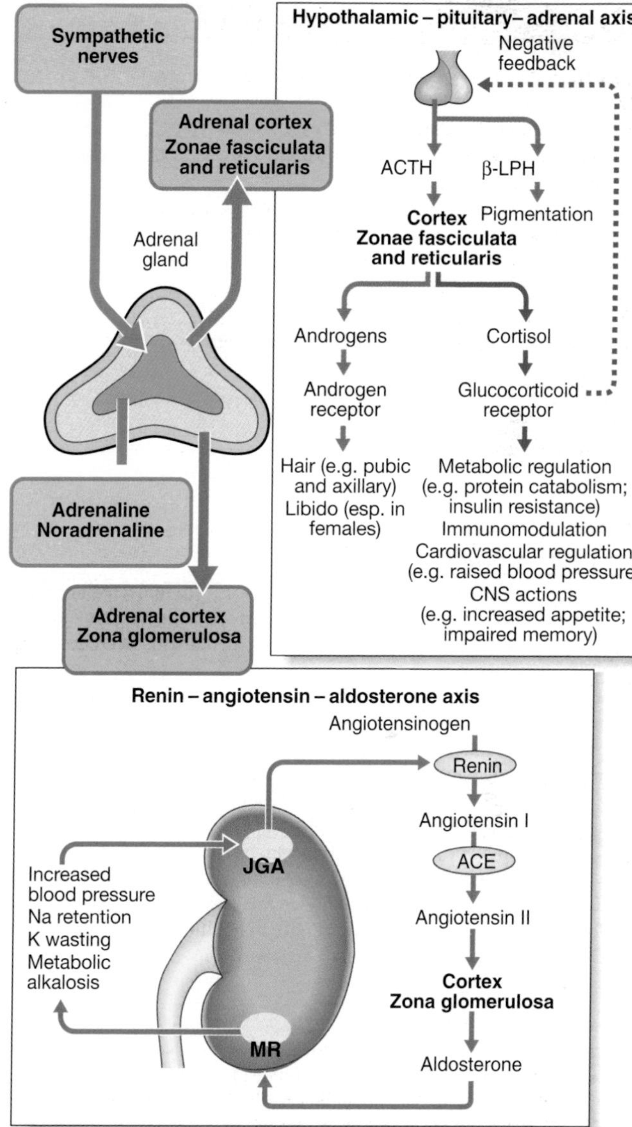

Fig. 10.5 Structure and function of the adrenal glands. (ACE = angiotensin-converting enzyme; JGA = juxtaglomerular apparatus; MR = mineralocorticoid receptor; β-LPH = β-lipotrophic hormone)

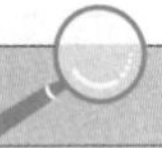

10.14 CLASSIFICATION OF CUSHING'S SYNDROME
ACTH-dependent
• Pituitary adenoma secreting ACTH (Cushing's disease) • Ectopic ACTH syndrome (e.g. bronchial carcinoid, small-cell lung carcinoma) • Iatrogenic (ACTH therapy)
Non-ACTH-dependent
• Iatrogenic (chronic glucocorticoid therapy) • Adrenal adenoma • Adrenal carcinoma
Pseudo-Cushing's syndrome (as part of another illness)
• Alcohol excess (clinical features) • Major depressive illness (biochemical features) • Primary obesity (mild biochemical features)

Clinical assessment

The diverse manifestations of glucocorticoid excess are indicated in Figure 10.6. Some common disorders can be confused with Cushing's syndrome because they are associated with alterations in cortisol secretion, e.g. obesity and depression.

A careful drug history is vital to exclude iatrogenic causes; even inhaled or topical glucocorticoids can induce Cushing's syndrome. Some clinical features are more common in ectopic ACTH syndrome. Ectopic tumours have no negative feedback sensitivity to cortisol. Very high ACTH levels are associated with marked pigmentation with hypokalaemic alkalosis, aggravating both myopathy and hyperglycaemia. When the tumour secreting ACTH is malignant (e.g. small-cell lung carcinoma), then the onset is usually rapid and may be associated with cachexia. In Cushing's disease, the pituitary tumour is usually a microadenoma (<10 mm diameter); hence other features of a pituitary macroadenoma (hypopituitarism, visual failure or disconnection hyperprolactinaemia) are rare.

Investigations

It is useful to divide investigations into those which establish whether the patient has Cushing's syndrome, and those which are used subsequently to elucidate the aetiology. Additional tests include plasma electrolytes, glucose, glycosylated haemoglobin and bone mineral density measurement. In iatrogenic Cushing's syndrome, cortisol levels are low unless the corticosteroid cross-reacts in immunoassays with cortisol (e.g. prednisolone).

Does the patient have Cushing's syndrome? Cushing's syndrome is confirmed by the demonstration of increased secretion of cortisol (24-hr

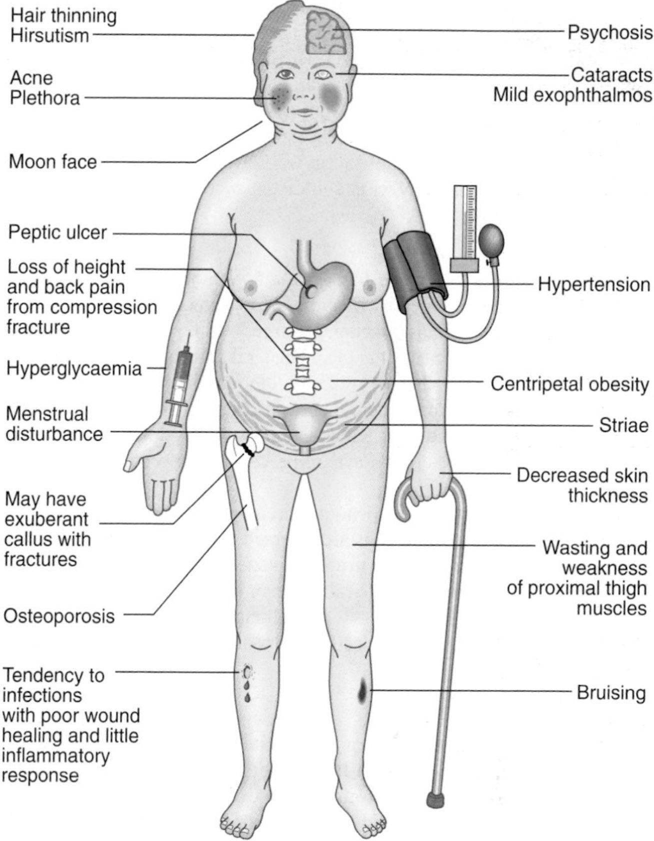

Fig. 10.6 Clinical features of Cushing's syndrome.

urinary cortisol) that fails to suppress either with a 1 mg overnight dexamethasone suppression test or with the 48-hr low-dose dexamethasone suppression test (0.5 mg 6-hourly for 48 hrs). Loss of diurnal variation, with elevated evening cortisol, is also characteristic of Cushing's syndrome.

What is the cause of the Cushing's syndrome? The following tests are available:

• Plasma ACTH: undetectable ACTH indicates an adrenal tumour, while any detectable ACTH indicates a pituitary or ectopic source. Tests to discriminate pituitary from ectopic ACTH rely on the fact that pituitary tumours, but not ectopic tumours, retain some features of normal regulation. Thus in pituitary disease ACTH and cortisol are stimulated by CRH injection and suppressed during a 48-hr high-dose dexamethasone suppression test (2 mg 6-hourly for 48 hrs). • CT/MRI: detects most adrenal adenomas. Adrenal carcinomas are usually large (>5 cm). Tumours not imaged are localised with selective adrenal vein catheterisation with cortisol sampling. • MRI with gadolinium enhancement: detects ~70% of pituitary microadenomas. Venous catheterisation with inferior petrosal sinus ACTH measurement is used if the MRI is non-diagnostic.

Management

Untreated Cushing's syndrome has a 50% 5-yr mortality. Corticosteroid biosynthesis can be inhibited by metyrapone or ketoconazole.

Cushing's disease: Trans-sphenoidal surgery with selective removal of the adenoma is the treatment of choice. Bilateral adrenalectomy is an alternative, but there is a risk that the pituitary tumour will grow in the absence of negative feedback suppression. This can result in Nelson's syndrome, with an aggressive pituitary macroadenoma and very high ACTH levels causing pigmentation. Nelson's syndrome can be prevented by pituitary irradiation.

Adrenal tumours: Adrenal adenomas are removed via laparoscopy or a loin incision. Adrenal carcinomas are resected if possible, the tumour bed is irradiated and the adrenolytic drug, mitotane, is given.

Ectopic ACTH syndrome: Localised tumours causing this syndrome should be removed. In unresectable malignancies, the severity of the Cushing's syndrome can be reduced with medical therapy (see above).

ADRENAL INSUFFICIENCY

Adrenal insufficiency results from inadequate secretion of cortisol and/or aldosterone. Causes are shown in Box 10.15. The most common is ACTH deficiency (secondary adrenocortical failure), usually because of withdrawal of chronic glucocorticoid therapy or a pituitary tumour. Congenital adrenal hyperplasia and Addison's disease are rare.

Clinical assessment

Patients may present with chronic features or in acute circulatory shock.
• With a chronic presentation, initial symptoms are often misdiagnosed (e.g. as depression or chronic fatigue); the diagnosis should be considered in all patients with hyponatraemia. • Features of an acute adrenal crisis include circulatory shock with severe hypotension, hyponatraemia, hyperkalaemia and, occasionally, hypoglycaemia and hypercalcaemia. Muscle cramps, vomiting, diarrhoea and fever may be present. The crisis is often precipitated by intercurrent disease, surgery or infection. • Pigmentation due to excess ACTH may be prominent, particularly in recent scars and pressure areas. Vitiligo occurs in 10–20% of patients with autoimmune Addison's disease.

10.15 CAUSES OF ADRENOCORTICAL INSUFFICIENCY
Secondary (↓ACTH)
• Withdrawal of glucocorticoid therapy • Hypothalamic/pituitary disease
Primary (↑ACTH)
Addison's disease • Autoimmune • TB • HIV/AIDS • Metastatic carcinoma • Intra-adrenal haemorrhage (Waterhouse–Friedrichsen syndrome in meningococcal septicaemia) • Rare causes: amyloidosis, haemochromatosis
Corticosteroid biosynthetic enzyme defects • Congenital adrenal hyperplasias • Drugs: metyrapone, ketoconazole

Investigations

In chronic illness, investigations may be performed before any treatment. In an acute crisis, a random blood sample should be stored for measurement of cortisol but other tests are deferred until treatment has been given.

Assessment of glucocorticoids: Random plasma cortisol is usually low in adrenal insufficiency, but may be inappropriately within the normal range for a seriously ill patient. The short ACTH stimulation test (tetracosactide, short Synacthen test) requires administration of 250 μg ACTH (Synacthen) i.m. with serum cortisol measured at 0 and 30 mins. A cortisol >460 nmol/l (~17 μg/dl) at either time excludes adrenal insufficiency. A cortisol level that fails to increase occurs with primary or secondary adrenal insufficiency. These can be distinguished by measurement of ACTH, which is low in ACTH deficiency and high in Addison's disease.

Assessment of mineralocorticoids: Hyponatraemia occurs in both aldosterone and cortisol deficiency. Hyperkalaemia is common in aldosterone deficiency. Plasma renin activity and aldosterone should be measured in the supine position. In mineralocorticoid deficiency, plasma renin activity is high, with a low or low normal plasma aldosterone.

Other tests to establish the cause: Patients with unexplained secondary adrenocortical insufficiency should be investigated for pituitary disease. In patients with elevated ACTH, further tests are required to establish the cause of Addison's disease. In autoimmune adrenal failure, adrenal antibodies can be measured. TFTs, FBC (pernicious anaemia screen), plasma calcium, glucose and gonadal function tests should be performed. Other tests include: CXR and AXR for TB (adrenal calcification), HIV test, and adrenal CT/MRI for metastatic malignancy.

Management

Glucocorticoid replacement: Hydrocortisone (i.e. cortisol) is the drug of choice. In the non-critically ill, cortisol is given 15 mg on waking and 5 mg at ~1800 hrs. Excess weight gain usually indicates over-replacement, whilst persistent lethargy or hyperpigmentation may indicate an inadequate dose. Replacement doses should not cause Cushingoid side-effects. Patients on glucocorticoid replacement should be advised:

• During intercurrent infection, double the dose of hydrocortisone. • Increase the dose perioperatively (major operation, 100 mg 6-hourly). • Keep parenteral hydrocortisone at home in case of vomiting. • Carry a steroid card and wear a medical bracelet.

An adrenal crisis is a medical emergency and requires i.v. hydrocortisone succinate 100 mg and i.v. fluid (normal saline and 10% dextrose for hypoglycaemia). Parenteral hydrocortisone should be continued (100 mg i.m. 6-hourly) until the patient is able to take oral therapy. The precipitating cause should be treated.

Mineralocorticoid replacement: Fludrocortisone is the mineralocorticoid used (0.05–0.2 mg daily). Adequacy of replacement can be assessed with measurement of BP, plasma electrolytes and plasma renin activity. In adrenal crisis, rapid infusion of i.v. saline to normalise haemodynamic indices is more important than fludrocortisone. In severe hyponatraemia (<125 mmol/l) rapid normalisation risks pontine demyelination.

PROBLEMS WITH GLUCOCORTICOID THERAPY

Glucocorticoids are widely used due to their anti-inflammatory properties. Equivalent doses of 5 mg prednisolone are:

• Hydrocortisone 20 mg. • Cortisone acetate 25 mg. • Dexamethasone 0.5 mg.

Side-effects of glucocorticoid therapy (see also p. 774)

The side-effects of glucocorticoid therapy are illustrated in Figure 10.5. These effects are related to dose, which should therefore be kept to a minimum.

• Diabetes mellitus or glucose intolerance can be worsened. • Rapid changes in cortisol levels can cause marked mood disturbance, either depression or mania, and insomnia. • Signs of perforation of a viscus may be masked and the patient may show no febrile response to an infection. • Gastric erosions are more common, probably because of impaired prostaglandin synthesis. Hence, the combination of corticosteroid with aspirin/NSAIDs may lead to haemorrhage from the stomach/duodenum. • Latent TB may be reactivated and contact with varicella zoster should be avoided if not immune. • Osteoporosis is a particularly important problem because the fracture risk is greater in glucocorticoid-induced osteoporosis than in post-menopausal osteoporosis. Therefore, people >65 or with previous osteoporotic fracture or with low bone mineral density should commence bone-protective therapy if the intended duration of steroid therapy is >3 mths with bisphosphonates, calcium/vitamin D and/or calcitonin.

Withdrawal of glucocorticoid therapy

All glucocorticoid therapy, even if inhaled or applied topically, can suppress the hypothalamic–pituitary–adrenal (HPA) axis. In practice, this is only a problem with systemic treatment >3 wks or repeated courses within the previous year, or if the dose is >40 mg prednisolone daily. In these circumstances, the drug must be withdrawn slowly, as it may take many months for the HPA axis to recover. All patients must be advised to avoid sudden drug withdrawal. They should be issued with a steroid card and/or wear an engraved bracelet.

ENDOCRINE HYPERTENSION

Investigation and management of hypertension are discussed on page 243. While there is no discernible cause in the majority of patients with hypertension (essential hypertension), a small percentage have an underlying endocrine disorder. Most cases of endocrine hypertension are related to mineralocorticoid excess. Phaeochromocytoma, Cushing's syndrome, hyperparathyroidism, acromegaly and thyroid dysfunction also raise BP.

MINERALOCORTICOID EXCESS

Indications to test for mineralocorticoid excess in hypertensive patients include:

• Hypokalaemia. • Poor control of BP with conventional therapy. • Presentation at a young age.

Causes of excessive activation of mineralocorticoid receptors can be differentiated by renin and aldosterone measurement.

Renin↑ and aldosterone↑ (secondary hyperaldosteronism): This is the most common cause. Enhanced renin secretion is in response to inadequate renal perfusion and hypotension, e.g. diuretic therapy, cardiac failure, liver failure or renal artery stenosis. Very rarely, renin-secreting renal tumours cause secondary hyperaldosteronism.

Renin↓ and aldosterone↑ (primary hyperaldosteronism): A small minority of patients with hypertension will be found to have primary hyperaldosteronism. Depending on the diagnostic criteria used, between 1 and 20% of these have an adrenal adenoma secreting aldosterone (Conn's syndrome) and the remainder have idiopathic bilateral adrenal hyperplasia.

Renin↓ and aldosterone↓: The mineralocorticoid receptor pathway in the distal nephron is activated, even though aldosterone levels are low. Either the receptors are activated by cortisol (ectopic ACTH syndrome) or

11-deoxycorticosterone (adrenal tumour), or post-receptor mechanisms are inappropriately activated (e.g. the epithelial sodium channel in Liddle's syndrome).

Clinical assessment

Many patients are asymptomatic but they may have features of sodium retention or potassium loss.

• Sodium retention may cause oedema. • Hypokalaemia causes muscle weakness (or even paralysis), polyuria (renal tubular damage producing nephrogenic diabetes insipidus) and occasionally tetany (associated metabolic alkalosis and low ionised calcium).

Investigations

Biochemical: Plasma electrolytes: hypokalaemia, ↑bicarbonate, sodium upper normal (primary hyperaldosteronism), hyponatraemia (secondary hyperaldosteronism: hypovolaemia stimulates antidiuretic hormone (ADH) release and high angiotensin II levels stimulate thirst). Renin and aldosterone should be measured.

Localisation: Abdominal CT/MRI can localise a Conn's adenoma but non-functioning adrenal adenomas are present in ~20% of patients with essential hypertension. If the scan is inconclusive, adrenal vein catheterisation with measurement of aldosterone may be helpful.

Management

• Spironolactone, an aldosterone antagonist, treats both hypokalaemia and hypertension due to mineralocorticoid excess (up to 400 mg daily). • Spironolactone can be changed to amiloride (10–40 mg/day) or eplerenone if gynaecomastia develops (~20%). • In patients with Conn's adenoma, pre-operative therapy to normalise whole-body electrolyte balance should be undertaken before unilateral adrenalectomy. • Post-operatively, hypertension remains in as many as 70% of cases.

INCIDENTAL ADRENAL MASS

Adrenal 'incidentalomas' are present in up to 10% of adults. They are identified on abdominal CT or MRI scan that has been performed for another indication. Around 85% are non-functioning adrenal adenomas. The remainder are functional tumours of the adrenal cortex, phaeochromocytomas, primary/secondary carcinomas or hamartomas.

• Investigations should include a 24-hr urine collection for catecholamines and urine free cortisol, plasma renin and aldosterone and, in women, serum androgens. • CT-guided biopsy may be performed if it is important to determine whether an adrenal mass is a metastatic lesion or not. • Functional lesions and tumours >5 cm in diameter are removed by laparoscopic adrenalectomy. • In non-functioning lesions <5 cm excision is only required if serial imaging suggests growth.

PHAEOCHROMOCYTOMA

This is a rare tumour of chromaffin tissue which is responsible for <0.1% of cases of hypertension. There is a useful 'rule of tens':

• ~10% are malignant. • ~10% are extra-adrenal. • ~10% are familial.

Clinical features

These can be paroxysmal and include:

• Hypertension (with postural hypotension). • Palpitations. • Pallor. • Sweating. • Headache. • Anxiety (with fear of death). • Abdominal pain. • Glucose intolerance.

Some patients present with a complication of hypertension, e.g. stroke. There may be features of familial syndromes, e.g. neurofibromatosis, von Hippel–Lindau syndrome and MEN type 2.

Investigations

• Excessive secretion of catecholamines can be confirmed by measuring them in serum (adrenaline/epinephrine, noradrenaline/norepinephrine and dopamine) and their metabolites in urine (e.g. vanillyl-mandelic acid, VMA; conjugated metanephrine and normetanephrine). False-negative results may be obtained due to intermittent catecholamine secretion. • Phaeochromocytomas are identified by abdominal CT/MRI. • To localise extra-adrenal tumours, scintigraphy using meta-iodobenzyl guanidine (MIBG) is used.

Management

Medical therapy is required pre-operatively, preferably for a minimum of 6 wks. The non-competitive α-antagonist phenoxybenzamine (10–20 mg orally 6–8-hourly) is used with a β-blocker (e.g. propranolol) or combined α- and β-antagonist (e.g. labetalol). β-antagonists must not be given before the α-antagonist as this may cause a paradoxical rise in BP.

THE ENDOCRINE PANCREAS AND GI TRACT

PRESENTING PROBLEMS

SPONTANEOUS HYPOGLYCAEMIA

Hypoglycaemia most commonly complicates treatment of diabetes mellitus with insulin or sulphonylureas. Spontaneous hypoglycaemia should only be diagnosed if all three conditions of Whipple's triad are met:

• Symptoms of hypoglycaemia. • Low blood glucose measured at the time of symptoms. • Symptoms resolve on correction of hypoglycaemia.

There is little evidence to support the existence of post-prandial hypoglycaemia (e.g. 'reactive' hypoglycaemia or 'late dumping syndrome' post-gastrectomy).

Clinical assessment

Clinical features of hypoglycaemia are described on page 397. Symptoms are episodic and key questions include symptom frequency on fasting/exercise and symptom relief by consumption of sugar. Hypoglycaemia should be considered in all comatose patients, even if there is an apparently obvious cause. In the acute setting, alcohol is the most likely cause.

Investigations

Does the patient have a hypoglycaemic disorder? In an acute presentation, hypoglycaemia is usually tested with capillary blood glucose strips. However, due to their relative inaccuracy, hypoglycaemia should be confirmed by formal laboratory measurement. Establishing the existence of a hypoglycaemic disorder in outpatient clinics requires a prolonged (72-hr) fast:

• If symptoms develop, blood samples are taken to confirm hypoglycaemia and for measurement of insulin and C-peptide. • If symptoms resolve with glucose, Whipple's triad is completed. • The absence of clinical and biochemical evidence of hypoglycaemia during the test excludes the diagnosis of hypoglycaemia.

What is the cause of the hypoglycaemia? Causes of spontaneous hypoglycaemia can be classified by the level of insulin and C-peptide measured in serum sampled during hypoglycaemia (see below):

• ↓Insulin and ↓C-peptide: impaired liver glucose release due to alcohol, drugs, critical illnesses (liver failure, renal failure, malaria), hypopituitarism, adrenocortical failure, non-islet cell tumours. • ↑Insulin and ↓C-peptide: exogenous insulin. • ↑Insulin and ↑C-peptide: insulinoma, drugs (sulphonylureas, pentamidine).

Insulinomas in the pancreas are usually small (<5 mm) and can be identified by CT, MRI or endoscopic/laparoscopic USS. About 10% of insulinomas are malignant. Rarely, tumours such as sarcomas may cause recurrent hypoglycaemia due to production of insulin-like growth factor-2.

Management

Acute hypoglycaemia should be treated as soon as blood samples have been taken.

• I.V. dextrose (10% or 50%) should be followed with oral carbohydrate. Continuous dextrose infusion may be necessary, especially in sulphonylurea poisoning. • I.M. glucagon (1 mg) stimulates hepatic glucose release, but is ineffective when glycogen reserves are depleted (alcohol excess, liver disease). • Chronic recurrent hypoglycaemia in insulin-secreting tumours can be treated by regular carbohydrate consumption combined with inhibitors of insulin secretion (diazoxide, thiazide diuretics or somatostatin analogues). • Insulinomas are usually resected.

NEUROENDOCRINE TUMOURS

Neuroendocrine tumours (NETs) constitute a heterogeneous group of neoplasms that originate from neuroendocrine cells. NETs arise in many different organs, including the pancreas, bowel, lung (carcinoid), adrenals (phaeochromocytoma) and thyroid (medullary carcinoma). They generally grow slowly and metastasise late. The majority of pancreatic NETs are non-secretory, but when hormones are produced, symptoms may ensue:

• Gastrinoma: Zollinger–Ellison syndrome. • Insulinoma: recurrent hypoglycaemia. • VIPoma: watery diarrhoea, hypokalaemia. • Glucagonoma: diabetes mellitus, necrolytic migratory erythema. • Somatostatinoma: diabetes mellitus, steatorrhoea. • Ectopic ACTH syndrome. • 5-HT: carcinoid syndrome.

The tumours may be single or multifocal (the latter typically occurring in the context of MEN 1).

Investigations

The investigation of suspected Cushing's syndrome and insulinoma are described above.

• Chromogranin A is produced by most NETs and may be measured in a fasting blood sample along with the other hormones specific to the tumours listed above. • NETs may be localised by USS, CT, MRI and, in the case of pancreatic tumours, endoscopic USS.

Management

• Treatment of solitary tumours is by surgical resection. • Diazoxide may reduce insulin secretion in insulinomas and high doses of proton pump inhibitors suppress acid production in gastrinomas. • Somatostatin analogues reduce the symptoms associated with 5-HT, glucagon and vasoactive intestinal peptide (VIP) excess. • Cytotoxic chemotherapy, targeted radionuclide therapy with ^{131}I-MIBG, and resection/embolisation of hepatic metastases have a more limited role.

THE HYPOTHALAMUS AND THE PITUITARY GLAND

Diseases of the hypothalamus and pituitary are rare (annual incidence ~1 : 50 000, the most common being adenoma of the anterior pituitary gland). The pituitary gland is enclosed in the sella turcica and bridged over by a fold of dura mater called the diaphragma sellae, with the sphenoidal air sinuses below and the optic chiasm above. The cavernous sinuses are lateral to the pituitary fossa and contain the 3rd, 4th and 6th cranial nerves

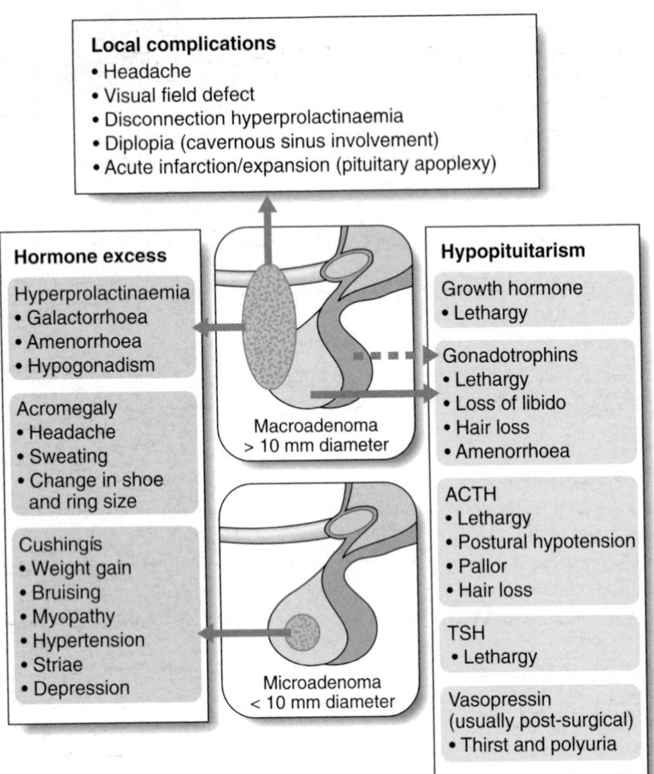

Fig. 10.7 Clinical effects of large and small pituitary tumours.

and the internal carotid arteries. The gland is composed of two lobes, anterior and posterior, and is connected to the hypothalamus by the infundibular stalk, which has portal vessels carrying blood from the median eminence of the hypothalamus to the anterior lobe and nerve fibres to the posterior lobe. (The functions of the pituitary are summarised in Fig. 10.1.)

PRESENTING PROBLEMS

Young women with pituitary disease most commonly present with secondary amenorrhoea or galactorrhoea (in hyperprolactinaemia). Men and post-menopausal women are less likely to report symptoms of hypogonadism and so are more likely to present late with larger tumours causing visual field defects. Pituitary tumours are increasingly discovered as an incidental finding on CT/MRI scan.

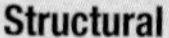

10.16 CAUSES OF ANTERIOR PITUITARY HORMONE DEFICIENCY
Structural
• Primary pituitary tumour: adenoma*, craniopharyngioma*, meningioma*, haemorrhage (apoplexy), Langerhans cell histiocytosis, arachnoid cyst
Inflammatory/infiltrative
• Sarcoidosis, haemochromatosis, infections (e.g. pituitary abscess, TB, syphilis, encephalitis)
Congenital deficiencies
• GnRH (Kallmann's syndrome)*, TRH, GHRH*, CRH
Functional*
• Chronic systemic illness, excessive exercise, anorexia nervosa
Other
• Head injury*, (para-)sellar radiotherapy*, (para-)sellar surgery*, post-partum necrosis (Sheehan's syndrome)
*Most common causes of pituitary hormone deficiency.

The presenting features depend on the size of the pituitary lesion (Fig. 10.7):

• Microadenomas (<10 mm diameter) are common incidental findings and should only be treated if they are secreting excess hormones (examples include Cushing's, acromegaly and hyperprolactinaemia). • In addition, macroadenomas may compress adjacent neural tissue and normal pituitary tissue causing neurological symptoms and hypopituitarism (Fig. 10.7).

ANTERIOR PITUITARY HORMONE DEFICIENCY

The term 'hypopituitarism' means the combined deficiency of any of the anterior pituitary hormones. This most commonly results from the destructive effects of a pituitary macroadenoma, but other causes are shown in Box 10.16.

Clinical assessment

With progressive pituitary lesions, onset of symptoms is insidious. Pituitary functions are lost in a characteristic sequence:

• Growth hormone: lethargy, muscle weakness and increased fat mass. • Gonadotrophins (LH and FSH): loss of libido, gynaecomastia, decreased shaving and, in the female, oligomenorrhoea or amenorrhoea. • ACTH: symptoms of cortisol insufficiency but aldosterone secretion is maintained. Serum K^+ is normal but postural hypotension and dilutional hyponatraemia may occur. Rather than the pigmentation of Addison's disease, pallor is usually present, due to lack of stimulation of melanocytes by β-lipotrophic

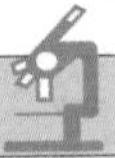

10.17 INVESTIGATION OF PITUITARY AND HYPOTHALAMIC DISEASE

Identify pituitary hormone deficiency

- ACTH deficiency: short ACTH stimulation test; insulin tolerance test (if uncertainty in interpretation of short ACTH stimulation test)
- LH/FSH deficiency: male: random serum testosterone, LH, FSH; pre-menopausal female: ask if menses are regular; post-menopausal female: random serum LH, FSH (usually >30 mU/l)
- TSH deficiency: serum thyroxine; TSH often detectable in secondary hypothyroidism (inactive circulating TSH isoforms)
- Growth hormone deficiency (only investigate if GH replacement contemplated): measure immediately after exercise; consider other stimulatory tests
- Cranial diabetes insipidus (may be masked by ACTH/TSH deficiency): exclude other causes of polyuria (blood glucose, potassium and calcium measurements); water deprivation test or 5% saline infusion test

Identify hormone excess

- Measure serum prolactin; investigate for acromegaly (glucose tolerance test) or Cushing's syndrome if indicated

Establish the anatomy and diagnosis

- Visual field testing; image pituitary/hypothalamus by MRI/CT

hormone (β-LPH, a fragment of the ACTH precursor). • TSH: secondary hypothyroidism contributes further to apathy and cold intolerance.

Investigations

The strategy of investigation of pituitary disease is described in Box 10.17. In acutely unwell patients, the priority is to diagnose and treat cortisol deficiency (see above). Other tests can be undertaken later. All patients with pituitary hormone deficiency should have an MRI or CT scan to identify pituitary or hypothalamic tumours. If no tumour is identified, further investigations are indicated to exclude infectious or infiltrative causes.

Management

Treatment of acutely ill patients is similar to that described for adrenocortical insufficiency (see above). Once the cause of hypopituitarism is established, specific treatment, e.g. of a pituitary macroadenoma, may be required.

Cortisol replacement: Hydrocortisone is used (see p. 368). Mineralocorticoid replacement is not required.

Thyroid hormone replacement: Thyroxine 100–150 μg once daily should be given. The aim is to maintain serum T_4 in the upper part of the reference range. It is dangerous to give thyroid replacement in adrenal

10.18 CAUSES OF DIABETES INSIPIDUS	
Cranial	
Structural hypothalamic or high stalk lesion	See Box 10.16
Idiopathic	
Genetic defect	Dominant. Recessive (DIDMOAD syndrome—diabetes insipidus with diabetes mellitus, optic atrophy, deafness)
Nephrogenic	
Genetic defect	V2 receptor mutation; aquaporin-2 mutation
Metabolic abnormality	Hypercalcaemia; hypokalaemia
Drug therapy	Lithium; demeclocycline
Poisoning	Heavy metals
Chronic kidney disease	Polycystic kidney disease, infiltrative disease, sickle-cell anaemia

insufficiency without first giving glucocorticoid therapy, since this may precipitate adrenal crisis.

Sex hormone replacement: This is indicated if there is gonadotrophin deficiency in men of any age and in women under the age of 50.

Growth hormone (GH) replacement: GH is administered to young patients with GH deficiency, renal failure or Turner's syndrome to assist them in attaining their growth potential. Until recently, GH was discontinued once the epiphyses had fused. There is now evidence that GH improves quality of life and exercise capacity in adults. It also helps young adults to achieve a higher peak bone mineral density. GH replacement is monitored by measurement of serum insulin-like growth factor-1 (IGF-1) levels.

DIABETES INSIPIDUS (DI)

This uncommon disorder is characterised by the excretion of excessive quantities of dilute urine and by thirst. It can be classified as cranial DI (deficient ADH production by hypothalamus) or nephrogenic DI (renal tubules unresponsive to ADH). Causes are listed in Box 10.18. The most marked symptoms are polyuria (5–20 litres/24 hrs) and polydipsia. Urine is of low specific gravity and osmolality. Adequate fluid intake can be maintained with an intact thirst mechanism in a conscious individual. However, in unconsciousness or hypothalamic thirst centre damage, DI is potentially lethal. The differential diagnosis includes diabetes mellitus and primary polydipsia (usually in patients with established psychiatric disease).

Investigations

DI is confirmed if, with an elevated plasma osmolality (>300 mOsm/kg), either serum ADH is not measurable or urine is not maximally concentrated (i.e. <600 mOsm/kg). Random simultaneous samples of blood and urine may exclude the diagnosis by demonstrating a urine osmolality >600 mOsm/kg. More often, the water deprivation test is required: no fluids are allowed for 8 hrs and body weight, plasma and urine osmolality are measured every 2 hrs; the test is stopped if >3% of body weight is lost. DI is confirmed by plasma osmolality >300 mOsm/kg with urine osmolality <600 mOsm/kg. DDAVP (see below) is then given to distinguish cranial and nephrogenic DI:

• Cranial DI is confirmed if urine osmolality rises by >50% after DDAVP.
• Nephrogenic DI is confirmed if DDAVP does not concentrate urine. • Primary polydipsia is suggested by low plasma osmolality at the start of the test.

Anterior pituitary function and suprasellar anatomy should be assessed in patients with cranial diabetes insipidus, as indicated in Box 10.17.

Management

• Treatment of cranial DI is with desmopressin (DDAVP), an analogue of ADH with a longer half-life. DDAVP is usually administered via the nasal mucous membrane as a spray, although it can be given orally or intramuscularly. The ideal dose prevents nocturia but avoids hyponatraemia, e.g. DDAVP nasal dose 5 µg in the morning and 10 µg at night. • Polyuria in nephrogenic DI is improved by thiazide diuretics (bendroflumethiazide 5 mg/day) or amiloride (5–10 mg/day).

PITUITARY AND (PARA-)SELLAR TUMOURS

Pituitary and hypothalamic disease may present as a space-occupying lesion that has been identified within the pituitary fossa or the suprasellar space by CT/MRI. Sellar and parasellar tumours produce a variety of mass effects. Compression of the optic chiasm causes a bitemporal hemianopia or upper quadrantanopia. Other types of visual field defect can result from suprasellar extension causing compression of the optic nerve (unilateral loss of acuity or scotoma) or optic tract (homonymous hemianopia). Optic atrophy may be apparent on ophthalmoscopy. Lateral extension into the cavernous sinus with subsequent compression of the 3rd, 4th or 6th cranial nerves may cause diplopia and strabismus.

Occasionally pituitary tumours infarct or there is bleeding into cystic lesions. This is termed 'pituitary apoplexy' and may result in sudden localised compression and acute-onset hypopituitarism. Non-haemorrhagic pituitary infarction may occur in obstetric haemorrhage (Sheehan's syndrome), diabetes mellitus and raised intracranial pressure.

A wide variety of disorders can present as a mass in the pituitary/hypothalamus region (see Box 10.16), but:

• The majority of intrasellar tumours are pituitary macroadenomas (most commonly non-functioning adenomas). • Most suprasellar masses are craniopharyngiomas. • Parasellar masses are most commonly meningiomas.

Investigations

A precise diagnosis requires surgical biopsy but this is usually performed as part of a therapeutic procedure. All patients should have pituitary function assessed (see Box 10.17). If serum prolactin is raised, dopamine agonists may shrink the lesion avoiding the need for surgery.

Management

Specific treatments are described in the sections on hyperprolactinaemia, acromegaly and Cushing's disease. Non-functioning pituitary macroadenomas and craniopharyngiomas should be managed surgically, if needed, with radiotherapy reserved for second-line treatment. If there is evidence of pressure on visual pathways, urgent treatment is required. Most operations on the pituitary are performed by the trans-sphenoidal approach from an incision under the upper lip or through the nose. Transfrontal surgery (craniotomy) is reserved for suprasellar tumours. All operations on the pituitary carry a risk of damaging endocrine function. Associated hypopituitarism should be treated as described above.

Pituitary function (see Box 10.17) should be retested 4–6 wks following surgery to detect the development of new hormone deficits. Imaging is repeated after a few months and, if there is any residual mass, external radiotherapy may reduce the risk of recurrence of radiosensitive tumours. Radiotherapy is not useful in patients requiring urgent therapy because it takes many months to be effective. It carries a lifelong risk of hypopituitarism (first 10 yrs 50–70%) and annual pituitary function tests are obligatory. Non-functioning tumours are followed up by repeated imaging. For smaller lesions therapeutic surgery may not be indicated and the lesion may be monitored by serial neuroimaging.

HYPERPROLACTINAEMIA

Cardinal features are galactorrhoea and hypogonadism. Galactorrhoea describes lactation without breastfeeding. Prolactin stimulates milk secretion but not breast development, so that galactorrhoea rarely occurs in men.

The causes of hyperprolactinaemia may be:

Physiological: Pregnancy, lactation, sleep, coitus, stress (e.g. post-seizure).

Drugs: Dopamine antagonists (phenothiazines, antidepressants, metoclopramide); dopamine-depleting drugs (reserpine, methyldopa); oestrogen (contraceptive pill).

Pathological: Pituitary tumours cause hyperprolactinaemia by secreting prolactin (prolactinoma), or by compressing the infundibular stalk, thus interrupting the tonic inhibitory effect of hypothalamic dopamine on prolactin secretion ('disconnection' hyperprolactinaemia). Prolactinomas are commonly microadenomas in pre-menopausal women, because the prolactin excess is symptomatic. In men and post-menopausal women, however, tumours are usually macroadenomas. Other causes of hyperprolactinaemia include primary hypothyroidism, PCOS, hypothalamic disease and macroprolactinaemia. Macroprolactin is prolactin bound to IgG antibodies, which cross-reacts with some prolactin assays. Macroprolactin cannot cross blood vessel walls to reach prolactin receptors in target tissues and so is less likely to cause pathology.

Clinical assessment

• In women, in addition to galactorrhoea, the associated hypogonadism causes secondary amenorrhoea and anovulation with infertility. • In men there is decreased libido, reduced shaving frequency and lethargy. • Important points in the history include drug use, recent pregnancy and menstrual history. • Further assessment should address the features of any pituitary disease (p. 374).

Investigations

Pregnancy should be excluded. Macroprolactin should be measured and, if present with a normal unbound prolactin concentration, then further investigation is not necessary in the absence of clinical features. Prolactin levels may indicate underlying pathology:

• Normal level: <500 mU/l (~14 ng/ml). • 500–1000 mU/l: stress or drugs most likely in non-pregnant/non-lactating. Repeat the measurement. • 1000–5000 mU/l: drugs, microprolactinoma or 'disconnection' hyperprolactinaemia. • >5000 mU/l: suggestive of macroprolactinoma. The higher the level, the bigger the tumour.

Other investigations include:

• TFTs to exclude primary hypothyroidism (TRH-induced prolactin excess). • MRI/CT of hypothalamus/pituitary if prolactin >1000 mU/l. • Patients with a macroadenoma need tests for hypopituitarism (see Box 10.17).

Management

The underlying cause should be corrected (stop offending drugs; give levothyroxine in primary hypothyroidism).

Medical: Dopamine agonist drugs are first-line therapy and are likely to be prescribed long-term. These include bromocriptine 2.5–15 mg/day, cabergoline 250–1000 μg/week and quinagolide 50–150 μg/day. In microprolactinomas, it may be possible to withdraw therapy without recurrence of hyperprolactinaemia after 5–10 yrs. In patients with macroadenomas, drugs can only be withdrawn after curative surgery or radiotherapy.

Surgical: Dopamine agonists shrink most prolactin-secreting macroadenomas. Thus, surgical decompression is not usually necessary. In those intolerant of dopamine agonists, trans-sphenoidal surgery cures 80% of microadenomas. Surgical cure rates in macroadenomas are substantially lower.

Radiotherapy: External irradiation may be required for some macroadenomas to prevent regrowth if dopamine agonists are stopped.

Pregnancy: Patients with microadenomas should have dopamine agonist therapy withdrawn as soon as pregnancy is confirmed. In contrast, macroprolactinomas may enlarge rapidly under oestrogen stimulation. Dopamine agonist therapy should be continued with monitoring of prolactin levels and visual fields during pregnancy. Bromocriptine has most safety data for use in pregnancy.

ACROMEGALY

Acromegaly is caused by growth hormone (GH) secretion, usually from a macroadenoma.

Clinical features

If GH hypersecretion occurs before epiphyseal fusion, then gigantism will result. More commonly, GH excess occurs after epiphyseal closure and acromegaly ensues. The most common complaints are headache and sweating. Other clinical features include: • skull growth with prominent supraorbital ridges, • prognathism, • enlargement of lips, nose and tongue, • enlargement of hands and feet, • carpal tunnel syndrome and • cardiomyopathy. In addition, the incidence of diabetes mellitus, hypertension, cardiovascular disease and colonic cancer is increased. Additional features include those of any pituitary tumour (p. 374).

Investigations

• An oral glucose tolerance test with GH measurement confirms the diagnosis. • In normal subjects, plasma GH suppresses to <2 mU/l. In acromegaly, it does not suppress, and in ~50% of patients there is a paradoxical rise. • Remaining pituitary function should be investigated (see Box 10.17). • Hyperprolactinaemia is present in ~30% due to tumour co-secretion of prolactin. • The diagnosis of acromegaly is more difficult in patients with insulin deficiency in diabetes mellitus. In diabetic patients without acromegaly, IGF-1 concentrations are low, while in acromegalic patients they are high. • Screening for colonic neoplasms with colonoscopy may also be undertaken.

Management

Surgical: Trans-sphenoidal surgery is first-line treatment and may result in cure of GH excess, especially in microadenomas. However, surgery usually debulks the tumour and further second-line therapy is required, according to post-operative imaging and glucose tolerance test results.

Radiotherapy: External radiotherapy is usually employed as second-line treatment if acromegaly persists after surgery, to stop tumour growth and lower GH levels. However, this works slowly (over many years) and there is a risk of hypopituitarism.

Medical: Medical therapy is used to lower GH levels to <5 mU/l following surgery. Medical therapy may be discontinued after several years in patients who have received radiotherapy. Somatostatin analogues (octreotide, lanreotide) are administered as slow-release injections. Dopamine agonists are less potent in lowering GH but may be helpful in patients with associated hyperprolactinaemia. A GH receptor antagonist (pegvisomant) is available for daily self-injection when GH concentrations fail to suppress following somatostatin analogue therapy.

DISEASES AFFECTING MULTIPLE ENDOCRINE GLANDS

MULTIPLE ENDOCRINE NEOPLASIA (MEN)

These are rare autosomal dominant syndromes characterised by hyperplasia and tumours in multiple glands.

• MEN 1 (Werner's syndrome) is the association of primary hyperparathyroidism, pituitary tumours and pancreatic neuroendocrine tumours. • In MEN 2 (Sipple's syndrome), primary hyperparathyroidism, thyroid medullary carcinoma and phaeochromocytoma are found. • In MEN 2b, additional phenotypic changes include marfanoid habitus, skeletal abnormalities and mucosal neuromas.

MEN 1 results from inactivating mutations in 'menin', a tumour suppressor gene on chromosome 11. In MEN 2, mutations are found in the *RET* proto-oncogene on chromosome 10. Genetic testing can be performed on relatives of affected individuals.

Individuals with MEN should have regular surveillance.

• In MEN 1, this involves annual measurements of calcium, GI hormones and prolactin; pituitary MRI is performed less frequently. • In MEN 2, measurement of calcium and urinary catecholamines is performed. The penetrance of thyroid medullary carcinoma is 100% in individuals with a *RET* mutation. Prophylactic thyroidectomy is therefore performed in childhood.

AUTOIMMUNE POLYENDOCRINE SYNDROMES (APS)

Two distinct autoimmune polyendocrine syndromes are known: APS types 1 and 2.

• APS type 2 (Schmidt's syndrome) is more common and is observed in women aged 20–60. It is defined as the occurrence of two or more autoimmune endocrine disorders, e.g. Addison's disease, hypoparathyroidism, type 1 diabetes, Graves' disease, coeliac disease and so on. Inheritance is autosomal dominant with incomplete penetrance and there is a strong association with HLA-DR3. • APS type 1 (autoimmune polyendocrinopathy—candidiasis—ectodermal dystrophy, APECED) is much rarer and displays autosomal recessive inheritance. In addition to autoimmune diseases, nail dystrophy, enamel hypoplasia and mucocutaneous candidiasis are seen.

11

Diabetes mellitus

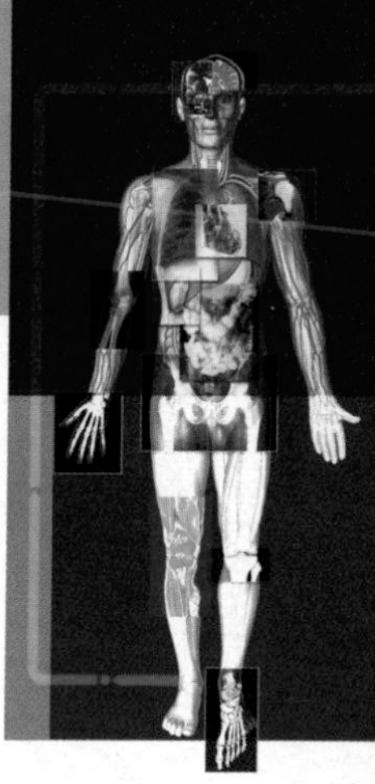

Diabetes mellitus is a clinical syndrome characterised by hyperglycaemia due to absolute or relative deficiency of insulin. Long-standing metabolic derangement can lead to the development of complications of diabetes, which characteristically affect the eye, kidney and nervous system. Diabetes occurs world-wide and its incidence is rising; 171 million people had diabetes in 2000, and this is expected to double by 2030. Diabetes is a major burden upon health-care facilities in all countries.

FUNCTIONAL ANATOMY, PHYSIOLOGY AND INVESTIGATIONS

NORMAL GLUCOSE AND FAT METABOLISM

Blood glucose is maintained within a narrow range by homeostatic mechanisms. Glucose enters the circulation from the liver and is taken up by peripheral tissues, particularly skeletal muscle. The brain relies upon glucose as its principal metabolic fuel as it cannot oxidise free fatty acids (FFAs).

When intestinal glucose absorption declines between meals, hepatic glucose output is increased in response to low insulin levels and increased levels of the counter-regulatory hormones, glucagon and adrenaline (epinephrine). The liver produces glucose by gluconeogenesis and glycogen breakdown.

After meals, blood insulin levels rise in response to a rise in blood glucose. Insulin is an anabolic hormone and is secreted from pancreatic β cells into the portal circulation. Insulin lowers blood glucose by suppressing

CLINICAL EXAMINATION OF THE PATIENT WITH DIABETES

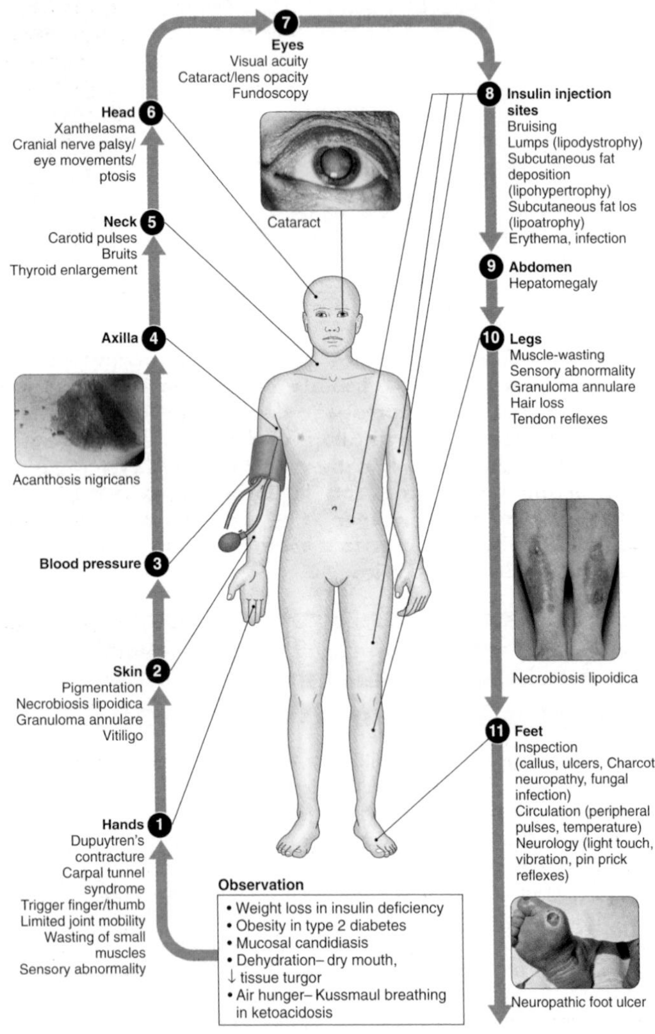

Observation

- Weight loss in insulin deficiency
- Obesity in type 2 diabetes
- Mucosal candidiasis
- Dehydration– dry mouth, ↓ tissue turgor
- Air hunger– Kussmaul breathing in ketoacidosis

hepatic glucose production and stimulating glucose uptake in skeletal muscle and fat.

Insulin stimulates lipogenesis and inhibits lipolysis. Lipolysis is stimulated by catecholamines and liberates FFAs, which can be oxidised by many tissues. Their partial oxidation in the liver produces ketone bodies, which can be oxidised and utilised as metabolic fuel. However, the rate of utilisation of ketone bodies by peripheral tissues is limited, and when production by the liver exceeds removal, hyperketonaemia results. Ketogenesis is enhanced by insulin deficiency and release of the counter-regulatory hormones that stimulate lipolysis.

AETIOLOGY AND PATHOGENESIS OF DIABETES

In both of the common types of diabetes, environmental factors interact with genetic susceptibility to determine which people develop the clinical syndrome, and the timing of its onset. However, the underlying genes, precipitating environmental factors and pathophysiology differ substantially between type 1 and type 2 diabetes.

TYPE 1 DIABETES

Type 1 diabetes (formerly 'insulin-dependent diabetes mellitus' (IDDM)) is invariably associated with profound insulin deficiency requiring replacement therapy.

Type 1 diabetes is a slowly progressive T cell-mediated autoimmune disease leading to destruction of the insulin-secreting β cells. Classical symptoms of diabetes occur only when 70–90% of β cells have been destroyed. Pathology shows insulitis (infiltration of the islets with mononuclear cells), in which β cells are destroyed, but cells secreting glucagon and other hormones remain intact. Islet cell antibodies can be detected before clinical diabetes develops and disappear with increasing duration of diabetes; however, they are not suitable for screening or diagnostic purposes. Glutamic acid decarboxylase (GAD) antibodies may have a role in identifying late-onset type 1 autoimmune diabetes in adults (LADA). Type 1 diabetes is associated with other autoimmune disorders, including thyroid disease (p. 342), coeliac disease (p. 446), Addison's disease (p. 366), pernicious anaemia (p. 539) and vitiligo (p. 709).

Genetic predisposition

Genetic factors account for about one-third of the susceptibility to type 1 diabetes, with 35% concordance between monozygotic twins. The human leucocyte antigen (HLA) haplotypes *DR3* and/or *DR4* on chromosome 6 are associated with increased susceptibility to type 1 diabetes. Defective presentation of autoantigens derived from β cells probably underlies the autoimmunity.

Environmental factors

Reduced exposure to microorganisms in early childhood may limit maturation of the immune system and increase susceptibility to autoimmune disease (the 'hygiene hypothesis'). Viral infections including mumps, Coxsackie B4, retroviruses, congenital rubella, cytomegalovirus and Epstein–Barr virus might cause some forms of type 1 diabetes. Bovine serum albumin (BSA—a constituent of cow's milk) has been implicated in triggering type 1 diabetes, since infants who are given cow's milk are more likely to develop type 1 diabetes in later life than those who are breastfed. Stress may precipitate type 1 diabetes by stimulating the secretion of counter-regulatory hormones and possibly by modulating immune activity.

Metabolic disturbances in type 1 diabetes

Patients with type 1 diabetes present when adequate insulin secretion can no longer be sustained. High glucose levels may be toxic to the remaining β cells so that profound insulin deficiency rapidly ensues. Insulin deficiency is associated with the metabolic sequelae shown in Figure 11.1. Hyperglycaemia leads to glycosuria and dehydration, which in turn induces secondary hyperaldosteronism. Unrestrained lipolysis and proteolysis result in weight loss, increased gluconeogenesis and ketogenesis. When generation of ketone bodies exceeds their metabolism, ketoacidosis results. Secondary hyperaldosteronism encourages urinary loss of K^+. Thus patients usually present with a short history of hyperglycaemic symptoms (thirst, polyuria, fatigue and infections) and weight loss, and may have developed ketoacidosis.

TYPE 2 DIABETES

In type 2 diabetes (formerly 'non-insulin-dependent diabetes mellitus' (NIDDM)), patients retain some capacity to secrete insulin but there is a combination of resistance to the actions of insulin followed by impaired pancreatic β-cell function, leading to 'relative' insulin deficiency.

Insulin resistance: Excessive production of glucose in the liver and under-utilisation of glucose in skeletal muscle result from resistance to the action of insulin. Type 2 diabetes is often associated with other medical disorders, which when they coexist are termed 'metabolic syndrome' (syndrome X, Box 11.1), with a predisposition to insulin resistance being the primary defect. It is strongly associated with macrovascular disease (coronary, cerebral, peripheral) and an excess mortality.

'Central' adipose tissue may amplify insulin resistance by releasing FFAs and hormones (adipokines). Sedentary people are more insulin-resistant than active people with the same degree of obesity. Inactivity down-regulates insulin-sensitive kinases and may also increase the accumulation of FFAs within skeletal muscle. Exercise also allows non-insulin-dependent glucose uptake into muscle, reducing the 'demand' on the pancreatic β cells to produce insulin.

Pancreatic β-cell failure: Deposition of amyloid in pancreatic islet cells is found in type 2 diabetes. While β-cell numbers are typically reduced by 20–30% in type 2 diabetes, β-cell mass is unchanged and glucagon secretion is increased, which may contribute to the hyperglycaemia.

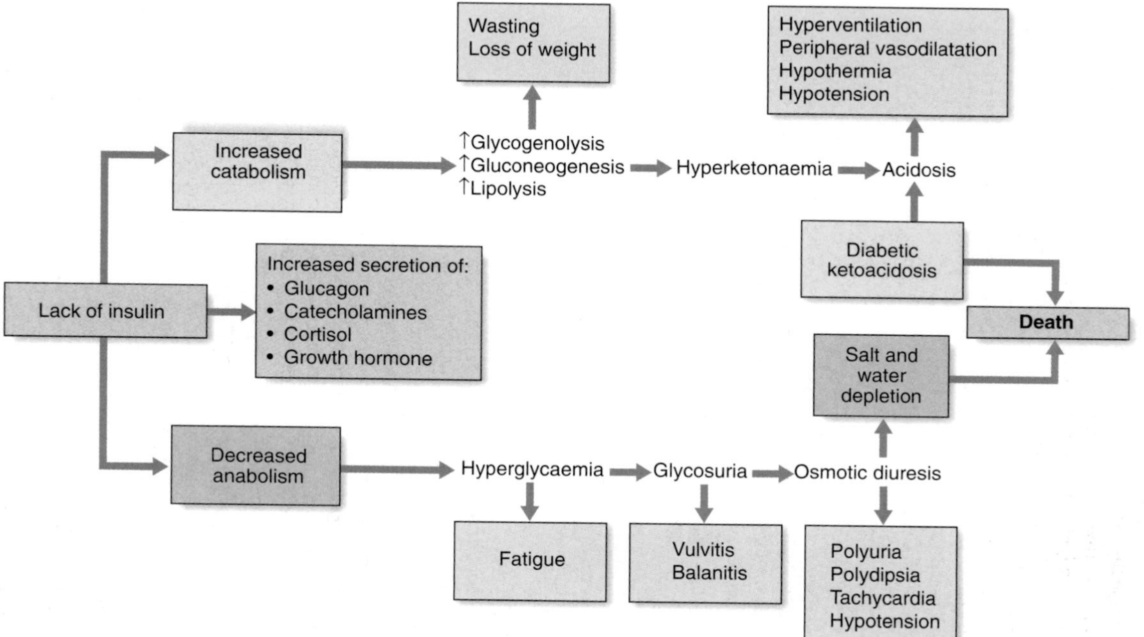

Fig. 11.1 Pathophysiological basis of the symptoms and signs of uncontrolled diabetes mellitus.

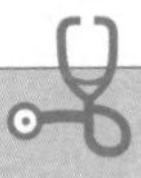

11.1 FEATURES OF THE INSULIN RESISTANCE (METABOLIC) SYNDROME

- Hyperinsulinaemia
- Type 2 diabetes or impaired glucose tolerance (IGT)
- Hypertension
- Low high-density lipoprotein (HDL) cholesterol; elevated triglycerides
- Microalbuminuria
- Increased fibrinogen, uric acid
- Central (visceral) obesity
- Increased sympathetic activity

Genetic predisposition

Genetic factors are important in the aetiology of type 2 diabetes; monozygotic twins have concordance rates approaching 100%. However, many genes are involved and the chance of developing diabetes is also influenced by environmental factors.

Environmental factors

Epidemiological studies indicate that type 2 diabetes is associated with overeating, especially when combined with obesity and under-activity. However, only a minority of obese people develop diabetes. Obesity probably acts as a diabetogenic factor in those who are genetically predisposed both to insulin resistance and to β-cell failure. The risk of developing type 2 diabetes increases tenfold in people with a body mass index (BMI) >30 kg/m^2.

Other risk factors

Age: Type 2 diabetes is principally a disease of the middle-aged and elderly. In the UK, it affects 10% of the population over 65, and over 70% of all cases of diabetes occur after the age of 50 yrs.

Pregnancy: During normal pregnancy, insulin sensitivity is reduced through the action of placental hormones. Repeated pregnancy may increase the likelihood of developing irreversible diabetes, particularly in obese women. Around 80% of women with gestational diabetes ultimately develop permanent diabetes.

Metabolic disturbances in type 2 diabetes

Relatively small amounts of insulin are required to suppress lipolysis, and some glucose uptake is maintained in muscle, so that weight loss and ketoacidosis are rare. Glycosuria occurs when the blood glucose concentration exceeds the renal threshold (10 mmol/l (180 mg/dl)). The severity of the classical 'osmotic' symptoms of polyuria and polydipsia is related to the degree of glycosuria. In type 2 diabetes, hyperglycaemia develops slowly and the renal threshold for glucose rises, so that osmotic symptoms are usually mild. Thus, patients are often asymptomatic, but usually present with a long history of fatigue, with or without osmotic symptoms.

In some patients, presentation is late and pancreatic β-cell function has declined to the point where there is profound insulin deficiency. These patients may present with weight loss, although ketoacidosis remains rare. Intercurrent illness, e.g. with infections, increases the production of counter-regulatory hormones (cortisol, growth hormone, catecholamines), resulting in more severe hyperglycaemia and dehydration (see hyperosmolar non-ketotic coma, p. 395). Dyslipidaemias are also common in patients with type 2 diabetes.

OTHER FORMS OF DIABETES

Other causes of diabetes are:

• Genetic defects of β-cell function (e.g. MODY—maturity-onset diabetes of the young, rare autosomal dominant, <5% of diabetes cases). • Genetic defects of insulin action. • Pancreatic disease (e.g. pancreatitis, haemochromatosis, cystic fibrosis). • Excess endogenous production of insulin antagonists (acromegaly, Cushing's disease, thyrotoxicosis). • Drug-induced (corticosteroids, thiazides, phenytoin). • Viral infections (congenital rubella, mumps, Coxsackie virus B). • Associated with genetic syndromes (e.g. Down's, DIDMOAD (diabetes insipidus, diabetes mellitus, optic atrophy, deafness)).

INVESTIGATIONS

URINE TESTING

Glucose

Sensitive glucose-specific dipsticks are used to detect glycosuria, ideally on urine passed 1–2 hrs after a meal, since this will detect more cases of diabetes. However, glycosuria can be due to a low renal threshold. This is a benign condition, common during pregnancy and in young people. Glycosuria always warrants further assessment by blood testing using an accurate laboratory method. In some individuals a rapid but transitory rise of blood glucose follows a meal and the concentration exceeds the normal renal threshold. This response is benign and is described as a 'lag storage' blood glucose curve or alimentary glycosuria. It may occur after gastric surgery or in hyperthyroidism, peptic ulceration or hepatic disease. Glycosuria is common in normal pregnancy (increased glomerular filtration rate). However, it should never be ignored and gestational diabetes should be excluded.

Ketones

Ketonuria may be found in normal people who have been fasting, exercising or vomiting repeatedly, or those on a high-fat, low-carbohydrate diet. Ketonuria is therefore not pathognomonic of diabetes but, if it is associated with glycosuria, diabetes is highly likely.

Protein

Dipstick testing will detect urinary albumin >300 mg/l and can indicate renal disease or urinary infection in people with diabetes.

BLOOD TESTING

Glucose

Laboratory blood glucose testing is cheap and highly reliable. Capillary blood glucose can also be measured with a portable electronic meter, used to monitor diabetes treatment. Glucose concentrations are lower in venous than in arterial or capillary (fingerprick) blood. Whole blood glucose concentrations are lower than plasma concentrations because red blood cells contain relatively little glucose. Venous plasma values are the most reliable for diagnostic purposes.

Glycated haemoglobin

Glycated haemoglobin (Hb) provides an accurate and objective measure of glycaemic control over a period of 2 mths. It is used to assess glycaemic control, but is not sufficiently sensitive to make a diagnosis of diabetes.

The non-enzymatic covalent attachment of glucose to Hb (glycation) increases the amount in the HbA_{1c} fraction relative to non-glycated adult Hb (HbA_0). The rate of formation of HbA_{1c} is directly proportional to the blood glucose concentration; a rise of 1% in HbA_{1c} corresponds to an increase of 2 mmol/l in blood glucose. HbA_{1c} concentration reflects blood glucose over the erythrocyte lifespan (120 days), but is affected more by recent events.

HbA_{1c} estimates may be erroneously diminished in anaemia and pregnancy, and may be difficult to interpret in uraemia and haemoglobinopathy. In clinical practice, HbA_{1c} is measured once or twice yearly to assess glycaemic control and provides an index of risk for developing diabetic complications.

Blood lipids

The concentration of serum lipids—total, LDL and HDL cholesterol and triglycerides—is another important index of metabolic control in diabetic patients and should be measured at diagnosis and regularly thereafter.

PRESENTING PROBLEMS

NEWLY DISCOVERED HYPERGLYCAEMIA

The key goals are to establish whether the patient has diabetes, what type of diabetes it is and how it should be treated.

Establishing the diagnosis of diabetes

In a symptomatic patient, the diagnosis may be confirmed by a random plasma glucose concentration ≥11.1 mmol/l (200 mg/dl) or a fasting plasma glucose concentration ≥7 mmol/l (126 mg/dl). In an asymptomatic patient two samples are required. An oral glucose tolerance test (OGTT) is indicated when plasma glucose levels are elevated but not diagnostic of diabetes: fasting range 6.1–7.0 mmol/l (110–126 mg/dl), or random plasma glucose range 7.8–11.0 mmol/l (140–199 mg/dl). The WHO criteria for

11.2 ORAL GLUCOSE TOLERANCE TEST: WHO DIAGNOSTIC CRITERIA		
	Glucose concentrations	
	Venous plasma mmol/l (mg/dl)	Capillary whole blood mmol/l (mg/dl)
Diabetes		
Fasting	≥7.0 (≥126)	≥6.1 (≥110)
2 hrs after glucose load	≥11.1 (≥200)	≥11.1 (≥200)
Impaired glucose tolerance		
Fasting	<7.0 (<126)	<6.1 (<110)
2 hrs after glucose load	7.8–11.0 (140–199)	7.8–11.0 (140–199)

diagnosing diabetes mellitus are shown in Box 11.2 and are based on the risk of developing microvascular disease. Patients who do not meet the criteria for diabetes may have 'impaired glucose tolerance' (IGT) or 'impaired fasting glucose' (fasting glucose 6.1–6.9 mmol/l (110–125 mg/dl)). These patients have an increased risk of progression to frank diabetes and of macrovascular disease.

Stress hyperglycaemia occurs when conditions impose a burden on the pancreatic β cells, e.g. during pregnancy, infection or treatment with corticosteroids. It usually disappears after the acute illness has resolved, but blood glucose should be remeasured.

When diabetes is confirmed, other investigations should include:

• U&Es. • Creatinine. • LFTs and TFTs. • Lipids. • Urine testing for protein or microalbuminuria.

Clinical assessment

Hyperglycaemia causes:

• Thirst. • Polyuria. • Fatigue. • Blurred vision. • Pruritus vulvae/balanitis. • Nausea. • Hyperphagia. • Irritability, poor concentration, headache.

Uncontrolled diabetes is associated with an increased susceptibility to infection and patients may present with skin infections. A history of pancreatic disease (particularly with alcohol excess) makes insulin deficiency more likely.

The clinical features of the two main types of diabetes are compared in Box 11.3. Overlap occurs particularly in age at onset, duration of symptoms and family history. Typical type 2 diabetes increasingly occurs in obese young people. Older adults may have evidence of autoimmune activity against β cells, a slowly evolving variant of type 1 diabetes (LADA). More than 70% of patients with type 2 diabetes are overweight, 50% have hypertension and hyperlipidaemia is common.

Management

• Dietary/lifestyle modification. • Oral anti-diabetic agents. • Insulin by injection (p. 406). • Suspected type 1 diabetes: urgent therapy with insulin

11.3 COMPARATIVE CLINICAL FEATURES OF TYPE 1 AND TYPE 2 DIABETES

	Type 1	Type 2
Typical age at onset	<40 yrs	>50 yrs
Duration of symptoms	Weeks	Months to years
Body weight	Normal or low	Obese
Ketonuria	Yes	No
Rapid death without treatment with insulin	Yes	No
Autoantibodies	Yes	No
Diabetic complications at diagnosis	No	25%
Family history of diabetes	Uncommon	Common
Other autoimmune disease	Common	Uncommon

and prompt referral to a specialist. • Suspected type 2 diabetes: advice about dietary and lifestyle modification, followed by initiation of oral anti-diabetic drugs if needed. • Hypertension, dyslipidaemia and smoking cessation need to be addressed.

Educating patients: This can be achieved by a multidisciplinary team (doctor, dietitian, specialist nurse and podiatrist) in the outpatient setting. However, patients requiring insulin initially need daily advice and possibly admission to hospital. They need to learn how to measure insulin doses, give their own injections, and adjust the dose depending on glucose monitoring, exercise, illness and hypoglycaemia. They must understand the principles of diabetes, recognise the symptoms of hypoglycaemia, and receive advice about risks of driving with diabetes.

Self-assessment of glycaemic control: Urine testing has limitations, as persistent hyperglycaemia may be masked and hypoglycaemia not detected. However, it is inexpensive and may suffice for those with well-controlled type 2 diabetes or those treated with diet alone. Those treated with insulin should be taught to perform capillary blood glucose measurements at home. This permits patients to make appropriate adjustments in treatment on a day-to-day basis. Thus changes in routine can be accommodated, ketoacidosis avoided and dietary compliance encouraged while avoiding hypoglycaemia. Blood glucose monitoring is expensive and may not be justified in many people with type 2 diabetes.

Advice to patients with IGT

• The same lifestyle advice recommended for type 2 diabetes may reduce the risk of progression of IGT to diabetes. • Treating other cardiovascular risk factors reduces the risk of macrovascular disease. • Patients with IGT should be monitored, e.g. with annual fasting blood glucose.

11.4 CHECKLIST FOR FOLLOW-UP OF PATIENTS WITH DIABETES MELLITUS	
Body weight (BMI)	
Urinalysis (fasting)	Glucose, ketones, macro- and microalbuminuria
Glycaemic control	HbA_{1c}, inspection of home blood glucose monitoring record
Hypoglycaemic episodes	Number and time of day of severe and mild episodes, nature of symptoms, awareness
BP	
Eye examination	Visual acuity, ophthalmoscopy, digital photography
Lower limbs	Peripheral pulses, tendon reflexes, sensory: proprioception, vibration, light touch
Feet	Callus skin indicating pressure areas, nails, podiatry, ulceration, deformity

LONG-TERM SUPERVISION OF DIABETES

Diabetes is a complex disorder, which progresses in severity with time. Patients with diabetes should therefore be seen at regular intervals for life. A checklist for follow-up visits is given in Box 11.4. The frequency of visits varies from weekly during pregnancy to annually in well-controlled type 2 diabetes.

Therapeutic goals

The aim of treatment is to achieve as near normal metabolism as is practicable. The recommended target HbA_{1c} is ≤7%, to minimise vascular complications. However, type 2 diabetes progresses in severity with time, making this target difficult to achieve. In addition, strict control in type 1 diabetes increases the risk of hypoglycaemia. Glycaemic targets should therefore be appropriate; strict control may be inappropriate in the very young, the elderly and people with cancer. Desirable blood glucose targets are:

• Fasting <6 mmol/l (108 mg/dl) in type 2 diabetes. • Pre-prandial 5–8 mmol/l (90–144 mg/dl) in type 1 diabetes (avoid values <4 mmol/l (72 mg/dl)).

Treatment of hypertension and dyslipidaemia is often required following assessment of cardiovascular risk. Targets are:

• BP <140/80 mmHg. • Total cholesterol <5.0 mmol/l (190 mg/dl). • LDL cholesterol <3.0 mmol/l (115 mg/dl).

DIABETIC KETOACIDOSIS (DKA)

Ketoacidosis is a major medical emergency, principally occurring in people with type 1 diabetes. A significant number of newly diagnosed diabetic

11.5 AVERAGE FLUID AND ELECTROLYTE LOSS IN ADULT DKA OF MODERATE SEVERITY

Water: 6 litres Sodium: 500 mmol Chloride: 400 mmol Potassium: 350 mmol	3 litres extracellular —replace with saline 3 litres intracellular —replace with dextrose

patients present in ketoacidosis. In established diabetes, any form of stress, particularly infection, can precipitate DKA. Patients lose their appetite, and stop or reduce their dose of insulin in the mistaken belief that less insulin is required. No obvious precipitating cause can be found in many cases. The average mortality in developed countries is 5–10% and is higher in the elderly. The cardinal biochemical features of DKA are:

• Hyperglycaemia. • Hyperketonaemia. • Metabolic acidosis.

Hyperglycaemia causes an osmotic diuresis leading to dehydration and electrolyte loss. Ketosis is caused by insulin deficiency, exacerbated by stress hormones (e.g. catecholamines) resulting in unrestrained lipolysis supplying FFAs for hepatic ketogenesis. When this exceeds the capacity to metabolise acidic ketones, these accumulate in blood. The resulting acidosis forces hydrogen ions into cells, displacing potassium ions, which are lost in urine or through vomiting. The average loss of fluid and electrolytes in moderately severe DKA in an adult is shown in Box 11.5. Patients with DKA have a total body potassium deficit but this is not reflected by plasma potassium levels, which may initially be raised due to disproportionate water loss. However, once insulin is started, plasma potassium can fall precipitously due to dilution by i.v. fluids, potassium movement into cells, and continuing renal loss of potassium.

Clinical assessment

Clinical features of DKA are listed in Box 11.6.

Investigations

The following are important but should not delay i.v. fluid and insulin replacement:

• U&Es, blood glucose, plasma bicarbonate (at admission and at 1, 2, 3, 6, 12 and 24 hrs). • Arterial blood gases to assess severity of acidosis (rapid assessment by plasma bicarbonate: <12 mmol/l is severe). • Urine and plasma for ketones. • ECG. • Infection screen: FBC, blood/urine culture, CRP, CXR. Leucocytosis invariably occurs, representing a stress response rather than infection. • Serum amylase may be elevated but rarely indicates pancreatitis.

Management

DKA should be treated in hospital, preferably in a high-dependency area. Regular clinical and biochemical monitoring is essential, particularly during the first 24 hrs. Guidelines for the management of ketoacidosis are shown

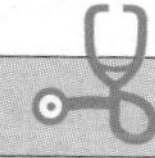

11.6 CLINICAL FEATURES OF DKA	
Symptoms	
• Polyuria, thirst • Weight loss • Weakness	• Nausea, vomiting • Blurred vision • Abdominal pain (especially children)
Signs	
• Dehydration • Tachycardia, hypotension (supine/erect) • Cold extremities/peripheral cyanosis • Air hunger (Kussmaul breathing)	• Smell of acetone • Hypothermia • Apathy, confusion, drowsiness, coma (10%)

in Box 11.7. The principal components of treatment are insulin, fluid and potassium.

• If i.v. insulin administration is not possible, 10–20 U can be given i.m., followed by 5 U i.m. hourly thereafter. • A rapid fall in blood glucose can cause cerebral oedema, particularly in children. • The half-life of i.v. insulin is short (2.5 mins) so the infusion should not be interrupted. • Restoration of the usual subcutaneous insulin regimen should be delayed until the patient is eating and drinking normally. • Plasma potassium is often high at presentation; treatment should be started cautiously and carefully monitored. Large amounts may be required (100–300 mmol in the first 24 hrs). • Cardiac rhythm should be monitored in severe cases because of the risk of arrhythmia.

In patients who are severely acidotic ($[H^+]$ >100 nmol/l (pH <7.0)) the infusion of sodium bicarbonate (with potassium) could be considered. Its use is controversial, however, and should only be considered in exceptional circumstances. Infections must be sought and treated. Complications of DKA include:

• Cerebral oedema. • Acute respiratory distress syndrome (p. 23). • Thromboembolism. • Disseminated intravascular coagulation. • Acute circulatory failure.

NON-KETOTIC HYPEROSMOLAR DIABETIC COMA

This condition is characterised by severe hyperglycaemia (>50 mmol/l (900 mg/dl)) without significant ketoacidosis. Severe dehydration and prerenal uraemia are common. It usually affects elderly patients who often have undiagnosed diabetes. Mortality is high (40%). Patients are sensitive to insulin and half the dose of insulin recommended for the treatment of

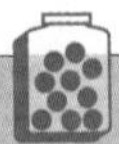

11.7 MANAGEMENT OF DKA

Fluid replacement

- 0.9% saline (NaCl) i.v.: 1 litre over 30 mins, 1 litre over 1 hr, 1 litre over 2 hrs, 1 litre over 2–4 hrs
- When blood glucose <15 mmol/l (270 mg/dl) switch to 5% dextrose, 1 litre 8-hourly
  If still dehydrated, continue 0.9% saline and add 5% dextrose 1 litre per 12 hrs
- Typical requirement is 6 litres in first 24 hrs (avoid overload in elderly)
- Subsequent fluid requirement should be based on clinical assessment

Insulin

- 50 U soluble insulin in 50 ml 0.9% saline i.v. via infusion pump
  6 U/hr initially, 3 U/hr when blood glucose <15 mmol/l (270 mg/dl), 2 U/hr if blood glucose <10 mmol/l (180 mg/dl)
- Check blood glucose hourly initially—if no reduction in first hr, increase insulin infusion rate
- Aim for fall in blood glucose of 3–6 mmol/l (~55–110 mg/dl)/hr

Potassium

- None in first litre of i.v fluid unless <3.0 mmol/l
- If plasma potassium <3.5 mmol/l, give 40 mmol added potassium in 1 litre fluid
  Avoid infusion rate >20 mmol/hr
- If plasma potassium is 3.5–5.0 mmol/l, give 20 mmol added potassium
- If plasma potassium is >5.0 mmol/l or patient is anuric, give no added potassium

Additional procedures

- Catheterisation if no urine passed after 3 hrs
- Nasogastric tube to keep stomach empty in unconscious patients or if vomiting is protracted
- Central venous line in cardiovascular-compromised (to guide fluid therapy more accurately)
- Plasma expander if systolic BP <90 mmHg
- Antibiotic if infection demonstrated or suspected
- ECG monitoring in severe cases

ketoacidosis is employed (3 U/hr). Plasma osmolality should be measured or calculated using the following formula:

$$\text{Plasma osmolality} = 2[Na^+] + 2[K^+] + [\text{glucose}] + [\text{urea}] \text{ (all mmol/l)}$$

The normal value is 280–300 mmol/kg and the conscious level is depressed when it is >340 mmol/kg. The patient should be given 0.45% saline until the osmolality approaches normal, when 0.9% saline is substituted. Replace fluid guided by central venous pressure, check plasma sodium frequently, and give prophylactic heparin (thromboembolic complications).

LACTIC ACIDOSIS

In coma due to lactic acidosis the patient is likely to be taking metformin for type 2 diabetes and is very ill and overbreathing, but not as dehydrated as in coma due to ketoacidosis. The patient's breath does not smell of acetone and ketonuria is mild/absent, yet pH is markedly reduced (H^+ >63 mmol/l (pH < 7.2)) and the anion gap is increased (p. 153). The diagnosis is confirmed by a high blood lactate (usually >5.0 mmol/l). Treatment is with i.v. sodium bicarbonate sufficient to raise the arterial pH to >7.2, along with insulin and glucose. Despite treatment, mortality remains >50%. Sodium dichloroacetate may lower blood lactate.

HYPOGLYCAEMIA

Hypoglycaemia (blood glucose <3.5 mmol/l (63 mg/dl)) occurs in a person with diabetes as a result of treatment with insulin and occasionally sulphonylureas. Hypoglycaemia in a non-diabetic person is called 'spontaneous' hypoglycaemia (p. 371). The risk of hypoglycaemia limits the attainment of near-normal glycaemia; fear of hypoglycaemia is common among patients and their relatives.

Clinical assessment

• Symptoms of autonomic nervous system activation: sweating, trembling, palpitation, hunger and anxiety. • Symptoms of glucose deprivation of the brain (neuroglycopenia), including confusion, drowsiness, poor coordination and speech difficulty.

Symptom recognition is an important aspect of patient education. Mood changes such as irritability or anger can occur, and behavioural changes are common in children. Elderly patients are more likely to experience neurological symptoms.

Impaired awareness of symptoms: Patients usually recognise the symptoms of hypoglycaemia and take appropriate remedial action. In certain circumstances (e.g. during sleep) warning symptoms of neuroglycopenia may not be perceived by the patient. In those who are chronically hyperglycaemic, awareness may develop at a higher blood glucose level; conversely, patients who have strict glycaemic control or frequent hypoglycaemic episodes may only be symptomatic if the blood glucose is <2.5 mmol/l (45 mg/dl). The prevalence of impaired hypoglycaemia awareness increases with the duration of insulin treatment; after 20 yrs 50% of patients with type 1 diabetes are affected. In patients with chronically impaired awareness, the frequency of severe hypoglycaemia is increased sixfold; intensive insulin therapy should be avoided and frequent blood glucose self-monitoring is mandatory.

11.8 HYPOGLYCAEMIA: COMMON CAUSES AND RISK FACTORS

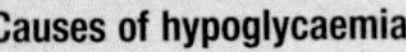

Causes of hypoglycaemia

- Missed/delayed meal
- Unexpected or unusual exercise
- Alcohol
- Error in insulin dose
- Lipohypertrophy causing variable insulin absorption
- Gastroparesis due to autonomic neuropathy
- Malabsorption, e.g. coeliac disease
- Unrecognised other endocrine disorder, e.g. Addison's disease
- Factitious (deliberately induced)

Risk factors for severe hypoglycaemia

- Strict glycaemic control
- Impaired awareness of hypoglycaemia
- Extremes of age
- Increasing duration of diabetes
- History of previous hypoglycaemia
- Renal impairment

Deficient counter-regulatory hormonal responses: In response to a falling blood glucose, there is normally suppression of endogenous insulin secretion (absent in type 1 diabetes) and a brisk secretion of counter-regulatory hormones (glucagon and adrenaline (epinephrine)) which antagonise the blood glucose-lowering effect of insulin. Hypoglycaemia-induced secretion of glucagon becomes impaired within 5 yrs of developing type 1 diabetes. After several years many also develop a defective adrenaline response, which autonomic neuropathy may exacerbate.

Causes, morbidity and prevention

Risk factors and causes of hypoglycaemia are listed in Box 11.8. Severe hypoglycaemia, defined as any episode requiring the assistance of another person for recovery, has a recognised mortality of 2–4% in insulin-treated patients. Complications include:

• Coma. • Convulsions. • Strokes. • Cardiac arrhythmias. • Myocardial ischaemia. • Hypothermia. • Accidents (e.g. road traffic accidents).

The frequency of hypoglycaemia can be reduced by patient education. People treated with insulin should carry glucose drinks or tablets at all times. Nocturnal hypoglycaemia in type 1 diabetes is common. It is a sensible precaution for patients to measure blood glucose before bed and to eat a carbohydrate snack if the reading is <6.0 mmol/l (~110 mg/dl).

Management

Treatment of acute hypoglycaemia depends on severity and on whether the patient is conscious.

• If it is recognised early, oral carbohydrate is sufficient. • In those unable to swallow, i.v. glucose (30–50 ml of 20–50% dextrose, 0.2 g/kg in children) or glucagon (1 mg i.m., 0.5 mg in children) should be administered. • Viscous glucose gel solution or jam can be applied into the buccal cavity but should not be used if the person is unconscious. • Full recovery may not occur immediately and reversal of cognitive impairment may take 60 mins. • The possibility of recurrence should be anticipated in those on long-acting insulins or sulphonylureas; a 10% dextrose infusion, titrated to the patient's blood glucose, may be necessary. • Cerebral oedema may have developed in patients who fail to regain consciousness after blood glucose is restored to normal. This has a high mortality and morbidity, and requires urgent treatment with mannitol and high-dose oxygen.

Following recovery, it is important to try to identify a cause, make appropriate adjustments to therapy and educate the patient. The management of self-poisoning with oral anti-diabetic agents is given on page 39.

DIABETES IN PREGNANCY

GESTATIONAL DIABETES

Glucose metabolism changes during normal pregnancy. Marked insulin resistance develops, particularly by the second half of pregnancy. Fasting glucose decreases slightly, while blood glucose may be increased post-prandially.

• Gestational diabetes is defined as diabetes with first onset or recognition during pregnancy. While this includes women with clinically undetected diabetes, the majority can expect to be restored to normal glucose tolerance immediately after pregnancy. • WHO definition: those meeting the criteria for IGT or diabetes after a 75 g OGTT. • European definition: fasting venous plasma glucose >5.5 mmol/l (99 mg/dl) or >9.0 mmol/l (162 mg/dl) at 2 hrs after a glucose load.

Risk factors for gestational diabetes include obesity, ethnicity (black, Hispanic or South Asian), family history of type 2 diabetes, and previous macrosomia or gestational diabetes.

Implications for the mother

Gestational diabetes is managed by dietary modification, blood glucose monitoring, and introduction of insulin if glycaemic control is unsatisfactory. Gestational diabetes is associated with an increased risk of later development of type 2 diabetes. Glucose tolerance is re-assessed at 6 wks post-partum. If this is normal, advice on lifestyle changes should be given to minimise the risk of later developing type 2 diabetes.

Implications for the fetus

Maternal glucose crosses the placenta, promoting fetal insulin production which stimulates growth. Maternal hyperglycaemia is therefore associated with increased fetal size (macrosomia), which may complicate labour and delivery, resulting in a higher caesarean section rate. Reduction of maternal blood glucose by insulin therapy can reduce fetal growth.

PREGNANCY IN WOMEN WITH ESTABLISHED TYPE 1 DIABETES

Maternal hyperglycaemia early in pregnancy has teratogenic effects. Fetal abnormalities include cardiac, renal and skeletal malformations, of which the caudal regression syndrome is the most characteristic. Diabetic women should receive pre-pregnancy counselling and be encouraged to achieve excellent glycaemic control before conceiving. Later in pregnancy maternal hyperglycaemia is associated with macrosomia. Fetal macrosomia increases the risk of birth injury during delivery, and of subsequent neonatal hypoglycaemia. Babies are also at increased risk of polycythaemia, hyperbilirubinaemia and hypocalcaemia.

Management

• Plan pregnancy. • Give folic acid supplementation. • Achieve strict glycaemic control (insulin requirements increase during pregnancy). • Avoid hypoglycaemia. • Avoid ketosis; ketoacidosis during pregnancy is associated with a high rate of fetal mortality (10–35%). • Arrange eye screening; retinopathy worsens during pregnancy.

Despite improvements, perinatal mortality rate remain 3–4 times that of the non-diabetic population (at around 30–40 per 1000 pregnancies) and the rate of congenital malformation is increased 5–6-fold.

SURGERY AND DIABETES

Surgery causes catabolic stress and secretion of counter-regulatory hormones. This results in increased glycogenolysis, gluconeogenesis, lipolysis, proteolysis and insulin resistance. This normally leads to increased secretion of insulin, which exerts a restraining and controlling influence. In diabetic patients, insulin deficiency leads to increased catabolism and ultimately metabolic decompensation. In addition, hyperglycaemia increases infection risk and impairs wound healing. Hypoglycaemia risk, particularly dangerous in the semiconscious patient, should be minimised.

Pre-operative assessment

This includes assessment of:

• Cardiovascular and renal function. • Neuropathy. • Glycaemic control (HbA_{1c} and pre-prandial glucose). • A review of diabetic treatments.

If significant alterations need to be made, patients may need admission prior to surgery. For emergency patients with significant hyperglycaemia or ketoacidosis, this should be corrected first with an i.v. infusion of saline and/or dextrose plus insulin, 6 U/hr, and potassium as required.

Perioperative management

The management of patients with diabetes undergoing surgery requiring general anaesthesia is summarised in Figure 11.2. Post-operatively, a glucose/insulin/potassium infusion should be continued until the patient's intake of food is adequate, when the normal regimen can be resumed. If

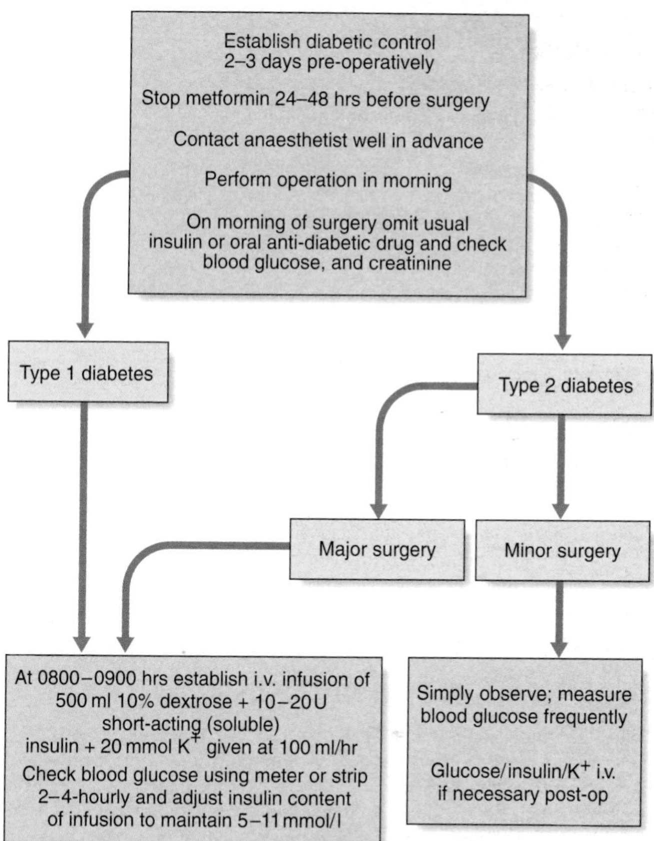

Fig. 11.2 Management of diabetic patients undergoing surgery and general anaesthesia. (Glucose of 5–11 mmol/l = 90–199 mg/dl.)

the infusion is prolonged, urea, electrolytes and urinary ketones should be checked daily. If fluids need to be restricted, e.g. in cardiovascular or renal disease, the rate of infusion can be halved by using a 20% dextrose solution and doubling the concentration of insulin and potassium.

CHILDREN, ADOLESCENTS AND YOUNG ADULTS

Children and teenagers are generally prone to insulin-deficient type 1 diabetes with ketosis, but cases of type 2 diabetes in obese children are now

11.9 COMPLICATIONS OF DIABETES	
Microvascular/neuropathic	
Retinopathy, cataract	Impaired vision
Nephropathy	Renal failure
Peripheral neuropathy	Sensory loss, motor weakness
Autonomic neuropathy	Postural hypotension, GI problems (gastroparesis; altered bowel habit)
Foot disease	Ulceration, arthropathy
Macrovascular	
Coronary circulation	Myocardial ischaemia/infarction
Cerebral circulation	Transient ischaemic attack, stroke
Peripheral circulation	Claudication, ischaemia

occurring and a diagnosis of MODY should be considered, especially when there is a strong family history of diabetes. Insulin therapy requires modification to accommodate physiological changes associated with growth and puberty. Deterioration in glycaemic control is common during adolescence as adherence to treatment may be erratic. Wide fluctuations in blood glucose and frequent metabolic emergencies are observed in a few adolescents and young adults, and may be due to self-manipulation of therapy.

COMPLICATIONS OF DIABETES

Diabetic complications (Box 11.9) may be the presenting finding in a patient not known to have diabetes. Around 20% of people with type 2 diabetes have established complications at the time of diagnosis. Patients presenting with hypertension or a vascular event should have coexistent diabetes excluded. See pages 407–414 for detailed investigation and management of diabetic complications.

MANAGEMENT OF DIABETES

Three methods of treatment are available for diabetic patients: diet and lifestyle advice alone, oral anti-diabetic drugs, and insulin. Approximately 50% of new cases of diabetes can be controlled adequately by diet alone, 20–30% will need oral anti-diabetic medication, and 20–30% will require insulin. Lifestyle changes such as taking regular exercise, observing a healthy diet, reducing alcohol consumption and stopping smoking are important. Ideal management allows the patient to lead a completely normal life, to remain symptom-free and to escape the long-term complications of diabetes. Although a few diabetic patients die from acute complications (ketoacidosis and hypoglycaemia), the major problem is the excess mortality and morbidity due to the long-term complications of diabetes. The factors associated with these are:

• Duration of diabetes. • Early age at onset of disease. • High glycated Hb (HbA_{1c}). • Raised BP. • Proteinuria; microalbuminuria. • Dyslipidaemia. • Obesity.

DIETARY MANAGEMENT

Dietary measures are required in the treatment of all people with diabetes. The aims are to improve glycaemic control, manage weight, and avoid both acute and long-term complications. People with diabetes should have access to dietitians at diagnosis, at review and at times of treatment change. Nutritional advice should be tailored to individuals and take account of their age and lifestyle.

COMPOSITION OF THE DIET

Carbohydrate

Traditionally, people with type 1 diabetes have been advised to maintain a regular intake of carbohydrate in meals throughout the day. It is now possible to match the amount of carbohydrate in a meal with a dose of short-acting insulin using methods such as DAFNE (dose adjustment for normal eating). Application of similar dietary principles enables motivated individuals with type 1 diabetes to achieve and maintain good glycaemic control, while avoiding post-prandial hyper- and hypoglycaemia. For people with type 2 diabetes, avoidance of refined carbohydrate and restriction of carbohydrate to 45–60% of total energy intake is recommended.

Glycaemic index (GI)

Both the amount and source of carbohydrate determine post-prandial glucose. Different foods can be ranked by their effect on post-prandial glycaemia (GI). Consumption of foods with a low GI is encouraged because they produce a slow, gradual rise in blood glucose. Examples include foods such as basmati rice, spaghetti and lentils. However, GI does not address the total amount consumed.

Fat

The intake of total fat should be restricted to <35% of energy intake, with <10% as saturated fat, 10–20% from monounsaturated fat and <10% from polyunsaturated fat. The ω-3 fatty acids, found predominantly in oily fish, have been shown to assist with secondary prevention of cardiovascular disease.

WEIGHT MANAGEMENT

A high percentage of people with type 2 diabetes are overweight or obese, and many anti-diabetic medications and insulin encourage weight gain. Abdominal obesity also predicts insulin resistance and cardiovascular risk. Weight loss is achieved through a reduction in energy intake and an increase in energy expenditure through physical activity. Overweight patients should be encouraged to reduce calorie intake and take regular exercise for approximately 30 mins daily, as this improves insulin sensitivity and the lipid profile, and lowers BP.

ALCOHOL

Alcohol can be consumed in moderation. As alcohol suppresses gluconeogenesis, it can precipitate or protract hypoglycaemia, particularly in patients taking insulin or sulphonylureas. Drinks containing alcohol can be a substantial source of calories and may have to be reduced to assist weight reduction.

SALT

People with diabetes should reduce sodium intake to no more than 6 g daily, or 3 g daily in the presence of hypertension.

ORAL ANTI-DIABETIC DRUGS

Most drugs used to treat type 2 diabetes depend upon a supply of endogenous insulin and therefore have no effect in patients with type 1 diabetes. The sulphonylureas and biguanides have been the mainstay of treatment in the past.

SULPHONYLUREAS

Sulphonylureas stimulate the release of insulin from the pancreatic β cell (insulin secretagogue). They are best used to treat non-obese people with type 2 diabetes who fail to respond to dietary measures, as treatment is often associated with weight gain.

• Chlorpropamide is rarely used, has a long half-life (~36 hrs) and is taken once daily, but may cause prolonged hypoglycaemia. • Gliclazide and glipizide cause few side-effects, but glibenclamide is prone to induce hypoglycaemia and should be avoided in the elderly. • Newer long-acting preparations such as glimepiride and modified-release gliclazide have no apparent increased risk of hypoglycaemia.

Those who fail to respond to initial treatment with sulphonylureas are considered 'primary treatment failures'. Patients with 'secondary failure' (after a period of satisfactory glycaemic control) include patients with LADA, those with type 2 diabetes and advanced β-cell failure, and, most commonly, those who are not adhering to the recommended diet. Secondary failure affects 3–10% of patients each year.

BIGUANIDES

In the UK Prospective Diabetes Study, metformin reduced myocardial infarctions, but its use is limited by side-effects, particularly gastrointestinal symptoms. It improves insulin sensitivity and peripheral glucose uptake, and impairs both glucose absorption by the gut and hepatic gluconeogenesis. Endogenous insulin is required for its glucose-lowering action, but it does not increase insulin secretion and seldom causes hypoglycaemia.

Metformin does not increase body weight and it is therefore preferred for obese patients. It acts synergistically with sulphonylureas, allowing the two to be combined. Metformin is given with food, 8- or 12-hourly. The usual starting dose is 500 mg 12-hourly (maximum 1 g 8-hourly). Its use is contraindicated in alcohol excess, and in impaired renal or hepatic function due to the increased risk of lactic acidosis. It should be discontinued temporarily if another serious medical condition develops (especially shock or hypoxaemia).

ALPHA-GLUCOSIDASE INHIBITORS

These delay carbohydrate absorption in the gut by selectively inhibiting disaccharidases. Acarbose or miglitol is taken with each meal and lowers post-prandial blood glucose. Side-effects are flatulence, abdominal bloating and diarrhoea.

THIAZOLIDINEDIONES

These drugs ('glitazones' or PPARγ agonists) bind and activate peroxisome proliferator-activated receptor-γ found in adipose tissue, and work by enhancing the actions of endogenous insulin. Plasma insulin concentrations are not increased and hypoglycaemia is not a problem. Rosiglitazone or pioglitazone are usually prescribed as second-line therapy with sulphonylureas in patients intolerant of metformin, or as third-line therapy in combination with sulphonylurea and metformin. They are effective in patients with the most severe insulin resistance (e.g. abdominal obesity) but body weight and total body fat are increased. Thiazolidinediones have few side-effects. They should be avoided in liver dysfunction (hepatic toxicity) and cardiac failure (sodium and fluid retention). Rosiglitazone should be avoided in patients with known coronary artery disease.

MEGLITINIDES AND AMINO ACID DERIVATIVES (PRANDIAL GLUCOSE REGULATORS)

Repaglinide and nateglinide directly stimulate endogenous insulin secretion and are taken immediately before food. They are less likely to cause hypoglycaemia than sulphonylureas.

COMBINED ORAL ANTI-DIABETIC THERAPY AND INSULIN

In diabetic patients who are requiring increasing doses of a sulphonylurea and/or biguanide (± thiazolidinedione), the introduction of a single dose of intermediate- or long-acting insulin at bedtime may improve glycaemic control and delay overt pancreatic β-cell failure. Isophane insulin with metformin is less likely to promote weight gain.

INCRETIN MIMETICS

Secretion of insulin is greater with oral rather than i.v. glucose. This is caused by secretion of gut hormones or incretins, e.g. glucagon-like peptide (GLP-1). GLP-1 analogues suppress glucagon secretion, delay gastric emptying, reduce appetite and encourage weight loss. They have to be given by injection. These preparations are used with other anti-diabetic medication and may

11.10 DURATION OF ACTION (HRS) OF INSULIN PREPARATIONS

Insulin	Onset	Peak	Duration
Rapid-acting (insulin analogues—lispro, aspart, glulisine)	<0.5	0.5–2.5	3–4.5
Short-acting (soluble (regular))	0.5–1	1–4	4–8
Intermediate-acting (isophane (NPH), lente)	1–3	3–8	7–14
Long-acting (bovine ultralente)	2–4	6–12	12–30
Long-acting (insulin analogues—glargine, detemir)	1–2	None	18–24

cause nausea and vomiting. As GLP-1 is rapidly degraded by dipeptidyl peptidase 4, inhibitors of this enzyme can be co-administered to prolong its effect.

INSULIN

The duration of action of the main groups of insulin preparation are given in Box 11.10.

Insulin delivery

Insulin is injected subcutaneously into the anterior abdominal wall, upper arms, outer thighs and buttocks. The rate of absorption of insulin may be influenced by the insulin formulation, the site, depth and volume of injection, skin temperature (warming), local massage and exercise. Absorption is delayed from areas of lipohypertrophy at injection sites.

Portable pumps infusing continuous subcutaneous or i.v. insulin can achieve excellent glycaemic control but will not be adopted for widespread use until they are less expensive and incorporate a miniaturised glucose sensor.

Short-acting insulin has to be injected at least 30 mins before a meal to allow adequate time for absorption. However, the rapidly absorbed fast-acting insulin analogues can be administered immediately before food, or even after meals, and their peak action coincides more closely with the post-prandial rise in blood glucose (Box 11.10). Once in the blood stream, insulin has a half-life of a few minutes. It is removed by the liver and kidneys; plasma insulin concentrations are elevated in patients with liver disease or renal failure. Clearance is also affected by binding to insulin antibodies (associated with the use of animal insulins).

Insulin regimens

Once-daily injections: Rarely achieve satisfactory glycaemic control; they are reserved either for elderly patients or for those who retain substantial endogenous insulin secretion.

Twice-daily injections: short-acting and intermediate-acting insulin (usually soluble and isophane insulins), given in combination before breakfast and the evening meal. Usually two-thirds of the total daily insulin requirement is given in the morning in a ratio of 1 : 2, short : intermediate-acting insulins. The remaining third is given in the evening. Pre-mixed formulations are available containing different proportions of soluble and isophane insulins (e.g. 30 : 70 and 50 : 50). These are useful in patients who have difficulty mixing insulins, but preclude adjustment of the individual components.

Multiple injections: short-acting insulin taken before each meal, and intermediate-acting insulin injected at bedtime (basal–bolus regimen). This allows greater freedom for timing of meals. Fast-acting insulin analogues may be used before meals, and are particularly useful if the evening meal is late, as they do not induce nocturnal hyperinsulinaemia. However, a long interval between meals allows the blood glucose to rise. A common problem is fasting hyperglycaemia (the 'dawn phenomenon') caused by the release of counter-regulatory hormones during the night, which increases insulin requirement before wakening.

Complications of insulin therapy

• Hypoglycaemia. • Weight gain. • Peripheral oedema (insulin treatment causes salt and water retention in the short term). • Insulin antibodies (animal insulins). • Local allergy (rare). • Lipodystrophy at injection sites.

FUTURE THERAPIES

Transplantation of isolated pancreatic islets (usually into the liver via the portal vein) has been achieved in a small number of humans. The development of methods of inducing tolerance to transplanted islets and the use of stem cells or transformation of hepatocytes to make insulin by genetic engineering mean that this may still prove the most promising approach in the long term.

Whole pancreas transplantation presents particular problems relating to the exocrine pancreatic secretions, and long-term immunosuppression is necessary. While results are steadily improving, they remain less favourable than for renal transplantation. However, it is questionable whether it will ever be considered justifiable to perform transplantation in young diabetic patients before vascular disease is clinically apparent.

Alternative methods and routes of insulin delivery other than subcutaneous injection are being sought. Inhaled, oral and transcutaneous (patch) routes of delivery are being explored.

LONG-TERM COMPLICATIONS OF DIABETES

People with diabetes have a mortality rate double that of age- and sex-matched controls. Large blood vessel disease accounts for 70% of all deaths. Atherosclerosis in diabetic patients occurs earlier and is more extensive and severe. Diabetes enhances the effects of the other major cardiovascular risk factors: smoking, hypertension and dyslipidaemia.

Microangiopathy (small blood vessel disease) is a specific complication of diabetes. It contributes to mortality by provoking renal failure (diabetic nephropathy) and causes substantial morbidity and disability: blindness, difficulty in walking, chronic foot ulceration, and bowel and bladder dysfunction. The risk of microangiopathy is related to the duration and degree of hyperglycaemia. Diabetic retinopathy, nephropathy, neuropathy and atherosclerosis are thought to result from the local response to the generalised vascular injury.

Preventing diabetes complications

No study has produced any evidence of improved glycaemic control reversing either retinopathy or nephropathy, and in some cases retinopathy worsened abruptly soon after control was improved. Despite this, in the long term the rate of progression of both retinopathy and nephropathy was reduced by continuing better control. The Diabetes Control and Complications Trial (DCCT) was a large study in type 1 diabetic patients to answer the question: are diabetic complications preventable? The trial demonstrated a 60% overall reduction in the risk of developing diabetic complications in those on intensive therapy with strict glycaemic control (mean HbA_{1c} 7%), compared with those on conventional therapy (HbA_{1c} 9%). This trial showed that diabetic complications are preventable and treatment aim should be 'near-normal' glycaemia. Strict glycaemic control was complicated by weight gain and severe hypoglycaemic episodes. This increased risk of hypoglycaemia may alter the risk : benefit ratio in patients who have impaired awareness of hypoglycaemia, have severe macrovascular disease (previous myocardial infarction/cerebrovascular accident), or are at the extremes of life.

The UK Prospective Diabetes Study (UKPDS) in type 2 diabetes found that diabetic complications were reduced and progression was slower with good glycaemic control (mean HbA_{1c} 7%) and effective treatment of hypertension, irrespective of the type of therapy used. RCTs have also shown that aggressive management of lipids and BP limits the complications of diabetes. ACE inhibitors are valuable in improving outcome in heart disease and in preventing diabetic nephropathy.

DIABETIC RETINOPATHY

Diabetic retinopathy is a common cause of blindness in adults in developed countries. Hyperglycaemia increases retinal blood flow and metabolism, and has direct effects on retinal endothelial cells, resulting in impaired vascular autoregulation. This leads to chronic retinal hypoxia which stimulates production of growth factors causing new vessel formation and increased vascular permeability.

Clinical features

Microaneurysms: Tiny, discrete, circular, dark red spots near to the retinal vessels (Fig. 11.3A) are the earliest abnormality detected.

Haemorrhages: These are found in the deeper layers of the retina and are round ('blot' haemorrhages, Fig. 11.3A). They are often grouped with microaneurysms as 'dots and blots'. Superficial flame-shaped haemorrhages in the nerve fibre layer also occur, particularly in hypertensive patients.

Exudates: Characteristic of diabetic retinopathy, these vary in size from specks to confluent patches, and tend to occur around the macula (Fig. 11.3B).

Cotton wool spots: Usually occurring within five disc diameters of the optic disc (Fig. 11.3E), these represent arteriolar occlusions causing retinal ischaemia and occur in pre-proliferative, often rapidly advancing retinopathy or uncontrolled hypertension.

Intraretinal microvascular abnormalities: These are dilated, tortuous capillaries representing patent capillaries in an area where most have been occluded (severe pre-proliferative retinopathy).

Neovascularisation: Vessels arise on the optic disc or retina in response to an ischaemic retina (Fig. 11.3F). They are fragile and leaky, causing haemorrhage which may be pre-retinal or vitreous. Leaking serous products stimulate a connective tissue reaction, called gliosis, by which retinal detachment can occur due to adhesions between the vitreous and the retina.

Venous changes: These range from venous dilatation (background) to venous beading and increased tortuosity ('oxbow lakes'/loops, pre-proliferative retinopathy).

Rubeosis iridis: This is the development of new vessels on the anterior surface of the iris. Vessels may obstruct the drainage angle, causing secondary glaucoma.

Classification

A classification based on prognosis is shown in Box 11.11. Background retinopathy does not threaten vision unless associated with macular disease. Macular oedema is suspected if there is impairment of visual acuity with peripheral non-proliferative retinopathy. New vessels may be symptomless until sudden visual loss occurs from pre-retinal or vitreous haemorrhage. This resolves, although recurrence is common. Fibrous tissue may interfere with vision by obscuring the retina or causing detachment.

Prevention

Good glycaemic control reduces the risk of retinopathy. Early diagnosis and treatment is important for patients with type 2 diabetes; 25% present with established retinopathy. A rapid reduction in blood glucose may cause an initial deterioration of retinopathy by causing relative ischaemia. Improvement in glycaemic control should therefore be effected gradually. BP lowering is of proven benefit. Elevated cholesterol is a risk factor, but

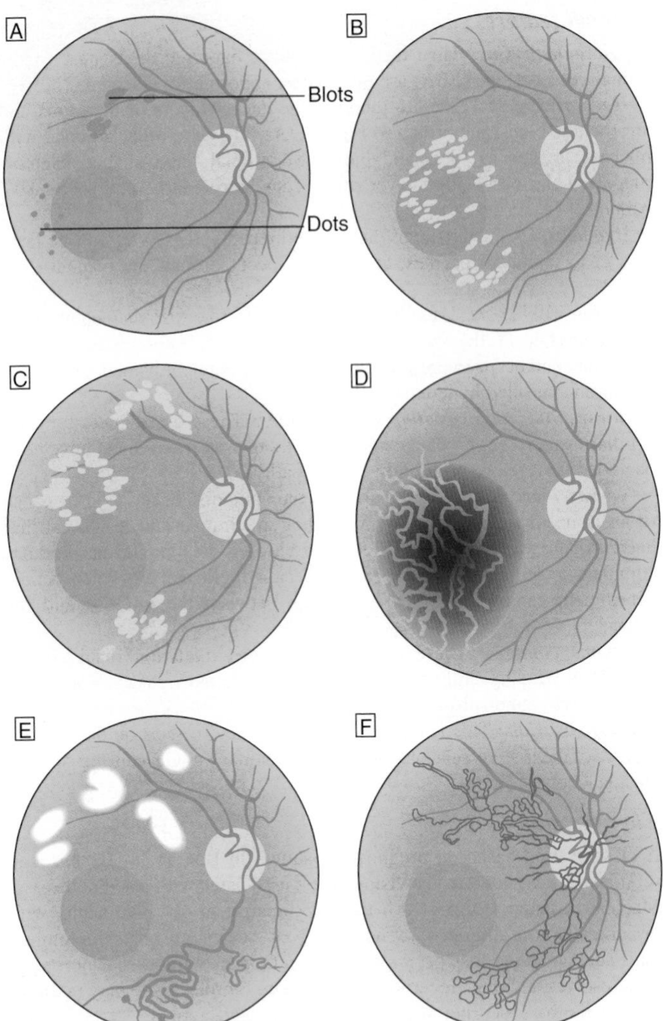

Fig. 11.3 Diagrammatic representation of diabetic eye disease. **A** Background diabetic retinopathy showing microaneurysms and blot haemorrhages. **B** Background retinopathy showing exudates. **C** Maculopathy with exudates. **D** Maculopathy showing oedema. **E** Pre-proliferative retinopathy showing venous changes and cotton wool spots. **F** Proliferative retinopathy showing neovascularisation.

11.11 CLASSIFICATION OF DIABETIC RETINOPATHY BY PROGNOSIS FOR VISION

Type of retinopathy	Prognosis/Action required
Background retinopathy Venous dilatation Peripheral microaneurysms, blot haemorrhages, exudates	No immediate threat to vision Control blood glucose, lipids and BP, advise to stop smoking Fundoscopy every 6–12 mths, refer if progression
Maculopathy Macular exudation, haemorrhage, ischaemia Macular oedema	Sight-threatening—refer for specialist opinion Review of risk factors, glycaemic control, BP and lipid levels
Pre-proliferative retinopathy Venous loops and beading Clusters of microaneurysms, blot haemorrhages, large retinal haemorrhages Intraretinal microvascular abnormalities, cotton wool spots Macular oedema Perimacular exudates ± haemorrhages	Sight-threatening—refer for specialist opinion Rapid lowering of blood glucose may worsen retinopathy (see text)
Proliferative retinopathy Pre-retinal haemorrhage Neovascularisation Fibrosis, exudative maculopathy	Sight-threatening—urgent review and treatment by specialist mandatory

evidence for statin use is awaited. Regular screening for retinopathy is essential in all diabetic patients, especially those with risk factors such as long duration of diabetes, hypertension, poor control, pregnancy, smoking, excess alcohol and evidence of microangiopathy. The preferred screening option is a digital imaging photographic system, with referral to an ophthalmologist when needed.

Management

Severe non-proliferative and proliferative retinopathy is treated with retinal photocoagulation, which has been shown to reduce severe visual loss by 85% (50% in maculopathy). Argon laser photocoagulation is used to:

• Destroy areas of retinal ischaemia. • Seal leaking microaneurysms. • Reduce macular oedema. • Gliose new vessels on the retinal surface.

Patients must be reviewed regularly to check for recurrence. Extensive bilateral photocoagulation can cause visual field loss, interfering with driving and night vision. Vitrectomy may be used where visual loss is due to recurrent vitreous haemorrhage which has failed to clear, or retinal detachment resulting from retinitis proliferans. Rubeosis iridis is managed by early pan-retinal photocoagulation.

OTHER CAUSES OF VISUAL LOSS IN DIABETES

Around 50% of visual loss in people with type 2 diabetes is due to causes other than diabetic retinopathy. These include:

• Cataract. • Macular degeneration. • Retinal vein occlusion. • Retinal arterial occlusion. • Ischaemic optic neuropathy. • Glaucoma.

Cataract occurs prematurely in people with diabetes due to the metabolic insult to the lens.

DIABETIC NEPHROPATHY

Diabetic nephropathy is among the most common causes of end-stage renal failure (ESRF) in developed countries. About 30% of patients with type 1 diabetes have developed diabetic nephropathy after 20 yrs, but the risk after this time falls to less than 1% per year. Risk factors for developing nephropathy include:

• Poor glycaemic control. • Duration of diabetes. • Asian ethnicity. • Hypertension. • Other microvascular complications. • A family history of nephropathy or hypertension.

Pathologically, thickening of the glomerular basement membrane is followed by nodular deposits (Kimmelstiel–Wilson nodules). As glomerulosclerosis worsens, heavy proteinuria develops, sometimes in the nephrotic range, and renal function progressively deteriorates.

Diagnosis and screening

Microalbuminuria (30–300 mg/24 hrs) is a risk factor for developing overt diabetic nephropathy, although it is also found in other conditions. Progressively increasing albuminuria, or albuminuria accompanied by hypertension, is more likely to be due to early diabetic nephropathy. Patients with type 1 diabetes should be screened annually from 5 yrs after diagnosis; those with type 2 diabetes should be screened annually from the time of diagnosis.

Management

If nephropathy is identified, progression can be reduced by improved blood glucose control, and aggressive reduction of BP and other cardiovascular risk factors.

• ACE inhibitors and angiotensin receptor blockers have been shown to provide greater benefit than equal BP reduction achieved with other drugs.
• Diabetic control becomes difficult in renal impairment. Metformin should be stopped when creatinine is >150 µmol/l (1.7 mg/dl; risk of lactic acido-

sis). Long-acting sulphonylureas should be replaced by short-acting agents. • Renal replacement therapy may benefit diabetic patients at an earlier stage than other ESRF patients. • Renal transplantation can improve quality of life, although macrovascular disease and neuropathy/retinopathy show continued progression. • Pancreatic transplantation can produce insulin independence and can reverse microvascular disease, but the supply of organs is limited.

DIABETIC NEUROPATHY

This complication affects approximately 30% of patients. It is symptomless in the majority and can occur in motor, sensory and autonomic nerves. Prevalence is related to the duration of diabetes and the degree of metabolic control.

Clinical features

Symmetrical sensory polyneuropathy: There is diminished perception of vibration sensation distally, 'glove-and-stocking' impairment of all other modalities of sensation, and loss of tendon reflexes in the lower limbs. Although frequently asymptomatic, it can cause paraesthesia in the feet or hands, pain on the anterior aspect of the legs (worse at night), burning sensations in the soles of the feet, hyperaesthesia and a wide-based gait. Toes may be clawed with wasting of the interosseous muscles. A diffuse small-fibre neuropathy causes altered pain and temperature sensation and is associated with symptomatic autonomic neuropathy; characteristic features include foot ulcers and Charcot neuroarthropathy. Management includes strict glycaemic control, tricyclic antidepressants (amitriptyline, imipramine), anticonvulsants (carbamazepine, gabapentin) and opioids (tramadol, oxycodone).

Asymmetrical motor diabetic neuropathy (diabetic amyotrophy): This presents as severe and progressive weakness and wasting of the proximal muscles of the lower (occasionally upper) limbs, accompanied by severe pain, hyperaesthesia and paraesthesia. There may also be marked loss of weight ('neuropathic cachexia'), tendon reflexes may be absent, and the CSF protein is often raised. This condition is thought to involve acute infarction of the lumbosacral plexus. Although recovery usually occurs within 12 mths, some deficits become permanent. Management is mainly supportive.

Mononeuropathy: Either motor or sensory function can be affected within a single peripheral or cranial nerve. Unlike other neuropathies, mononeuropathies are severe and of rapid onset; the patient usually recovers. Most commonly affected nerves are 3rd and 6th cranial nerves, femoral and sciatic nerves. Multiple nerves are affected in mononeuritis multiplex. Nerve compression palsies commonly affect the median nerve and lateral popliteal nerve (foot drop).

Autonomic neuropathy: This is less clearly related to poor metabolic control, and improved control rarely improves symptoms. Clinical features

11.12 CLINICAL FEATURES AND MANAGEMENT OF AUTONOMIC NEUROPATHY	
Feature	**Management**
Postural hypotension (drop in systolic pressure of ≥20 mmHg)	Fludrocortisone, support stockings
Gastroparesis	Metoclopramide, erythromycin
Diarrhoea/constipation	Loperamide, stimulant laxatives
Atonic bladder	Intermittent self-catheterisation
Hyperhydrosis	Topical/oral anti-muscarinics
Erectile dysfunction (30% of males)	Phosphodiesterase inhibitors, prostaglandin injections

and management are shown in Box 11.12. Within 10 yrs of developing autonomic neuropathy, 30–50% of patients are dead. Those with postural hypotension have the highest subsequent mortality.

THE DIABETIC FOOT

Tissue necrosis in the feet is a common reason for hospital admission in diabetic patients. Foot ulceration occurs as a result of often trivial trauma in the presence of neuropathy (peripheral and autonomic) and/or peripheral vascular disease; infection occurs as a secondary phenomenon. In most cases all three components are involved in producing tissue necrosis. Most ulcers are neuropathic or neuro-ischaemic in type. The most common cause of ulceration is a plaque of callus skin beneath which tissue necrosis occurs, eventually breaking through to the surface.

Management

Preventative management is the most effective method of dealing with the diabetic foot. Regular podiatry, patient education and orthotic footwear (preventing recurrence and protecting deformed feet) are required. Medical management includes:

• Removal of callus skin (podiatrist only). • Treatment of infection (often protracted courses, especially in the presence of osteomyelitis). • Avoidance of weight-bearing. • Good glycaemic control. • Control of oedema. • Angiography if the foot is ischaemic: to assess feasibility of vascular reconstruction. • Amputation: if there is extensive tissue/bony destruction or intractable ischaemic pain when vascular reconstruction is not possible or has failed.

12

Gastrointestinal and nutritional disorders

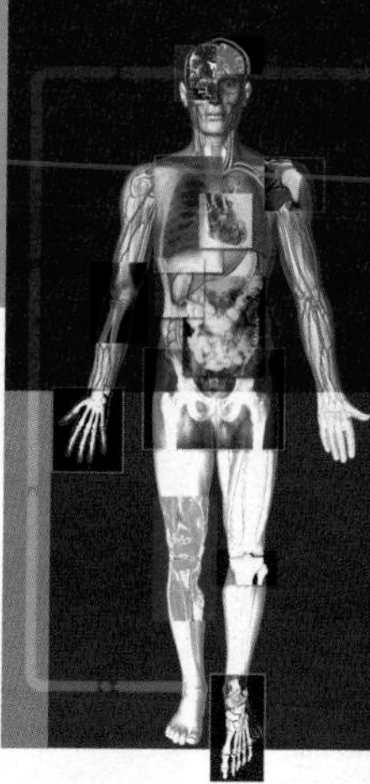

Diseases of the GI tract are a major cause of morbidity and mortality. Approximately 10% of all GP consultations in the UK are for indigestion, and 1 in 14 is for diarrhoea. Infective diarrhoea and malabsorption are responsible for much ill health and many deaths in the developing world.

PRESENTING PROBLEMS

DYSPHAGIA

Dysphagia means difficulty in swallowing, as distinct from globus sensation (a 'lump' in the throat without organic cause) and odynophagia (pain during swallowing). Oropharyngeal dysphagia results from neuromuscular dysfunction that affects swallowing, causing choking, nasal regurgitation or tracheal aspiration. Drooling, dysarthria, hoarseness and other neurological signs may be present. Oesophageal causes include benign or malignant strictures and oesophageal dysmotility. Patients complain of food 'sticking' after swallowing, although swallowing of liquids is normal until strictures become extreme.

- Endoscopy is preferred to facilitate biopsy and dilatation of strictures.
- Videofluoroscopic barium swallow will detect most motility disorders.
- Oesophageal manometry is occasionally required.

DYSPEPSIA

Dyspepsia ('indigestion') may arise from causes within or outside the gut (Box 12.1). Heartburn and other 'reflux' symptoms are separate and are considered elsewhere. Although symptoms correlate poorly with diagnosis,

CLINICAL EXAMINATION OF THE GASTROINTESTINAL TRACT

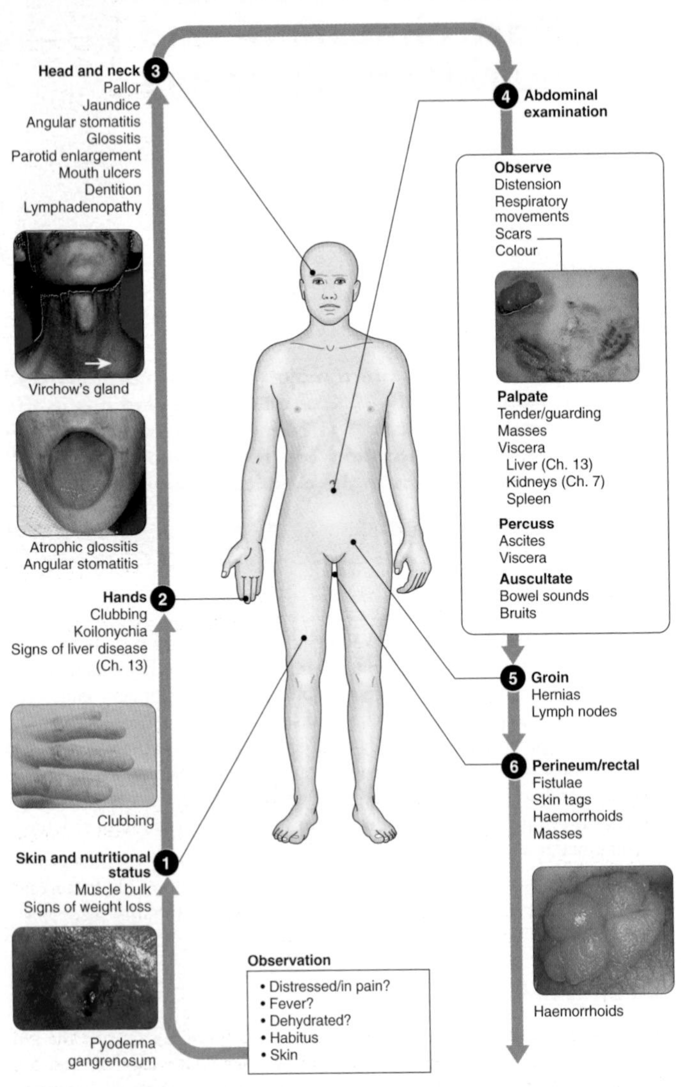

12.1 CAUSES OF DYSPEPSIA	
GI disorders	
• Peptic ulcer disease • Acute gastritis • Gallstones • Motility disorders, e.g. oesophageal spasm • Colonic carcinoma	• 'Functional' (non-ulcer dyspepsia and irritable bowel syndrome) • Pancreatic disease (cancer, chronic pancreatitis) • Hepatic disease (hepatitis, metastases)
Systemic disease	
• Renal failure	• Hypercalcaemia
Drugs	
• NSAIDs • Iron and potassium supplements	• Corticosteroids • Digoxin
Others	
• Alcohol	• Psychological, e.g. anxiety, depression

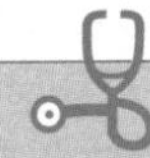

12.2 ALARM' FEATURES IN DYSPEPSIA	
• Weight loss • Anaemia • Vomiting	• Haematemesis and/or melaena • Dysphagia • Palpable abdominal mass

careful history may reveal classical symptoms of peptic ulcer, 'alarm' features requiring urgent investigation (Box 12.2) or symptoms of other disorders. Dyspepsia affects up to 80% of the population at some time, often with no abnormality on investigation, especially in younger patients.

• Examination may reveal anaemia, weight loss, lymphadenopathy, abdominal masses or liver disease. • Patients with 'alarm' symptoms, and those >55 with new dyspepsia require prompt endoscopy. • Younger patients should be tested for *Helicobacter pylori*; if symptoms persist after treatment, these patients should have endoscopy.

VOMITING

Vomiting is a complex reflex involving contraction of the diaphragm and intercostal and abdominal muscles, and simultaneous relaxation of the lower oesophageal sphincter, causing forcible ejection of gastric contents.

The history should reveal associated abdominal pain, fever, diarrhoea, relationship to food, drugs, headache, vertigo and weight loss. Pregnancy, alcoholism or bulimia should be considered. Examination may reveal:
• Dehydration. • Fever. • Abdominal masses. • Peritonitis or intestinal obstruction. • Papilloedema. • Nystagmus. • Photophobia. • Neck stiffness.

The diagnostic approach will be dictated by the history and examination.

GI BLEEDING

ACUTE UPPER GI HAEMORRHAGE

This is the most common GI emergency, accounting for 50–120 hospital admissions per 100 000 each year in the UK.

Haematemesis may be red with clots when bleeding is profuse, or black ('coffee grounds') when less severe. Syncope may occur with rapid bleeding. Anaemia suggests chronic bleeding. Melaena is the passage of black, tarry stools containing altered blood. This is usually due to upper GI bleeding, although the ascending colon is occasionally responsible. Severe acute upper GI bleeding occasionally causes maroon or bright red stool. Causes of acute upper GI haemorrhage are shown in Box 12.3.

Management

I.V. access: Should be secured with a large-bore cannula.

Clinical assessment: Should be made for circulatory status (tachycardia, hypotension and oliguria indicating severe bleeding), liver disease (jaundice, cutaneous stigmata, hepatosplenomegaly and ascites) and comorbidity (cardiorespiratory, cerebrovascular or renal disease, which increases the hazards of endoscopy and surgery).

Blood tests: FBC (slow bleeding causes anaemia; haemoglobin may be normal after sudden, major bleeding); cross-matching of at least 2 U of blood; U&Es (shock may cause renal failure; the urea also rises as the luminal blood is digested); LFTs and prothrombin time, if there is clinical suggestion of liver disease or in anticoagulated patients.

Resuscitation: Oxygen should be given to all patients in shock. I.V. crystalloid or colloid infusion restores blood pressure. Normal saline should be avoided in liver disease because it can cause ascites. Blood transfusion should be given if there is shock or the haemoglobin is <100 g/litre. CVP monitoring helps to reveal rebleeding and guide fluid replacement.

12.3 CAUSES OF ACUTE UPPER GI HAEMORRHAGE

- Peptic ulcer (*H. pylori* or NSAID) (35–50%)
- Gastric erosions (10–20%)
- Oesophagitis (10%)
- Varices (2–9%)
- Mallory–Weiss tear (5%)
- Vascular malformation (5%)
- Carcinoma of stomach or oesophagus (2%)

Endoscopy: After resuscitation, this will reveal a diagnosis in 80% of cases. Patients with spurting haemorrhage or a visible vessel can be treated by thermal probe, adrenaline (epinephrine) injection or metal clips. This may stop bleeding and, combined with i.v. proton pump inhibitor (PPI) therapy, prevent rebleeding, thus avoiding surgery.

Monitoring: Hourly pulse, BP and urine output.

Surgery: Indicated when endoscopic haemostasis fails to stop the bleeding, or rebleeding occurs once in an elderly or frail patient/twice in younger, fitter patients. Following successful surgery for ulcer bleeding, all patients should be treated with *H. pylori* eradication therapy if positive and should avoid NSAIDs.

LOWER GI BLEEDING

This may be due to haemorrhage from the small bowel, colon or anal canal.

Severe acute lower GI bleeding

Diverticular disease: The most common cause. Patients present with profuse red or maroon diarrhoea and shock. Bleeding almost always stops spontaneously, but if not, the diseased segment is located by angiography or colonoscopy and resected.

Angiodysplasia: Characterised by vascular malformations resembling spider naevi in the proximal colon of elderly patients. Bleeding usually stops spontaneously but commonly recurs. Treatment is by colonoscopic thermal ablation, or resection if bleeding continues.

Ischaemia due to inferior mesenteric artery occlusion: Presents with abdominal colic and rectal bleeding. It occurs in elderly patients with atherosclerosis and is diagnosed by colonoscopy. Resection is required only in the presence of peritonitis.

Meckel's diverticulum: May erode into a major artery and cause profuse lower GI bleeding in children or adolescents. The diagnosis is commonly made only by resection at laparotomy.

Subacute or chronic lower GI bleeding

This is extremely common and is usually due to haemorrhoids or anal fissure. Proctoscopy reveals the diagnosis but if there is altered bowel habit and in all patients presenting at age 40 and over, colonoscopy or barium enema is necessary to exclude colorectal cancer.

OBSCURE MAJOR GI BLEEDING

If upper endoscopy and colonoscopy are inconclusive, mesenteric angiography usually identifies the site and embolisation can be used to stop the bleeding. If angiography is negative, enteroscopy or wireless capsule endoscopy can be used to identify a bleeding source in the small intestine. When all else fails, laparotomy with on-table endoscopy is indicated.

OCCULT GI BLEEDING

Occult bleeding (no visible blood) may reach 200 ml/day, cause iron deficiency anaemia and signify serious disease. The most important cause is colorectal cancer, which may have no GI symptoms. GI investigations should be considered in any patient with unexplained iron deficiency anaemia. A negative faecal occult blood (FOB) test does not exclude important GI disease.

DIARRHOEA

'Diarrhoea' most commonly means increased stool frequency and loose or watery stools. Normal bowel frequency ranges from three movements/day to one every third day. Gastroenterologists define diarrhoea as the passage of >200 g of stool daily. In severe cases, urgency of defecation and faecal incontinence occur.

ACUTE DIARRHOEA

Infective diarrhoea is usually due to faecal–oral transmission and is normally short-lived. Diarrhoea lasting >10 days is rarely caused by infection. Drugs including antibiotics, cytotoxics, PPIs and NSAIDs may cause acute diarrhoea.

CHRONIC OR RELAPSING DIARRHOEA

The most common cause is irritable bowel syndrome, in which diarrhoea is most severe before and after breakfast and rarely occurs at night. At other times the patient is constipated. The stool often contains mucus but never blood, and 24-hr stool volume is <200 g. Chronic diarrhoea can also be due to inflammatory or neoplastic disease of the colon or small bowel, or to malabsorption. Negative investigations suggest irritable bowel syndrome.

MALABSORPTION

Diarrhoea and weight loss in patients with a normal diet suggest malabsorption. Bulky, pale and offensive stools which float (steatorrhoea) signify fat malabsorption. Abdominal distension, borborygmi, cramps and undigested food in the stool may be present. Malaise, lethargy, peripheral neuropathy and symptoms related to vitamin or mineral deficiencies may occur.

Malabsorption results from abnormalities of the three components of normal digestion:

• Intraluminal maldigestion due to deficiency of bile or pancreatic enzymes. • Mucosal malabsorption from small bowel resection or damage to the small intestinal epithelium. • 'Post-mucosal' lymphatic obstruction preventing the uptake of absorbed lipids into lymphatic vessels.

An approach to investigations is shown in Figure 12.1.

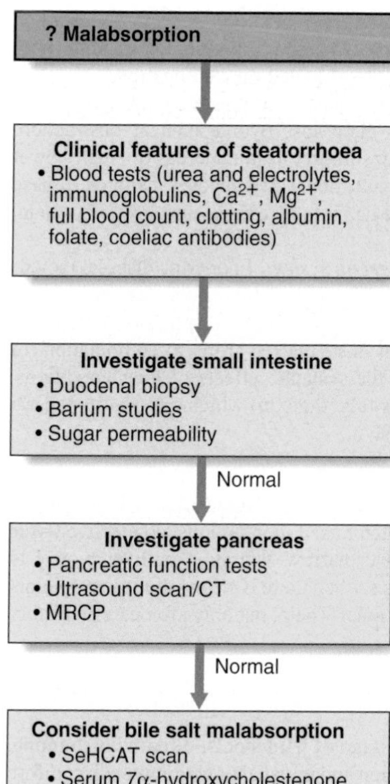

Fig. 12.1 Investigation for suspected malabsorption.

WEIGHT LOSS

Unplanned weight loss of >3 kg over 6 mths is significant. Previous weight records may be valuable. Pathological weight loss can be due to psychiatric illness, systemic disease, GI causes or advanced disease of any specific organ system.

History and examination

'Physiological' weight loss: Should be obvious from the history but may be more difficult to determine in older patients when nutritional history may be unreliable; a dietitian's opinion is often valuable.

Psychiatric illness: Features of anorexia nervosa, bulimia and affective disorders may only be apparent after formal psychiatric input. Alcoholic patients lose weight through self-neglect and poor diet.

Systemic diseases: Chronic infections lead to weight loss, and a history of foreign travel, fever, night sweats, rigors, productive cough and dysuria must be sought. Sensitive questions regarding lifestyle (promiscuous sexual activity and drug misuse) may suggest HIV infection. Weight loss is a late feature of disseminated malignancy (carcinoma, lymphoma or other haematological disorders), which may be revealed on examination.

GI disease: Dysphagia and gastric outflow obstruction cause defective intake. Malignancy may cause weight loss by mechanical obstruction, anorexia or systemic effects. Malabsorption from pancreas or small bowel causes profound weight loss and nutritional deficiencies. Crohn's disease and ulcerative colitis cause anorexia, fear of eating, and loss of protein, blood and nutrients from the gut.

Specific diseases of any major organ system: Endocrine disease, including diabetes mellitus, Addison's disease and thyrotoxicosis, may cause weight loss. In patients with disabling end-stage respiratory, cardiac or rheumatological diseases, weight loss occurs from a combination of anorexia, physical disability and the systemic effects of their conditions, often compounded by drug effects (e.g. digoxin) which may cause nausea, dyspepsia, constipation or depression.

Investigations

• Urinalysis for glucose, protein and blood. • Blood tests: LFTs, random blood glucose and TFTs; ESR (often raised in infections, connective tissue disorders and malignancy). • Bone marrow aspiration or liver biopsy to identify cryptic miliary tuberculosis when there is strong clinical suspicion. • Abdominal and pelvic CT: occasionally help, but only after careful history and reweighing.

CONSTIPATION

Constipation is the infrequent passage of hard stools, often with straining, a sensation of incomplete evacuation and perianal or abdominal discomfort. It may be the end result of many disorders.

In the absence of a history suggesting a specific cause (Box 12.4), it is not necessary to investigate every person with constipation. Most respond

12.4 CAUSES OF CONSTIPATION
GI
• Lack of dietary fibre • Altered motility, e.g. irritable bowel syndrome • Structural, e.g. colonic carcinoma, Hirschsprung's • Obstructed defecation, e.g. anal fissure
Non-GI
• Drugs, e.g. opiates, anticholinergics • Neurological, e.g. multiple sclerosis, paraplegia • Metabolic/endocrine, e.g. hypothyroidism • Others: any serious illness, especially in the elderly

to dietary fibre supplementation and the judicious use of laxatives. Middle-aged or elderly patients with a short history or worrying symptoms (rectal bleeding, pain or weight loss) must be investigated promptly, by either barium enema or colonoscopy. Others should be investigated as follows:

• Initially, digital rectal examination, proctoscopy and sigmoidoscopy, routine biochemistry, including serum calcium and thyroid function, and an FBC should be carried out. • If these are normal, a 1-mth trial of dietary fibre and/or laxatives is justified. • If symptoms persist, then examination of the colon by barium enema or colonoscopy is indicated to look for structural disease.

ABDOMINAL PAIN

Abdominal pain may be:

• Visceral: usually midline, due to stretching or torsion of a viscus. • Parietal: usually sharp, lateralised and localised, due to peritoneal irritation. • Referred: e.g. gallbladder pain referred to the back or shoulder tip. • Psychogenic: cultural, emotional and psychosocial factors influence the experience of pain. In some patients, no organic cause is found despite investigation.

THE ACUTE ABDOMEN

This accounts for ~50% of all urgent admissions to general surgical units. It is a consequence of one or more pathological processes:

Inflammation (e.g. appendicitis, pancreatitis, diverticulitis): Diffuse pain develops gradually, over hours. If the parietal peritoneum is involved, pain becomes localised. Movement exacerbates it; rigidity and guarding occur.

Perforation (e.g. peptic ulcer, ovarian cyst, diverticular disease): Pain starts abruptly, is severe and leads to generalised peritonitis.

Obstruction (intestinal, biliary or ureteric): Pain is colicky, with spasms causing the patient to writhe around. If it does not disappear between spasms, this suggests complicating inflammation.

If there are signs of peritonitis (i.e. guarding and rebound tenderness with rigidity), adequate resuscitation is needed. In other circumstances further investigations are required:

• FBC may reveal leucocytosis. • U&Es reveal dehydration. • Serum amylase is raised in acute pancreatitis. • Erect CXR reveals air under the diaphragm and an AXR reveals obstruction. • USS may help if gallstones, ureteric colic or a soft tissue mass is suspected, and may also reveal free fluid or intra-abdominal abscess. • Contrast studies, by either mouth or anus, are useful to evaluate obstruction, and essential to distinguish pseudo-obstruction from mechanical large bowel obstruction. • CT is useful for pancreatitis, retroperitoneal collections or masses, and aortic aneurysm. • Angiography or multi-slice CT angiography is used in mesenteric ischaemia. • Diagnostic laparoscopy may be advised if the cause remains obscure.

Management

Perforations are closed, inflammatory conditions are treated with antibiotics or resection, and obstructions are relieved. Most but not all patients require surgery. The speed of intervention and the need for surgery depend on several factors, particularly the presence or absence of peritonitis.

Acute appendicitis: Although conservative treatment can be successful, the risk of perforation or recurrence is high, so surgery is advisable.

Small bowel obstruction: If the suspected cause is adhesions from previous surgery, only patients who do not settle within 48 hrs with i.v. fluids, fasting and nasogastric aspiration, or who develop signs of strangulation (colicky pain becoming constant, peritonitis, tachycardia, fever, leucocytosis) will require surgery.

Large bowel obstruction: Pseudo-obstruction is treated non-operatively. Some patients benefit from colonoscopic decompression, but mechanical obstruction merits surgery. Differentiation between the two is by a water-soluble contrast enema.

Acute cholecystitis: See page 521.

Acute diverticulitis: See page 473.

Perforated peptic ulcer: See page 442.

CHRONIC OR RECURRENT ABDOMINAL PAIN

A detailed history, including associated symptoms, is essential. If abdominal and rectal examination is normal, a careful search should be made for disease affecting other structures, particularly the vertebral column, spinal cord, lungs and cardiovascular system.

The choice of investigations depends on the history and examination (Box 12.5). Persistent symptoms require exclusion of colonic or small

12.5 INVESTIGATION OF CHRONIC OR RECURRENT ABDOMINAL PAIN

Symptom	Probable diagnosis	Investigation
Epigastric pain; dyspepsia; relationship to food	Gastroduodenal or biliary disease	Endoscopy and USS
Altered bowel habit; rectal bleeding; features of obstruction	Colonic disease	Barium enema and sigmoidoscopy/ colonoscopy
Pain provoked by food in widespread atherosclerosis	Mesenteric ischaemia	Mesenteric angiography
Upper abdominal pain radiating to the back; history of alcohol misuse; weight loss; diarrhoea	Chronic pancreatitis or pancreatic cancer	USS, CT and pancreatic function tests
Recurrent loin or flank pain with urinary symptoms	Renal or ureteric stones	USS and i.v. urography

bowel disease. A history of psychiatric disturbance, repeated negative investigations or vague symptoms not fitting any particular disease or organ pattern may point to a psychological origin.

CONSTANT ABDOMINAL PAIN

Patients with constant abdominal pain usually have features to suggest the underlying diagnosis, e.g. malignancy, chronic pancreatitis or intra-abdominal abscess. Occasionally no cause will be found, leading to the diagnosis of 'chronic functional abdominal pain'. In these patients a psychological cause is highly likely and treatment is aimed at symptom control, psychological support and minimising disease impact.

DISORDERS OF NUTRITION

VITAMIN DEFICIENCY

Vitamins are categorised as fat-soluble or water-soluble. Deficiency of fat-soluble vitamins occurs in fat malabsorption.

• In developed countries, older people and alcoholic patients are particularly at risk of vitamin deficiency. • In developing countries, vitamin deficiency diseases are more prevalent.

Box 12.6 summarises the sources of vitamins and their deficiency states.

MALNUTRITION

STARVATION AND FAMINE

There remain regions of the world, particularly in Africa, where the prevalence of BMI <18.5 in adults remains as high as 20%. In adults, the predominant form of protein–energy malnutrition is undernutrition, i.e. a sustained negative energy (calorie) balance.

Decreased energy intake: Causes include:

• Famine. • Persistent regurgitation or vomiting. • Anorexia. • Malabsorption (e.g. small intestinal disease). • Maldigestion (e.g. pancreatic exocrine insufficiency).

Increased energy expenditure: Causes include:

• Increased basal metabolic rate (BMR) (thyrotoxicosis, trauma, fever, cancer cachexia). • Excessive physical activity (e.g. marathon runners). • Energy loss (e.g. glycosuria in diabetes). • Impaired energy storage (e.g. Addison's disease, phaeochromocytoma).

Clinical features

The severity of malnutrition can be assessed by measurements of BMI, mid-arm circumference and skinfold thickness. The clinical features of severe undernutrition in adults include:

• Loss of weight. • Thirst, weakness, feeling cold, nocturia, amenorrhoea, impotence. • Lax, pale, dry skin. • Hair thinning or loss. • Cold, cyanosed

12.6 CLINICALLY IMPORTANT VITAMINS AND VITAMIN DEFICIENCY STATES

Name	Sources	Deficiency	Investigations
Fat-soluble			
Vitamin A	Liver, milk, butter, fish oils	Xerophthalmia, night blindness, keratomalacia, follicular hyperkeratosis	Serum retinol
Vitamin D	Synthesised in skin	Rickets, osteomalacia	Plasma 25(OH)D/1,25$(OH)_2$D
Vitamin E	Vegetables, seed oils	Haemolytic anaemia, ataxia	Plasma vitamin E
Vitamin K	Green vegetables, dairy products	Coagulation disorder	Coagulation assay $\pm$ plasma vitamin K
Water-soluble			
Thiamine (B_1)	Cereals, grains, beans, pork	Beri-beri, Wernicke–Korsakoff syndrome	RBC transketolase, whole blood vitamin B_1
Riboflavin (B_2)	Milk	Glossitis, stomatitis	RBC glutathione reductase, whole blood B_2
Niacin (B_3)	Meat, cereals	Pellagra	Urinary metabolites
Pyridoxine (B_6)	Meat, fish, potatoes, bananas	Polyneuropathy	Plasma pyridoxal phosphate or RBC transaminase activation coefficient
Biotin	Liver, egg yolk, cereals	Dermatitis, alopecia, paraesthesiae	Whole blood or urine biotin
Folate	Liver, milk	Anaemia, neural tube defects during gestation	RBC folate
Vitamin B_{12}	Animal products	Anaemia, neurological degeneration	Plasma B_{12}
Vitamin C	Fresh fruit, vegetables	Scurvy	Ascorbic acid (plasma: daily intake; leucocyte: tissue stores)

extremities, pressure sores. • Muscle-wasting. • Loss of subcutaneous fat. • Oedema (even without hypoalbuminaemia). • Subnormal body temperature, slow pulse, low BP. • Distended abdomen, with diarrhoea. • Diminished tendon jerks. • Apathy, loss of initiative, depression, introversion, aggression if food is nearby. • Susceptibility to infections.

Undernutrition often leads to vitamin deficiencies, especially of thiamine, folate and vitamin C. Diarrhoea leads to sodium, potassium and magnesium depletion. The high mortality is often due to infections, e.g. typhus or cholera, but the usual signs may not appear. In advanced starvation, patients become completely inactive and may assume a flexed, fetal position; death comes quietly and often quite suddenly.

Investigations

• Plasma free fatty acids are increased, with ketosis and a mild metabolic acidosis. • Plasma glucose is low but albumin is often maintained. • Insulin secretion is diminished, glucagon and cortisol increase, and reverse T_3 replaces normal triiodothyronine. • Resting metabolic rate falls, due to reduced lean body mass and hypothalamic compensation. • There may be mild anaemia, leucopenia and thrombocytopenia.

Management

Patients should be graded according to BMI. Those with moderate starvation need extra feeding, while those who are severely underweight need hospital care. In severe starvation there is atrophy of the intestinal epithelium and the exocrine pancreas.

• Small amounts of food should be given at first; it should be palatable and similar to the usual staple meal, e.g. cereal with some sugar, milk powder and oil. • Salt should be restricted and micronutrient supplements may be essential (e.g. potassium, magnesium, zinc and multivitamins). • Between 6.3 and 8.4 MJ/day (1500–2000 kcal/day) will prevent deterioration, but additional calories are required for regain of weight. During refeeding, a gain of 5% body weight per month indicates satisfactory progress. • Other measures are supportive, and include care for the skin, adequate hydration, treatment of infections, and careful monitoring of body temperature since thermoregulation may be impaired.

MALNUTRITION IN HOSPITAL

One-third of hospital patients in the UK (particularly the elderly) are affected by moderate or severe malnutrition on admission. Once in hospital, many lose weight due to poor appetite, concurrent illness and being kept 'nil by mouth' for investigations. Malnutrition leads to impaired immunity and muscle weakness, and to increased morbidity, mortality and length of stay.

Nutritional support of the hospital patient

Normal diet: Inadequate intake may be due to unpalatability of food, cultural and religious factors restricting diet, or simple problems such as difficulty with hand dexterity (arthritis, stroke) or immobility in bed. Patients at risk of malnutrition should have food intake charted.

Dietary supplements: If a patient is unable to achieve sufficient nutritional intake from normal diet alone, then liquid dietary supplements with high energy and protein content should be used.

Enteral tube feeding: Patients who cannot swallow may require artificial nutritional support. The enteral route should be used if possible, as this preserves the integrity of the mucosal barrier, prevents bacteraemia and, in intensive care patients, reduces the risk of multi-organ failure.

• For short-term support, liquid feeds are given by fine-bore nasogastric tube. Tube position should be checked prior to use; gastric aspirate has a pH <4. A CXR can confirm tube position if in doubt. • A nasojejunal tube can be placed in cases of gastric stasis or outlet obstruction. • For long-term enteral feeding, a percutaneous endoscopic gastrostomy (PEG) is more comfortable and less likely to become displaced. However, inserting a gastrostomy is an invasive procedure and complications include local infection (30%) and perforation of intra-abdominal organs.

Parenteral nutrition: IV feeding is expensive, carries higher risks of complications and should only be used when enteral feeding is impossible. Less than 1 wk of parenteral feeding confers little benefit. There are a number of possible routes:

• Peripheral venous cannula: this can only be used for low osmolality solutions due to the risk of thrombophlebitis. • Peripherally inserted central catheter (PICC): a 60 cm cannula is inserted into a vein in the antecubital fossa. The distal end lies in a central vein, allowing hyperosmolar solutions to be used. • Central line: a single-lumen subclavian catheter in the internal jugular vein is preferred, due to lower infection rates. Hyperosmolar solutions can be used. The main energy source in total parenteral nutrition (TPN) is provided by carbohydrate, usually as glucose. TPN also contains amino acids, lipid emulsion, electrolytes, trace elements and vitamins, mixed as a large bag in a sterile environment. Constituents are adjusted according to the results of regular blood monitoring. Fever indicates a likely line infection.

Refeeding syndrome

When nutritional support is given to a malnourished patient, anabolic hormones are released. Insulin causes cellular uptake of phosphate, potassium and magnesium. Falling levels can lead to serious consequences, such as cardiac arrhythmias. Electrolyte levels should be corrected before refeeding is commenced. Wernicke's encephalopathy may be precipitated by refeeding with carbohydrates in thiamine deficiency. This can be countered by giving thiamine before feeding.

ANOREXIA NERVOSA

Anorexia nervosa is a well-defined eating disorder, although a much higher prevalence of abnormal eating behaviour in the population does not meet the diagnostic criteria. There is marked weight loss, arising from food avoidance, in combination with bingeing, purging, excessive exercise, or the use of diuretics and laxatives. Despite their emaciation, patients feel overweight due to body image disturbance. Downy hair (lanugo) develops on the back, forearms and cheeks. Extreme starvation is associated with a range of pathophysiological changes, such as cardiac arrhythmias (prolonged QT and ventricular tachycardia), anaemia and osteoporosis. The condition usually emerges in adolescence, and 90% of cases are female.

Diagnostic criteria are:

• Loss of at least 15% of total body weight. • Avoidance of high-calorie foods. • Distortion of body image. • Amenorrhoea for at least 3 mths.

Differential diagnosis includes:

• Depression. • Inflammatory bowel disease. • Malabsorption. • Hypopituitarism. • Cancer.

Management and prognosis

• The aim is to increase weight into the normal range by addressing abnormal beliefs and behaviour. • Treatment is given on an outpatient basis, inpatient treatment being indicated only if weight loss is intractable or if there is a risk of death. • Measures include cognitive behavioural therapy (CBT) and family therapy. • Compulsory admission and tube feeding are resorted to when patients are at risk of death and other measures have failed. • About 20% of patients have a good outcome, 20% develop a chronic disorder and the remainder have an intermediate outcome. Long-term mortality is 10–20%.

OBESITY

Obesity is a pandemic with potentially disastrous consequences for health. More than 20% of adults in the UK and more than 30% in USA are obese. The prevalence of obesity is increasing.

The pandemic reflects changes in both energy intake and expenditure. The estimated average global daily supply of food energy per person increased from ~2350 kcal in the 1960s to ~2800 kcal in the 1990s. Portion sizes, particularly of sugary drinks and high-fat snacks, have increased. Corresponding changes in energy expenditure are important; obesity is correlated positively with hours spent watching television, and inversely with physical activity.

Although obese people were ridiculed in the past when they bemoaned their inability to control their weight, it is likely that susceptibility does vary between individuals. Twin studies confirm a genetic pattern of inheritance, suggesting a polygenic disorder. In a few cases, specific causal factors can be identified, such as hypothyroidism, Cushing's syndrome or insulinoma. Drugs implicated include: tricyclic antidepressants, sulphonylureas, sodium valproate and β-blockers.

Complications of obesity

Health consequences of obesity include:

• Metabolic syndrome (p. 388). • Non-alcoholic steatohepatitis. • Cirrhosis. • Sleep apnoea. • Osteoarthritis.

Obesity has adverse effects on both mortality and morbidity; life expectancy is reduced by 13 yrs amongst obese smokers. Coronary heart disease is the major cause of death but cancer rates are also increased.

Clinical features and investigations

Obesity can be quantified using the body mass index (BMI = weight in kilograms divided by the height in metres squared (kg/m^2)):
• Normal 18.5–25. • Overweight 25–30. • Obese >30.

A dietary history may be helpful in guiding dietary advice, but is susceptible to under-reporting of consumption. Alcohol consumption is an important source of energy intake.

• All obese patients should have thyroid function tests performed, and an overnight dexamethasone suppression test or 24-hr urine free cortisol if Cushing's syndrome is suspected. • Assessment of other cardiovascular risk factors is important. • BP should be measured, and type 2 diabetes and dyslipidaemia detected by measuring blood glucose and serum lipids. • Elevated transaminases suggest non-alcoholic fatty liver disease.

Management

The health risks of obesity are largely reversible. Interventions which reduce weight in studies in obese patients have also been shown to ameliorate cardiovascular risk factors. Lifestyle advice which lowers body weight and increases physical exercise reduces the incidence of type 2 diabetes.

Most patients seeking assistance will have attempted weight loss previously, sometimes repeatedly. An empathetic explanation of energy balance, recognising that some individuals are more susceptible to obesity, is important. Appropriate weight loss goals (e.g. 10% of body weight) should be agreed.

Lifestyle advice: All patients should be advised to maximise their physical activity by incorporating it into the daily routine (e.g. walking rather than driving to work). Changes in eating behaviour (including portion size control, avoidance of snacking, regular meals to encourage satiety, and use of artificial sweeteners) should be discussed.

Weight loss diets: In overweight people, the lifestyle advice given above may gradually succeed. In obese patients, more active intervention is usually required. Weight loss diets require a reduction in daily total energy intake of ~2.5 MJ (600 kcal) from the patient's normal consumption. The goal is to lose ~0.5 kg/week. Patient compliance is the major determinant of success. In some patients more rapid weight loss is required, e.g. in preparation for surgery. There is no role for starvation diets, which carry a risk of sudden death from heart disease. Very low calorie diets produce weight loss of 1.5–2.5 kg/week, but require the supervision of a physician and nutritionist.

Drugs: Drug therapy is usually reserved for obese patients with a high risk of complications. Patients who continue to take anti-obesity drugs tend to regain weight with time. This has led to the recommendation that anti-obesity drugs are used short-term to maximise the weight loss in patients who are demonstrating their adherence to a low calorie diet by current weight loss.

• Orlistat: inhibits pancreatic and gastric lipases, reducing dietary fat absorption by ~30%. Side-effects relate to the resultant fat malabsorption: namely, loose stools, oily spotting, faecal urgency, flatus and malabsorption of fat-soluble vitamins. • Sibutramine: reduces food intake by blocking re-uptake of both noradrenaline and 5-HT in the CNS. Side-effects include dry mouth, constipation, insomnia, tachycardia and hypertension. It is therefore a second choice after orlistat and cannot be used in those with hypertension or cardiovascular disease.

Surgery: Surgery to reduce the size of the stomach is the most effective long-term treatment for obesity. It should be contemplated in patients with a very high risk of developing the complications of obesity, in whom dietary and drug therapy has been ineffective. The mechanism of weight loss may not relate to limiting the stomach capacity per se, but rather in disrupting the release of ghrelin from the stomach, which signals hunger in the hypothalamus. Mortality is low in experienced centres but post-operative complications are common.

DISEASES OF THE MOUTH AND SALIVARY GLANDS

Aphthous ulceration: Common, superficial, painful and idiopathic. In severe cases other causes, such as infection, drug reaction or Behçet's syndrome, must be considered. Topical triamcinolone in Orabase or choline salicylate gel can aid healing.

Squamous carcinoma of the oral cavity: Common world-wide and increasing in the UK. Mortality is ~50%, largely as a result of late diagnosis. Poor diet, alcohol excess, smoking or tobacco chewing, or chewing areca nuts wrapped in betel leaves ('betel nuts') are the main risk factors. Suspicious lesions should be biopsied if treatment for local trauma or infection fails to produce improvement after 2 wks. Treatment is by resection, radiotherapy or both.

Vincent's angina: Deep, sloughing gum ulcers, caused by invasion of the mucous membranes by organisms such as *Borrelia vincentii*. Poor oral hygiene, malnutrition, debility and AIDS predispose. Symptoms include halitosis and fever, and treatment with hydrogen peroxide mouthwashes and broad-spectrum antibiotics is indicated.

Candida albicans: A normal mouth commensal which proliferates to cause thrush in babies, patients receiving corticosteroids, antibiotic or cytotoxic therapy, people with diabetes and the immunosuppressed. White patches are seen on the tongue and buccal mucosa. Dysphagia suggests pharyngeal and oesophageal candidiasis. A clinical diagnosis is sufficient to instigate therapy, using nystatin or amphotericin suspensions or lozenges.

Parotitis: Due to viral or bacterial infection. Mumps causes a self-limiting acute parotitis. Bacterial parotitis usually occurs as a complication of major surgery and can be avoided by good post-operative care. Broad-spectrum antibiotics are required, whilst surgical drainage is necessary if abscesses are present.

DISEASES OF THE OESOPHAGUS

GASTRO-OESOPHAGEAL REFLUX DISEASE (GORD)

Gastro-oesophageal reflux resulting in heartburn affects ~30% of the general population.

GORD develops when the oesophageal mucosa is exposed to gastric contents for prolonged periods, resulting in symptoms and, in a proportion of cases, oesophagitis. Reflux may occur if there is reduced oesophageal sphincter tone or frequent inappropriate sphincter relaxation. Herniation of the stomach through the diaphragm (hiatus hernia) occurs in 30% of the population >50 and is often asymptomatic. It causes reflux because of loss of the oblique angle between the cardia and oesophagus. Almost all patients who develop oesophagitis, Barrett's oesophagus or peptic strictures have a hiatus hernia. Defective oesophageal peristaltic activity is common in patients with oesophagitis, and persists after oesophagitis has been healed by acid-suppressing drugs.

Gastric acid is the most important oesophageal irritant and there is a close relationship between acid exposure time and symptoms. Gastric emptying is delayed in patients with GORD. Increased intra-abdominal pressure due to pregnancy and obesity may contribute. Weight loss may improve symptoms. Dietary fat, chocolate, alcohol and coffee relax the lower oesophageal sphincter and may provoke symptoms.

Clinical features

• The major symptoms are heartburn and regurgitation, often provoked by bending, straining or lying down. • 'Waterbrash', reflex salivation on acid reflux, is often present. • Recent weight gain is common. • Some patients are woken at night by choking as refluxed fluid irritates the larynx. • Others develop odynophagia, dysphagia or atypical chest pain which may mimic angina and is probably due to reflux-induced oesophageal spasm.

Complications

Oesophagitis: Features a range of endoscopic findings, from mild redness to severe, bleeding ulceration with stricture formation, with a poor correlation between symptoms and appearances. A normal endoscopy and normal histology do not exclude significant reflux disease.

Barrett's oesophagus ('columnar lined oesophagus', CLO): A premalignant condition in which the squamous lining of the lower oesophagus is replaced by columnar mucosa with areas of metaplasia. It occurs in response to chronic reflux and is seen in 10% of endoscopies for reflux. The true prevalence may be up to 20 times greater, as it is often asymptomatic or first discovered when the patient develops oesophageal cancer. CLO carries a lifetime risk of oesophageal adenocarcinoma of ~10%. The absolute risk is low and >95% of patients with CLO die of causes other than oesophageal cancer. Prevalence is increasing, especially in white men aged >50. It is weakly associated with smoking but not alcohol. Duodenogastro-oesophageal reflux, containing bile, pancreatic enzymes and pepsin in addition to acid, may be important.

Diagnosis requires multiple biopsies to detect intestinal metaplasia and/or dysplasia.

Neither acid suppression nor antireflux surgery stops progression of CLO, and treatment is only indicated for symptoms of reflux or complications such as stricture. Endoscopic ablation or photodynamic therapy can induce regression but islands of glandular mucosa remain and cancer risk is not eliminated. Regular endoscopic surveillance is controversial; it can detect dysplasia and early malignancy but, because most CLO is undetected until cancer develops, will not reduce overall oesophageal cancer mortality.

Oesophagectomy is widely recommended for those with high-grade dysplasia (HGD), as the resected specimen harbours cancer in up to 40%. Close follow-up with biopsies every 3 mths is an alternative for those with HGD.

Iron deficiency anaemia: Occurs as a consequence of chronic blood loss from oesophagitis. Many such patients have bleeding from erosions in a hiatus hernia. Nevertheless, hiatus hernia is very common and other causes of blood loss, particularly colorectal cancer, must be considered even when endoscopy reveals oesophagitis and a hiatus hernia.

Benign oesophageal stricture: Develops as a consequence of longstanding oesophagitis, usually in elderly patients presenting with dysphagia for solids. A history of heartburn is common but not invariable in the elderly. Diagnosis is by endoscopy, when biopsies can be taken to exclude malignancy. Endoscopic balloon dilatation or bouginage is helpful, followed by long-term therapy with a PPI to reduce the risk of recurrence. Dentition should be checked and the patient advised to chew food thoroughly.

Gastric volvulus: Occasionally a massive intrathoracic hiatus hernia twists upon itself (gastric volvulus), causing complete obstruction, severe chest pain, vomiting and dysphagia. The diagnosis is made by CXR and barium swallow. Most resolve spontaneously but recur and surgery is usually advised.

Investigations

Young patients with typical symptoms of GORD can be treated empirically without investigation.

Endoscopy: Advisable if patients present in middle or old age, if symptoms are atypical or if complications are suspected. A normal endoscopy in a patient with typical symptoms should not preclude treatment for reflux.

24-hr pH monitoring: If the diagnosis is unclear after endoscopy or if surgery is considered. Intraluminal pH and symptoms are recorded during normal activities. A pH of <4 for more than 6–7% of the study is diagnostic of reflux.

Management

• Lifestyle advice should cover weight loss, avoidance of dietary triggers, elevation of the bed head, avoidance of late meals and giving up smoking. • Antacids, alginates and H_2-receptor antagonists relieve symptoms without healing oesophagitis. • PPIs relieve symptoms and heal oesophagitis in the majority, and are the treatment of choice for severe symptoms and complicated reflux disease. Recurrence is common and some patients require life-long treatment. • Surgery should be considered in patients who fail to respond, are unwilling to take long-term PPIs or have severe regurgitation. Although heartburn and regurgitation are alleviated in most patients, a few develop complications.

OTHER CAUSES OF OESOPHAGITIS

Infection: Oesophageal candidiasis is mentioned above (p. 431).

Corrosives: Suicide attempt by bleach or acid causes painful burns of the mouth and pharynx and erosive oesophagitis. Complications include perforation, mediastinitis and stricture. Early treatment is conservative (analgesia and nutritional support); vomiting and endoscopy are avoided to prevent perforation. Later, endoscopic dilatation of strictures is usually necessary, although hazardous.

Drugs: Potassium supplements and NSAIDs may cause oesophageal ulcers if tablets are trapped above a stricture. Bisphosphonates cause oesophageal ulceration and should be used with caution in patients with oesophageal disorders.

MOTILITY DISORDERS

PHARYNGEAL POUCH

Incoordination of swallowing leads to herniation of a pouch through the cricopharyngeus muscle. Most patients are elderly and asymptomatic, but regurgitation, halitosis and dysphagia can occur. A barium swallow demonstrates the pouch and may show pulmonary aspiration. Endoscopy may perforate the pouch. Surgical resection is indicated in symptomatic patients.

ACHALASIA OF THE OESOPHAGUS

Achalasia is characterised by a hypertonic lower oesophageal sphincter which fails to relax during swallowing and failure of propagated oesophageal contraction, with progressive dilatation. The cause is unknown, although failure of the local nerve supply is implicated. Chagas disease (infestation with *Trypanosoma cruzi*) is endemic in South America and causes an indistinguishable clinical syndrome (p. 112).

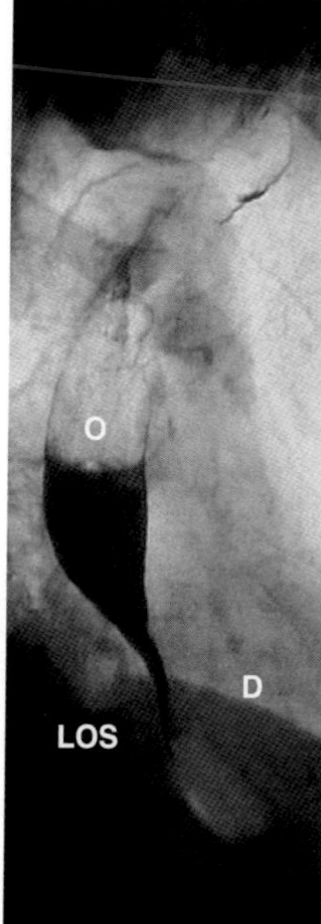

Fig. 12.2 Achalasia. X-ray showing a dilated, barium-filled oesophagus (O) with fluid level and distal tapering, and a closed lower oesophageal sphincter (LOS). (D = diaphragm).

Clinical features and investigations

Achalasia is rare, affecting 1 : 100 000 people. It usually develops slowly in middle age with intermittent dysphagia for solids, which is eased by drinking, standing and moving around. Heartburn is absent, but some patients experience severe chest pain due to oesophageal spasm. As dysphagia progresses, nocturnal pulmonary aspiration develops. Achalasia predisposes to squamous carcinoma of the oesophagus.

• CXR shows widening of the mediastinum and features of aspiration. • Barium swallow (Fig. 12.2) shows tapered narrowing of the lower oesophagus and a dilated, aperistaltic and food-filled oesophageal body. • Endoscopy is essential to rule out carcinoma. • Manometry confirms the non-relaxing lower oesophageal sphincter and poor contractility of the oesophageal body.

Management

Endoscopic dilatation: Dilatation of the oesophageal sphincter using a fluoroscopically positioned balloon improves symptoms in 80% of patients. Some require repeat dilatation but frequent recurrence is best treated surgically. Endoscopic injection of botulinum toxin into the sphincter induces remission, but relapse is common.

Surgical myotomy: Performed either as an open operation or laparoscopically, this is extremely effective. Both dilatation and myotomy may be complicated by gastro-oesophageal reflux, and for this reason myotomy is often augmented by an anti-reflux procedure and a PPI is given.

OTHER OESOPHAGEAL MOTILITY DISORDERS

Oesophageal spasm or abnormally forceful peristaltic activity: May lead to episodic chest pain mimicking angina. Oral or sublingual nitrates or nifedipine may relieve attacks of pain.

Systemic sclerosis: The oesophageal muscle is replaced by fibrous tissue, leading to heartburn, dysphagia, oesophagitis and benign strictures. Such patients require long-term therapy with PPIs. Dermatomyositis, rheumatoid arthritis and myasthenia gravis may also cause dysphagia.

Rings of submucosal fibrosis at the oesophago-gastric junction: Cause intermittent dysphagia, often in middle age.

Post-cricoid web: A rare complication of iron deficiency anaemia, which may predispose to squamous carcinoma. Benign strictures are treated by endoscopic balloon dilatation.

TUMOURS OF THE OESOPHAGUS

CARCINOMA OF THE OESOPHAGUS

Almost all are adenocarcinoma or squamous cancers. Small-cell cancer is a rare third type.

Squamous cancer: Rare in the West (approx. 4 : 100 000) but common in Iran, parts of Africa and China (200 : 100 000). Squamous cancer can arise anywhere in the oesophagus but almost all tumours above the lower third of the oesophagus are squamous.

Adenocarcinoma: Arises in the lower third of the oesophagus from Barrett's oesophagus or from the cardia of the stomach. Incidence is increasing in the UK (approx. 5 : 100 000).

Clinical features and investigations

• There is progressive, painless dysphagia for solids. • Food bolus obstruction may occur acutely. • Chest pain or hoarseness suggests mediastinal invasion. • Weight loss is common. • Fistulation between the oesophagus and the airway leads to coughing after swallowing, pneumonia and pleural effusion. • Physical signs include cachexia and cervical lymphadenopathy but these may be absent.

Endoscopy with biopsy is the investigation of choice. Subsequent investigations are performed to TNM-stage the tumour and define operability. Thoracic and abdominal CT define metastatic spread and local invasion, which may preclude surgery. Endoscopic ultrasound (EUS) with nodal sampling is the most sensitive technique.

Management and prognosis

Approximately 70% of patients have extensive disease at presentation. In these, treatment is palliative and based upon relief of dysphagia and pain.

Endoscopic laser ablation or stenting may improve swallowing, while palliative radiotherapy may shrink both squamous cancers and adenocarcinomas.

Despite treatment, the 5-yr survival of patients with oesophageal cancer is 6–9%. Tumours which have breached the oesophageal wall and involve lymph nodes (T3, N1) have a 5-yr survival of ~10% after surgery. This figure improves significantly for less extensive disease. Five-yr survival following 'potentially curative' surgery (all visible tumour removed) is 30%, and may be improved further by pre-operative chemotherapy. Although squamous carcinomas are radiosensitive, radiotherapy alone is associated with a 5-yr survival of only 5%.

PERFORATION OF THE OESOPHAGUS

The most common cause is endoscopic perforation complicating dilatation or intubation. A perforated peptic stricture is usually managed conservatively using broad-spectrum antibiotics and parenteral nutrition; most heal within days. Malignant, caustic and radiotherapy stricture perforations require surgery.

Spontaneous oesophageal perforation results from forceful vomiting. Patients present with severe chest pain, shock, subcutaneous emphysema, pleural effusions and pneumothorax. The diagnosis is made using a water-soluble contrast swallow. Treatment is surgical and mortality is high.

DISEASES OF THE STOMACH AND DUODENUM

GASTRITIS

Acute gastritis: Most commonly results from alcohol, aspirin or NSAID ingestion. It is often asymptomatic and self-limiting, but may cause dyspepsia, anorexia, nausea, vomiting, haematemesis or melaena. In persistent cases, endoscopy is necessary to exclude peptic ulcer or cancer. Treatment involves avoiding the cause; symptomatic therapy with antacids, and acid suppression using PPIs or antiemetics may also be necessary.

Chronic gastritis: The most common cause of chronic gastritis is *H. pylori* infection. Correlation between symptoms and endoscopic and pathological findings is poor. Most patients are asymptomatic and do not require treatment but patients with dyspepsia may benefit from *H. pylori* eradication.

Autoimmune chronic gastritis: Usually asymptomatic and results from autoimmune activity against parietal cells in the body of the stomach. Circulating parietal cell and intrinsic factor antibodies may be present. In some patients gastric atrophy leads to loss of intrinsic factor secretion and pernicious anaemia. Other autoimmune conditions, particularly thyroid disease, may be present. There is a fourfold increase in gastric cancer.

PEPTIC ULCER DISEASE

'Peptic ulcer' means an ulcer in the lower oesophagus, stomach or duodenum, in the jejunum after gastrojejunostomy or, rarely, in the ileum adjacent to a Meckel's diverticulum. Ulcers in the stomach or duodenum may be acute or chronic; both penetrate the muscularis mucosae but acute ulcers show no evidence of fibrosis. Erosions do not penetrate the muscularis mucosae.

GASTRIC AND DUODENAL ULCER

The prevalence of peptic ulcer is decreasing in many Western communities as a result of *H. pylori* eradication therapy but it remains high in developing countries. The male to female ratio for duodenal ulcer varies from 5:1 to 2:1, whilst that for gastric ulcer is 2:1 or less.

Chronic gastric ulcer is usually single; most are situated on the lesser curve within the antrum. Duodenal ulcer usually occurs in the first part of the duodenum just distal to the junction of pyloric and duodenal mucosa. Gastric and duodenal ulcers coexist in 10% of patients and multiple ulcers occur in 10–15%.

H. pylori: In the UK the prevalence of *H. pylori* infection rises with age (reaching 50% in those aged >50); in the developing world it affects up to 90%. The bacteria spread by contact with gastric refluxate or vomit and, although infection is usually acquired in childhood, most colonised people remain healthy. Around 90% of duodenal ulcer patients and 70% of gastric ulcer patients are infected with *H. pylori*; the remaining 30% of gastric ulcers are due to NSAIDs.

H. pylori is a motile Gram-negative organism which uses multiple flagellae to burrow beneath the epithelial mucus layer. Here the pH is nearly neutral and any acidity is buffered by the organism's production of ammonia from urea. *H. pylori* exclusively colonises gastric-type epithelium and is only found in the duodenum at patches of gastric metaplasia. It stimulates chronic gastritis by provoking an inflammatory response in the epithelium.

In most people *H. pylori* causes antral gastritis with depletion of somatostatin. The subsequent hypergastrinaemia stimulates parietal cell acid production, but usually without clinical consequences. In a few patients, particularly smokers, this process is exaggerated, leading to duodenal ulceration. The pathogenesis of gastric ulcer is less clear but *H. pylori* probably acts by reducing gastric mucosal resistance to acid and pepsin. Occasionally, *H. pylori* causes a pan-gastritis, leading to gastric atrophy and hypochlorhydria, with bacterial proliferation in the stomach, predisposing to gastric cancer.

Many diagnostic tests for *H. pylori* infection are available (Box 12.7). Some require endoscopy; others are non-invasive. Overall, breath tests are best because of their accuracy, simplicity and non-invasiveness.

NSAIDs: See page 776.

Smoking: Increases the risk of gastric and, to a lesser extent, duodenal ulcer. Once the ulcer has formed, it is more likely to cause complications and less likely to heal if the patient smokes.

Acid-pepsin versus mucosal resistance: An ulcer forms when there is an imbalance between the digestive power of acid and pepsin, and the

12.7 METHODS FOR THE DIAGNOSIS OF *H. PYLORI* INFECTION		
Test	**Advantages**	**Disadvantages**
Non-invasive		
Serology	Rapid office kits available; good for population studies	Lacks sensitivity and specificity; cannot differentiate current from past infection
Urea breath tests	High sensitivity and specificity	^{14}C uses radioactivity; ^{13}C requires expensive mass spectrometer
Faecal antigen test	Cheap, accurate	Acceptability
Invasive (antral biopsy)		
Histology	Sensitivity and specificity	False negatives occur; takes several days to process
Rapid urease tests, e.g. CLO, Pyloritek	Cheap, quick; specificity	Lack sensitivity
Microbiological culture	'Gold standard'; defines antibiotic sensitivity	Slow and laborious; lacks sensitivity

ability of the mucosa to resist digestion. Ulcers occur only in the presence of acid and pepsin. Severe peptic ulceration nearly always occurs in patients with the Zollinger–Ellison syndrome (p. 443), who have very high acid secretion.

Most duodenal ulcer patients have markedly exaggerated acid secretion in response to gastrin stimulation. In gastric ulcer patients, impaired mucosal defence due to *H. pylori* infection, NSAIDs and smoking may be more important.

Clinical features and investigations

Peptic ulcer disease is a chronic condition with spontaneous relapse and remission extending over decades. Duodenal and gastric ulcers share common symptoms:

• Recurrent episodes of epigastric pain occur in relation to meals. • Vomiting occasionally occurs; persistent daily vomiting suggests gastric outlet obstruction.

In one-third of patients, especially elderly subjects taking NSAIDs, the history is less characteristic:

• Pain may be absent or experienced only as vague epigastric unease. Occasionally, the only symptoms are anorexia and nausea, or a sense of undue repletion after meals. • The ulcer may even be 'silent', presenting with anaemia from chronic undetected blood loss, haematemesis or acute perforation. • The diagnostic value of individual symptoms of ulcer disease is poor.

Endoscopy is the preferred investigation. Gastric ulcers may occasionally be malignant and therefore must always be biopsied and followed up to ensure healing.

Management

The aims of management are to relieve symptoms, induce healing and prevent recurrence.

H. pylori eradication: All patients with acute or chronic duodenal ulcer disease and those with gastric ulcers who are *H. pylori*-positive should receive eradication. This heals ulcers, prevents relapse and eliminates the need for long-term therapy in >90% of patients. A PPI is taken with two antibiotics (from amoxicillin, clarithromycin and metronidazole) for 7 days. First-line therapy is a PPI (12-hourly), clarithromycin 500 mg 12-hourly, and amoxicillin 1 g 12-hourly or metronidazole 400 mg 12-hourly, for 7 days. Second-line therapy is a PPI (12-hourly), bismuth 120 mg 6-hourly, metronidazole 400 mg 12-hourly, and tetracycline 500 mg 6-hourly, for 7 days. Compliance, side-effects and metronidazole resistance influence success rates.

Patients who remain infected after initial therapy should be offered second-line therapy. For those who are still colonised after two treatments, the choice lies between a third attempt with quadruple therapy (bismuth, PPI and two antibiotics) or long-term acid suppression.

H. pylori and NSAIDs are independent risk factors for ulcer but it is not clear whether patients requiring long-term NSAID therapy should first undergo eradication therapy to reduce ulcer risk. This is probably not necessary in young, fit patients with no history of ulcer or dyspepsia, but a 'test and treat' strategy for older patients with major comorbidity or previous ulcer history is recommended. Subsequent co-prescription of a PPI with the NSAID is advised but is not always necessary for patients being given low-dose aspirin.

General measures: Cigarette smoking, aspirin and NSAIDs should be avoided. Alcohol in moderation is not harmful and no special dietary advice is required.

Short-term management: Many drugs are available for the short-term management of acid peptic symptoms (Box 12.8).

Maintenance treatment: Should not be necessary after successful *H. pylori* eradication.

Surgical treatment: The cure of most ulcers by *H. pylori* eradication therapy and the availability of safe, potent acid-suppressing drugs have made elective surgery for peptic ulcer disease uncommon. Non-healing gastric ulcer is treated by partial gastrectomy in which the ulcer and the ulcer-bearing area of the stomach are resected to exclude an underlying cancer. In the emergency situation biopsies are taken, then 'under-running' the ulcer for bleeding or 'oversewing' (patch repair) for perforation is sufficient.

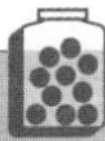

12.8 DRUGS USED IN THE SHORT-TERM MANAGEMENT OF PEPTIC ULCERS		
Group	**Examples**	**Mechanism**
Antacids and alginates	Aluminium hydroxide, magnesium trisilicate, alginic acid	Antacids; alginates form protective mucosal 'raft'
H_2-antagonists	Ranitidine, cimetidine, famotidine, nizatidine	Competitive inhibitors of H_2-receptors on parietal and ECL cells
Proton pump inhibitors (PPIs)	Omeprazole, esomeprazole, lansoprazole, pantoprazole, rabeprazole	Irreversible inhibitors of H^+/K^+ ATPase on parietal cell surface
Chelates	Tripotassium dicitratobismuthate	Ammoniacal suspension of complex bismuth salt; has anti-*H. pylori* activity and enhances mucosal protection
Complex salts	Sucralfate	Aluminium salt of sucrose octasulphate; little effect on acid—may protect ulcer base from peptic activity and enhance epithelial cell turnover
Prostaglandin analogues	Misoprostol	Enhance mucosal blood flow, stimulate mucus and bicarbonate secretion; stimulate epithelial proliferation

Complications of gastric resection or vagotomy

Although gastric surgery is now rarely needed for benign disease, many patients underwent operations in the pre-*H. pylori* era and some degree of disability is seen in up to 50% of these.

Dumping: Rapid gastric emptying leads to distension of the proximal small intestine as the hypertonic contents draw fluid into the lumen. This causes abdominal discomfort, flushing, palpitations, sweating, tachycardia, hypotension and diarrhoea after eating. Patients should avoid large meals with high carbohydrate content.

Bile reflux gastritis: Duodenogastric bile reflux leads to chronic gastritis. This is usually asymptomatic but dyspepsia can occur. Symptomatic treatment with aluminium-containing antacids or sucralfate may be effective. A few patients require revisional surgery.

Diarrhoea and maldigestion: Diarrhoea 1–2 hrs after eating may develop after any peptic ulcer operation. Rapid stomach emptying, inadequate mixing with pancreatic and biliary secretions, reduced small intestinal transit times and bacterial overgrowth may lead to malabsorption. Dietary advice should be given to eat small, dry meals with reduced refined carbohydrates; drugs such as codeine phosphate or loperamide are also helpful.

Weight loss: Most patients lose weight after surgery and 30–40% are unable to regain the lost weight. The usual cause is reduced intake because of a small gastric remnant, but diarrhoea and mild steatorrhoea also contribute.

Anaemia: Common many years after subtotal gastrectomy. Iron deficiency is the most common cause; folic acid and B_{12} deficiency are much less frequent. Inadequate dietary iron and folate, lack of acid and intrinsic factor secretion, mild chronic low-grade blood loss from the gastric remnant and recurrent ulceration are responsible.

Metabolic bone disease: Both osteoporosis and osteomalacia occur as a consequence of calcium and vitamin D malabsorption.

Gastric cancer: An increased risk of gastric cancer has been reported. The risk is highest in those with hypochlorhydria, duodenogastric reflux of bile, smoking and *H. pylori* infection. Although the relative risk is increased, the absolute risk of cancer remains low and endoscopic surveillance is not indicated following gastric surgery.

Complications of peptic ulcer

Perforation: Allows stomach contents to escape into the peritoneum, causing peritonitis. It is more common in duodenal than in gastric ulcers. About one-quarter of cases occur in acute ulcers, often with NSAIDs. It causes:

• Sudden, severe pain of perforation, often the first sign of ulcer. It starts in the upper abdomen and becomes generalised. Shoulder tip pain due to diaphragmatic irritation, shallow respiration due to pain and shock are common. • Generalised rigidity. • Absent bowel sounds. • Loss of liver dullness due to gas under the diaphragm.

Rigidity persists, and although pain may temporarily improve, the patient's condition later deteriorates with general peritonitis. In at least 50% of cases an erect CXR shows free air beneath the diaphragm. If not, a water-soluble contrast swallow will confirm perforation.

After resuscitation, the acute perforation is closed surgically. Following surgery *H. pylori* should be treated (if present) and NSAIDs avoided. The mortality from perforation is 25%, reflecting the age and comorbidity of the patients.

Gastric outlet obstruction: The most common cause is an ulcer near the pylorus, but occasional cases are due to antral cancer or adult hypertrophic pyloric stenosis.

Clinical features include:

• Nausea. • Vomiting of large quantities of gastric content. • Abdominal distension.

Examination reveals wasting, dehydration and a succussion splash persisting 4 hrs or more after the last meal. Visible gastric peristalsis is diagnostic.

Investigations are as follows:

• Low serum chloride and potassium. • Bicarbonate and urea are raised; dehydration results in enhanced renal absorption of Na^+ in exchange for H^+ and paradoxical aciduria. • Nasogastric aspiration of at least 200 ml after an overnight fast suggests the diagnosis. • Endoscopy is performed after the stomach has been emptied by nasogastric tube. Balloon dilatation of benign stenoses may be possible. • Barium studies fail to distinguish between peptic ulcer and cancer, and barium may be retained in the stomach.

Management includes:

• Nasogastric suction and the administration of large volumes of i.v. fluids with potassium. Correction of metabolic alkalosis is not required. • PPIs may heal ulcers, relieve pyloric oedema and overcome the need for surgery. • In other patients partial gastrectomy after a 7-day period of nasogastric aspiration is necessary.

Bleeding: See pages 418–420.

ZOLLINGER–ELLISON SYNDROME

This rare disorder (0.1% of duodenal ulcers) is characterised by the triad of severe peptic ulceration, gastric acid hypersecretion and a non-beta cell islet tumour of the pancreas ('gastrinoma'). It is most common between 30 and 50 yrs of age. The gastrinoma secretes large amounts of gastrin, which stimulates and increases the parietal cell mass. The high acid output inactivates pancreatic lipase and precipitates bile acids. Diarrhoea and steatorrhoea result. Most tumours occur in the proximal duodenal wall or the pancreatic head. Half are multiple, and over half are malignant but slow-growing. Multiple endocrine neoplasia (MEN) type 1 (p. 382) is present in 20–60%.

Multiple, severe peptic ulcers unresponsive to standard therapy are usual. The history is usually short; bleeding and perforations are common. Diarrhoea occurs in one-third of patients and can be the presenting feature.

Hypersecretion of acid under basal conditions with little increase following pentagastrin may be confirmed by gastric aspiration. Serum gastrin is grossly elevated (10- to 1000-fold). Tumour localisation is by endoscopic USS and radio-labelled somatostatin receptor scintigraphy.

Approximately 30% of small and single tumours can be localised and resected. In the majority of patients continuous therapy with high-dose omeprazole heals ulcers and alleviates diarrhoea. Subcutaneous octreotide reduces gastrin secretion and is sometimes used. All patients should be monitored for the development of other manifestations of MEN 1.

FUNCTIONAL DISORDERS

NON-ULCER DYSPEPSIA

This is defined as chronic dyspepsia (pain or upper abdominal discomfort) in the absence of organic disease. Other commonly reported symptoms include fullness, bloating and nausea. The aetiology covers a spectrum of mucosal, motility and psychiatric disorders.

Patients are usually young (<40 yrs) and women are affected twice as commonly as men.

Clinical features and investigations

• Abdominal pain is associated with a combination of other 'dyspeptic' symptoms, the most common being nausea, early satiety and bloating after meals. • Pain or nausea on waking is characteristic, and direct enquiry may elicit symptoms of irritable bowel syndrome. • Peptic ulcer disease and intra-abdominal malignancy must be considered. • Patients often appear anxious, but there are no diagnostic signs and no weight loss. • A drug history should be taken and depression considered. • Alcohol misuse should be suspected when early morning nausea and retching are prominent.

The history will often suggest the diagnosis but in older subjects an endoscopy is necessary to exclude mucosal disease.

Management

The most important elements are explanation and reassurance. Possible psychological factors should be explored and the concept of psychological influences on gut function should be explained. Idiosyncratic diets are of little benefit, but fat restriction may help.

Drug treatment is not especially successful but trials of antacids, metoclopramide, domperidone or H_2-receptor antagonists may be helpful according to symptoms. Low-dose amitriptyline sometimes helps. The role of *H. pylori* eradication remains controversial. Counselling or psychotherapy may help in those with major stress.

FUNCTIONAL VOMITING

This disorder typically occurs on wakening or immediately after breakfast and is probably a reaction to facing up to the worries of everyday life; in the young it can be due to school phobia. Early morning vomiting also occurs in pregnancy, alcohol misuse and depression. There is little or no weight loss.

In all patients it is essential to exclude other common causes. Tranquillisers and antiemetic drugs have only a secondary place in management. Antidepressants may be effective.

GASTROPARESIS

Defective gastric emptying without obstruction can be due to inherited or acquired disorders of the gastric pacemaker, or secondary to disorders of autonomic nerves (particularly diabetic neuropathy) or the gastroduodenal musculature (e.g. systemic sclerosis and amyloidosis). Early satiety and vomiting are typical symptoms; abdominal fullness and a succussion splash may be present on examination. Treatment is with metoclopramide and domperidone.

TUMOURS OF THE STOMACH

GASTRIC CARCINOMA

Gastric cancer is extremely common in China, Japan and parts of South America, less common in the UK and uncommon in the USA. Second-generation Japanese migrants in the USA have a much lower incidence than recent migrants, confirming the importance of environmental factors. Gastric cancer is more common in men and the incidence rises after 50 yrs of age.

H. pylori infection is associated with gastric cancer and may be responsible for 60–70% of cases. Infection at an early age may be important. A few *H. pylori*-infected individuals become hypo- or achlorhydric and these people are thought to be at greatest risk.

Diets rich in salted, smoked or pickled foods and lacking fresh fruit and vegetables as well as vitamins C and A may predispose. Carcinogenic compounds formed by nitrite-reducing bacteria which colonise the achlorhydric stomach may also contribute. No predominant genetic abnormality has been identified, although cancer risk is increased two- to threefold in first-degree relatives of patients.

Virtually all tumours are adenocarcinomas arising from mucus-secreting cells in the base of the gastric crypts. In the developing world 50% of gastric cancers develop in the antrum, 20–30% in the gastric body, and 20% in the cardia. In Western populations, however, proximal gastric tumours are becoming more common than those arising in the body and distal stomach. This may reflect changes in lifestyle or the decreasing prevalence of *H. pylori* in the West. Diffuse submucosal infiltration by a scirrhous cancer (linitis plastica) is uncommon. Early gastric cancer is defined as cancer confined to the mucosa or submucosa, regardless of lymph node involvement. It is common in Japan, where widespread screening is practised. Over 80% of patients in the West present with advanced gastric cancer.

Clinical features

• Early gastric cancer is usually asymptomatic but may be discovered during endoscopy for dyspepsia. • Weight loss occurs in two-thirds of patients with advanced cancers. • Ulcer-like pain occurs in 50%. • Anaemia from occult bleeding is also common. • Anorexia and nausea occur in one-third. • Early satiety, haematemesis, melaena and dyspepsia are less common features. • Dysphagia occurs in tumours which obstruct the gastro-oesophageal junction.

Examination may reveal no abnormalities, but signs of weight loss, anaemia or a palpable epigastric mass are not infrequent. Jaundice or ascites may signify metastatic spread. Occasionally, tumour spread occurs to the supraclavicular lymph nodes, umbilicus or ovaries. Paraneoplastic phenomena, such as acanthosis nigricans, thrombophlebitis and dermatomyositis, occur rarely. Metastases occur most commonly in the liver, lungs, peritoneum and bone marrow.

Investigations

• For diagnosis and staging endoscopy is the investigation of choice and should be performed promptly in any dyspeptic patient with 'alarm features' (Box 12.2). • Multiple biopsies from the edge and base of a gastric ulcer are required and brush cytology also improves the diagnostic yield. • Once the diagnosis is made, CT is necessary for accurate staging and assessment of resectability, but may miss small involved lymph nodes. • Even with these techniques, laparoscopy is required to determine whether the tumour is resectable.

Management and prognosis

Surgery: Resection offers the only hope of cure, which can be achieved in 90% of patients with early gastric cancer. Extensive lymph node resection may increase survival rates but carries greater morbidity. Even for those who cannot be cured, palliative resection may be necessary when presentation is with bleeding or gastric outflow obstruction. Complete removal of all macroscopic tumour combined with lymphadenectomy will achieve a 50–60% 5-yr survival. There is no current evidence to suggest that chemotherapy improves survival rates, and post-operative radiotherapy has no value.

Unresectable tumours: Modest palliation of symptoms can be achieved in some patients with chemotherapy. Endoscopic insertion of stents or laser ablation of tumour for control of dysphagia or bleeding benefits some patients.

The overall prognosis remains very poor, with <30% surviving 5 yrs. Earlier detection of tumours offers the best hope of improved survival.

GASTRIC LYMPHOMA

Primary gastric lymphoma accounts for <5% of all gastric malignancies, but 60% of primary GI lymphomas occur at this site. Lymphoid tissue is not found in the normal stomach but lymphoid aggregates develop in the presence of *H. pylori* infection.

The clinical presentation is similar to that of gastric cancer and endoscopically the tumour appears as a polypoid or ulcerating mass. High-grade B-cell lymphomas are treated by a combination of chemotherapy, surgery and radiotherapy. The prognosis depends on the stage at diagnosis. Features predicting a favourable prognosis are:

• Stage I or II disease. • Small resectable tumours. • Tumours with low-grade histology • Age <60 yrs.

DISEASES OF THE SMALL INTESTINE

DISORDERS CAUSING MALABSORPTION

COELIAC DISEASE

Coeliac disease is an immunologically mediated inflammatory disorder of the small bowel occurring in genetically susceptible individuals. It is caused by intolerance to wheat gluten and similar proteins in rye, barley and oats. It can result in malabsorption and responds to a gluten-free diet. The condition occurs world-wide but is more common in northern Europe.

The precise pathogenesis is unclear but immunological responses to gluten play a key role. Tissue transglutaminase (TTG) is now recognised as the autoantigen for anti-endomysial antibodies. Coeliac disease is associated with other HLA-linked autoimmune disorders and with certain other diseases (Box 12.9).

Clinical features

• Infancy: failure to thrive, malabsorption. • Older children: delayed growth and puberty, malnutrition, mild abdominal distension. • Adults: peak onset in fifth decade. • Florid malabsorption in some; others present with tiredness, weight loss, iron or folate deficiency. • Oral ulceration, dyspepsia and bloating.

Investigations

Duodenal or jejunal biopsy: Villous atrophy is characteristic but other causes should also be considered (Box 12.10 and Fig. 12.3).

12.9 DISEASE ASSOCIATIONS OF COELIAC DISEASE

- Insulin-dependent diabetes mellitus (2–8%)
- Thyroid disease (5%)
- Primary biliary cirrhosis (3%)
- Sjögren's syndrome (3%)
- IgA deficiency (2%)
- Pernicious anaemia
- Inflammatory bowel disease
- Sarcoidosis
- Neurological complications—encephalopathy, cerebellar atrophy, peripheral neuropathy, epilepsy
- Myasthenia gravis
- Dermatitis herpetiformis
- Down's syndrome
- Enteropathy-associated T-cell lymphoma
- Small bowel carcinoma
- Squamous carcinoma of oesophagus
- Ulcerative jejunitis
- Pancreatic insufficiency
- Microscopic colitis
- Splenic atrophy

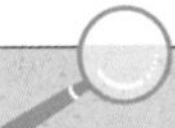

12.10 IMPORTANT CAUSES OF SUBTOTAL VILLOUS ATROPHY

- Coeliac disease
- Tropical sprue
- Dermatitis herpetiformis
- Lymphoma
- AIDS enteropathy
- Giardiasis
- Hypogammaglobulinaemia
- Radiation
- Whipple's disease
- Zollinger–Ellison syndrome

A 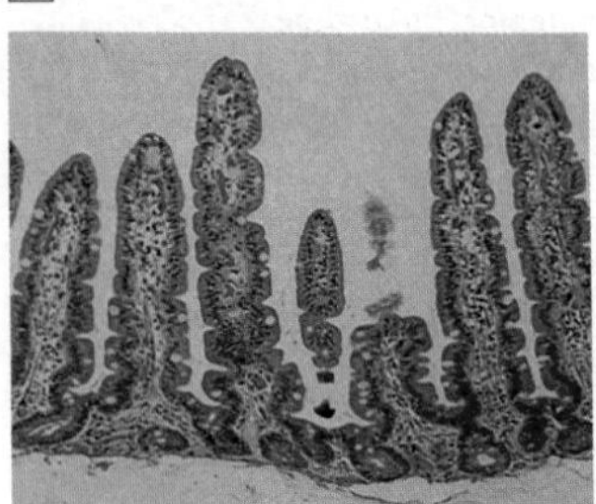

B 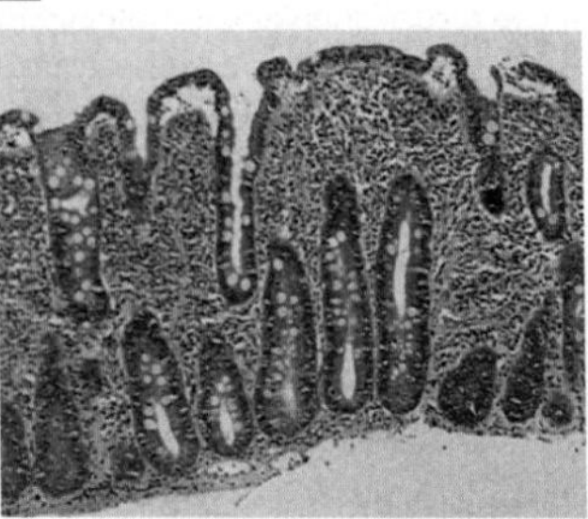

Fig. 12.3 Jejunal mucosa. A Normal. B Jejunum in coeliac disease showing subtotal villous atrophy and marked inflammatory infiltrate.

Antibodies: Serum antigliadin (especially IgA) and anti-endomysial antibodies are detectable in most untreated cases. IgG antibodies must be analysed in patients with coexisting IgA deficiency. TTG assays are easier to perform, semi-quantitative and more accurate in patients with IgA deficiency. These antibody tests are not a substitute for small bowel biopsy; they usually become negative with successful treatment.

Haematology and biochemistry: There is microcytic or macrocytic anaemia from iron or folate deficiency. Target cells, spherocytes and Howell–Jolly bodies are due to hyposplenism. Calcium, magnesium, total protein, albumin and vitamin D are reduced.

Measurement of bone density by DEXA scanning: To look for evidence of metabolic bone disease.

Management

• Life-long gluten-free diet. • Correction of deficiencies of iron, folate, calcium and vitamin D. • Regular monitoring of symptoms, weight and nutrition. • Repeat jejunal biopsies: should be reserved for patients who do not symptomatically improve or whose antibodies remain persistently positive.

Rarely, patients are 'refractory' and require corticosteroids or immunosuppressive drugs to induce remission. Dietary compliance should be carefully assessed, but if this is satisfactory, other conditions such as pancreatic insufficiency or microscopic colitis should be sought, as should complications of coeliac disease such as ulcerative jejunitis or enteropathy-associated T-cell lymphoma.

Complications

There is an increased risk of malignancy, particularly of enteropathy-associated T-cell lymphoma, small bowel carcinoma and squamous carcinoma of the oesophagus.

Ulcerative jejunoileitis may occur; fever, pain, obstruction or perforation may then supervene. The diagnosis is made by laparotomy and full-thickness biopsy. Corticosteroids are used with mixed success and some patients require surgical resection and parenteral nutrition.

Metabolic bone disease occurs, but is less common in patients who adhere strictly to a gluten-free diet.

DERMATITIS HERPETIFORMIS

This is characterised by crops of intensely itchy blisters over the elbows, knees, back and buttocks. Almost all patients have partial villous atrophy on jejunal biopsy, even though they usually have no GI symptoms. The rash usually responds to a gluten-free diet but some patients require additional treatment with dapsone.

TROPICAL SPRUE

Tropical sprue is a chronic, progressive malabsorption with abnormalities of small intestinal structure and function occurring in patients in or from the tropics. The disease occurs mainly in the West Indies and in Asia, including southern India, Malaysia and Indonesia. It often begins after an acute diarrhoeal illness. Small bowel bacterial overgrowth with *Escherichia coli*, *Enterobacter* and *Klebsiella* is frequently seen. Partial villous atrophy is more common than subtotal villous atrophy.

Clinical features include:

• Diarrhoea, abdominal distension, anorexia, fatigue and weight loss. • Onset of severe diarrhoea: may be sudden and accompanied by fever.

When chronic:

• Megaloblastic anaemia (folic acid malabsorption). • Ankle oedema, glossitis and stomatitis: common. • Remissions and relapses: may occur.

The differential diagnosis is infective diarrhoea, including giardiasis (p. 116).

Tetracycline (250 mg 6-hourly for 28 days) brings about long-term remission or cure. Folic acid (5 mg daily) improves symptoms and jejunal morphology.

SMALL BOWEL BACTERIAL OVERGROWTH ('BLIND LOOP SYNDROME')

The normal duodenum and jejunum contain coliform organisms, but numbers never exceed 10^3/ml. In bacterial overgrowth there may be 10^8–10^{10}/ml organisms, most of which are normally found only in the colon. Disorders which predispose to bacterial overgrowth include hypochlorhydria, impaired motility (e.g. systemic sclerosis, diabetes), surgical resection, fistulae and hypogammaglobulinaemia.

Clinical features include:

• Watery diarrhoea and/or steatorrhoea. • Anaemia due to B_{12} deficiency.

There may also be symptoms from the underlying intestinal cause.

Investigations are as follows:

• Serum vitamin B_{12} concentration is low, whilst folate levels are normal or elevated. • Barium follow-through or small bowel enema may reveal blind loops or fistulae. • Endoscopic duodenal biopsies exclude mucosal disease such as coeliac disease. • Endoscopic aspiration of jejunal contents is carried out for anaerobic and aerobic culture. • In glucose, hydrogen or ^{14}C-glycocholic acid breath tests serial breath samples are measured after oral ingestion of the test material. Bacteria in the small bowel cause an early rise in breath hydrogen or ^{14}C.

Management is of the underlying cause. Tetracycline is the treatment of choice, although up to 50% of patients do not respond. Metronidazole or ciprofloxacin is an alternative. Some patients require up to 4 wks of treatment and a few cases become chronic. Intramuscular vitamin B_{12} supplementation is needed in the latter.

WHIPPLE'S DISEASE

This rare condition is characterised by infiltration of small intestinal mucosa by 'foamy' macrophages which stain positive with periodic acid–Schiff (PAS) reagent. Electron microscopy reveals small Gram-positive bacilli (*Tropheryma whipplei*) within the macrophages.

This is a multisystem disease (Box 12.11). Middle-aged men are most commonly affected and the presentation depends on the pattern of organ involvement. Low-grade fever is common.

Whipple's disease is often fatal if untreated but responds well to co-trimoxazole, and to a lesser degree, to tetracycline. Relapse occurs in up to one-third of patients, often within the CNS, in which case 2 wks of parenteral ceftriaxone, followed by 6–12 mths of oral co-trimoxazole are necessary.

ILEAL RESECTION

Ileal resection is usually performed as treatment for Crohn's disease. The long-term effects depend on the site and the amount of intestine resected, and vary from trivial to life-threatening.

Clinical features include:

• Diarrhoea. • Fat malabsorption due to loss of bile salts. • Gallstones due to lithogenic bile. • Oxalate renal calculi. • Vitamin B_{12} deficiency.

Contrast studies of the small bowel and tests of B_{12} and bile acid absorption are useful.

12.11 CLINICAL FEATURES OF WHIPPLE'S DISEASE	
GI	Diarrhoea, steatorrhoea, protein-losing enteropathy
Musculoskeletal	Seronegative large joint arthritis
Cardiac	Pericarditis, myocarditis, endocarditis
Pulmonary	Pleurisy, cough, infiltrates
Haematological	Anaemia, lymphadenopathy
Other	Fever, pigmentation, fits

Parenteral vitamin B_{12} supplementation is necessary. Diarrhoea usually responds well to colestyramine or aluminium hydroxide therapy.

SHORT BOWEL SYNDROME

Short bowel syndrome is defined as malabsorption resulting from extensive small intestinal resection or disease. Loss of surface area for digestion and absorption is the key problem.

Clinical features include:

• Large-volume jejunostomy fluid loss. • If colon is preserved: diarrhoea and steatorrhoea. • Dehydration and signs of hypovolaemia. • Weight loss, loss of muscle bulk and malnutrition.

Management entails:

• Total parenteral nutrition (TPN – see p. 428). • PPI therapy to reduce gastric secretions. • Enteral feeding, to be cautiously introduced after 1–2 wks and slowly increased as tolerated.

The principles of long-term management are:

• Detailed nutritional assessments at regular intervals. • Monitoring of fluid and electrolyte balance. Patients can usually be taught how to do this for themselves. A readily available supply of oral rehydration solution is useful for intercurrent illness. • Adequate calorie and protein intake. Fats and medium-chain triglyceride supplements should be taken as tolerated. • Replacement of B_{12}, calcium, vitamin D, magnesium, zinc and folic acid. • Antidiarrhoeal agents, e.g. loperamide or codeine phosphate.

In patients who are unable to maintain positive fluid balance, octreotide to reduce GI secretions is useful, but some patients require long-term TPN. Small bowel transplantation may be an option.

RADIATION ENTERITIS AND PROCTOCOLITIS

Intestinal damage occurs in 10–15% of patients undergoing radiotherapy for abdominal or pelvic malignancy. The risk varies with total dose, dosing schedule and the use of concomitant chemotherapy.

Acutely, there is nausea, vomiting, cramping abdominal pain and diarrhoea. When the rectum and colon are involved, mucus, bleeding and tenesmus occur. The chronic phase develops after 5–10 yrs in some patients and may feature bleeding from telangiectasis, fistulae, adhesions, strictures or malabsorption.

Sigmoidoscopy appearances resemble ulcerative proctitis. Colonoscopy shows the extent of the lesion. Barium follow-through shows small bowel strictures, ulcers and fistulae.

Management entails:

• Acute phase: codeine, loperamide, corticosteroid enemas for proctitis and antibiotics for bacterial overgrowth. • Nutritional supplements for malabsorption; colestyramine for bile salt malabsorption may be necessary. • Endoscopic laser or argon plasma coagulation therapy: may reduce bleeding from proctitis. • Surgery: should be avoided, because the injured intestine is difficult to resect and anastomose, but it may be necessary for obstruction, perforation or fistula.

MISCELLANEOUS DISORDERS OF THE SMALL INTESTINE

PROTEIN-LOSING ENTEROPATHY

Defined as excessive loss of protein into the gut lumen, sufficient to cause hypoproteinaemia, protein-losing enteropathy occurs in a variety of inflammatory and neoplastic gut disorders but is most common in ulcerating conditions. In other disorders protein loss results from increased mucosal permeability or obstruction of intestinal lymphatic vessels.

Patients present with peripheral oedema and hypoproteinaemia in the presence of normal liver function and without proteinuria. The diagnosis is confirmed by measurement of faecal clearance of α_1-antitrypsin or ^{51}Cr-labelled albumin after i.v. injection. Treatment is that of the underlying disorder, with nutritional support and measures to control peripheral oedema.

MECKEL'S DIVERTICULUM

This is the most common congenital anomaly of the GI tract and occurs in 0.3–3% of people. Most patients are asymptomatic. The diverticulum results from failure of closure of the vitelline duct, with persistence of a blind-ending sac, usually within 100 cm of the ileocaecal valve and up to 5 cm long. Approximately 50% contain ectopic gastric mucosa.

Complications usually occur in the first 2 yrs of life but occasionally in young adults. Bleeding results from ulceration of ileal mucosa adjacent to the ectopic parietal cells and presents as recurrent melaena or altered blood per rectum. Diagnosis can be made by gamma scanning following i.v. ^{99m}Tc-pertechnate, which is concentrated by ectopic parietal cells. Other complications include intestinal obstruction, diverticulitis, intussusception and perforation. Surgery is unnecessary unless complications occur.

INFECTIONS OF THE SMALL INTESTINE

TRAVELLERS' DIARRHOEA, GIARDIASIS AND AMOEBIASIS

See pages 92, 116 and 114.

ABDOMINAL TUBERCULOSIS

Mycobacterium tuberculosis rarely causes abdominal disease in Caucasians but must be considered in the developing world and in AIDS patients. Gut infection usually results from human *M. tuberculosis* which is swallowed after coughing. Many patients have no pulmonary symptoms and a normal CXR. It most commonly affects the ileocaecal region; presentation and radiological findings may resemble Crohn's disease. Abdominal pain can be acute or chronic, but diarrhoea is less common in TB than in Crohn's disease. Low-grade fever is common. TB can affect any part of the GI tract, including perianal disease with fistula. Peritoneal TB may result in peritonitis with exudative ascites, abdominal pain and fever. Granulomatous hepatitis also occurs.

Useful investigations include:

• ESR: elevated. • Alkaline phosphatase: raised, suggesting hepatic involvement. • Endoscopy, laparoscopy or liver biopsy: for histological confirmation. • Culture of biopsies: may take 6 wks but faster diagnosis is now possible using rapid PCR techniques.

When the presentation is very suggestive of abdominal TB, chemotherapy with isoniazid, rifampicin, pyrazinamide and ethambutol should be commenced, even if bacteriological or histological proof is lacking.

TUMOURS OF THE SMALL INTESTINE

The small intestine is rarely affected by neoplasia, and <5% of all GI tumours occur here.

Benign tumours

The most common are peri-ampullary adenomas, GI stromal tumours (GIST), lipomas and hamartomas. Multiple adenomas are common in the duodenum of patients with familial adenomatous polyposis (FAP), who merit regular endoscopic surveillance. Hamartomatous polyps with almost no malignant potential occur in Peutz–Jeghers syndrome (p. 470).

Malignant tumours

These are rare and include adenocarcinoma, carcinoid tumour, malignant GIST and lymphoma. The majority occur in middle age or later. Kaposi's sarcoma is seen in patients with AIDS.

Adenocarcinomas occur with increased frequency in patients with FAP, coeliac disease and Peutz–Jeghers syndrome. Barium follow-through examination or small bowel enema studies will demonstrate most lesions. Enteroscopy, capsule endoscopy, mesenteric angiography and CT are also used. Treatment is by surgical resection.

CARCINOID TUMOURS

These are derived from enterochromaffin cells. They are most common in the ileum, but also occur in the rectum and in the appendix. Localised spread and the potential for metastasis to the liver increase with primary lesions >2 cm in diameter. These tumours grow slowly and are less aggressive than carcinomas.

'Carcinoid syndrome': Refers to systemic symptoms produced when secretory products of carcinoid tumours reach the systemic circulation (Box 12.12). Substances produced by the primary tumour are usually metabolised in the liver before reaching the systemic circulation. The syndrome is therefore only seen with hepatic metastases.

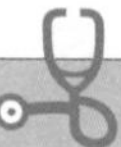

12.12 CLINICAL FEATURES OF CARCINOID TUMOURS

- Small-bowel obstruction due to the tumour mass
- Intestinal ischaemia (due to mesenteric infiltration or vasospasm)
- Hepatic metastases causing pain, hepatomegaly and jaundice
- Flushing and wheezing
- Diarrhoea
- Cardiac involvement (tricuspid regurgitation, pulmonary stenosis, right ventricular endocardial plaques) leading to heart failure
- Facial telangiectasia

The diagnosis is made by detecting excess levels of the 5-HT metabolite, 5-HIAA, in a 24-hr urine collection.

Treatment of carcinoid tumour is by surgical resection. The treatment of carcinoid syndrome is palliative because hepatic metastases have occurred, although prolonged survival is common. Removal of the primary tumour is usually attempted and the hepatic metastases can be excised as reduction of tumour mass improves symptoms. Hepatic artery embolisation retards growth of metastases. Octreotide may reduce tumour release of secretagogues.

LYMPHOMA

Non-Hodgkin lymphoma may involve the GI tract as part of generalised disease or may rarely arise in the gut, most commonly in the small intestine. Lymphomas are more common in patients with coeliac disease, AIDS and other immunodeficiencies.

Colicky abdominal pain, obstruction and weight loss are the usual presenting features, and diagnosis is by small bowel biopsy, contrast studies and CT. After staging, surgical resection is performed where possible, with radiotherapy and chemotherapy reserved for advanced disease.

DISEASES OF THE PANCREAS

ACUTE PANCREATITIS

Acute pancreatitis accounts for 3% of all cases of abdominal pain admitted to hospital. It affects 2–28 per 100 000 of the population and may be increasing in incidence.

The condition results from premature activation of zymogen granules, releasing proteases which digest the pancreas and surrounding tissue. Causes of acute pancreatitis are given in Box 12.13. It is usually mild and self-limiting, with minimal organ dysfunction and uneventful recovery. In some patients, however, it is severe, with complications such as necrosis, pseudocyst or abscess, and multi-organ failure. The mortality in this severe group is ~30%.

12.13 CAUSES OF ACUTE PANCREATITIS	
Common (90% of cases)	
• Gallstones • Alcohol	• Idiopathic • Post-endoscopic retrograde cholangiopancreatography (ERCP)
Rare	
• Post-surgical • Trauma • Drugs (e.g. azathioprine) • Infection (e.g. mumps)	• Renal failure • Hypothermia • Sphincter of Oddi dysfunction • Petrochemical exposure

Clinical features and complications

• Severe, constant upper abdominal pain: builds up over 15–60 mins, radiating to the back in 65%. • Nausea and vomiting. • Epigastric tenderness, but in the early stages guarding and rebound tenderness are absent because inflammation is mainly retroperitoneal. • Bowel sounds: become quiet or absent as paralytic ileus develops. • Hypoxia and hypovolaemic shock with oliguria in severe cases. • Discoloration of the flanks (Grey Turner's sign) or the periumbilical region (Cullen's sign): a feature of severe pancreatitis with haemorrhage.

Complications are listed in Box 12.14.

Investigations

• Serum amylase or lipase is elevated, although amylase may return to normal in 24–48 hrs. Amylase is also elevated (but less so) in intestinal ischaemia, perforated ulcer and ruptured ovarian cyst, whilst salivary amylase is elevated in parotitis. Persistently elevated serum amylase suggests pseudocyst formation. Peritoneal amylase is massively elevated in pancreatic ascites. • Elevated urinary amylase : creatinine ratio is helpful if serum amylase has returned to normal. • USS evidence of pancreatic swelling. This may also show gallstones, biliary obstruction or pseudocyst formation. • Plain X-rays help to exclude perforation, obstruction and pulmonary complications. • CT 3–10 days after admission helps to define the viability of the pancreas; decreased contrast enhancement indicates necrotising pancreatitis. Gas within necrotic material suggests infection and impending abscess formation, in which case percutaneous aspiration for bacterial culture is carried out and appropriate antibiotics prescribed. CT also reveals involvement of the colon, blood vessels and other adjacent structures by the inflammatory process.

Management and prognosis

Adverse prognostic factors are shown in Box 12.15. Serial CRP is a useful indicator of progress. A peak CRP >210 mg/l in the first 4 days predicts

12.14 COMPLICATIONS OF ACUTE PANCREATITIS

Complication	Cause
Systemic	
Systemic inflammatory response syndrome (SIRS)	Increased vascular permeability from cytokine, platelet aggregating factor and kinin release, paralytic ileus, vomiting; renal failure
Hypoxia	ARDS due to microthrombi in pulmonary vessels
Hyperglycaemia	Disruption of islets of Langerhans with altered insulin/glucagon axis
Hypocalcaemia	Sequestration of calcium in fat necrosis, fall in ionised calcium
Reduced serum albumin	Increased capillary permeability
Pancreatic	
Necrosis	Non-viable pancreatic tissue and peripancreatic tissue death; frequently infected
Abscess	Circumscribed collection of pus close to the pancreas and containing little or no pancreatic necrotic tissue
Pseudocyst	Disruption of pancreatic ducts
Pancreatic ascites or pleural effusion	Disruption of pancreatic ducts
GI	
Upper GI bleeding	Gastric or duodenal erosions
Variceal haemorrhage	Splenic or portal vein thrombosis
Erosion into colon	
Duodenal obstruction	Compression by pancreatic mass
Obstructive jaundice	Compression of common bile duct

12.15 ADVERSE PROGNOSTIC FACTORS IN ACUTE PANCREATITIS (GLASGOW CRITERIA)*

- Age >55 yrs
- PO_2 <8 kPa (60 mmHg)
- WBC >15 × 10^9/litre
- Albumin <32 g/l (3.2 g/dl)
- Serum calcium <2 mmol/l (8 mg/dl) (corrected)
- Glucose >10 mmol/l (180 mg/dl)
- Urea >16 mmol/l (45 mg/dl) (after rehydration)
- ALT >200 U/l
- LDH >600 U/l

*Severity and prognosis worsen as the number of these factors increases. More than three implies severe disease.

severe acute pancreatitis with 80% accuracy. Serum amylase has no prognostic value.

Management comprises diagnosis, resuscitation, detection and treatment of complications, and treating the underlying cause—specifically gallstones.

• Analgesia using pethidine. • Correction of hypovolaemia using normal saline and/or colloids. • Nasogastric aspiration: only necessary if paralytic ileus is present. • Enteral feeding via a nasoenteral tube: should be started early in severe pancreatitis. It decreases endotoxaemia and thereby may reduce systemic complications. • Insulin to correct hyperglycaemia. • Oxygen for hypoxic patients; those with acute respiratory distress syndrome (ARDS) may require ventilatory support. • Calcium: only needed if hypocalcaemic tetany occurs. • Prophylaxis of thromboembolism with low-dose subcutaneous heparin: advisable. • Prophylactic broad-spectrum i.v. antibiotics such as imipenem or cefuroxime: may improve outcome in severe cases.

Severe cases should be managed in a high-dependency or intensive care unit. A central venous line or Swan–Ganz catheter and urinary catheter are used to monitor patients with shock.

Patients with cholangitis or jaundice in association with severe acute pancreatitis should undergo urgent ERCP to diagnose and treat choledocholithiasis. In less severe cases of gallstone pancreatitis, biliary imaging (using MRCP) can be carried out after the acute phase has resolved. Cholecystectomy with an on-table cholangiogram should be undertaken within 2 wks of resolution of pancreatitis to prevent further potentially fatal attacks.

Patients with necrotising pancreatitis or pancreatic abscess require urgent surgical débridement followed by drainage of the pancreatic bed. Pancreatic pseudocysts are treated by delayed drainage into the stomach, duodenum or jejunum.

Mortality is 10–15%. About 80% of all cases are mild with a mortality <5%; 98% of deaths occur in the 20% of severe cases. One-third occur within the first week, usually from multi-organ failure.

CHRONIC PANCREATITIS

Chronic pancreatitis is a chronic inflammatory disease characterised by fibrosis and destruction of exocrine pancreatic tissue. Diabetes mellitus occurs in advanced cases because the islets of Langerhans are involved. Around 80% of cases in Western countries result from alcohol misuse. Other causes include malnutrition, cystic fibrosis and cassava consumption, while some cases are idiopathic. Chronic pancreatitis predominantly affects middle-aged alcoholic men.

Clinical features and complications

• Abdominal pain: in 50% this occurs as episodes of 'acute pancreatitis', although each attack results in further pancreatic damage. Relentless, slowly progressive pain without acute exacerbations affects 35% of patients. Pain may be relieved by leaning forwards or by alcohol. • Diarrhoea without pain is an uncommon presentation. • Weight loss. • Steatorrhoea: indicates that >90% of the exocrine tissue has been destroyed; protein malabsorption develops in the most advanced cases. • Diabetes mellitus in 30%, rising to 70% in those with chronic calcific pancreatitis. • Epigastric tenderness, sometimes with erythema ab igne over the abdomen and back due to chronic use of a hot water bottle. • Features of other alcohol- and smoking-related diseases.

Complications include:

• Pseudocysts and pancreatic ascites, which occur in both acute and chronic pancreatitis. • Extrahepatic obstructive jaundice due to a benign stricture of the common bile duct as it passes through the diseased pancreas. • Duodenal stenosis. • Portal or splenic vein thrombosis leading to segmental portal hypertension and gastric varices. • Peptic ulcer.

Investigations

Investigations are shown in Box 12.16 and Figure 12.4.

Management

Alcohol avoidance: Crucial in halting disease progression and reducing pain. Unfortunately, most patients continue to drink.

Pain relief: NSAIDs are valuable, but the severe, unremitting pain often leads to opiate use with the risk of addiction. Oral pancreatic enzyme supplements suppress pancreatic secretion and reduce analgesic requirement in some patients.

Surgery: Abstinent patients with severe chronic pain resistant to conservative measures may benefit from surgical or endoscopic pancreatic therapy.

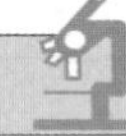

12.16 INVESTIGATIONS IN CHRONIC PANCREATITIS	
Tests to establish the diagnosis	
• USS • CT (may show atrophy, calcification or ductal dilatation) • AXR (may show calcification)	• MRCP • Endoscopic USS
Tests of pancreatic function	
• Collection of pure pancreatic juice after secretin injection (gold standard but invasive and seldom used) • Pancreolauryl or PABA test	• Faecal pancreatic chymotrypsin or elastase • Oral glucose tolerance test
Tests of anatomy prior to surgery	
• MRCP	

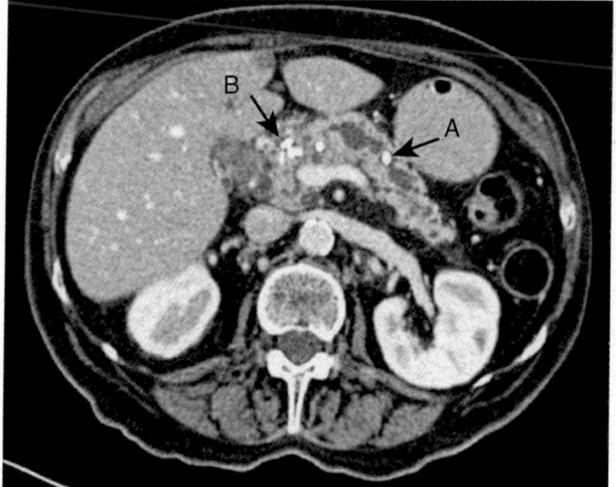

Fig. 12.4 Imaging in chronic pancreatitis. CT scan showing a grossly dilated and irregular duct with a calcified stone (arrow A). Note the calcification in the head of the gland (arrow B).

Patients without a surgically or endoscopically correctable abnormality require total pancreatectomy. Unfortunately, even after this, some patients continue to experience pain. Moreover, the procedure causes diabetes which may be difficult to control.

Fat restriction and oral pancreatic enzyme supplements: Used to treat steatorrhoea. A PPI is added to optimise duodenal pH for pancreatic enzyme activity.

Surgical or endoscopic therapy may be necessary for the management of pseudocysts, pancreatic ascites, common bile duct or duodenal stricture, and the consequences of portal hypertension.

CONGENITAL ABNORMALITIES OF THE PANCREAS

ANNULAR PANCREAS

In this congenital anomaly, the pancreas encircles the second/third part of the duodenum, leading to gastric outlet obstruction.

CYSTIC FIBROSIS

See page 290.

TUMOURS OF THE PANCREAS

Pancreatic carcinoma affects 10–15 per 100 000 in Western populations, rising to 100 per 100 000 in those over the age of 70. Men are affected twice as often as women. The disease is associated with smoking and chronic pancreatitis. Between 5 and 10% of patients have a genetic predisposition.

Approximately 90% of pancreatic neoplasms are adenocarcinomas which arise from the pancreatic ducts and spread early to involve local structures and regional lymph nodes.

Clinical features

• Pain: incessant, boring, with radiation to the back; may be eased by bending forward. • Weight loss due to anorexia, steatorrhoea and metabolic effects of the tumour. • Obstructive jaundice: 60% of tumours arise from the head of the pancreas, with obstruction of the common bile duct and associated severe pruritus. • Less common: diarrhoea, vomiting from duodenal obstruction, diabetes mellitus, recurrent venous thrombosis, acute pancreatitis or depression.

Examination reveals evidence of weight loss, abdominal mass due to the tumour itself, a palpable gallbladder or hepatic metastasis. A palpable gallbladder in a jaundiced patient is usually due to biliary obstruction by a pancreatic cancer (Courvoisier's sign).

Investigations

• LFTs for cholestatic jaundice. • USS and CT: demonstrate a pancreatic mass. • MRCP or ERCP when diagnosis is in doubt. • Staging to define operability: entails laparoscopy with laparoscopic USS to define tumour size, involvement of blood vessels and metastatic spread.

In patients unsuitable for surgery because of advanced disease, frailty or comorbidity, USS or CT-guided cytology or biopsy can be used. EUS with fine needle aspiration is used to define vascular invasion and obtain cytological proof of diagnosis.

Management

Surgical resection: The only curative treatment; 5-yr survival after complete resection is ~20%. Survival may be improved with adjuvant chemotherapy. Only 15% of tumours are amenable to curative resection since most are locally advanced at diagnosis. For the great majority therapy is based on palliation.

Pain relief: Analgesics with or without coeliac plexus neurolysis by a percutaneous or EUS-guided alcohol injection.

Jaundice: Choledochojejunostomy in fit patients; percutaneous or endoscopic stenting is used in the elderly or in patients who have very advanced disease. Overall survival is only 3–5%.

ENDOCRINE TUMOURS

These arise from neuroendocrine tissue within the pancreas. They may occur in association with parathyroid and pituitary adenomas (p. 382). The majority of endocrine tumours are non-secretory and, although malignant, grow slowly and metastasise late. Other tumours secrete hormones and present because of their endocrine effects.

INFLAMMATORY BOWEL DISEASE

Ulcerative colitis and Crohn's disease are chronic inflammatory bowel diseases which relapse and remit over years. The diseases have many similarities and it is sometimes impossible to distinguish them (Box 12.17). However, ulcerative colitis only involves the colon, while Crohn's disease can involve any part of the GI tract.

The incidence of inflammatory bowel disease (IBD) varies widely between populations. Crohn's disease is rare in the developing world yet ulcerative colitis is becoming more common. In the West, the prevalence of ulcerative colitis is stable at 100–200 per 100 000, while Crohn's disease

12.17 COMPARISON OF ULCERATIVE COLITIS AND CROHN'S DISEASE

	Ulcerative colitis	Crohn's disease
Age group	Any	Any
Gender	M = F	M = F
Ethnic group	Any	Any; more common in Ashkenazi Jews
Genetic factors	HLA-DR103 associated with severe disease	CARD 15/NOD-2 mutations predispose
Risk factors	More common in non-/ ex-smokers; appendicectomy protects	More common in smokers
Anatomical distribution	Colon only; begins at anorectal margin with variable proximal extension	Any part of GI tract; perianal disease common; patchy distribution—'skip lesions'
Extraintestinal manifestations	Common	Common
Presentation	Bloody diarrhoea	Variable; pain, diarrhoea, weight loss all common
Histology	Inflammation limited to mucosa; crypt distortion, cryptitis, crypt abscesses, loss of goblet cells	Submucosal or transmural inflammation common; deep fissuring ulcers, fistulae; patchy changes; granulomas
Management	5-ASA; corticosteroids; azathioprine; colectomy is curative	Corticosteroids; azathioprine; methotrexate; infliximab; nutritional therapy; surgery for complications is not curative

is increasing and now affects 50–100 per 100 000. Both diseases most commonly start in young adults.

IBD develops as a response to an environmental trigger in genetically susceptible individuals. There is activation of macrophages, lymphocytes and polymorphonuclear cells with release of inflammatory mediators, events which represent targets for future therapies.

Clinical features of ulcerative colitis

These depend upon the site and activity of the disease. The first attack is usually the most severe and thereafter is followed by relapses and remissions; a few have unremitting symptoms. Emotional stress, intercurrent infection, gastroenteritis, antibiotics or NSAIDs may provoke relapse.

Proctitis: Rectal bleeding and mucus discharge, sometimes with tenesmus. Some pass frequent, small-volume fluid stools, while others are constipated. Constitutional symptoms do not occur.

Proctosigmoiditis: Bloody diarrhoea with mucus. Almost all patients are constitutionally well.

Extensive colitis: Bloody diarrhoea with mucus, anorexia, malaise, weight loss and abdominal pain. The patient is toxic with fever, tachycardia and peritoneal inflammation (Box 12.18).

Clinical features of Crohn's disease

Ileal Crohn's disease: The features are:

• Abdominal pain, because of subacute intestinal obstruction, an inflammatory mass, intra-abdominal abscess or acute obstruction. • Diarrhoea which

12.18 FACTORS CONSIDERED FOR DISEASE SEVERITY ASSESSMENT IN ULCERATIVE COLITIS

	Mild	**Severe**
Daily bowel frequency	<4	>6
Blood in stools	+/–	+++
Stool volume (g/24 hrs)	<200	>400
Pulse (bpm)	<90	>90
Temperature (°C)	Normal	>37.8, 2 days out of 4
Sigmoidoscopy	Normal or granular mucosa	Blood in lumen
AXR	Normal	Dilated bowel and/or mucosal islands
Hb (g/l)	Normal	<100
ESR (mm/hr)	Normal	>30
Serum albumin (g/l)	>35	<30

is watery without blood or mucus. • Weight loss due to anorexia or malabsorption; some patients present with features of fat, protein or vitamin deficiencies.

Crohn's colitis: Presents exactly like ulcerative colitis, with bloody diarrhoea, mucus, lethargy, malaise, anorexia and weight loss. Rectal sparing and perianal disease suggest Crohn's disease rather than ulcerative colitis.

Many patients present with both small bowel and colonic disease. A few have isolated perianal disease, vomiting from jejunal strictures or severe oral ulceration.

Physical examination reveals:

• Weight loss, anaemia, glossitis and angular stomatitis. • Abdominal tenderness most marked over the inflamed area. • Abdominal mass due to matted loops of thickened bowel or an intra-abdominal abscess. • Perianal skin tags, fissures or fistulae in at least 50% of patients.

Complications

Life-threatening inflammation of the colon: Occurs in both ulcerative colitis and Crohn's disease. The colon dilates (toxic megacolon) and bacterial toxins cross the diseased mucosa into the circulation. This occurs most commonly during the first attack of colitis and is recognised by the features in Box 12.18. If an AXR shows the transverse colon is dilated to >6 cm there is a high risk of perforation. Perforation of the small intestine or colon can occur without the development of toxic megacolon. Life-threatening acute haemorrhage due to erosion of a major artery occurs rarely.

Fistulae and perianal disease: Occur only in Crohn's disease and not in ulcerative colitis. Enteroenteric fistulae cause diarrhoea and malabsorption. Enterovesical fistulation causes recurrent urinary infections and pneumaturia. Enterovaginal fistula causes feculent vaginal discharge. Fistulation from the bowel may also cause perianal or ischiorectal abscesses, and fissures.

Cancer: Extensive active colitis lasting >8 yrs increases the risk of cancer. The cumulative risk for ulcerative colitis reaches 20% after 30 yrs but is lower for Crohn's colitis. Small bowel adenocarcinoma occasionally complicates long-standing small bowel Crohn's disease. Patients with chronic colitis should start surveillance colonoscopy 8–10 yrs after diagnosis. Patients with no or only low-grade dysplasia are screened every 1–2 yrs, while those with high-grade dysplasia should be considered for panproctocolectomy.

Extraintestinal complications: IBD can be considered as a systemic illness and in some patients extraintestinal complications dominate the clinical picture. Some of these occur during relapse of intestinal disease; others appear unrelated to intestinal disease activity (Box 12.19).

The differential diagnosis is shown in Boxes 12.20 and 12.21.

Investigations

FBC: May show anaemia from bleeding or malabsorption of iron, folic acid or vitamin B_{12}. Serum albumin is low due to protein-losing enteropathy or because of poor nutrition.

ESR: Raised in exacerbations or because of abscess.

12.19 SYSTEMIC MANIFESTATIONS OF IBD	
Eyes	Conjunctivitis, iritis, episcleritis
Mouth	Ulcers
Liver	Abscess, fatty change, hepatitis, sclerosing cholangitis
Vascular	Mesenteric, portal or deep vein thrombosis
Skin	Erythema nodosum, pyoderma gangrenosum (see p. 416)
Bone/joint	Metabolic bone disease, sacroiliitis

12.20 CONDITIONS MIMICKING CROHN'S DISEASE AND ULCERATIVE OR COLITIS	
Infective	E.g. *Salmonella*, *Shigella*, *Campylobacter*, *E. coli* 0157, diverticulitis, amoebiasis
Vascular	Radiation proctitis, ischaemic colitis
Neoplastic	Colonic carcinoma
Inflammatory	Behçet's disease
Drugs	NSAIDs

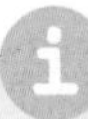

12.21 DIFFERENTIAL DIAGNOSIS OF SMALL BOWEL CROHN'S DISEASE

- Other causes of right iliac fossa mass: caecal carcinoma*, appendix abscess*, infection (TB, *Yersinia*, actinomycosis)
- Mesenteric adenitis
- Pelvic inflammatory disease
- Lymphoma

*Common; other causes are rare.

CRP: Helpful in monitoring Crohn's disease activity.

Stool cultures: Help to exclude superimposed enteric infection in patients with exacerbations.

Blood cultures: Also advisable in febrile patients with known colitis or Crohn's disease.

Sigmoidoscopy: Should be performed in those with diarrhoea. In ulcerative colitis sigmoidoscopy shows loss of vascular pattern, granularity, friability and ulceration. In Crohn's disease patchy inflammation with discrete, deep ulcers, perianal disease or rectal sparing occurs.

Colonoscopy: May show active inflammation with pseudopolyps or a complicating carcinoma. Biopsies are taken to define disease extent and to seek dysplasia in long-standing colitis. In ulcerative colitis the abnormalities are confluent and most severe in the distal colon and rectum. Stricture formation does not occur in the absence of a carcinoma. In Crohn's colitis the endoscopic abnormalities are patchy, with intervening normal mucosa, and ulcers and strictures are common.

Barium enema: Less sensitive than colonoscopy. Loss of haustration, pseudopolyps and dilatation are seen in ulcerative colitis; in Crohn's disease strictures and ulcers are also seen. Small bowel contrast studies are normal in ulcerative colitis, but in Crohn's disease may show areas of narrowing, ulceration and strictures.

AXR: May show dilatation of the colon, mucosal oedema or evidence of perforation. In small bowel Crohn's disease there may be intestinal obstruction or displacement of bowel loops by a mass.

USS: May identify thickened small bowel and abscess in Crohn's disease.

Radio-labelled white cell scans: Show areas of active inflammation and may be useful in severely ill patients in whom invasive tests are best avoided.

MRI: Delineates pelvic or perineal involvement by Crohn's disease.

General management

Multidisciplinary management by physicians, surgeons, radiologists and dietitians is advantageous. Ulcerative colitis and Crohn's disease are lifelong conditions and counsellors and patient support groups have important roles. The key aims are to:

• Treat acute attacks. • Prevent relapses. • Detect carcinoma at an early stage. • Select patients for surgery.

Medical management of ulcerative colitis

Treatment depends upon the extent and activity of colitis. Aminosalicylates (e.g. mesalazine, sulfasalazine, olsalazine) modulate cytokine release from the mucosa and are widely used.

Active proctitis: In mild to moderate disease mesalazine enemas or suppositories combined with oral mesalazine are effective. Topical corticosteroids are less effective but are used in patients intolerant of topical mesalazine. Patients who fail to respond are treated with oral prednisolone.

Active left-sided or extensive ulcerative colitis: In mild cases, high-dose aminosalicylates combined with topical aminosalicylate and corticosteroids are effective. Oral prednisolone is indicated for severe or unresponsive cases.

Severe ulcerative colitis: Patients with severe colitis unresponsive to maximal oral therapy should be monitored in hospital:

• Clinically, for abdominal pain, temperature, pulse rate, stool blood and frequency. • To check Hb, WCC, albumin, electrolytes, ESR and CRP. • For colonic dilatation on plain AXR.

I.v. fluids and enteral nutritional support are often needed. I.v. corticosteroids are given as a constant infusion. Topical and oral aminosalicylates are also used. In patients unresponsive to corticosteroids, i.v. ciclosporin or infliximab avoids the need for colectomy in 30%. Patients who deteriorate despite 7–10 days' maximal medical therapy, and those with colonic dilatation (>6 cm) require urgent colectomy.

Maintenance of remission: Life-long maintenance therapy is recommended for all patients with extensive disease and patients with distal disease who relapse more than once a year. Oral aminosalicylates—either mesalazine or balsalazide—are first-line agents. Patients who relapse frequently despite aminosalicylates are treated with thiopurines, e.g. azathioprine.

Medical management of Crohn's disease

Active disease: Colitis or ileocolitis is initially treated in the same way as active ulcerative colitis. In severe disease i.v. prednisolone is indicated, but abscess or fistulating disease should be excluded first. Nutritional therapy using polymeric or elemental diets induces remission, but relapse rates are higher and primary nutritional therapy is rarely used.

Isolated ileal disease is treated with corticosteroids. Poorly responding patients should be considered early for resection, which usually leads to prolonged remission.

For disease in any site, infliximab given as an i.v. infusion 4–8-weekly on three occasions induces remission in patients with active GI Crohn's disease and is also effective for pyoderma gangrenosum and some forms of arthritis. Contraindications include infection, such as TB, and allergic reactions. Relapse commonly occurs ~12 wks after treatment, so it is usually combined with either thiopurines or methotrexate, to maintain remission. Infliximab causes remarkable mucosal healing, but this can lead to scarring and stricturing, and is used with caution in patients with stenosing disease.

For extensive ileocolonic disease, a combination of drug therapies, nutritional support, sometimes including parenteral nutrition, surgery and endoscopic dilatation of strictures may be needed.

Fistulating and perianal disease: The site of fistulation is defined using barium radiology, CT and MRI. Examination under anaesthetic and surgical intervention are usually required, although treatment of underlying active disease with corticosteroids and nutritional support (TPN) are also required in many. For simple perianal disease, metronidazole or ciprofloxacin (or both) is used. Thiopurines are used in chronic disease. Infliximab, infused 4–8-weekly, helps to heal enterocutaneous fistulae and perianal disease.

Maintenance of remission: The most effective step is smoking cessation. Aminosalicylates have minimal efficacy. Patients who relapse more than once a year are treated with thiopurines. Those who are intolerant or resistant to these drugs should receive methotrexate with folic acid. Patients with aggressive disease are managed with both immunomodulating agents and infliximab. Chronic use of corticosteroids is avoided because of side-effects and because they do not prevent relapse.

Surgical treatment of ulcerative colitis

Up to 60% of patients with extensive ulcerative colitis eventually require surgery. Indications include impaired quality of life, failure of medical therapy, fulminant colitis, cancer or severe dysplasia. Panproctocolectomy with ileostomy or proctocolectomy with ileal–anal pouch anastomosis cures the patient. Before surgery, patients must be counselled both by staff and by patients who have had surgery.

Surgical treatment of Crohn's disease

The indications for surgery are similar to those for ulcerative colitis. Operations are often necessary to deal with fistulae, abscesses and perianal disease, or to relieve small or large bowel obstruction. In contrast to ulcerative colitis, surgery is not curative and disease recurrence is the rule, so a conservative approach is used. Those with extensive colitis require total colectomy but ileal–anal pouch formation should be avoided because of the high risk of recurrence within the pouch with fistulae, abscess formation and pouch failure.

Prognosis

Life expectancy in patients with IBD is now similar to that of the general population, and despite the burden of treatment the majority are able to work and pursue a normal life.

IRRITABLE BOWEL SYNDROME

Irritable bowel syndrome (IBS) is a common functional bowel disorder in which abdominal pain is associated with defecation or a change in bowel habit in the absence of structural pathology.

Approximately 20% of the general population fulfil diagnostic criteria for IBS but only 10% of these consult their doctors with symptoms. IBS is the most common cause of GI referral, and causes frequent absence from work and impaired quality of life. Young women are affected 2–3 times more often than men. There is wide overlap with non-ulcer dyspepsia, chronic fatigue syndrome, dysmenorrhoea and urinary frequency. A significant proportion of patients have a history of physical or sexual abuse.

Most patients seen in general practice do not have psychological problems but ~50% of patients referred to hospital have significant anxiety, depression, somatisation, panic attacks and neurosis. Acute psychological stress and overt psychiatric disease alter visceral perception and GI motility. These factors, coupled with abnormal illness behaviour, contribute to but do not cause IBS.

A range of motility disorders from diarrhoea to constipation is found but none is diagnostic. IBS is associated with increased visceral sensitivity to intestinal distension induced by inflation of balloons in the ileum, colon and rectum. This is more common in women and in diarrhoea-predominant IBS.

Some patients develop IBS following an episode of gastroenteritis, more commonly young women and those with existing background psychological problems. Others may be intolerant of specific dietary components, particularly lactose and wheat.

Clinical features and investigations

• Recurrent colicky pain in the lower abdomen relieved by defecation. • Abdominal bloating that worsens throughout the day; the cause is unknown but it is not due to excessive intestinal gas. • Abnormal bowel habit. It is useful to classify patients as having predominantly constipation or predominantly diarrhoea. The constipated type tends to pass infrequent pellety stools, usually with abdominal pain or proctalgia. Those with diarrhoea have frequent defecation but produce low-volume stools and rarely have nocturnal symptoms. • Passage of mucus is common but rectal bleeding does not occur.

Patients do not lose weight and are constitutionally well. Examination does not reveal any abnormalities, although bloating and tenderness to palpation are common.

Investigations are normal. An FBC, ESR and sigmoidoscopy are usually done routinely, but barium enema or colonoscopy should only be undertaken in older patients to exclude colorectal cancer. Atypical presentations require investigations to exclude organic GI disease. All patients with rectal bleeding should undergo colonoscopy to exclude colonic cancer or IBD.

Management

Many patients are concerned that they have developed cancer, and a cycle of anxiety leading to colonic symptoms, which further heighten anxiety, can be broken by explanation that symptoms are not due to organic disease but are the result of altered bowel motility and sensation. In patients who fail to respond to reassurance, symptomatic treatment should be tried. Elimination diets are generally unhelpful but some may benefit from exclusion of wheat, lactose, excess caffeine or artificial sweeteners such as sorbitol. The role of probiotics is uncertain.

Patients with intractable symptoms sometimes benefit from several months of therapy with low-dose amitriptyline. Active anxiety or affective disorders should be separately treated. Psychological interventions such as cognitive behavioural therapy, relaxation and gut-directed hypnotherapy are reserved for the most difficult cases. Most patients have a relapsing and remitting course.

ISCHAEMIC GUT INJURY

Ischaemic gut injury is usually the result of arterial occlusion. The presentation is variable and the diagnosis is difficult.

ACUTE SMALL BOWEL ISCHAEMIA

Superior mesenteric blood flow may be compromised by embolism from the heart or aorta (40–50%), thrombosis on underlying atheroma (25%), or hypotension (25%). Vasculitis and venous occlusion are rare causes. Patients usually have evidence of cardiac disease and arrhythmia.

Abdominal pain develops, which is more impressive than the physical findings. In the early stages the abdomen may be distended, with absent or diminished bowel sounds, and peritonitis is a later feature.

Investigations reveal:

• Leucocytosis. • Metabolic acidosis. • Raised phosphate and amylase. • 'Thumb-printing' on AXR due to mucosal oedema. • An occluded or narrowed major artery on mesenteric or CT angiography.

Management

• Resuscitation, management of cardiac disease and i.v. antibiotic therapy should be followed by laparotomy, embolectomy and vascular reconstruction. • In patients at high surgical risk thrombolysis may sometimes be effective. • Survivors often develop short bowel syndrome requiring nutritional support, sometimes including home parenteral nutrition, as well as anticoagulation. • Small bowel transplantation is promising in selected patients.

ACUTE COLONIC ISCHAEMIA

The splenic flexure and descending colon lie in 'watershed' areas of arterial supply. Arterial thromboembolism is usually responsible but colonic ischaemia can also follow severe hypotension, colonic volvulus, strangulated hernia, systemic vasculitis, aortic aneurysm surgery or hypercoagulable states. The patient is usually elderly and presents with sudden cramping left-sided lower abdominal pain and rectal bleeding. The diagnosis is established by colonoscopy or barium enema. Symptoms usually resolve spontaneously over 24–48 hrs and healing occurs within 2 wks. Some have a residual fibrous stricture or segment of colitis.

CHRONIC MESENTERIC ISCHAEMIA

This results from atherosclerotic stenosis affecting at least two of the coeliac axis, superior mesenteric and inferior mesenteric arteries. Patients present with dull but severe mid- or upper abdominal pain about 30 mins after eating, with weight loss and sometimes with diarrhoea. Examination reveals generalised arterial disease and sometimes an audible abdominal bruit. Mesenteric angiography confirms at least two affected arteries. Vascular reconstruction or percutaneous angioplasty is sometimes possible. Left untreated, many patients develop intestinal infarction.

DISORDERS OF THE COLON AND RECTUM

TUMOURS OF THE COLON AND RECTUM

POLYPS AND POLYPOSIS SYNDROMES

Polyps may be neoplastic or non-neoplastic, single or multiple, and vary from a few mm to several cm in size.

Colorectal adenomas: Extremely common in the Western world; 50% of people >60 yrs of age have adenomas, usually in the rectum and distal colon. Nearly all colorectal carcinomas develop from adenomatous polyps. Large, multiple, villous or dysplastic polyps carry a higher risk of malignancy. Adenomas are usually asymptomatic and discovered incidentally. Occasionally, they cause bleeding and anaemia. Villous adenomas sometimes secrete large amounts of mucus, causing diarrhoea and hypokalaemia.

Discovery of a polyp at sigmoidoscopy is an indication for colonoscopy and polypectomy, which considerably reduce subsequent cancer risk. Very large or sessile polyps sometimes require surgery. Once all polyps have been removed, patients <75 should undergo surveillance colonoscopy at 3–5-yr intervals, as new polyps develop in 50%.

Between 10 and 20% of polyps show evidence of malignancy. When cancer cells are found within 2 mm of the resection margin, and when the polyp cancer is poorly differentiated or invading lymphatics, segmental colonic resection is recommended. Others can be followed up by surveillance colonoscopy.

The polyposis syndromes are classified by histopathology. They include neoplastic familial adenomatous polyposis and several non-neoplastic syndromes, including Peutz–Jeghers syndrome.

Familial adenomatous polyposis (FAP): An uncommon (1 in 13 000) autosomal dominant disorder. Around 20% are new mutations with no family history. By age 15, 80% of patients will develop up to several thousand adenomatous colonic polyps, with symptoms such as rectal bleeding beginning a few years later. Within 10–15 yrs of the appearance of adenomas, colorectal cancer will develop, affecting 90% by the age of 50. Malignant transformation of duodenal adenomas occurs in 10% and is the leading cause of death after prophylactic colectomy. Extra-intestinal features include subcutaneous epidermoid cysts, benign osteomas, dental abnormalities and lipomas. Dark, round, pigmented retinal lesions (congenital hypertrophy of the retinal pigment epithelium) occur in some patients; in at-risk individuals these are 100% predictive of FAP.

Investigations and management:
• Early identification is essential. • Sigmoidoscopy, if normal, excludes the diagnosis. • Genetic testing confirms the diagnosis, and first-degree relatives should also be tested. • Children of FAP families should undergo mutation testing at 13–14 yrs of age, followed by regular sigmoidoscopy in those carrying the mutation. • Affected individuals should undergo colectomy on leaving school or college. • Periodic upper GI endoscopy is recommended to detect duodenal adenomas.

Peutz–Jeghers syndrome: Comprises multiple hamartomatous polyps in the small intestine and colon and melanin pigmentation of the lips, mouth and digits, and is usually asymptomatic. There is a small but significant risk of small bowel or colonic adenocarcinoma and of cancer of the pancreas, lung, ovary, breast and endometrium. Colonoscopy with biopsies should be performed every 1–3 yrs.

COLORECTAL CANCER

Although relatively rare in the developing world, colorectal cancer is the second most common internal malignancy and the second leading cause of cancer deaths in Western countries. In the UK the incidence is 50–60 per 100 000 per year. The condition becomes increasingly common over the age of 50.

Around 80% are 'sporadic', 10% are hereditary non-polyposis colon cancer (HNPCC), and 1% are associated with FAP and 1% with inflammatory bowel disease.

Environmental factors account for >80% of all 'sporadic' colorectal cancers. The risk declines in migrants who move from high- to low-risk countries. Dietary factors increasing risk are red meat and saturated fat, while fibre, fruit, vegetables, folic acid and calcium appear to protect.

Colorectal cancer development results from the accumulation of multiple genetic mutations. HNPCC accounts for 10% of cancers; it occurs in those with a family history and often at a young age. The lifetime risk of colorectal cancer in affected individuals is 80%. Those who fulfil the criteria for diagnosis should be referred for pedigree assessment, genetic testing and colonoscopy, which needs to be repeated every 1–2 yrs, and despite which interval cancers still occur. The lifetime risk of developing cancer with one or two affected first-degree relatives is 1 in 12 and 1 in 6, respectively. The risk is even higher if relatives were affected at an early age.

Most tumours arise from malignant transformation of a benign adenomatous polyp. Over 65% occur in the rectosigmoid and a further 15% recur in the caecum or ascending colon. Rectal cancers may invade the pelvic viscera and side walls. Lymphatic invasion is common at presentation, as is hepatic spread. Tumour stage at diagnosis determines prognosis.

Clinical features

• In tumours of the left colon, fresh rectal bleeding is common and obstruction occurs early. • Tumours of the right colon present with anaemia from occult bleeding, or with altered bowel habit, but obstruction is a late feature. • Colicky lower abdominal pain is present in two-thirds of patients and rectal bleeding occurs in 50%. • A minority present with either obstruction or perforation. • Carcinoma of the rectum usually causes early bleeding, mucus discharge or a feeling of incomplete emptying.

On examination there may be a palpable mass, signs of anaemia or hepatomegaly from metastases. Low rectal tumours may be palpable on digital examination.

Investigations and management

• Colonoscopy is more sensitive and specific than barium enema and permits biopsy (Fig. 12.5). Rigid sigmoidoscopy will detect < one-third of tumours. • CT colography detects tumours and polyps >1 cm and can be used if colonoscopy is incomplete or high-risk. • CT is valuable for detecting hepatic metastases. • Intraoperative USS is increasingly being used for this purpose. • Carcinoembryonic antigen (CEA) is raised in only a propor-

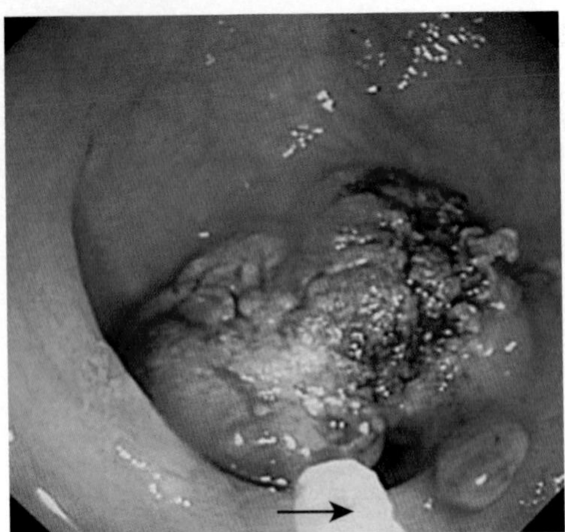

Fig. 12.5 Colonoscopic view of a polypoid rectal carcinoma undergoing laser therapy (arrow) in a patient unfit for surgery.

tion of patients and so of little use in diagnosis. Serial CEA can help to detect early recurrence during follow-up.

Surgery: The tumour is removed, along with pericolic lymph nodes. Direct anastomosis is performed wherever possible or colostomy if not. Solitary hepatic or lung metastases are sometimes resected at a later stage. Post-operatively, patients should undergo colonoscopy after 6–12 mths and periodically thereafter to search for local recurrence or development of new 'metachronous' lesions, which occur in 6% of cases.

Adjuvant therapy: Two-thirds of patients have lymph node or distant spread at presentation and are, therefore, beyond cure with surgery alone (Box 12.22). Most recurrences are within 3 yrs, either at the site of resection or in lymph nodes, liver or peritoneum. Adjuvant chemotherapy improves survival in patients with Dukes C colon cancer by ~4–13%. Pre-operative radiotherapy is used to 'down-stage' large rectal cancers, making them resectable. Dukes C and some Dukes B rectal cancers are given post-operative radiotherapy to reduce the risk of local recurrence if resection margins are involved.

Palliation: Surgical resection of the primary tumour is appropriate for some patients with metastases to treat obstruction, bleeding or pain. Palliative chemotherapy with 5-fluorouracil and folinic acid improves survival, and second-line therapy with irinotecan is used when this fails. Pelvic radiotherapy is sometimes useful for rectal pain, bleeding or severe tenesmus. Endoscopic laser therapy or insertion of an expandable metal stent can be used to relieve obstruction.

Secondary prevention (screening): Aims to detect and remove lesions at an early or pre-malignant stage. Several potential methods exist:

12.22 STAGING AND SURVIVAL IN COLORECTAL CANCER				
	Dukes stage			
	A	B	C	D
Definition	Tumour confined within bowel wall	Extension through bowel wall	Tumour involving lymph nodes	Distant metastases
Prevalence at diagnosis (%)	10	35	30	25
5-yr survival rate (%)	>90	65	30–35	<5

• Widespread screening by regular FOB testing reduces colorectal cancer mortality and increases early detection. In the USA, annual FOB screening is recommended after the age of 50 yrs. • Colonoscopy remains the gold standard but requires expertise, is expensive and carries risks. • Flexible sigmoidoscopy has been shown to reduce overall colorectal cancer mortality by ~35% (70% for cases arising in the rectosigmoid). It is recommended in the USA every 5 yrs in all persons over the age of 50.

DIVERTICULOSIS

Asymptomatic diverticula ('diverticulosis') occur in the sigmoid and descending colon in >50% of people over 70. Symptomatic ('diverticular disease') or complicated diverticulosis ('diverticulitis') is uncommon, occurring in 10–25% of cases.

Dietary fibre deficiency is thought to be responsible and diverticulosis is rare in populations with a high dietary fibre. Small-volume stools require high intracolonic pressures for propulsion, leading to herniation of mucosa.

Diverticula are protrusions of mucosa covered by peritoneum, which become impacted with faecoliths then inflamed. This may resolve or progress with haemorrhage, perforation, abscess formation, fistula and peritonitis. Repeated attacks may lead to fibrotic strictures.

Clinical features

• Colicky pain in the suprapubic area or left iliac fossa from associated constipation or spasm. • Palpable sigmoid colon or iliac fossa mass. • Local tenderness, guarding, rigidity ('left-sided appendicitis') with diverticulitis. • Diarrhoea, rectal bleeding or fever. • Complications occur in ~5%; they are more common in patients who take NSAIDs or aspirin.

Investigations and management

• Barium enema shows diverticula, strictures and fistulae. • Flexible sigmoidoscopy excludes coexisting neoplasm, which is easily missed radiologically. • CT is used to assess complications.

Asymptomatic diverticulosis requires no treatment. Constipation is relieved by a high-fibre diet with or without a bulking laxative and plenty of fluids. Stimulants should be avoided, but antispasmodics sometimes help.

Acute diverticulitis requires 7 days of metronidazole, with either a cephalosporin or ampicillin. Trials show no benefit from acute resection compared to conservative management, except for severe haemorrhage or perforation. Percutaneous drainage of acute abscesses can be effective. Elective resection of the affected segment is indicated after repeated acute obstruction.

CONSTIPATION AND DISORDERS OF DEFECATION

Simple constipation: Extremely common and usually responds to increased dietary fibre or bulking agents with an adequate fluid intake.

Severe idiopathic constipation: Occurs almost exclusively in young women and often begins in childhood or adolescence. The cause is unknown and the condition is often resistant to treatment. Bulking agents may exacerbate symptoms but prokinetic agents or balanced solutions of polyethylene glycol 3350 benefit some patients with slow transit.

Faecal impaction: Tends to occur in frail, disabled, immobile or institutionalised patients. Drugs, autonomic neuropathy and painful anal conditions also contribute. Obstruction, perforation and bleeding may supervene. Treatment involves softening the stool with arachis oil enemas, hydration and careful digital disimpaction.

Melanosis coli and laxative misuse syndromes: Long-term stimulant laxative use causes brown discoloration of the colonic mucosa ('tiger skin'), which is benign and resolves with laxative withdrawal. Surreptitious laxative misuse is a psychiatric condition seen in young women, who may have a history of bulimia or anorexia nervosa. They complain of refractory watery diarrhoea and deny laxative use. Screening of urine for laxatives may be helpful.

MEGACOLON

Hirschsprung's disease: Congenital absence of ganglion cells causes the internal anal sphincter to fail to relax. Constipation, abdominal distension and vomiting usually develop immediately after birth but occasionally in childhood or adolescence. A family history is present in one-third. The rectum is empty on digital examination.

Barium enema shows a small rectum and colonic dilatation above the narrowed segment. Full-thickness biopsies confirm the absence of ganglion cells. Treatment involves resection of the affected segment.

Acquired megacolon: In childhood this is a result of voluntary withholding of stool during toilet training. It presents after the first year and is distinguished from Hirschsprung's disease by the urge to defecate and the presence of stool in the rectum. It usually responds to osmotic laxatives.

In adults, acquired megacolon may occur in depressed or demented patients, either as part of the condition or as a side-effect of antidepressant drugs. Prolonged misuse of stimulant laxatives may cause megacolon, as may neurological disorders, scleroderma and hypothyroidism. Patients are managed by treating the underlying cause, and with high-residue diets, laxatives and enemas.

Acute colonic pseudo-obstruction (Ogilvie's syndrome): Can be caused by trauma, surgery, respiratory or renal failure, or diabetes mellitus. There is sudden painless, massive enlargement of the proximal colon without features of mechanical obstruction. Bowel sounds are normal or high-pitched rather than absent. The condition may progress to perforation and peritonitis.

X-rays show colonic dilatation with air extending to the rectum. A caecal diameter >10–12 cm is associated with a high risk of perforation. Barium enemas demonstrate the absence of mechanical obstruction. Management consists of treating the underlying disorder and correcting any biochemical abnormalities. Neostigmine is used to enhance gut motility. Decompression either with a rectal tube or by careful colonoscopy may be effective.

Clostridium difficile infection: Antibiotic-associated diarrhoea, colitis and pseudomembranous colitis are part of a spectrum caused by disturbance of the normal intestinal flora. *Cl. difficile,* a Gram-positive, anaerobic, spore-forming bacterium, is found in a variable proportion and is thought to be the cause in most.

Around 5% of healthy adults and up to 20% of elderly patients in long-term care carry *Cl. difficile.* Infection is usually hospital-acquired and usually occurs when the normal colonic flora is disrupted by antibiotics, most commonly cephalosporins, penicillins and clindamycin.

The organism produces exotoxins which contribute to virulence. Host antibody responses may influence why some people are asymptomatic whilst others develop fulminant colitis. The mucosa shows inflammation and ulceration, which may become covered by a creamy-white fibrinous 'pseudomembrane'.

Symptoms usually begin in the first week of antibiotic therapy but can occur up to 6 wks later. Lower abdominal pain and diarrhoea, which may become profuse and watery, may progress to bloody diarrhoea, fever, toxic dilatation and perforation. Ileus may also be seen.

The diagnosis should be suspected in any patient recently treated with antibiotics. Sigmoidoscopy may show characteristic erythema, white plaques or an adherent pseudomembrane, or appearances may resemble ulcerative colitis. Occasionally the rectum is spared. As some healthy people may harbour *Cl. difficile*, isolation of toxins A and B by cell cytotoxicity assays is required to prove the diagnosis.

Causative antibiotics should be stopped and the patient isolated. I.V. fluids and bowel rest are often needed. Sick patients with ileus, dilatation or pseudomembranous colitis should receive 7–10 days of oral metronidazole or vancomycin. Relapses occur in 5–20%. I.V. immunoglobulin is sometimes given in the most severe cases. Preventative measures include hygiene, hand-washing and disinfection.

ENDOMETRIOSIS

Ectopic endometrial tissue can become embedded on the serosal aspect of the sigmoid and rectum. Cyclical engorgement and inflammation causes low backache, bleeding, diarrhoea, constipation, adhesions or obstruction. It usually affects nulliparous women between 20 and 45 yrs old. Bimanual examination may reveal tender nodules in the pouch of Douglas. Sigmoidoscopy during menstruation reveals a bluish mass with intact overlying mucosa. Treatment options include laparoscopic diathermy and hormonal therapy with progestogens.

ANORECTAL DISORDERS

FAECAL INCONTINENCE

Common causes include severe diarrhoea, impaction, anorectal or neurological disease and obstetric trauma. A careful history and examination, especially of the anorectum and perineum, may help to establish the underlying cause. Endoanal USS is valuable for defining the integrity of the anal sphincters, while manometry and electrophysiology are also useful.

Management involves treating underlying disorders. Pelvic floor exercises, biofeedback techniques and sphincter repair operations help some patients.

HAEMORRHOIDS ('PILES')

Haemorrhoids are extremely common and arise from congestion of the venous plexuses around the anal canal. They are associated with constipation and straining and may develop during pregnancy. First-degree piles bleed, second-degree piles prolapse but retract spontaneously, and third-degree piles require manual replacement. Symptoms include bright red bleeding after defecation, pain, pruritus ani and mucus discharge. Treatment involves preventing constipation, injection sclerotherapy or band ligation. A minority require haemorrhoidectomy, which is usually curative.

PRURITUS ANI

This is common and can result from contamination of the perianal skin with faecal contents. An itch-scratch-itch cycle may exacerbate the problem. Good personal hygiene is essential, with careful washing after defecation. The perineal area must be kept dry and clean.

SOLITARY RECTAL ULCER SYNDROME

This occurs in young adults who develop an ulcer with mucosal prolapse on the anterior rectal wall. Symptoms include minor bleeding and mucus per rectum, tenesmus and perineal pain. Treatment is often difficult but avoidance of straining at defecation is important.

ANAL FISSURE

This is a superficial tear in the anal mucosa, most commonly in the midline posteriorly, with spasm of the internal anal sphincter. Severe pain occurs on defecation with minor bleeding, mucus discharge and pruritus. The skin may be indurated and an oedematous skin tag, or 'sentinel pile', is common.

Avoidance of constipation with bulk-forming laxatives and increased fluid intake is important. Relaxation of the internal sphincter, using glyceryl trinitrate or diltiazem ointment, is effective in 60–80% of patients. Resistant cases may respond to injection of botulinum toxin into the internal anal sphincter to induce sphincter relaxation. Manual dilatation under anaesthesia leads to long-term incontinence and should not be considered.

ANORECTAL ABSCESSES AND FISTULAE

Perianal abscesses develop between the anal sphincters and may point at the perianal skin. Ischiorectal abscesses occur in the ischiorectal fossa. Crohn's disease is sometimes responsible.

Patients complain of extreme perianal pain, fever and/or discharge of pus. Spontaneous rupture may also lead to the development of fistulae. Abscesses and fistulae are treated surgically.

DISEASES OF THE PERITONEAL CAVITY

PERITONITIS

Peritonitis usually occurs as the result of a ruptured viscus, but may also complicate ascites or occur in children without ascites, due to pneumococcal or streptococcal infection. Chlamydial peritonitis is a complication of pelvic inflammatory disease, and presents with right upper quadrant pain, pyrexia and a hepatic rub. TB may cause peritonitis and ascites.

TUMOURS

The most common is secondary adenocarcinoma from the ovary or GI tract. Mesothelioma is a rare tumour complicating asbestos exposure. The prognosis is extremely poor.

13 Liver and biliary tract disease

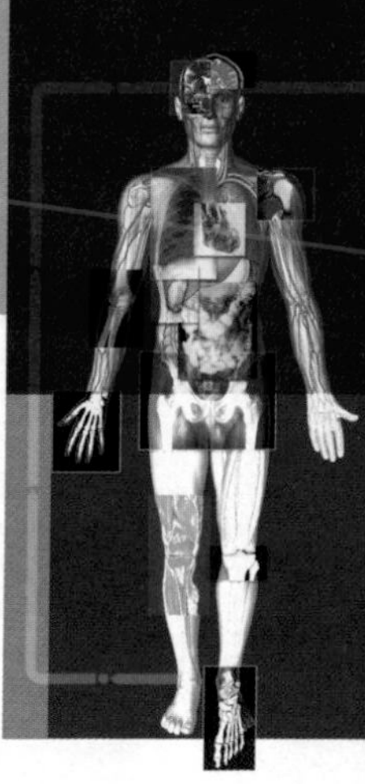

The liver is the largest organ in the body and performs many important functions (Fig. 13.1). Cirrhosis caused more than 25 000 deaths in the USA in 2003. In the developed world, the most common cause of liver disease is alcohol abuse. In contrast, in the developing world, infections caused by hepatitis viruses and parasites are responsible for most chronic liver disease and hepatobiliary cancer.

PRESENTING PROBLEMS

'ASYMPTOMATIC' ABNORMAL LIVER FUNCTION TESTS (LFTs)

When LFTs are measured routinely prior to elective surgery, 3.5% of patients will have some elevation of transaminase concentrations. The majority of patients with persistently abnormal LFTs have significant liver disease. The most common abnormality is alcoholic or non-alcoholic fatty liver disease (pp. 506 and 507). Most hepatologists investigate patients with LFT results greater than twice the limit of normal. The investigations that make up a standard liver screen and additional or confirmatory tests are shown in Box 13.1. An algorithm for investigating abnormal LFTs is illustrated in Figure 13.2. The presence or absence of stigmata of chronic liver disease (p. 492) does not reliably identify patients with significant chronic liver disease. Also, normal LFTs do not exclude significant chronic liver disease, which might progress to cirrhosis, e.g. primary sclerosing cholangitis, haemochromatosis and chronic hepatitis C.

CLINICAL EXAMINATION OF THE ABDOMEN FOR LIVER AND BILIARY DISEASE

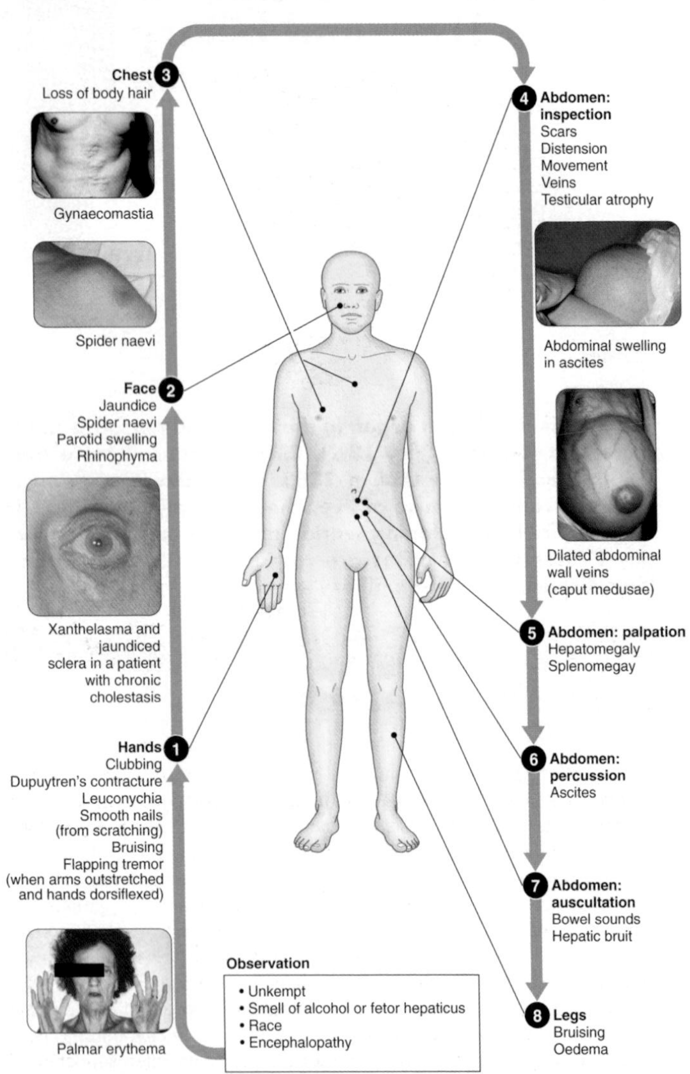

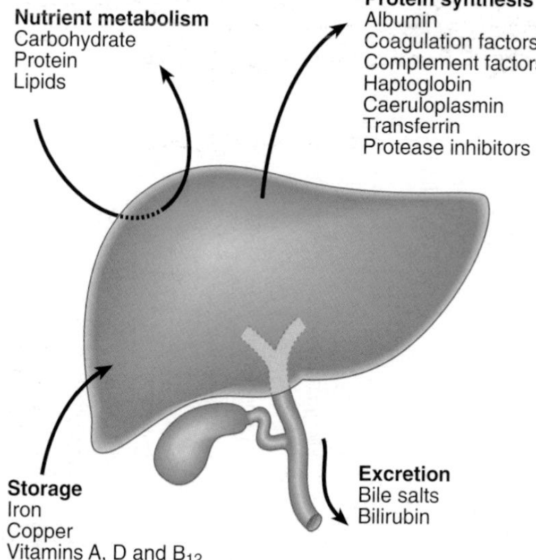

Fig. 13.1 Important liver functions.

JAUNDICE

Jaundice is the yellow appearance of the skin, sclerae and mucous membranes resulting from an increased bilirubin concentration in the body fluids. It is usually detectable clinically when the plasma bilirubin exceeds 50 µmol/l (~3 mg/dl).

Bilirubin metabolism

Bilirubin in the blood is normally almost all unconjugated and, because it is not water-soluble, it is bound to albumin and does not enter the urine. Unconjugated bilirubin is conjugated by glucuronyl transferase into water-soluble conjugates which are exported into the bile. The excretion pathways for bilirubin are shown in Figure 13.3.

HAEMOLYTIC JAUNDICE

This results from increased destruction of red blood cells or their precursors, causing increased bilirubin production. Jaundice due to haemolysis is usually mild because (except in the newborn) a healthy liver can excrete a bilirubin load six times greater than normal before unconjugated bilirubin accumulates in the plasma. Increased excretion of bilirubin and hence stercobilinogen leads to normal-coloured or dark stools, and increased urobilinogen excretion causes the urine to turn dark on standing as urobilin

13.1 TESTS TO IDENTIFY THE CAUSE OF LFT ABNORMALITY

Diagnosis	Clinical clue	Initial test	Additional tests
Alcoholic liver disease	AST > ALT; high MCV	Random blood alcohol	
Non-alcoholic fatty liver disease (NAFLD)	Metabolic syndrome (central obesity, diabetes, hypertension)	Transaminases up to 300 U/l	
Chronic hepatitis B	Injection drug use, blood transfusion	Transaminases up to 300 U/l HBsAg	HBeAg, HBeAb HBV-DNA
Chronic hepatitis C		HCV antibody	HCV-RNA
Primary biliary cirrhosis	Raised alkaline phosphatase	AMA	
Primary sclerosing cholangitis	Inflammatory bowel disease	MRCP	ANCA antibody
Autoimmune hepatitis	Other autoimmune diseases	ASMA, ANA, LKM, transaminases 100–300 U/l	Immunoglobulin
Haemochromatosis	Diabetes/joint pain	Transferrin saturation, ferritin	HFE gene test
Wilson's disease	Neurological signs	Caeruloplasmin, transaminases 100–300 U/l	24-hr urinary copper
Alpha$_1$-antitrypsin	Lung disease	Alpha$_1$-antitrypsin level	Alpha$_1$-antitrypsin phenotype
Drug-induced liver disease	Drug/herbal remedy history	Transaminases >300 U/l	
Coeliac disease	Malabsorption	Endomysial antibody	

(ALT = alanine aminotransferase; AMA = antimitochondrial antibody; ANA = antinuclear antibody; ANCA = antineutrophil cytoplasmic antibodies; ASMA = anti-smooth muscle antibody; AST = aspartate aminotransferase; HBeAb = antibody to hepatitis B e antigen; HBeAg = hepatitis B e antigen; HBsAg = hepatitis B surface antigen; HBV = hepatitis B virus; HCV = hepatitis C virus; LKM = liver-kidney microsomal antibody; MCV = mean cell volume; MRCP = magnetic resonance cholangiopancreatography)

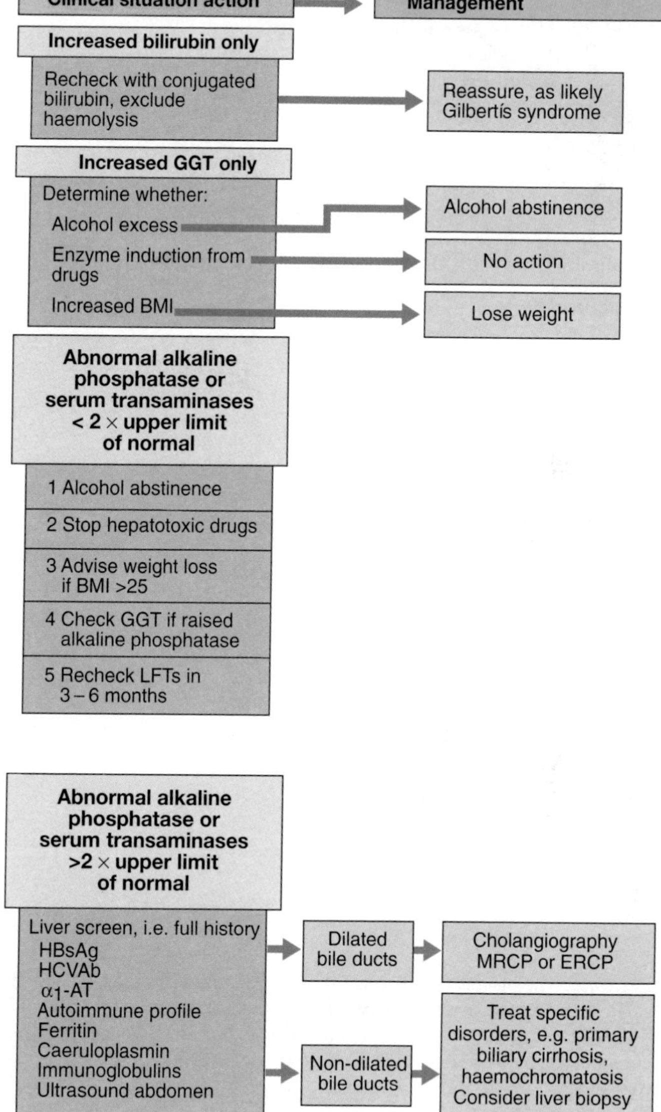

Fig. 13.2 Suggested management of abnormal LFTs in asymptomatic patients.
(ERCP = endoscopic retrograde cholangiopancreatography; GGT = γ-glutamyl transferase; MRCP = magnetic resonance cholangiopancreatography)

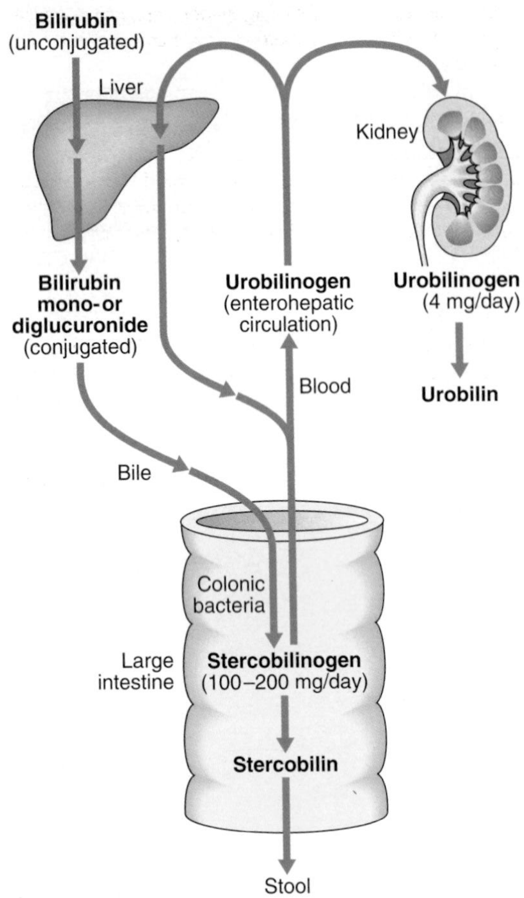

Fig. 13.3 Pathway of bilirubin excretion.

is formed. The plasma bilirubin is usually <100 µmol/l (~6 mg/dl) and the LFTs are otherwise normal. There is no bilirubinuria because the hyperbilirubinaemia is predominantly unconjugated. Pallor and splenomegaly are common and blood examination may show evidence of haemolytic anaemia (p. 543).

CONGENITAL NON-HAEMOLYTIC HYPERBILIRUBINAEMIA

Familial Gilbert's syndrome is the only common cause, resulting from an autosomal dominant mutation reducing expression of UDP-glucuronyl transferase. This causes decreased bilirubin conjugation, with isolated accumulation of unconjugated bilirubin in the blood. It has an excellent prognosis and needs no treatment.

HEPATOCELLULAR JAUNDICE

Hepatocellular jaundice results from an inability of the liver to transport bilirubin into the bile, as a consequence of parenchymal liver disease. In hepatocellular jaundice the concentrations of both unconjugated and conjugated bilirubin in the blood increase, perhaps because of the variable way in which bilirubin transport is disturbed.

CHOLESTATIC JAUNDICE

In unrelieved cholestasis jaundice increases progressively because conjugated bilirubin cannot enter the bile canaliculi and passes back into the blood, and also because there is a failure of clearance of unconjugated bilirubin arriving at the liver.

Intrahepatic causes include:

• Primary biliary cirrhosis. • Alcohol. • Drugs. • Viral or autoimmune hepatitis. • Severe bacterial infections.

Extrahepatic causes include:

• Choledocholithiasis. • Carcinoma. • Parasitic infestation. • Biliary strictures.

Clinical assessment

Early features include:

• Jaundice. • Dark urine. • Pale stools. • Pruritus.

Late features include:

• Xanthelasma and xanthomas. • Malabsorption. • Weight loss. • Steatorrhoea. • Osteomalacia. • Bleeding tendency.

ASCITES

Ascites means the accumulation of free fluid in the peritoneal cavity and is usually due to malignant disease, cirrhosis or heart failure; however, primary disorders of the peritoneum and visceral organs can produce ascites, and these need to be considered, even in a patient with chronic liver disease (Box 13.2).

Clinical assessment

• Ascites causes abdominal distension with fullness in the flanks, shifting dullness on percussion and, when the ascites is marked, a fluid thrill. • These signs do not appear until the ascites volume exceeds 1 litre, even in thin patients. • Pleural effusions are found in ~10% of patients, usually on the right side (hepatic hydrothorax); most are small and only identified on CXR.

13.2 CAUSES OF ASCITES

Common causes	
• Malignant disease Hepatic Peritoneal	• Cardiac failure • Hepatic cirrhosis
Other causes	
• Hypoproteinaemia Nephrotic syndrome Protein-losing enteropathy Malnutrition • Hepatic venous occlusion Budd–Chiari syndrome Veno-occlusive disease • Pancreatitis • Lymphatic obstruction	• Infection TB Spontaneous bacterial peritonitis • Rare Meigs' syndrome Vasculitis Hypothyroidism Renal dialysis

Pathogenesis of ascites in cirrhosis

Splanchnic vasodilatation, mediated mainly by nitric oxide, is thought to be the main factor leading to ascites in cirrhosis. Systemic arterial pressure falls due to splanchnic vasodilatation as cirrhosis advances, with activation of the renin–angiotensin system, secondary aldosteronism, increased sympathetic nervous activity, increased atrial natriuretic hormone secretion and altered activity of the kallikrein–kinin system (Fig. 13.4). These systems tend to normalise arterial pressure but produce salt and water retention. The combination of splanchnic arterial vasodilatation and portal hypertension alter intestinal capillary permeability, promoting fluid accumulation within the peritoneum.

Investigations

• USS is the best means of confirming ascites. • Paracentesis may point to the underlying cause (Box 13.3). • If the total protein concentration is <25 g/l and ascites albumen lower than serum albumin by 11 g/l or more, this indicates ascites due to transudation rather than exudation. • Transudates strongly suggest portal hypertension and cirrhosis. • Exudative ascites (total protein concentration >25 g/l or a serum–ascites albumin gradient <11 g/l) raises the possibility of infection (especially TB), malignancy, hepatic venous obstruction, pancreatic ascites or, rarely, hypothyroidism. • Ascites amylase activity >1000 U/l identifies pancreatic ascites, and low ascites glucose suggests malignancy or TB. • Cytology may reveal malignant cells (one-third of cirrhotic patients with a bloody tap have a hepatoma). • Polymorphonuclear leucocyte counts $>250 \times 10^6$/l strongly suggest infection (spontaneous bacterial peritonitis, see below).

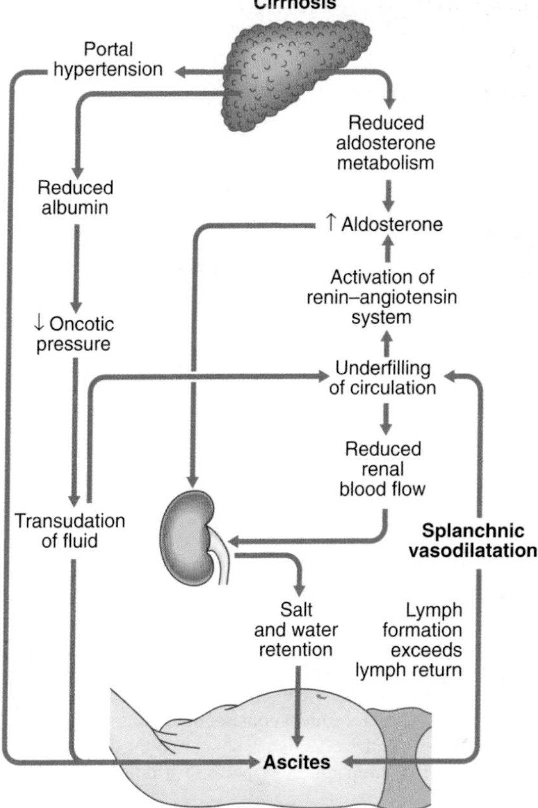

Fig. 13.4 Pathogenesis of ascites.

Management

Successful treatment of ascites relieves discomfort but does not prolong life, and if over-vigorous, can produce serious disorders of fluid and electrolyte balance and precipitate hepatic encephalopathy (p. 489).

Sodium restriction: Restriction to 100 mmol/day ('no added salt diet') is normally adequate. Avoid sodium-rich drugs (e.g. many antibiotics, antacids) and those promoting sodium retention (e.g. steroids, NSAIDs).

Diuretics: Most patients require diuretics in addition to sodium restriction. Spironolactone (100–400 mg/day) is the drug of choice for long-term therapy. Some patients will also require loop diuretics, e.g. furosemide.

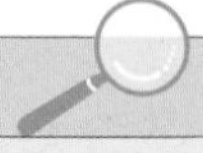

13.3 ASCITIC FLUID: APPEARANCE AND ANALYSIS	
Cause/appearance	
• Cirrhosis: clear, straw-coloured or light green • Malignant disease: bloody • Infection: cloudy • Biliary communication: heavy bile staining • Lymphatic obstruction: milky-white (chylous)	
Useful investigations	
• Total albumin (plus serum albumin) • Amylase • WCC	• Cytology • Microscopy and culture

Paracentesis: Large-volume paracentesis with i.v. albumin can be used as first-line treatment of refractory ascites or when other treatments fail.

Transjugular intrahepatic portosystemic stent shunts (TIPSS, p. 497): Can relieve resistant ascites but do not prolong life.

HEPATORENAL SYNDROME

Ten per cent of patients with advanced cirrhosis and ascites develop the hepatorenal syndrome, which is mediated by severe renal vasoconstriction due to extreme underfilling of the arterial circulation.

Type 1 hepatorenal syndrome: Characterised by progressive oliguria, a rapid rise of the serum creatinine and a very poor prognosis. There is usually no proteinuria, urine sodium excretion is <10 mmol/day and urine/plasma osmolarity ratio is >1.5. Treatment consists of albumin infusions in combination with terlipressin and is effective in about two-thirds of patients. Haemodialysis should not be used routinely because it does not improve the outcome.

Type 2 hepatorenal syndrome: Usually occurs in patients with refractory ascites, is characterised by a moderate and stable increase in serum creatinine, and has a better prognosis.

SPONTANEOUS BACTERIAL PERITONITIS (SBP)

Patients with cirrhosis are very susceptible to ascitic fluid infection.

• SBP usually presents suddenly with abdominal pain, rebound tenderness, absent bowel sounds and fever in a patient with obvious cirrhosis and ascites. • Abdominal signs are mild or absent in about one-third of patients, in whom hepatic encephalopathy and fever dominate. • The source of infection cannot usually be determined, but most organisms isolated from ascitic fluid or blood cultures are of enteric origin; *Escherichia coli* is the most frequently found. • SBP needs to be differentiated from other intra-abdominal emergencies, and the finding of multiple organisms on culture should arouse suspicion of a perforated viscus.

Treatment should be started immediately with broad-spectrum antibiotics, such as cefotaxime. Recurrence of SBP is common and may be reduced by prophylactic quinolones such as norfloxacin (400 mg daily) or ciprofloxacin (250 mg daily).

HEPATIC (PORTOSYSTEMIC) ENCEPHALOPATHY

Hepatic encephalopathy is a neuropsychiatric syndrome caused by liver disease which progresses from confusion to coma. Confusion needs to be differentiated from delirium tremens and Wernicke's encephalopathy, and coma from subdural haematoma which can occur in alcoholics after a fall. Liver failure and portosystemic shunting of blood are two important factors underlying hepatic encephalopathy and the balance between these varies in different patients. The 'neurotoxins' causing the encephalopathy are thought to be mainly nitrogenous substances produced by bacterial action in the gut, which are normally metabolised by the healthy liver and therefore excluded from the systemic circulation. Ammonia has long been considered an important factor but much interest has centred recently on γ-aminobutyric acid.

Clinical assessment

The earliest features are very mild and easily overlooked but mental impairment increases as the condition becomes more severe (Box 13.4). Precipitating causes include trauma, drugs, infection, protein load (including GI bleeding) and constipation. Examination usually shows:

• A flapping tremor (asterixis). • Inability to perform simple mental arithmetic. • Inability to draw objects such as a star (constructional apraxia). • Hyper-reflexia. • Bilateral extensor plantar responses.

An EEG shows diffuse slowing of the normal alpha waves with eventual development of delta waves. Convulsions sometimes occur.

Management

Episodes of encephalopathy are common in cirrhosis and are usually readily reversible until the terminal stages are reached. The principles of manage-

13.4 CLINICAL GRADING OF HEPATIC ENCEPHALOPATHY

Clinical grade	Clinical signs
Grade 1	Poor concentration, slurred speech, slow mentation, disordered sleep rhythm
Grade 2	Drowsy but easily rousable, occasional aggressive behaviour, lethargic
Grade 3	Marked confusion, drowsy, sleepy but responds to pain and voice, gross disorientation
Grade 4	Unresponsive to voice, may or may not respond to painful stimuli, unconscious

ment are to treat or remove precipitating causes and to suppress production of neurotoxins by bacteria in the bowel. Lactulose (15–30 ml 8-hourly) is a disaccharide which is taken orally and produces an osmotic laxative effect. It reduces the colonic pH, thereby limiting colonic ammonia absorption, and promotes the incorporation of nitrogen into bacteria. Neomycin (1–4 g 4–6-hourly) acts by reducing the bacterial content of the bowel. Dietary protein restriction is rarely needed and can lead to worsening nutritional state in already malnourished patients.

ACUTE LIVER FAILURE

Acute liver failure is an uncommon syndrome in which hepatic encephalopathy, characterised by mental changes progressing from confusion to stupor and coma, results from a sudden severe impairment of hepatic function (Box 13.5). Any cause of liver damage can produce acute liver failure, provided it is sufficiently severe.

Acute viral hepatitis is the most common cause world-wide. Paracetamol toxicity (p. 37) is the most frequent cause in the UK. Acute liver failure occurs occasionally with other drugs, or from *Amanita phalloides* (mushroom) poisoning, in pregnancy, in Wilson's disease, or following shock (p. 22). The cause remains unknown in others; these patients are often labelled as having non-A–E viral hepatitis or cryptogenic acute liver failure.

Clinical assessment

• Cerebral disturbance (hepatic encephalopathy) is the cardinal manifestation of acute liver failure, but in the early stages this can be mild and episodic. • The initial clinical features are described above. • Cerebral oedema may occur and can produce increased intracranial pressure causing unequal or abnormally reacting pupils, fixed pupils, hypertensive episodes, bradycardia, hyperventilation, profuse sweating, local or general myoclonus, focal fits or decerebrate posturing. • Papilloedema occurs rarely and is a late sign. • More general symptoms include weakness, nausea and vomiting. • Right hypochondrial discomfort is an occasional feature.

Examination shows:

• Jaundice, which develops rapidly and is usually deep in subsequently fatal cases. However, jaundice is not seen in Reye's syndrome, and death in other

13.5 CLASSIFICATION OF ACUTE LIVER FAILURE

Type	Time: jaundice to encephalopathy	Cerebral oedema	Common causes
Hyperacute	<7 days	Common	Viral, paracetamol
Acute	8 wks	Common	Cryptogenic, drugs
Subacute	8–12 wks	Uncommon	Cryptogenic, drugs

causes of acute liver failure occasionally occurs before jaundice develops. • Hepatomegaly is unusual and, in the presence of a sudden onset of ascites, suggests venous outflow obstruction (Budd–Chiari). • Splenomegaly is uncommon and never prominent. • Ascites and oedema are late developments and may be a consequence of fluid therapy.

Investigations

Investigations are used to determine the cause of the liver failure and the prognosis (Boxes 13.6 and 13.7).

• The prothrombin time rapidly becomes prolonged as coagulation factor synthesis fails; this is the laboratory test of greatest prognostic value and should be carried out at least twice daily. • Plasma aminotransferase activity

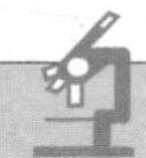

13.6 INVESTIGATIONS TO DETERMINE THE CAUSE OF ACUTE LIVER FAILURE

- Toxicology screen of blood and urine
- IgM anti-HBc
- IgM anti-HAV
- Anti-HEV, HCV, cytomegalovirus, herpes simplex, Epstein–Barr virus
- Caeruloplasmin, serum copper, urinary copper, slit-lamp eye examination
- Autoantibodies: ANF, ASMA, LKM
- Immunoglobulins
- USS of liver and Doppler of hepatic veins

(ANF = antinuclear factor; ASMA = anti-smooth muscle antibody; LKM = liver-kidney microsomal antibody)

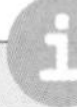

13.7 ADVERSE PROGNOSTIC CRITERIA IN ACUTE LIVER FAILURE*

Paracetamol overdose

- H^+ >50 nmol/l (pH <7.3) at or beyond 24 hrs following the overdose
  or
- Serum creatinine >300 μmol/l + prothrombin time >100 secs + encephalopathy grade 3 or 4

Non-paracetamol cases

- Prothrombin time >100 secs
  or
- Any three of the following: jaundice to encephalopathy time >7 days; age <10 or >40 yrs; indeterminate or drug-induced causes; bilirubin >300 μmol/l; prothrombin time >50 secs
  or
- Factor V level <15% and encephalopathy grade 3 or 4

*Predict a mortality rate of ≥90%.
Creatinine of 300 μmol/l = 3.39 mg/dl. Bilirubin of 300 μmol/l = 17.6 mg/dl.

is particularly high after paracetamol overdose, reaching 100–500 times normal, but falls as liver damage progresses and is not helpful in determining prognosis.

Management

A patient with acute hepatic damage should be observed in a high-dependency or intensive care unit as soon as a progressive prolongation of the prothrombin time or hepatic encephalopathy is identified, so that prompt treatment of complications (hypoglycaemia, infections, renal failure, metabolic acidosis) can be initiated. Treatment is supportive in the hope that hepatic regeneration will occur. *N*-acetylcysteine therapy may improve outcome, particularly in patients with acute liver failure due to paracetamol poisoning. Liver transplantation is an increasingly important treatment option. Patients with a poor prognosis (Box 13.7) should, wherever possible, be transferred to a transplant centre early to allow time for assessment and to maximise the time for a donor liver to become available. Survival following liver transplantation for acute liver failure is improving and 1-yr survival rates of ~60% can be expected.

CHRONIC LIVER FAILURE

Chronic liver failure develops when the functional capacity of the liver can no longer maintain normal physiological conditions and is characterised by the presence of encephalopathy and/or ascites. The term 'hepatic decompensation' or 'decompensated liver disease' is often used when chronic liver failure occurs. The most common cause is cirrhosis, which is usually the result of chronic liver injury occurring over many years. In addition to encephalopathy and/or ascites, patients may develop peripheral oedema, variceal bleeding, renal failure, jaundice, and hypoalbuminaemia and coagulation abnormalities due to defective protein synthesis.

CHRONIC LIVER DISEASE

CIRRHOSIS

Any condition leading to persistent or recurrent hepatocyte death may lead to hepatic cirrhosis (Box 13.8). World-wide, the most common causes are viral hepatitis and alcohol. Prolonged biliary damage or obstruction, as can occur in primary biliary cirrhosis, sclerosing cholangitis and post-surgical biliary strictures, will also result in cirrhosis.

Clinical features

Cirrhosis may be entirely asymptomatic; in life it may be found incidentally at surgery or may be associated with minimal features such as isolated hepatomegaly. Frequent symptoms include weakness, fatigue, muscle cramps, weight loss and non-specific digestive symptoms such as anorexia, nausea, vomiting and upper abdominal discomfort. Otherwise, clinical features are due mainly to hepatic insufficiency and portal hypertension.

13.8 CAUSES OF CIRRHOSIS

- Alcohol
- Chronic viral hepatitis (B or C)
- Non-alcoholic fatty liver disease
- Immune
  - Primary sclerosing cholangitis
  - Autoimmune liver disease
- Biliary
  - Primary biliary cirrhosis
  - Cystic fibrosis
- Genetic
  - Haemochromatosis
  - Alpha$_1$-antitrypsin deficiency
  - Wilson's disease
- Cryptogenic (unknown)

• Hepatomegaly is common in alcoholic liver disease and haemochromatosis. In other causes of cirrhosis (e.g. viral hepatitis or autoimmune liver disease), progressive hepatocyte destruction and fibrosis gradually reduce liver size. The liver is often hard, irregular and painless. • Jaundice is usually mild when it first appears and is due primarily to a failure to excrete bilirubin. • Palmar erythema can be seen early in the disease but is of limited value as it occurs in many other conditions and in some normal people. • One or two small spider telangiectasia are found in ~2% of healthy people and can occur transiently in greater numbers in the third trimester of pregnancy, but otherwise they are a strong indicator of liver disease. • Endocrine changes are noticed more readily in men, who show loss of male hair distribution and testicular atrophy. Gynaecomastia is common and can be due to drugs such as spironolactone. • Easy bruising becomes more frequent as cirrhosis advances. • Epistaxis is common and sometimes severe; it can mimic upper GI bleeding if the blood is swallowed. • Splenomegaly and collateral vessel formation are features of portal hypertension, which occurs in more advanced disease. • Ascites is due to a combination of liver failure and portal hypertension (p. 493) and signifies advanced disease. • Evidence of hepatic encephalopathy also becomes increasingly common with advancing disease. • Non-specific features include finger and toe clubbing. • Dupuytren's contracture is traditionally regarded as being associated with cirrhosis, especially that due to alcohol, but the evidence for this association is weak.

Management and prognosis

Management of cirrhosis is by treatment of the underlying cause and its complications, or by liver transplantation in selected cases of advanced cirrhosis. Prognosis is linked to severity (Box 13.9).

PORTAL HYPERTENSION

Portal hypertension is characterised by prolonged elevation of the portal venous pressure (normally 2–5 mmHg). Patients developing clinical features or complications of portal hypertension usually have portal venous pressures >12 mmHg.

13.9 CHILD–PUGH CLASSIFICATION OF PROGNOSIS IN CIRRHOSIS			
Score	**1**	**2**	**3**
Encephalopathy	None	Mild	Marked
Bilirubin (μmol/l)* In primary biliary cirrhosis and sclerosing cholangitis	<34 <68	34–50 68–170	>50 >170
Albumin (g/l)	>35	28–35	<28
Prothrombin time (secs prolonged)	<4	4–6	>6
Ascites	None	Mild	Marked
Add the individual scores:	<7 = Child's A; 1-yr survival 82% 7–9 = Child's B; 1-yr survival 62% >9 = Child's C; 1-yr survival 42%		
*To convert bilirubin in μmol/l to mg/dl, divide by 17.1.			

Extrahepatic portal vein obstruction is the usual cause of portal hypertension in childhood and adolescence, while cirrhosis causes 90% or more of portal hypertension in adults in developed countries. Schistosomiasis is a common cause of portal hypertension world-wide but it is infrequent outside endemic areas. Other causes are shown in Box 13.10 and Figure 13.5. Increased portal vascular resistance leads to a gradual reduction in the flow of portal blood to the liver and simultaneously to the development of collateral vessels, allowing half or more of the portal blood to bypass the liver and enter the systemic circulation directly.

Clinical features

• Splenomegaly is a cardinal finding, and a diagnosis of portal hypertension is unlikely when splenomegaly cannot be detected clinically or by USS. The spleen is rarely enlarged >5 cm below the left costal margin in adults. • Hypersplenism is common and frequently results in thrombocytopenia. Platelet counts are usually ~100×10^9/l. Leucopenia occurs occasionally but anaemia can hardly ever be attributed directly to hypersplenism. • Collateral vessels may be visible on the anterior abdominal wall and occasionally several radiate from the umbilicus to form a caput medusae. The most important collateral vessels occur in the oesophagus and stomach, where they can cause severe bleeding. Rectal varices also cause bleeding and are often mistaken for haemorrhoids. • Fetor hepaticus results from portosystemic shunting of blood, which allows mercaptans to pass directly to the lungs.

Investigations

• Radiological and endoscopic examination of the upper GI tract can show varices. • Imaging, particularly USS, can show splenomegaly and collateral

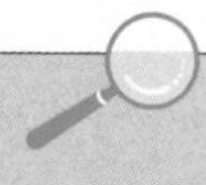

13.10 CAUSES OF PORTAL HYPERTENSION ACCORDING TO SITE OF ABNORMALITY
Extrahepatic post-sinusoidal 1
• Budd–Chiari syndrome
Intrahepatic post-sinusoidal 2
• Veno-occlusive disease
Sinusoidal 3
• Cirrhosis* • Cystic liver disease • Partial nodular transformation of the liver • Metastatic malignant disease
Intrahepatic pre-sinusoidal 4
• Schistosomiasis* • Sarcoidosis • Congenital hepatic fibrosis • Vinyl chloride • Drugs
Extrahepatic pre-sinusoidal 5
• Portal vein thrombosis due to sepsis* (umbilical, portal pyaemia) or procoagulopathy (thrombotic diseases, oral contraceptives, pregnancy), or secondary to cirrhosis • Abdominal trauma, including surgery • Malignant disease of pancreas or liver • Pancreatitis • Congenital
*Most common causes. Numbers refer to Figure 13.5.

vessels, and can sometimes indicate the cause, such as liver disease or portal vein thrombosis. • Portal venography demonstrates the site and often the cause of portal venous obstruction and is performed prior to surgical intervention.

VARICEAL BLEEDING

Bleeding usually occurs from varices near the gastro-oesophageal junction or in the stomach. It is often severe, and recurs if preventative treatment is not given. The mortality from bleeding oesophageal varices is high (up to 50% in those with advanced liver disease), and is largely dependent on the severity of liver dysfunction.

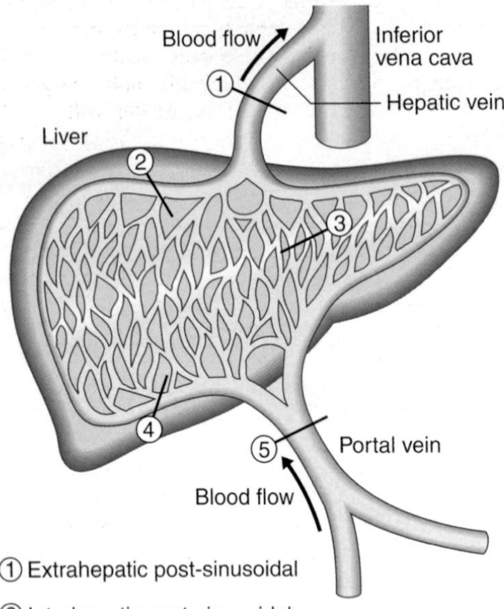

① Extrahepatic post-sinusoidal

② Intrahepatic post-sinusoidal

③ Sinusoidal

④ Intrahepatic pre-sinusoidal

⑤ Extrahepatic pre-sinusoidal

Fig. 13.5 Classification of portal hypertension according to site of vascular obstruction.

Management of acute variceal bleeding

See also acute upper GI haemorrhage (p. 418).

The priority in acute bleeding from oesophageal varices is to restore the circulation with blood and plasma. All patients with cirrhosis and GI bleeding should receive prophylactic broad-spectrum antibiotics such as ciprofloxacin.

Diagnostic endoscopy with banding or sclerotherapy: The most widely used initial treatment, which should be undertaken as soon as possible. It stops variceal bleeding in 80% of patients and can be repeated if bleeding recurs. Banding can be less easy to apply than sclerotherapy. Active bleeding at endoscopy may make endoscopic therapy difficult; in such cases bleeding should be controlled by balloon tamponade prior to endoscopic therapy.

Balloon tamponade: Employs a Sengstaken–Blakemore tube possessing two balloons which exert pressure in the fundus of the stomach and in the lower oesophagus respectively. Current modifications, such as the Minnesota tube, have additional lumens to allow aspiration from the stomach and from the oesophagus above the oesophageal balloon. Gentle traction is essential to maintain pressure on the varices. Initially, only the gastric balloon should be inflated with 200–250 ml of air, as this will usually control bleeding. Inadvertent inflation of the gastric balloon in the oesophagus causes pain and can lead to oesophageal rupture. If the oesophageal balloon needs to be used because of continued bleeding, it should be deflated for 10 mins every 3 hrs to avoid oesophageal mucosal damage. Pressure in the oesophageal balloon is maintained at <40 mmHg using a sphygmomanometer. Balloon tamponade will almost always stop variceal bleeding, but only creates time for the use of definitive therapy. Patients unable to protect their airway should be intubated to avoid pulmonary aspiration whilst the tube is inserted.

Reduction of portal venous pressure

Pharmacological reduction of portal pressure is less important than sclerotherapy or banding, is expensive and is not always used. Terlipressin (which releases vasopressin) and octreotide (the synthetic form of somatostatin) reduce portal pressure and can stop variceal bleeding. TIPSS, described below, can be used for acute bleeding not responding to sclerotherapy or banding.

Prevention of recurrent bleeding

Recurrent bleeding is the rule rather than the exception in patients who have previously bled from oesophageal varices, and treatment is needed to prevent this.

Band ligation: This is a technique in which varices are sucked into an endoscope accessory, allowing them to be occluded with a tight rubber band. Banding is repeated every 1–2 wks until the varices are obliterated.

Sclerotherapy: The injection of varices with a sclerosing agent may cause chest or abdominal pain, fever, dysphagia and even perforation or stricture, and has now been largely abandoned in favour of banding ligation.

TIPSS: A stent is placed between the portal and hepatic veins in the liver to form a portosystemic shunt and reduce portal pressure. The procedure is carried out under radiological control via the internal jugular vein; prior patency of the portal vein must be determined angiographically, coagulation deficiencies may require correction with fresh frozen plasma, and antibiotic cover is provided. Successful TIPSS stops and prevents variceal bleeding.

Portosystemic shunt surgery: Surgical portosystemic shunts carry a high mortality and often cause encephalopathy; they are now reserved for patients with good liver function in whom other treatments have failed.

Beta-adrenoceptor antagonists (β-blockers): Propranolol (80–160 mg/day) reduces portal venous pressure in portal hypertension and can be used in secondary prevention to prevent recurrent variceal bleeding.

Primary prophylaxis of initial variceal bleeding

Propranolol or nadolol, at a dose which reduces heart rate by 25%, have given beneficial results and should be used for primary prevention. Prophylactic banding is probably as effective as a β-blocker.

CONGESTIVE GASTROPATHY

Long-standing portal hypertension causes chronic gastric congestion recognisable at endoscopy as multiple areas of punctate erythema. These areas may become eroded, causing bleeding from multiple sites. Acute bleeding can occur, but repeated minor bleeding causing iron-deficiency anaemia is more common. Reduction of the portal pressure using propranolol is the best initial treatment. If this is ineffective, TIPSS can be undertaken.

PULMONARY MANIFESTATIONS OF CHRONIC LIVER DISEASE

HEPATOPULMONARY SYNDROME

Many patients with cirrhosis are hypoxaemic due to a variety of factors, including pulmonary hypertension, pleural effusions and the hepatopulmonary syndrome. The latter occurs in patients with chronic liver disease and portal hypertension, and is characterised by intrapulmonary shunting through direct arteriovenous communications causing resistant hypoxaemia (PaO_2 <9.3 kPa or 70 mmHg) that worsens on standing.

VIRAL HEPATITIS

This is a common cause of jaundice and must be considered in anyone presenting with hepatitic liver blood tests (high transaminases). Hepatitis viruses (Box 13.11) are the most common cause, with cytomegalovirus, Epstein–Barr, herpes simplex and yellow fever causing occasional cases. All these viruses cause illnesses with similar clinical and pathological features, which are frequently anicteric or even asymptomatic. They differ in their tendency to cause acute and chronic infections.

Clinical features of acute infection

• Prodromal symptoms (headache, myalgia, arthralgia, nausea and anorexia) usually precede jaundice by a few days to 2 wks. • Vomiting and diarrhoea may follow and abdominal discomfort is common. • Dark urine and pale stools may precede jaundice. • There are usually few physical signs. • The liver is often tender but only minimally enlarged. • Occasionally, mild splenomegaly and cervical lymphadenopathy are seen. • Jaundice may be

13.11 FEATURES OF THE MAIN HEPATITIS VIRUSES

	Hepatitis A	Hepatitis B	Hepatitis C	Hepatitis D	Hepatitis E
Virus					
Group	Enterovirus	Hepadna	Flavivirus	Incomplete virus	Calicivirus
Nucleic acid	RNA	DNA	RNA	RNA	RNA
Size (diameter)	27 nm	42 nm	30–38 nm	35 nm	27 nm
Incubation (wks)	2–4	4–20	2–26	6–9	3–8
Spread					
Faeces	Yes	No	No	No	Yes
Blood	Uncommon	Yes	Yes	Yes	No
Saliva	Yes	Yes	Yes	?	?
Sexual	Uncommon	Yes	Uncommon	Yes	?
Vertical	No	Yes	Uncommon	Yes	No
Chronic infection	No	Yes	Yes	Yes	No
Prevention					
Active	Vaccine	Vaccine	No	Prevented by hepatitis B vaccination	No
Passive	Immune serum globulin	Hyperimmune serum globulin	No		No

Note All body fluids are potentially infectious, although some (e.g. urine) are less infectious than others.

mild and the diagnosis may be suspected only after finding abnormal liver blood tests in the setting of non-specific symptoms. • Symptoms rarely last longer than 3–6 wks.

Investigations

• A hepatitic pattern of LFTs develops, with serum transaminases typically between 200 and 2000 U/l. • The plasma bilirubin reflects the degree of liver damage. • The alkaline phosphatase rarely exceeds twice the upper limit of normal. • Prolongation of the prothrombin time indicates the severity of the hepatitis but rarely exceeds 25 secs. • The WCC is usually normal with a relative lymphocytosis. • Serological tests confirm the aetiology of the infection.

Management

• Most individuals do not need hospital care. • Drugs such as sedatives and narcotics, which are metabolised in the liver, should be avoided. • No specific dietary modifications are needed. • Alcohol should be avoided during the acute illness. • Elective surgery should be avoided in cases of acute viral hepatitis as there is a risk of post-operative liver failure.

SPECIFIC VIRAL HEPATITIS

Although the hepatitis viruses all cause similar hepatic illnesses, they belong to distinct viral groups.

HEPATITIS A

The hepatitis A virus (HAV) is highly infectious and is spread by the faecal–oral route. Infection is common in children but often asymptomatic, and so up to 30% of adults will have serological evidence of past infection but give no history of jaundice. Infection is also more common in areas of overcrowding and poor sanitation. In occasional outbreaks water and shellfish have been the vehicles of transmission. A chronic carrier state does not occur.

Anti-HAV IgM antibodies are diagnostic of acute HAV infection, and are present from the onset of symptoms until up to 3 mths after recovery.

Infection in the community is best prevented by improving overcrowding and poor sanitation. Individuals can be given substantial protection by active immunisation with an inactivated virus vaccine. Immunisation should be considered for individuals with chronic hepatitis B or C infections and for close contacts, the elderly, those with other major disease, people travelling to endemic areas and perhaps pregnant women. Immediate protection can be provided by immune serum globulin if given soon after exposure to the virus.

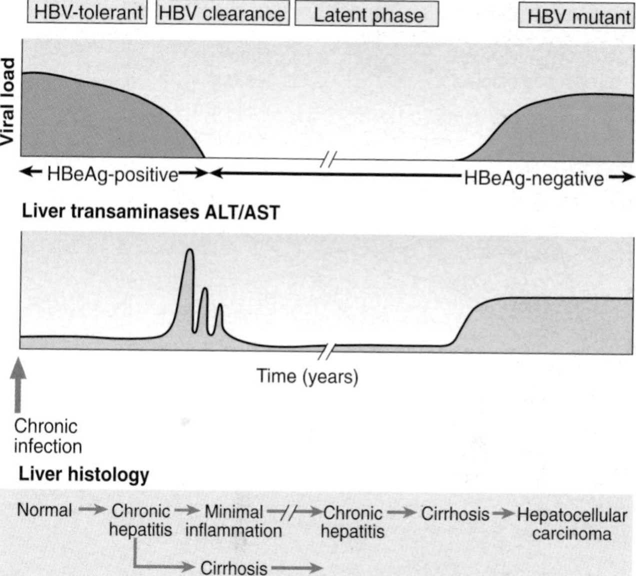

Fig. 13.6 Natural history of chronic hepatitis B infection. There is an initial immunotolerant phase with high levels of virus and normal liver biochemistry. An immunological response to the virus then occurs, with elevation in serum transaminases which causes liver damage: chronic hepatitis. If this response is sustained over many years and viral clearance does not occur promptly, chronic hepatitis may result in cirrhosis. In individuals where the immunological response is successful, viral load falls, HBe antibody develops and there is no further liver damage. Some individuals may subsequently develop HBV-DNA mutants, which escape from immune regulation, and viral load again rises with further chronic hepatitis. Mutations in the core protein result in the virus's inability to secrete HBe antigen despite high levels of viral replication; such individuals have HBeAg-negative chronic hepatitis. (ALT = alanine aminotransferase; AST = aspartate aminotransferase)

Acute liver failure complicates acute hepatitis A in only 0.1% of cases; however, HAV infection in patients with chronic liver disease may cause serious or life-threatening disease.

HEPATITIS B

The hepatitis B virus (HBV) consists of a core surrounded by surface protein. The virus and an excess of its surface protein (known as hepatitis B surface antigen, HBsAg) circulate in the blood. Humans are the only source of infection. Hepatitis B infection affects 300 million people and is one of the most common causes of chronic liver disease and hepatocellular carcinoma world-wide. The natural history of HBV infection is shown in Figure 13.6.

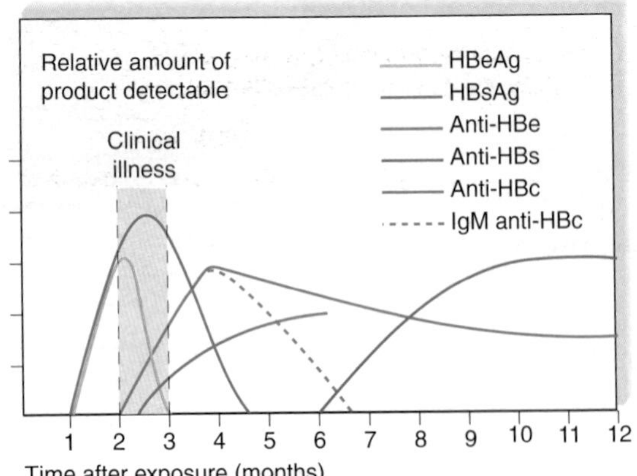

Fig. 13.7 Serological responses to hepatitis B virus infection. (HBsAg = hepatitis B surface antigen; anti-HBs = antibody to HBsAg; HBeAg = hepatitis B e antigen; anti-HBe = antibody to HBeAg; anti-HBc = antibody to hepatitis B core antigen)

Investigations

Serology: In acute infection HBsAg is a reliable marker of HBV infection (Fig. 13.7). Antibody to HBsAg (anti-HBs) appears after about 3–6 mths and persists for many years or even permanently. Anti-HBs implies either a previous infection, in which case anti-HBc (see below) is usually also present, or previous vaccination, when anti-HBc is not present.

The hepatitis B core antigen (HBcAg) is not found in the blood, but antibody to it (anti-HBc) appears early in the illness. Anti-HBc is initially of IgM type with IgG antibody appearing later.

The hepatitis B e antigen (HBeAg) appears only transiently at the outset of the illness and is followed by the production of antibody (anti-HBe). HBeAg reflects active replication of the virus in the liver. Chronic HBV infection (see below) is marked by the presence of HBsAg and anti-HBc (IgG) in the blood. Usually, HBeAg or anti-HBe is also present. Interpretation of serological tests is shown in Box 13.12.

Viral load: HBV-DNA can be measured by polymerase chain reaction (PCR) in the blood. Viral loads are usually $>10^5$ copies/ml in the presence of active viral replication, as indicated by the presence of e antigen. In contrast, in those with low viral replication, HBsAg- and anti-HBe-positive, viral loads are usually $<10^5$ copies/ml.

Management

Acute hepatitis B: Treatment is supportive with monitoring for acute liver failure, which occurs in <1% of cases.

13.12 INTERPRETATION OF MAIN INVESTIGATIONS USED IN THE SEROLOGICAL DIAGNOSIS OF HEPATITIS B VIRUS INFECTION				
		Anti-HBc		
Interpretation	**HBsAg**	**IgM**	**IgG**	**Anti-HBs**
Incubation period	+	+	–	–
Acute hepatitis				
Early	+	+	–	–
Established	+	+	+	–
Established (occasional)	–	+	+	–
Convalescence				
(3–6 mths)	–	±	+	±
(6–9 mths)	–	–	+	+
Post-infection				
>1 yr	–	–	+	+
Uncertain	–	–	+	–
Chronic infection				
Usual	+	–	+	–
Occasional	–	–	+	–
Immunisation without infection	–	–	–	+
+ positive; – negative; ± present at low titre or absent.				

Chronic hepatitis B:
• Alfa-interferon: this is most effective in patients with low viral load and high transaminases in whom it acts by augmenting a native immune response. Interferon is contraindicated in the presence of cirrhosis as it may precipitate liver failure. Longer-acting pegylated interferons which can be given once weekly have been evaluated in both HBeAg-positive and HBeAg-negative chronic hepatitis. • Other drugs: lamivudine and adefovir both inhibit DNA polymerase and suppress HBV-DNA levels. Other drugs which are currently being studied in chronic hepatitis B include tenofovir, which has anti-HIV efficacy, and L-deoxythymidine. • Liver transplantation: the use of post-liver transplant prophylaxis with lamivudine and hepatitis B immunoglobulins has reduced the reinfection rate to 10% and increased 5-yr survival to 80%, making transplantation an acceptable treatment option in selected cases.

Prevention

Individuals are most infectious when markers of continuing viral replication, such as HBeAg, and high levels of HBV-DNA are present in the blood.

HBV-DNA can be found in saliva, urine, semen and vaginal secretions. The virus is about ten times more infectious than hepatitis C, which in turn is about ten times more infectious than HIV. A recombinant hepatitis B vaccine containing HBsAg is available (Engerix) and is capable of producing active immunisation in 95% of normal individuals. Infection can also be prevented or minimised by the i.m. injection of hyperimmune serum globulin prepared from blood containing anti-HBs. This should be given within 24 hrs, or at most a week, of exposure to infected blood in circumstances likely to cause infection (e.g. needlestick injury, contamination of cuts or mucous membranes).

Prognosis

Acute hepatitis: Full recovery occurs in 90–95% of adults following acute HBV infection. The remaining 5–10% develop a chronic infection which usually continues for life, although later recovery occasionally occurs. Recovery from acute HBV infection occurs within 6 mths, with the appearance of antibody to viral antigens. Persistence of HBsAg beyond this time indicates chronic infection. Combined HBV and HDV infection causes more aggressive disease.

Chronic infection: Most patients with chronic hepatitis B are asymptomatic and develop complications such as cirrhosis and hepatocellular carcinoma only after many years (Fig. 13.6). Cirrhosis develops in 15–20% of patients with chronic HBV over 5–20 yrs.

HEPATITIS D (DELTA VIRUS)

The hepatitis D virus (HDV) is an RNA-defective virus which has no independent existence; it requires HBV for replication. It can infect individuals simultaneously with HBV, or can superinfect those who are already chronic carriers of HBV. Simultaneous infections give rise to acute hepatitis, which is often severe but is limited by recovery from the HBV infection. Infections in individuals who are chronic carriers of HBV can cause acute hepatitis with spontaneous recovery, and occasionally simultaneous cessation of the chronic HBV infection takes place. Chronic infection with HBV and HDV can also occur, and this frequently causes rapidly progressive chronic hepatitis and eventually cirrhosis.

HDV has a world-wide distribution. It is endemic in parts of the Mediterranean basin, Africa and South America, where transmission is mainly by close personal contact; occasionally, vertical transmission occurs from mothers who also carry HBV. In non-endemic areas, transmission is mainly a consequence of parenteral drug misuse.

HDV contains a single antigen to which infected individuals make an antibody (anti-HDV). Diagnosis depends on detecting anti-HDV. This antibody generally disappears within 2 mths but persists in a few patients.

HEPATITIS C

This is caused by an RNA flavivirus. Acute symptomatic infection with hepatitis C virus (HCV) is rare. Infection occurs with i.v. drug misuse, needlestick injury, transfusion prior to donor screening or through sharing toothbrushes or razors. Most individuals will be unaware of becoming infected and are only identified when they develop chronic liver disease. Eighty per cent of individuals exposed to the virus will become chronically infected.

Investigations

It may take 6–12 wks for antibodies to appear in the blood following acute infection such as a needlestick injury. In these cases hepatitis C RNA can be identified in the blood as early as 2–4 wks after infection. Active infection is confirmed by the presence of serum hepatitis C RNA in anyone who is antibody-positive. LFTs may be normal or show fluctuating serum transaminases with ALT between 50 and 200 U/l. Jaundice only usually appears in end-stage cirrhosis. Serum transaminase levels in hepatitis C are a poor predictor of the degree of liver fibrosis that has developed as a result of chronic viral hepatitis, and so a liver biopsy is often required to stage the degree of liver damage.

Management

The aim of treatment is to eradicate infection.

• The treatment of choice is pegylated α-interferon given weekly subcutaneously, together with oral ribavirin, a synthetic nucleotide analogue. The length of treatment and efficacy depend on viral genotype. • The main side-effect of ribavirin is haemolytic anaemia. Side-effects of interferon are significant and include flu-like symptoms, irritability and depression. • Virological relapse can occur in the first 3 mths after stopping treatment and cure is defined as loss of virus from serum 6 mths after completing therapy. • Liver transplantation should be considered when complications of cirrhosis occur. Unfortunately, hepatitis C almost always recurs in the transplanted liver.

Prevention and prognosis

There is no active or passive protection against HCV. Not everyone with hepatitis C infection will necessarily develop cirrhosis but ~20% do so within 20 yrs. Once cirrhosis is present, 2–5%/yr will develop primary hepatocellular carcinoma.

HEPATITIS E

Hepatitis E is caused by an RNA virus which is endemic in India and the Middle East. The clinical presentation of hepatitis E is similar to hepatitis A. It is spread via the faecal–oral route; in most cases it presents as a self-limiting acute hepatitis and does not cause chronic liver disease. It differs from hepatitis A in that infection during pregnancy is associated with the development of acute liver failure, which has a high mortality. In acute infection IgM antibodies to HEV are positive. There is no active or passive immune therapy for hepatitis E.

OTHER FORMS OF VIRAL HEPATITIS

Cytomegalovirus and Epstein–Barr virus infection causes abnormal LFTs in most patients, and occasionally icteric hepatitis occurs. Herpes simplex may cause hepatitis in immunocompromised adults. Abnormal LFTs are also common in chickenpox, measles, rubella and acute HIV infection.

ALCOHOLIC LIVER DISEASE

The risk of alcoholic liver disease is variable; not everyone who drinks heavily will develop it, and it does not occur below 21 U/wk in women and 28 U/wk in men. Only 10% of alcoholics have cirrhosis at postmortem. Although the average alcohol consumption of an individual with cirrhosis is 160 g/day for 8 yrs, there is no clear linear relationship between dose and liver damage.

Risk factors are:

• Drinking patterns: liver damage is more likely to occur in continuous rather than binge drinkers. • Genetics: alcoholism is more common in monozygotic than dizygotic twins. • Nutrition: animals given a choline-deficient diet are more likely to develop alcoholic liver disease.

Clinical features

Clinical syndromes include:

• Fatty liver: abnormal liver biochemistry and hepatomegaly. • Alcoholic hepatitis: jaundice, malnutrition, hepatomegaly, portal hypertension • Cirrhosis: spider naevi, Dupuytren's contracture, palmar erythema, ascites, varices, encephalopathy and increased risk of hepatocellular carcinoma.

Investigations

• Macrocytosis without anaemia may suggest alcohol misuse. • Raised γ-glutamyl transferase (GGT): not specific for alcohol misuse, also elevated in hepatic steatosis and fibrosis. May not return to normal with abstinence. • Jaundice suggests alcoholic hepatitis. • Prothrombin time and bilirubin can be used to give a 'discriminant function' (DF, Maddrey's score), which predicts prognosis in alcoholic hepatitis:

$$DF = [4.6 \times \text{Increase in prothrombin time (sec)}] + \text{bilirubin (mg/dl)}$$

A value >32 implies severe liver disease with a poor prognosis. (Divide bilirubin in μmol/l by 17.1 to convert to mg/dl.)

Management

• Cessation of alcohol consumption is the most important treatment; without this other therapies are of limited value. Abstinence is even effective at preventing progression of liver disease and death when cirrhosis is present. • Good nutrition is very important and enteral feeding via a fine-bore nasogastric tube may be needed in severely ill patients. • Corticosteroids increase survival in patients with severe alcoholic hepatitis (Maddrey's score >32).

• Pentoxifylline, which has a weak anti-tumour necrosis factor (TNF) action, may be beneficial in severe alcoholic hepatitis. It appears to reduce the incidence of hepatorenal failure and its use is not complicated by sepsis.
• In many centres alcoholic liver disease is a common indication for liver transplantation. The challenge is to identify patients with an unacceptable risk of returning to harmful alcohol consumption. Many programmes require a 6-mth period of abstinence from alcohol before a patient is considered for transplantation. Although this relates poorly to the incidence of alcohol relapse after transplantation, liver function may improve to the extent that transplantation is no longer necessary. Transplantation for alcoholic hepatitis has a poorer outcome than for complications of alcoholic cirrhosis.

Prognosis

Alcoholic fatty liver disease: Has a good prognosis, and steatosis usually disappears after 3 mths of abstinence.

Alcoholic hepatitis: About one-third of patients die in the acute episode. In patients presenting with jaundice who subsequently abstain, the 3- and 5-yr survival is 70%.

Alcoholic cirrhosis: Often presents with a serious complication such as variceal haemorrhage or ascites, and only half of such patients survive 5 yrs from presentation.

NON-ALCOHOLIC FATTY LIVER DISEASE (NAFLD)

This a disease of affluent societies and its prevalence is increasing in proportion to the rise in obesity. It can be classified into simple fatty liver disease (or steatosis) and non-alcoholic steatohepatitis (NASH). The former has a benign prognosis but the latter is associated with fibrosis and progression to cirrhosis. Dietary factors and insulin resistance cause fatty liver and then a 'second hit' from inflammation or oxidative stress is required to produce NASH.

NAFLD affects 15–20% of the population in the USA. The prevalence is higher in those with diabetes and those with the metabolic syndrome (hypertriglyceridaemia, hypertension, diabetes mellitus, an elevated BMI >25 and especially truncal obesity, p. 386).

Clinical features

Most patients present with asymptomatic abnormal LFTs, particularly elevation of the transaminases or isolated elevation of the GGT. Occasionally, disease presents with a complication of cirrhosis such as variceal bleeding.

Investigations

LFTs: Unlike in alcoholic liver disease, ALT is normally higher than AST. It is important to differentiate simple fatty liver disease, which does not require follow-up, from NASH. Elevated serum transaminases greater than twice the upper limit of normal and the presence of the metabolic syndrome are useful predictors of NASH, whereas USS cannot distinguish steatosis from NASH.

Liver biopsy: Individuals with serum transaminases greater than twice the upper limit of normal and features of the metabolic syndrome should be offered a liver biopsy to determine whether inflammation and fibrosis are present.

Management and prognosis

Current treatments are aimed at reducing BMI and insulin resistance. Metformin has been shown to improve LFTs and should be the first-line treatment in type 2 diabetes with NAFLD. Weight loss reduces transaminase levels and insulin resistance and improves liver fibrosis.

Once cirrhosis has occurred, 5- and 10-yr survival rates are 90% and 84% respectively. Hepatocellular carcinoma frequently complicates NAFLD cirrhosis. Although <5% of liver transplants are currently performed for NAFLD, this is likely to increase.

HEPATOTOXIC DRUG REACTIONS

TYPES OF LIVER INJURY

Cholestasis: Chlorpromazine and antibiotics such as flucloxacillin cause cholestatic hepatitis, with inflammation and canalicular injury. Co-amoxiclav is the most common antibiotic to cause abnormal LFTs but it may not produce symptoms until 10–42 days after it is stopped.

Hepatocyte necrosis: Paracetamol (p. 37) is the best-known cause. Inflammation is not always present but does accompany necrosis in liver injury due to diclofenac (an NSAID) and isoniazid (an anti-tuberculous drug). Acute hepatocellular necrosis has also been described following the use of cocaine, ecstasy and several herbal remedies including germander, comfrey and jin bu huan.

Steatosis: Tetracyclines and sodium valproate cause microvesicular steatosis; amiodarone toxicity can produce a similar histological picture to NASH (p. 507).

Hepatic fibrosis: Most drugs cause reversible liver injury and hepatic fibrosis is very uncommon. Methotrexate, however, as well as causing acute liver injury when it is started, can lead to cirrhosis when used in high doses over a long period of time.

INHERITED LIVER DISEASES

HAEMOCHROMATOSIS

In haemochromatosis, total body iron is increased and excess iron is deposited in and damages several organs including the liver. It may be primary, or secondary to iatrogenic or dietary iron overload or other rare diseases.

HEREDITARY (PRIMARY) HAEMOCHROMATOSIS

Hereditary haemochromatosis (HHC) is caused by increased absorption of dietary iron and is inherited as an autosomal recessive gene on chromosome 6. Approximately 90% of patients have a single-point mutation (C282Y) in a protein (HFE). Iron loss in menstruation and pregnancy may protect females, as 90% of patients are male.

Clinical features

The important organs involved are the liver, pancreatic islets, endocrine glands and heart.

• Symptomatic disease usually presents in men aged 40 yrs or over with features of hepatic cirrhosis (especially hepatomegaly), diabetes mellitus or heart failure. • Tiredness, fatigue and arthropathy are early symptoms. • Leaden-grey skin pigmentation due to excess melanin occurs, especially in exposed parts, axillae, groins and genitalia: 'bronzed diabetes'. • Impotence, loss of libido, testicular atrophy and arthritis are common. • Cardiac failure or dysrhythmia may complicate heart muscle disease.

Investigations

• Serum ferritin is greatly increased • Plasma iron is also increased, with a highly saturated plasma iron-binding capacity. • Liver biopsy is used to confirm the diagnosis. The iron content of the liver can be measured directly. • Genetic testing identifies the common mutations.

Management and prognosis

Weekly venesection of 500 ml blood (250 mg iron) is performed until the serum iron is normal; this may take 2 yrs or more. Thereafter, venesection is continued as required to keep the serum ferritin normal. Liver and cardiac problems improve after iron removal, but diabetes mellitus does not resolve. First-degree relatives should be screened.

Pre-cirrhotic patients with HHC have a normal life expectancy and three-quarters of cirrhotic patients are alive 5 yrs after diagnosis. Screening for hepatocellular carcinoma (p. 517) is mandatory because this affects about one-third of patients with cirrhosis irrespective of therapy.

ACQUIRED IRON OVERLOAD (SECONDARY HAEMOCHROMATOSIS)

Many conditions, including chronic haemolytic disorders, sideroblastic anaemia, other conditions requiring multiple blood transfusion (generally >50 litres), porphyria cutanea tarda, dietary iron overload and occasionally alcoholic cirrhosis, are associated with widespread secondary siderosis.

WILSON'S DISEASE (HEPATOLENTICULAR DEGENERATION)

Wilson's disease is a rare but important autosomal recessive disorder of copper metabolism. Normally, dietary copper is absorbed from the stomach and proximal small intestine and is rapidly taken into the liver, where it is stored and incorporated into caeruloplasmin, which is secreted into the blood. The accumulation of excessive copper in the body is prevented by its excretion, most importantly via the bile. Wilson's disease is usually caused by a failure of synthesis of caeruloplasmin. The amount of copper in the body at birth is normal, but thereafter it increases steadily; the organs most affected are the liver, basal ganglia of the brain, eyes, kidneys and skeleton.

Clinical features

Symptoms usually appear between the ages of 5 and 45 yrs.

• Acute hepatitis, sometimes recurrent, can occur, especially in children, and may progress to acute fulminant liver failure. • Chronic hepatitis can develop insidiously and eventually present with established cirrhosis. • Neurological effects include extrapyramidal features, particularly tremor, choreoathetosis, dystonia, parkinsonism and dementia (p. 630). Unusual clumsiness for age may be an early symptom. • Kayser–Fleischer rings (greenish-brown discoloration of the corneal margin appearing first at the upper periphery, Fig. 13.8) are the most important single clinical clue to the diagnosis and are seen in 60% of adults with Wilson's disease. They eventually disappear with treatment.

Investigations

• Low serum caeruloplasmin: the best single laboratory clue to the diagnosis. • High free serum copper concentration. • High urine copper excretion. • Very high hepatic copper content.

Management

• The copper-binding agent penicillamine is the drug of choice. • Liver transplantation is indicated for fulminant liver failure or for advanced

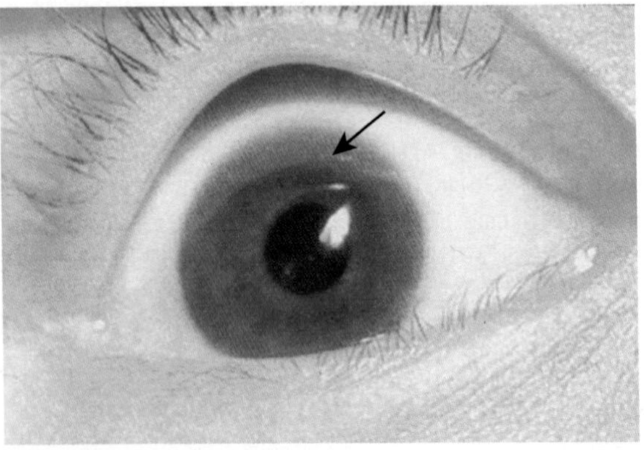

Fig. 13.8 Kayser–Fleischer rings at the junction of the cornea and sclera (arrow) in a patient with Wilson's disease.

cirrhosis with liver failure. • The prognosis is excellent, provided treatment is started before there is irreversible damage.

ALPHA$_1$-ANTITRYPSIN DEFICIENCY

Alpha$_1$-antitrypsin (α_1-AT) is a serine protease inhibitor (Pi) produced by the liver. Homozygotes for the PiZ variant have low plasma α_1-AT concentrations and they may develop hepatic and pulmonary disease (p. 285). Liver disease includes cholestatic jaundice in the neonatal period (neonatal hepatitis) which can resolve spontaneously, chronic hepatitis and cirrhosis in adults, and ultimately hepatocellular carcinoma. There are no clinical features to distinguish from other causes of liver disease, and the diagnosis is made from the low plasma α_1-AT concentration and the genotype. No specific treatment is available; the concurrent risk of severe early-onset emphysema means that all patients should be advised to abandon cigarette smoking.

CYSTIC FIBROSIS

Cystic fibrosis (p. 290) is sometimes associated with biliary cirrhosis, which leads to portal hypertension in a small percentage of cases.

AUTOIMMUNE LIVER DISEASES

AUTOIMMUNE HEPATITIS

Autoimmune hepatitis is a liver disease of unknown aetiology characterised by a strong association with other autoimmune diseases (Box 13.13), hypergammaglobulinaemia and autoantibodies in the serum. It occurs most often in women, particularly in the second and third decades of life, but may develop in either sex at any age.

Clinical features

• Onset is usually insidious, with fatigue, anorexia and jaundice. • Fever, arthralgia, vitiligo and epistaxis may occur, and signs of chronic liver disease are usually present. • Some patients have a 'Cushingoid' face with

13.13 CONDITIONS ASSOCIATED WITH AUTOIMMUNE HEPATITIS

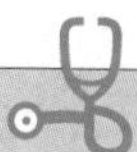

- Migrating polyarthritis
- Urticarial rashes
- Lymphadenopathy
- Hashimoto's thyroiditis
- Thyrotoxicosis
- Myxoedema
- Coombs-positive haemolytic anaemia
- Pleurisy
- Transient pulmonary infiltrates
- Ulcerative colitis
- Glomerulonephritis
- Nephrotic syndrome

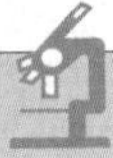

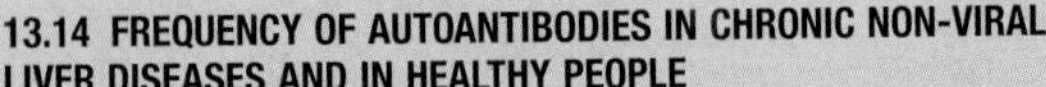

13.14 FREQUENCY OF AUTOANTIBODIES IN CHRONIC NON-VIRAL LIVER DISEASES AND IN HEALTHY PEOPLE

Disease	Antinuclear antibody (%)	Anti-smooth muscle antibody (%)	Antimitochondrial antibody*
Healthy controls	5	1.5	0.01
Autoimmune hepatitis	80	70	15
Primary biliary cirrhosis	25	35	95
Cryptogenic cirrhosis	40	30	15

*Patients with antimitochondrial antibody frequently have cholestatic LFTs and may have primary biliary cirrhosis (see text).

acne, hirsutism and pink cutaneous striae, especially on the thighs and abdomen. • In ~25%, the onset is acute, resembling viral hepatitis, but resolution does not occur, and it may progress to extensive liver necrosis and liver failure. • Approximately two-thirds of patients have associated autoimmune disease such as Hashimoto's thyroiditis, renal tubular acidosis and rheumatoid arthritis.

Diagnosis and investigations

• Serological testing for specific autoantibodies may suggest autoimmune hepatitis (Box 13.14) but is not specific. Antimicrosomal antibodies (anti-LKM) occur, particularly in children and adolescents. • Elevated serum IgG is invariable and is an important diagnostic feature. • Liver biopsy typically shows interface hepatitis, with or without cirrhosis.

Management

• Treatment with corticosteroids is life-saving in autoimmune hepatitis. Initially, prednisolone 40 mg/day is given orally; the dose is then gradually reduced as the patient and LFTs improve. • Withdrawal of treatment should not be considered unless a liver biopsy is normal. • Azathioprine may allow the dose of prednisolone to be reduced. • Approximately 50% of symptomatic patients will die of liver failure within 5 yrs without treatment, but with therapy only 10% will die.

PRIMARY BILIARY CIRRHOSIS (PBC)

PBC is a chronic, progressive cholestatic liver disease of unknown cause which predominantly affects middle-aged women. It is strongly associated with serum antibodies to mitochondria (AMA), which are diagnostic. Granulomatous inflammation of the portal tracts occurs, leading to progressive fibrosis and cirrhosis.

Clinical features

• Non-specific symptoms, such as lethargy and arthralgia, are common and may precede diagnosis for years. Pruritus is the most common initial complaint and may precede jaundice by months or years. Bone pain or fractures can rarely result from osteomalacia (fat-soluble vitamin malabsorption) or from accelerated osteoporosis (hepatic osteodystrophy). • Initially, patients are well nourished but considerable weight loss can occur as the disease progresses. • Scratch marks may be found. • Jaundice is a late feature and can become intense. • Xanthomatous deposits occur in a minority, especially around the eyes, in the hand creases and over the elbows, knees and buttocks. • Hepatomegaly is virtually constant, and splenomegaly becomes increasingly common as portal hypertension develops. • Liver failure may supervene. • Autoimmune and connective tissue diseases occur with increased frequency in PBC, particularly Sjögren's syndrome (p. 608), systemic sclerosis, coeliac disease (p. 446) and thyroid diseases.

Diagnosis and investigations

• LFTs show the pattern of cholestasis. • Hypercholesterolaemia is common but non-specific. • AMA is present in >95% of patients, and when it is absent the diagnosis should not be made without biopsy and cholangiography (MRCP or ERCP) to exclude other biliary disease. • USS examination shows no sign of biliary obstruction.

Management

The hydrophilic bile acid, ursodeoxycholic acid (UDCA), improves bile flow, replaces toxic hydrophobic bile acids in the bile acid pool, and reduces apoptosis of the biliary epithelium. It improves LFTs, may slow down histological and clinical progression, and has few side-effects.

Liver transplantation should be considered once liver failure has developed and may be indicated in patients with intractable pruritus. Transplantation is associated with an excellent 5-yr survival of >80%.

Pruritus: Best treated with the anion-binding resin colestyramine, which probably acts by binding potential pruritogens in the intestine and increasing their excretion in the stool. Alternative treatments for pruritus include rifampicin, naltrexone (an opioid antagonist), plasmapheresis and a liver support device (e.g. a molecular adsorbent recirculating system (MARS) machine).

Lethargy: Affects about one-third of patients with PBC. Unfortunately, once depression and hypothroidism have been excluded, there is no treatment.

Prolonged cholestasis: Associated with steatorrhoea and malabsorption of fat-soluble vitamins, which should be replaced as necessary.

Osteopenia and osteoporosis: Common and should be treated with replacement calcium and vitamin D_3. Bisphosphonates such as risedronate should be used if there is evidence of osteopenia.

SECONDARY BILIARY CIRRHOSIS

This develops after prolonged large duct biliary obstruction due to gallstones, benign bile duct strictures or sclerosing cholangitis (see below). The clinical features are of chronic cholestasis with episodes of ascending cholangitis or even liver abscess (p. 518). Cirrhosis, ascites and portal hypertension are late features. Cholangitis requires treatment with antibiotics, which can be given continuously if attacks recur frequently.

PRIMARY SCLEROSING CHOLANGITIS (PSC)

PSC is a cholestatic liver disease caused by diffuse inflammation and fibrosis that can involve the entire biliary tree. It leads to the gradual obliteration of intrahepatic and extrahepatic bile ducts, and ultimately biliary cirrhosis, portal hypertension and hepatic failure. Cholangiocarcinoma develops in ~10–30% of patients during the course of the disease.

PSC occurs mainly in young men (male : female ratio 2 : 1). There is a close association with inflammatory bowel disease, particularly ulcerative colitis (Box 13.15). Most patients present at age 25–40 yrs.

The diagnostic criteria are:

• Generalised beading and stenosis of the biliary system on cholangiography. • Absence of choledocholithiasis (or history of bile duct surgery). • Exclusion of bile duct cancer, usually by prolonged follow-up.

Clinical features

• The diagnosis is often made incidentally when persistently raised serum alkaline phosphatase is discovered in an individual with ulcerative colitis. • Symptoms include fatigue, intermittent jaundice, weight loss, right upper quadrant abdominal pain and pruritus. • Physical signs, most commonly jaundice and hepatomegaly/splenomegaly, are present in only 50% of symptomatic patients.

Investigations

Serum biochemical tests: Usually indicate cholestasis. However, alkaline phosphatase and bilirubin levels vary widely in individual patients during the course of the disease, sometimes spontaneously, sometimes with therapy. In addition to ANCA, low titres of serum ANA and ASMA have been found in PSC but have no diagnostic significance.

13.15 DISEASES ASSOCIATED WITH PRIMARY SCLEROSING CHOLANGITIS

- Ulcerative colitis
- Crohn's colitis
- Chronic pancreatitis
- Retroperitoneal fibrosis
- Reidel's thyroiditis
- Retro-orbital tumours
- Immune deficiency states
- Sjögren's syndrome
- Angio-immunoplastic lymphadenopathy
- Histiocytosis X
- Autoimmune haemolytic anaemia

Radiology: ERCP is usually diagnostic and may reveal multiple irregular stricturing and dilatation. MRCP is a non-invasive method of imaging the biliary tree; it is being assessed and will probably become the standard method of diagnosis.

Histology: The characteristic early features of PSC are periductal 'onion-skin' fibrosis and inflammation.

Management and prognosis

• Pruritus is best managed initially with colestyramine. • Broad-spectrum antibiotics (e.g. ciprofloxacin) should be given for acute attacks of cholangitis. • If cholangiography shows a well-defined obstruction to the extrahepatic bile ducts, mechanical relief can be obtained by placement of a prosthesis or by balloon dilatation performed at ERCP. • Fat-soluble vitamin replacement is necessary in jaundiced patients. • Metabolic bone disease (usually osteoporosis) is a common complication that requires treatment (p. 598). • UDCA reduces levels of cholestatic liver enzymes and in large doses (20–25 mg/kg daily) has beneficial effects on liver histology and cholangiographic appearance. • Immunosuppressive agents have been tried but generally results have been disappointing. • Transplantation is the only option in young patients with PSC and advanced liver disease; 5-yr survival is 80–90% in most centres. Unfortunately, the condition may recur in the graft.

The course of PSC is variable. In symptomatic patients, median survival from presentation to death or liver transplantation is ~12 yrs.

VASCULAR LIVER DISEASES

HEPATIC ARTERIAL DISEASE

Hepatic artery occlusion may result from inadvertent injury during biliary surgery or may be caused by emboli, neoplasms, polyarteritis nodosa, blunt trauma or radiation. It usually causes severe upper abdominal pain with or without signs of circulatory shock. LFTs show a high transaminase activity. Patients usually survive if the liver and portal blood supply are otherwise normal.

PORTAL VENOUS DISEASE

Portal venous thrombosis is rare but can occur in any condition predisposing to thrombosis. Acute portal venous thrombosis causes abdominal pain and diarrhoea, and may lead to bowel infarction. Treatment is surgical, although patients will require anticoagulation if an underlying thrombotic condition is diagnosed. Subacute thrombosis can be asymptomatic but may lead to extrahepatic portal hypertension (p. 493) later on.

HEPATIC VENOUS OUTFLOW OBSTRUCTION

Obstruction to hepatic venous blood flow can occur in the small central hepatic veins, the large hepatic veins, the inferior vena cava or the heart.

BUDD–CHIARI SYNDROME

This uncommon condition is characterised by thrombosis of the larger hepatic veins and sometimes the inferior vena cava. The cause cannot be found in about half of patients. Some have haematological disorders such as primary polycythaemia, paroxysmal nocturnal haemoglobinuria and antithrombin III, protein C or protein S deficiencies (p. 564).

Clinical features

• Sudden venous occlusion causes the rapid development of upper abdominal pain, marked ascites and occasionally acute liver failure. • More gradual occlusion causes gross ascites and often upper abdominal discomfort. • Hepatomegaly, often with tenderness over the liver, is almost always present. • Hepatic congestion is the initial consequence. • Centrilobular fibrosis develops later and eventually cirrhosis supervenes in those who survive long enough.

Investigations

• LFTs vary considerably depending on the presentation and can show the features of acute hepatitis (p. 500) when the onset is rapid. Ascitic fluid analysis typically shows a protein concentration >25 g/l (exudate) in the early stages. • USS, CT, MRI or venography may demonstrate occlusion of the hepatic veins and inferior vena cava.

Management

• Where recent thrombosis is suspected, thrombolysis with streptokinase followed by heparin and oral anticoagulation should be considered. • Short hepatic venous strictures can be treated with angioplasty; more extensive hepatic vein occlusion can be managed by TIPSS.

VENO-OCCLUSIVE DISEASE

Widespread occlusion of central hepatic veins is the characteristic of this rare condition. Pyrrolizidine alkaloids in *Senecio* and *Heliotropium* plants used to make teas, cytotoxic drugs and hepatic irradiation are all recognised causes. The clinical features are similar to those of the Budd–Chiari syndrome (see above).

CARDIAC DISEASE

Hepatic damage due primarily to congestion may develop in all forms of right heart failure (p. 250); the clinical features are usually dominated by the cardiac disease. Very rarely, long-standing cardiac failure and hepatic congestion cause cardiac cirrhosis.

Acute heart failure sometimes causes a syndrome similar to acute hepatitis. This is usually mediated by a reduction in hepatic perfusion and is termed 'shock liver'. The patient is generally very ill with an enlarged tender liver, jaundice and LFTs showing very high serum transaminases (often >2000 U/l).

TUMOURS OF THE LIVER

HEPATOCELLULAR CARCINOMA

This is the most common primary liver tumour. There is an increased risk in chronic hepatitis B without cirrhosis, and in cirrhosis due to hepatitis B and C, haemochromatosis, alcohol, NAFLD and α_1-antitrypsin deficiency. The risk is higher in men and rises with age.

Clinical features

• Many tumours are asymptomatic and discovered on screening. • In patients with underlying cirrhosis there may be ascites, jaundice, worsening synthetic LFTs and variceal haemorrhage. • Other symptoms include weight loss, anorexia and abdominal pain. • Examination may reveal hepatomegaly or a right hypochondrial mass.

Investigations

• Alpha-fetoprotein (AFP) is produced by 60% of hepatocellular carcinomas, but is also raised in active hepatitis B and C viral replication and in acute hepatic necrosis such as that following paracetamol toxicity. • Combinations of USS scanning and CT or MRI are often helpful but may underestimate the multifocality of the tumour. • Biopsy is advisable to confirm the diagnosis and exclude metastatic tumour in patients with large tumours who do not have cirrhosis or hepatitis B. Biopsy is usually avoided in patients eligible for transplantation or surgical resection because of a small risk of tumour seeding along the needle tract.

Management

Hepatic resection: The treatment of choice for non-cirrhotic patients. The 5-yr survival in this group is ~50%. However, there is a 50% recurrence rate at 5 yrs.

Liver transplantation: In the presence of cirrhosis transplantation has the benefit of curing the cirrhosis and removing the risk of a second de novo tumour.

Percutaneous ablation: Percutaneous ethanol injection into the tumour under USS guidance is efficacious (80% cure rate) for tumours 3 cm or smaller. Recurrence rates (50% at 3 yrs) are similar to those following surgical resection.

Chemoembolisation: Hepatic artery embolisation with Gelfoam and adriamycin yields survival rates of 60% in cirrhotic patients with unresectable hepatocellular carcinoma and good liver function (compared with 20% in untreated patients) at 2 yrs. Unfortunately, any survival benefit is lost at 4 yrs.

FIBROLAMELLAR HEPATOCELLULAR CARCINOMA

This rare variant occurs in young adults, in the absence of hepatitis B infection and cirrhosis. The tumours are often large at presentation and the AFP is usually normal. Treatment is by surgical resection.

SECONDARY MALIGNANT TUMOURS

The primary neoplasm (most commonly lung, breast or abdominal) is asymptomatic in about half of patients. There is usually liver enlargement and weight loss; jaundice may be present. Ascitic fluid, if present, has a high protein content and may be blood-stained; cytology sometimes reveals malignant cells. Hepatic resection can improve survival for slow-growing tumours such as colonic carcinomas.

LIVER ABSCESSES

Liver abscesses can be classified as pyogenic, hydatid or amoebic.

PYOGENIC LIVER ABSCESS

Pyogenic liver abscesses are uncommon but important because they are potentially curable, inevitably fatal if untreated, and readily overlooked.

Infection reaches the liver through the hepatic or portal circulation, up the biliary tree, via injury or by direct spread from adjacent organs. Abscesses most commonly occur in older patients through ascending infection due to biliary obstruction (cholangitis) or contiguous spread from an empyema of the gallbladder. Immunocompromised patients are particularly likely to develop liver abscesses. *E. coli* and various streptococci, particularly *Strep. milleri*, are the most common organisms; anaerobes, including streptococci and *Bacteroides*, may be found when infection has spread from large bowel pathology via the portal vein.

Clinical features

• Patients are generally ill with fever, sometimes rigors and weight loss. • Abdominal pain in the right upper quadrant, sometimes radiating to the right shoulder is the most common symptom. The pain may be pleuritic in nature. • Hepatomegaly, often with tenderness to percussion, occurs in more than half of patients. • Mild jaundice may be present but is severe only when large abscesses cause biliary obstruction. • Atypical presentations are common and a gradual onset of pyrexia of unknown origin without localising features may lead to the diagnosis being missed.

Investigations

• USS reveals 90% or more of symptomatic abscesses and is also used to guide needle aspiration of pus for culture. • Leucocytosis is frequently found. • Plasma alkaline phosphatase activity is usually increased. • Serum albumin is often low. • CXR may show a raised right diaphragm and lung collapse or an effusion at the base of the right lung. • Blood culture should always be carried out.

Management and prognosis

• Pending the results of culture of blood and pus from the abscess, treatment should commence with a combination of antibiotics such as ampicillin, gentamicin and metronidazole. • Aspiration or drainage with a catheter placed in the abscess under USS guidance is required if the abscess is large or if it does not respond to antibiotics. • Surgical drainage is rarely required.

The mortality of liver abscesses is 20–40%; failure to make the diagnosis is the most common cause of death. Older patients and those with multiple abscesses also have a higher mortality.

HYDATID CYSTS AND AMOEBIC LIVER ABSCESSES

These are covered elsewhere (pp. 125 and 115).

PREGNANCY-ASSOCIATED LIVER DISEASE

INTRAHEPATIC CHOLESTASIS OF PREGNANCY

• Usually occurs in the third trimester and is associated with intrauterine growth retardation and premature birth. • Presents with itching and cholestatic or hepatitic LFTs. • UDCA (15 mg/kg daily) prevents premature birth.

ACUTE FATTY LIVER OF PREGNANCY

• More common in twin and first pregnancies. • Typically presents between 31 and 38 wks of pregnancy with vomiting and abdominal pain followed by jaundice. • In severe cases lactic acidosis, a coagulopathy, encephalopathy, hypoglycaemia and renal failure may occur. • Differentiation from toxaemia of pregnancy (which is more common) can be made by the finding of high serum uric acid levels and the absence of haemolysis. • Early diagnosis and delivery of the fetus has led to a fall in maternal mortality to 1–15%.

TOXAEMIA OF PREGNANCY AND HELP

The HELP syndrome (haemolysis, elevated liver enzymes and thrombocytopenia) is a variant of pre-eclampsia that tends to affect multiparous women. Serum transaminases are high and the condition can be complicated by hepatic infarction and rupture.

LIVER TRANSPLANTATION

The outcome following liver transplantation has improved significantly over the last decade and it is now an effective treatment for end-stage liver disease.

Indications: 71% are performed for cirrhosis, 11% for hepatocellular carcinoma, 10% for acute liver failure and 6% for metabolic diseases.

Contraindications: The main contraindications to transplantation are sepsis, extrahepatic malignancy, active alcohol or other substance misuse, and marked cardiorespiratory dysfunction.

Complications: Include acute rejection, hepatic artery thrombosis, anastomotic biliary strictures, and infections.

Outcomes: The outcome following transplantation for acute liver failure is worse than for chronic liver disease because most patients have coexisting multi-organ failure. The 1-yr survival is 65%, falling to 59% at 5 yrs. The 1-yr survival for patients with cirrhosis is 80–90%, falling to 70–75% at 5 yrs.

GALLBLADDER AND EXTRAHEPATIC BILIARY DISEASE

GALLSTONES

Gallstones are conveniently classified into cholesterol or pigment stones, although the majority are of mixed composition. Cholesterol stones are most common in developed countries, whereas pigment stones are more frequent in developing countries.

Cholesterol gallstones: Cholesterol is held in solution in bile by its association with bile acids and phospholipids in the form of micelles and vesicles. In gallstone disease the liver produces bile which contains a relative excess of cholesterol ('lithogenic bile').

Pigment stones: Brown crumbly pigment stones are almost always the consequence of bacterial or parasitic infection in the biliary tree. They are found commonly in the Far East, where infection of the biliary tree allows bacterial β-glucuronidase to hydrolyse conjugated bilirubin to its free form, which then precipitates as calcium bilirubinate. The mechanism of black pigment gallstone formation in developed countries is not satisfactorily explained but haemolysis is important.

Clinical features

• Only about 10% of people with gallstones develop clinical evidence of gallstone disease. • Symptomatic gallstones (Box 13.16) cause either biliary

13.16 CLINICAL FEATURES AND COMPLICATIONS OF GALLSTONES 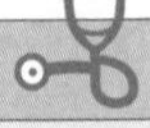

Clinical features	
• Asymptomatic • Biliary colic	• Acute cholecystitis • Chronic cholecystitis
Complications	
• Empyema of the gallbladder • Porcelain gallbladder • Choledocholithiasis • Pancreatitis • Fistulae between the gallbladder and duodenum or colon	• Pressure on/inflammation of the common bile duct by a gallstone in the cystic duct (Mirizzi's syndrome) • Gallstone ileus • Cancer of the gallbladder

pain ('biliary colic') or cholecystitis (see below). • Typically, the pain occurs suddenly and persists for about 2 hrs; if it continues for more than 6 hrs, a complication such as cholecystitis or pancreatitis may be present. • Pain is usually felt in the epigastrium (70% of patients) or right upper quadrant (20% of patients) and radiates to the interscapular region or the tip of the right scapula.

Investigations

• USS is the method of choice for diagnosing gallstones. • MRCP is becoming increasingly available and can demonstrate gallstones and their complications.

Management

• Asymptomatic gallstones found incidentally are not usually treated because the majority will never give symptoms. • Symptomatic gallstones are best treated surgically using minimal access techniques. • Radiolucent stones <15 mm diameter causing mild symptoms may be dissolved by oral administration of the bile acid UDCA. • Extracorporeal shock-wave lithotripsy can be used in about 30% of patients, but is expensive and not widely available and must be followed by UDCA therapy. • All therapeutic regimens which retain the gallbladder have a 50% recurrence of stones after 5 yrs.

CHOLECYSTITIS

ACUTE CHOLECYSTITIS

Acute cholecystitis is almost always associated with obstruction of the gallbladder neck or cystic duct by a gallstone. Occasionally, obstruction may be by mucus, parasitic worms or a tumour. Acalculous cholecystitis can occur in the intensive care setting.

Clinical features

• The cardinal feature is severe and prolonged pain in the right upper quadrant but also in the epigastrium, the right shoulder tip or interscapular region. • There is usually fever and leucocytosis. • Examination shows right hypochondrial tenderness, and rigidity worse on inspiration (Murphy's sign). • Jaundice occurs in less than 10% of patients and is usually due to the presence or recent passage of stones in the common bile duct.

Investigations

• Leucocytosis is common. • USS detects gallstones and gallbladder thickening due to cholecystitis. • Plasma amylase should be measured to detect acute pancreatitis (p. 454). • Plain X-rays of the abdomen and chest may show radio-opaque gallstones, and rarely intrabiliary gas due to fistulation of a gallstone into the intestine, and are important in excluding lower lobe pneumonia and a perforated viscus.

Management

Medical: This consists of bed rest, pain relief, antibiotics (e.g. cefuroxime) and maintenance of fluid balance.

Surgical: Urgent surgery is required when cholecystitis progresses in spite of medical therapy and when complications such as empyema or perforation develop. Operation should be carried out within 5 days of the onset of symptoms. Delayed surgery after 2–3 mths is no longer favoured. Recurrent biliary colic or cholecystitis is frequent if the gallbladder is not removed.

CHRONIC CHOLECYSTITIS

Chronic inflammation of the gallbladder is almost invariably associated with gallstones. The usual symptoms are those of recurrent attacks of upper abdominal pain, often at night and following a heavy meal. The clinical features are similar to those of acute calculous cholecystitis but milder. The patient may recover spontaneously or following analgesia and antibiotics. Patients are usually advised to undergo elective laparoscopic cholecystectomy.

ACUTE CHOLANGITIS

Acute cholangitis is caused by bacterial infection of bile ducts and occurs in patients with other biliary problems such as choledocholithiasis (see below), biliary strictures or tumours, or after ERCP. Jaundice, rigors and abdominal pain are the cardinal presenting features. Treatment is with antibiotics and removal (if possible) of the underlying cause.

CHOLEDOCHOLITHIASIS

Stones in the common bile duct (choledocholithiasis) occur in 10–15% of patients with gallstones and have usually migrated from the gallbladder. In Far Eastern countries, where bile duct infection is common, primary common bile duct stones are thought to follow bacterial infection secondary to parasitic infections with *Clonorchis sinensis, Ascaris lumbricoides* or *Fasciola hepatica* (p. 117). Common bile duct stones can cause partial or complete bile duct obstruction and may be complicated by cholangitis due to secondary bacterial infection, septicaemia, liver abscess and biliary stricture.

Clinical features

• Choledocholithiasis may be asymptomatic, may be found incidentally by operative cholangiography at cholecystectomy, or may manifest as recurrent abdominal pain with or without jaundice. • The pain is usually in the right upper quadrant and fever, pruritus and dark urine may be present. • Rigors may be a feature; painless jaundice is uncommon.

Investigations

• USS is the most convenient method of demonstrating obstruction to the common bile duct. • LFTs show a cholestatic pattern and there is bilirubinuria. • If cholangitis is present, the patient usually has a leucocytosis.

Management

• Urgent endoscopic sphincterotomy and stone extraction is the treatment of choice, particularly in patients over the age of 60, and is successful in about 90% of patients. • Analgesia, i.v. fluids and broad-spectrum antibiotics such as cefuroxime and metronidazole should be given. • Surgical treatment of choledocholithiasis is performed less frequently than ERCP because of higher morbidity and mortality. • Recurrence should be prevented by elective cholecystectomy.

TUMOURS OF THE GALLBLADDER AND BILE DUCT

CARCINOMA OF THE GALLBLADDER

This is uncommon, occurring more often in females and usually encountered above the age of 70. More than 90% of such tumours are adenocarcinomas; the remainder are anaplastic or, rarely, squamous tumours. Gallstones are usually present and are thought to be important in the aetiology of the tumour.

CHOLANGIOCARCINOMA

This uncommon tumour can arise anywhere in the biliary tree from the small intrahepatic bile ducts to the papilla of Vater. The cause is unknown but the tumour is associated with gallstones, primary and secondary sclerosing cholangitis, and choledochal cysts. In the Far East chronic liver fluke infection is a major risk factor. The patient presents with obstructive jaundice. The diagnosis is made by a combination of USS and cholangiography, but can be difficult to confirm in patients with sclerosing cholangitis. The prognosis is poor.

CARCINOMA AT THE PAPILLA OF VATER

Nearly 40% of all adenocarcinomas of the small intestine arise in relationship to the papilla of Vater and present with pain, anaemia, vomiting and weight loss. Jaundice may be intermittent or persistent. Diagnosis is by duodenal endoscopy and biopsy. Ampullary carcinoma must be differentiated from carcinoma of the head of the pancreas and cholangiocarcinoma because both have a worse prognosis.

MISCELLANEOUS BILIARY DISORDERS

POST-CHOLECYSTECTOMY SYNDROME

Dyspeptic symptoms following cholecystectomy (post-cholecystectomy syndrome) occur in ~30% of patients. The usual complaints include right upper quadrant abdominal pain, flatulence, fatty food intolerance, and occasionally jaundice and cholangitis. USS is used to detect biliary obstruction, and ERCP or MRCP to detect common bile duct stones. If retained bile duct stones are excluded, sphincter of Oddi dysfunction should be considered (see below).

SPHINCTER OF ODDI DYSFUNCTION (SOD)

The sphincter of Oddi is a small smooth muscle sphincter situated at the junction of the bile duct and pancreatic duct in the duodenum. SOD is characterised by an increase in contractility that produces a benign non-calculous obstruction to the flow of bile or pancreatic juice. This may cause pancreatico-biliary pain, deranged LFTs or recurrent pancreatitis. Patients are predominantly female. Patients with biliary-type SOD experience recurrent episodic biliary-type pain. Patients with pancreatic SOD usually present with unexplained recurrent attacks of pancreatitis. The diagnosis is established by excluding gallstones and demonstrating a dilated or slowly draining bile duct.

Patients with biliary pain, who also have deranged liver enzymes and/or radiological abnormality due to SOD, are treated with endoscopic sphincterotomy. The results are good but patients should be warned that there is a high risk of complications, particularly acute pancreatitis.

14

Blood disorders

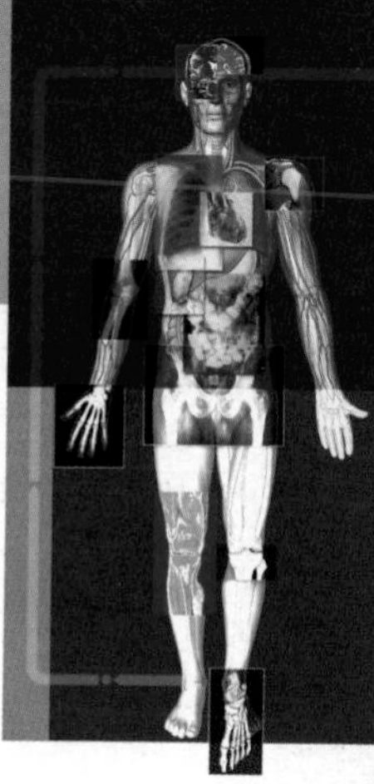

Blood diseases cover a wide spectrum of illnesses, ranging from common anaemias to rare conditions such as leukaemias and congenital coagulation disorders. Haematological change may occur as a consequence of disease affecting any system, and measurement of haematological parameters is an important part of routine clinical assessment.

PRESENTING PROBLEMS

ANAEMIA

Anaemia refers to a state in which the level of haemoglobin (Hb) in the blood is below the normal range appropriate for age and sex. Other factors, including pregnancy and altitude, also affect Hb levels. The clinical features of anaemia reflect diminished oxygen supply to the tissues. The symptoms of anaemia will be more severe if the onset is rapid or if there is coexisting cardiorespiratory disease.

Clinical assessment

Many clinical features are non-specific but together they should raise suspicion of anaemia.

Symptoms include:

• Tiredness. • Lethargy. • Breathlessness. • Ankle swelling. • Worsening of coexisting disease, e.g. angina.

Signs include:

• Mucous membrane pallor. • Tachypnoea. • Raised JVP. • Flow murmurs. • Ankle oedema. • Postural hypotension. • Tachycardia.

CLINICAL EXAMINATION IN BLOOD DISORDERS

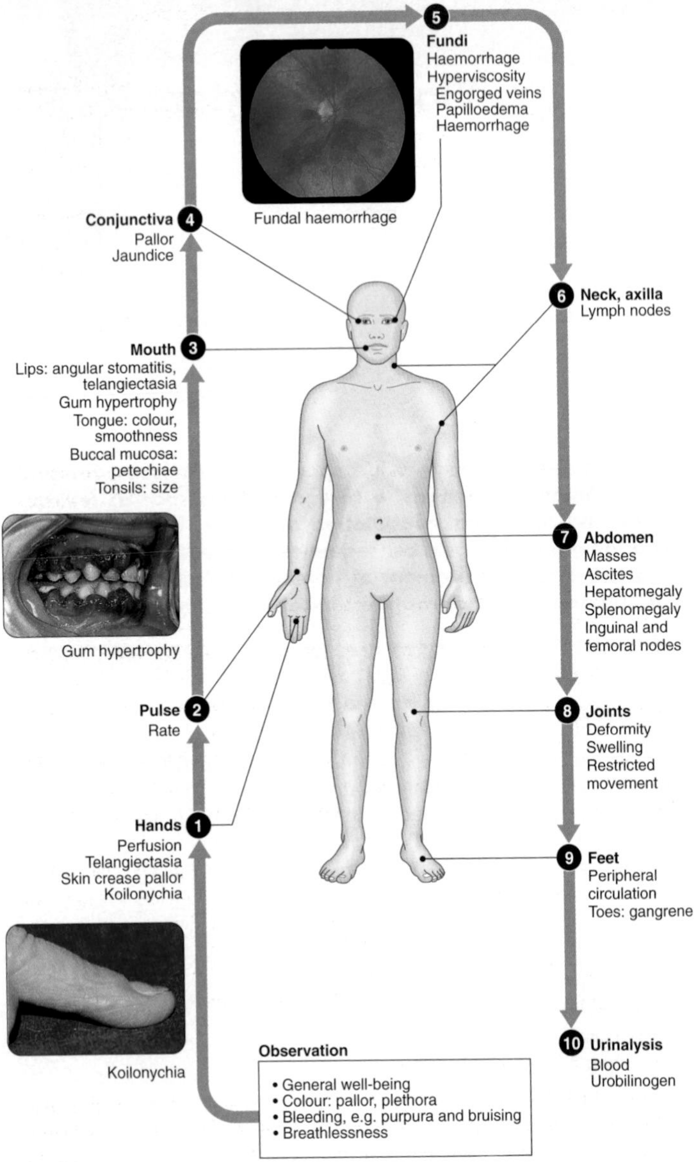

5 Fundi
Haemorrhage
Hyperviscosity
- Engorged veins
- Papilloedema
- Haemorrhage

Fundal haemorrhage

4 Conjunctiva
Pallor
Jaundice

3 Mouth
Lips: angular stomatitis, telangiectasia
Gum hypertrophy
Tongue: colour, smoothness
Buccal mucosa: petechiae
Tonsils: size

Gum hypertrophy

2 Pulse
Rate

1 Hands
Perfusion
Telangiectasia
Skin crease pallor
Koilonychia

Koilonychia

6 Neck, axilla
Lymph nodes

7 Abdomen
Masses
Ascites
Hepatomegaly
Splenomegaly
Inguinal and femoral nodes

8 Joints
Deformity
Swelling
Restricted movement

9 Feet
Peripheral circulation
Toes: gangrene

10 Urinalysis
Blood
Urobilinogen

Observation
- General well-being
- Colour: pallor, plethora
- Bleeding, e.g. purpura and bruising
- Breathlessness

The diagnosis of anaemia not only includes an assessment of its clinical severity but must also define the underlying cause. This rests on history and examination, FBC and blood film, and further investigations.

History

Iron deficiency anaemia: The most common type of anaemia world-wide. Seek symptoms indicating GI blood loss and menorrhagia in females.

Dietary history: Should assess the intake of iron and folate, which may become deficient in comparison to needs (e.g. in pregnancy or during periods of rapid growth).

Past medical history: May reveal disease known to be associated with anaemia (e.g. rheumatoid arthritis), or previous surgery (e.g. stomach or small bowel resection which may lead to malabsorption of iron and/or vitamin B_{12}).

Family history: May be relevant in haemolytic anaemias and pernicious anaemia.

Drug history: Many drugs can be associated with blood loss (e.g. NSAIDs) and others may cause haemolysis or aplasia.

Physical examination

The general physical findings of anaemia (see above) may be accompanied by specific findings related to the underlying aetiology. Examples include a right iliac fossa mass in a patient with caecal carcinoma; jaundice in patients with haemolytic anaemia; and neurological signs, including peripheral neuropathy and subacute combined degeneration of the cord, in individuals with vitamin B_{12} deficiency.

Schemes for the investigation of anaemias are often based on the size of the red cells, which is most accurately indicated by the mean cell volume (MCV) in the FBC. Commonly:

• A normal MCV (normocytic anaemia) suggests acute blood loss or anaemia of chronic disease (ACD). • A low MCV (microcytic anaemia) suggests iron deficiency or thalassaemia. • A high MCV (macrocytic anaemia) suggests vitamin B_{12} or folate deficiency. A high MCV (in the absence of anaemia) may also be caused by liver disease, hypothyroidism, hyperlipidaemia and pregnancy.

Supplementary investigations are often required for a precise diagnosis. • A raised reticulocyte count in microcytic anaemia suggests bleeding or haemolysis. • A low ferritin is characteristic of iron deficiency. • In macrocytic anaemia, the blood film may show typical abnormalities, e.g. a dimorphic picture in sideroblastic anaemia, target cells in liver disease, or hypersegmented neutrophils due to B_{12} or folate deficiency or drug toxicity.

HIGH HAEMOGLOBIN

A Hb level > the upper limit of normal (adult females 165 g/l, adult males 180 g/l) may be due to an increase in the number of red blood cells (true polycythaemia) or a reduction in the plasma volume (relative or apparent

14.1 CAUSES OF TRUE POLYCYTHAEMIA		
	Aetiology	**Examples**
Primary	Myeloproliferative disorder	Polycythaemia rubra vera (PRV)
Secondary	Appropriately increased Epo due to tissue hypoxia	High altitude Lung disease Cyanotic heart disease
	Inappropriately increased Epo	Renal disease (hydronephrosis, cysts, carcinoma) Other tumours (e.g. hepatoma, bronchogenic carcinoma, cerebellar haemangioblastoma)

polycythaemia); these can be distinguished by isotope measures of red cell mass.

True polycythaemia: Caused by increased erythropoiesis in the bone marrow. This may be due to a primary increase in marrow activity (polycythaemia rubra vera, PRV) or secondary to increased erythropoietin (Epo) production, either as a consequence of chronic hypoxaemia or because of inappropriate erythropoietin secretion (e.g. lung or renal disorders) (Box 14.1). History and examination will provide clues to the aetiology of true polycythaemia. Those with PRV may have arterial thromboses, pruritus, gout due to high red cell turnover and hepatosplenomegaly. The cardiovascular and respiratory systems should be assessed for causes of hypoxaemia, and further investigations to exclude inappropriate erythropoietin secretion should be performed.

Relative polycythaemia with a reduction in plasma volume: Usually a consequence of dehydration, diuretic use or alcohol consumption.

LEUCOPENIA (LOW WHITE COUNT)

Leucopenia may be due to a reduction in all types of white cell or in individual cell types. A reduction in neutrophil count ($<1.5 \times 10^9$/l) is called neutropenia. Causes of neutropenia include:

• Infection. • Connective tissue disease. • Alcohol. • Bone marrow infiltration (e.g. leukaemia, myelodysplasia).

A number of drugs can also result in neutropenia. Examples include:

• Antirheumatic drugs (e.g. gold, penicillamine). • Antithyroid drugs (e.g. carbimazole). • Anticonvulsants (e.g. phenytoin, sodium valproate). • Antibiotics.

Clinical manifestations of neutropenia range from no symptoms to overwhelming sepsis. Fever may be the only manifestation of infection, and immediate antibiotic therapy is required to prevent rapid development of septic shock.

LEUCOCYTOSIS (HIGH WHITE COUNT)

Leucocytosis is usually due to an increase in a specific type of white blood cell. Neutrophilia (an increase in circulating neutrophils) is caused by:
• Infection. • Trauma. • Myocardial infarction (MI). • Inflammation. • Malignancy. • Myeloproliferative disorders.

Neutrophils are physiologically raised in pregnancy and in the healthy neonate. The most common cause of an elevated lymphocyte count (lymphocytosis, $>3.5 \times 10^9$/l in adults) is viral infection.

LYMPHADENOPATHY

Enlarged lymph nodes may be an indicator of haematological disease but can also occur in reaction to infection or inflammation (Box 14.2). Reactive nodes usually expand rapidly and are painful, whereas those due to haematological disease are frequently painless and may be generalised. Initial investigations in lymphadenopathy should include:
• FBC (to detect neutrophilia in infection or evidence of haematological disease). • CXR (to detect mediastinal lymphadenopathy).

If the findings suggest malignancy, lymph node biopsy is required.

SPLENOMEGALY

Causes of splenic enlargement are listed in Box 14.3.
• Massive splenomegaly occurs in chronic myeloid leukaemia, myelofibrosis, malaria and leishmaniasis. • Hepatosplenomegaly is more suggestive of lympho- or myeloproliferative disease or liver disease. • The presence of lymphadenopathy makes a diagnosis of lymphoproliferative disease more likely.

An enlarged spleen may cause abdominal discomfort; splenic infarction causes severe pain radiating to the shoulder tip. In rare cases, spontaneous or traumatic rupture may occur.

14.2 CAUSES OF LYMPHADENOPATHY

Infective	Bacterial, e.g. streptococcal, TB Viral, e.g. Epstein–Barr, HIV Protozoal, e.g. toxoplasmosis Fungal, e.g. histoplasmosis
Neoplastic	Primary, e.g. lymphomas, leukaemias Secondary, e.g. lung, breast, thyroid, stomach
Inflammatory	Connective tissue disorders, e.g. rheumatoid arthritis, SLE Sarcoidosis
Miscellaneous	Amyloidosis

14.3 CAUSES OF SPLENOMEGALY	
Congestive	Portal hypertension, e.g. cirrhosis, portal vein thrombosis Cardiac, e.g. congestive cardiac failure
Infective	Bacterial, e.g. endocarditis, septicaemia, TB Viral, e.g. hepatitis, Epstein–Barr Protozoal, e.g. malaria, leishmaniasis (kala-azar) Fungal, e.g. histoplasmosis
Inflammatory/ granulomatous disorders	e.g. Felty's syndrome, SLE, sarcoidosis
Haematological	Red cell disorders, e.g. megaloblastic anaemia, haemoglobinopathies Autoimmune haemolytic anaemias Myeloproliferative disorders, e.g. chronic myeloid leukaemia, myelofibrosis, PRV, essential thrombocythaemia Neoplastic, e.g. leukaemias, lymphomas

• USS or CT will detect splenomegaly, and will also allow imaging of the liver and abdominal lymph nodes. • FBC, blood film examination and CXR are required in all patients. • Further investigations may include lymph node biopsy and bone marrow examination.

BLEEDING

Normal haemostasis

Haemostasis depends upon interactions between the vessel wall, platelets and clotting factors. In the initial primary phase, the damaged vessel constricts and platelets aggregate to form a plug. This is followed by activation of the coagulation cascade, resulting in the formation of a cross-linked fibrin clot (Fig. 14.1). Clotting factors are synthesised by the liver and several are dependent on vitamin K for their activation; activated factors are designated by the suffix 'a'. The extrinsic pathway is the main physiological mechanism in vivo.

Excessive coagulation is prevented by natural inhibitors of the clotting system. Antithrombin is a protein with inhibitory activity against thrombin and factor Xa. Its inhibitory activity is markedly increased by heparin. Protein C inactivates factors Va and VIIIa; protein S is a co-factor for protein C. Any reduction in the function of these inhibitors results in a tendency to thrombosis.

History

• Abnormal or excessive bleeding may be due to deficiency of coagulation factors, thrombocytopenia, or occasionally excessive fibrinolysis following

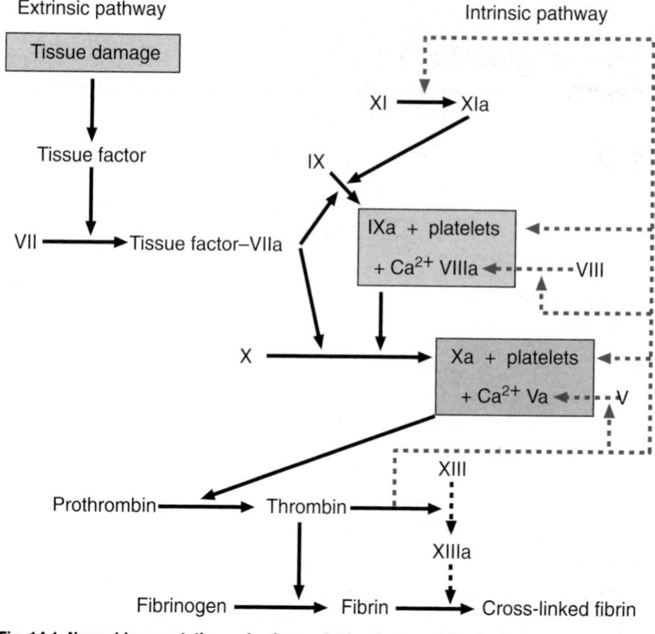

Fig. 14.1 Normal haemostatic mechanisms: clotting factors of the intrinsic and extrinsic pathways. The reactions of IXa/VIIIa and Xa/Va (in the boxes) take place on the platelet surface. The dotted lines represent positive feedback effects from small amounts of thrombin.

therapeutic fibrinolytic therapy. • Muscle and joint bleeds indicate a coagulation defect, whereas purpura, prolonged bleeding from cuts, epistaxis, GI haemorrhage and menorrhagia indicate a platelet disorder, thrombocytopenia or von Willebrand disease.

The duration of the history may help determine whether the disorder is congenital or acquired. Family history may be relevant in genetic disorders such as haemophilia. Coexisting illness or drug therapy predisposing to bleeding should be noted.

Examination

Check for:

• Bruising. • Purpura. • Telangiectasia on lips (indicates hereditary haemorrhagic telangiectasia). • Swollen joints/haemarthrosis. • Hepatomegaly. • Splenomegaly.

Investigations

Initial screening tests comprise:

• Platelet count. • Blood film. • Coagulation tests including the prothrombin time (PT), activated partial thromboplastin time (APTT) and fibrinogen.

PT: Assesses the extrinsic system and is prolonged by deficiencies of factors II, V, VII and X and by liver disease.

International normalised ratio (INR): Used to assess the control of warfarin treatment, and is the ratio of the patient's PT to a normal control using an international reference thromboplastin.

APTT: Assesses the intrinsic system and is sensitive to deficiencies in factors V, VIII, IX, X, XI and XII.

Bleeding time: Assesses platelet function.

THROMBOCYTOPENIA (LOW PLATELETS)

Causes of thrombocytopenia are listed in Box 14.4. Purpura, bruising and spontaneous oral, nasal, GI or GU bleeding may occur but not usually until the platelet count falls below 30×10^9/l. Blood film may be diagnostic (e.g. acute leukaemia). Bone marrow examination may reveal:

• A reduced number of megakaryocytes (platelet precursors) in cases of decreased platelet formation (e.g. hypoplastic anaemia). • An increased number of megakaryocytes indicating excessive platelet destruction (e.g. idiopathic thrombocytopenic purpura).

THROMBOCYTOSIS (HIGH PLATELETS)

The platelet count may be raised as part of the inflammatory response (reactive thrombocytosis), as with infection, malignancy or GI bleeding. Alternatively, it may be a feature of myeloproliferative disorders such as primary thrombocythaemia, PRV and chronic myeloid leukaemia.

VENOUS THROMBOSIS

Deep venous thrombosis (DVT) must be excluded in patients presenting with unilateral leg-swelling. Other causes include a calf haematoma, cel-

14.4 CAUSES OF THROMBOCYTOPENIA	
Marrow disorders	Hypoplasia Infiltration, e.g. leukaemia, myeloma, carcinoma, myelofibrosis Vitamin B_{12}/folate deficiency
Increased platelet consumption	Disseminated intravascular coagulation (DIC) Idiopathic thrombocytopenic purpura (ITP) Infections, e.g. Epstein–Barr virus, Gram-negative septicaemia Hypersplenism Thrombotic thrombocytopenic purpura Liver disease Connective tissue diseases, e.g. SLE

14.5 PROCEDURE FOR PREDICTING THE PRE-TEST PROBABILITY OF DVT

Clinical characteristic	Score
Active cancer (patient receiving treatment for cancer within the previous 6 mths or currently receiving palliative treatment)	1
Paralysis, paresis or recent plaster immobilisation of the lower extremities	1
Recently bedridden for 3 days or more, or major surgery within the previous 12 wks requiring general or regional anaesthesia	1
Localised tenderness along the distribution of the deep venous system	1
Entire leg swollen	1
Calf swelling at least 3 cm larger than that on the asymptomatic side (measured 10 cm below tibial tuberosity)	1
Pitting oedema confined to the symptomatic leg	1
Collateral superficial veins (non-varicose)	1
Previously documented DVT	1
Alternative diagnosis at least as likely as DVT	–2
Clinical probability	**Total score**
DVT unlikely	<2
DVT likely	≥2

lulitis and a ruptured Baker's cyst (which normally occurs in rheumatoid arthritis of the knee). Bilateral leg-swelling may result from extensive proximal DVT extending into the inferior vena cava, impaired venous or lymphatic return due to obstruction in the pelvis, right-sided heart failure and hypoalbuminaemia.

Using the patient's symptoms, the probability of DVT can be established using the Well's score (Box 14.5). Those with a medium or high risk should undergo further investigation.

USS is a reliable, non-invasive method of demonstrating thrombus between the popliteal fossa and the inguinal ligament, but venography remains the most accurate and reliable way of demonstrating DVT. For those with a low Well's score, plasma D-dimer level should be measured; if low, DVT is excluded, but if raised, USS or venography is required.

ELEVATED MARKERS OF INFLAMMATION (Box 14.6)

C-REACTIVE PROTEIN (CRP)

CRP is an acute phase reactant which opsonises invading pathogens. Levels of CRP increase within 6 hrs of an inflammatory stimulus. The short plasma half-life of CRP (19 hrs) means it can be used to monitor disease activity. Some diseases (e.g. SLE, systemic sclerosis, ulcerative colitis and leukaemia) are associated with only minor elevations of CRP despite the presence of inflammation. Intercurrent infection, however, does provoke a significant CRP response in these conditions.

ERYTHROCYTE SEDIMENTATION RATE (ESR)

The rate of fall of erythrocytes through plasma (ESR) is an indirect measure of the acute phase response. Normal erythrocytes repel each other because of their negative charge. Plasma proteins are positively charged, and raised levels overcome the repulsion between erythrocytes, causing rouleau formation and increased sedimentation rate.

The most common cause of an increased ESR (and CRP) is an increase in acute phase proteins. Increased monoclonal or polyclonal immunoglobulin levels also increase the ESR. In addition, changes in erythrocyte size, morphology and density influence sedimentation. For these reasons, an abnormally low ESR occurs in spherocytosis, sickle cell anaemia and microcytic anaemia, and with low plasma protein levels.

Clinical assessment

A comprehensive history and examination are crucial. Extreme elevations in the ESR (>100 mm/hr) rarely occur in the absence of significant disease.

Investigations

• CRP, serum immunoglobulins and urine electrophoresis measurements will help determine if the elevation in ESR is due to an acute inflammatory process. • An FBC may show a normocytic, normochromic anaemia signifying chronic inflammation. • Leucocytosis may reflect infection, inflammatory disease or tissue necrosis. • Neutrophilia suggests infection or acute inflammation. • Atypical lymphocytes may occur in CMV and EBV infection. • Abnormalities in liver function suggest either a local infective process (hepatitis, hepatic abscess or biliary sepsis) or a systemic disease, including malignancy. • Blood and urine cultures should be performed.

Imaging

• CXR/abdominal CT may identify a source of unknown infection or malignancy. • Abdominal/pelvic USS may identify hepatic lesions and abscesses/collections. • MRI is used for soft tissue or bone/joint infections. • Echocardiography images vegetations in suspected bacterial endocarditis. • White cell scans may identify the site of pyogenic infection. • Isotope bone scans identify malignancy or focal bone infection.

BLOOD PRODUCTS AND TRANSFUSION

BLOOD PRODUCTS

Transfusion may be needed in patients with deficiency of a certain blood constituent. Blood products are obtained from donations by healthy individuals. Every blood donation must be reliably tested to exclude those containing transmissible agents. In the developed world, this includes:

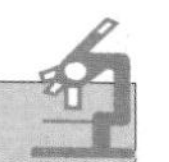

14.6 COMMON CONDITIONS ASSOCIATED WITH ABNORMAL CRP AND/OR ESR

Condition	Consequence	Effect on CRP[1]	Effect on ESR[2]
Acute bacterial, fungal or viral infection	Stimulates acute phase response	↑	↑
Necrotising bacterial infection	Stimulates profound acute inflammatory response	↑↑↑ (>300 mg/l)	↑
Chronic bacterial or fungal infection, e.g. localised abscess, SBE or TB	Stimulates acute and chronic inflammatory response with ↑ polyclonal Ig and ↑ acute phase proteins	↑ (50–150 mg/l)	↑ disproportionate to CRP
Acute inflammatory diseases, e.g. Crohn's, systemic vasculitides, PMR, GCA	Stimulates acute phase response	↑ (50–150 mg/l)	↑
SLE, Sjögren's syndrome	Chronic inflammatory response	Normal (paradoxically)	↑
Myeloma	Monoclonal increase in serum Ig without acute inflammation	Normal	↑
Pregnancy, old age, ESRD	Increased fibrinogen	Normal	Moderate ↑
Macrocytic anaemia	Increased red cell viscosity	Normal	Moderate ↑

[1]Normal range <10 mg/l. [2]Normal range: adult males <10 mm/hr, adult females <20 mm/hr.

ESRD = end-stage renal disease; GCA = giant cell arteritis; Ig = immunoglobulin; PMR = polymyalgia rheumatica; SBE = subacute bacterial endocarditis; SLE = systemic lupus erythmatosus; TB = tuberculosis.

• Hepatitis B. • Hepatitis C. • HIV. • Human T lymphotrophic virus (HTLV).

In the UK, in order to minimise the risk of passing on variant Creutzfeldt–Jakob disease (vCJD, p. 674), all blood components are processed to remove white cells, and in addition transfusion recipients are not subsequently accepted as blood donors.

Red cell concentrate: Used to increase red cell mass in patients with anaemia and in acute blood loss. Red cell components must be compatible with the patient's ABO blood group.

Platelet concentrate: Used to treat and prevent bleeding due to thrombocytopenia.

Fresh frozen plasma (FFP): Used to replace coagulation factors.

Cryoprecipitate: Obtained from plasma and contains proteins including fibrinogen, factor VIII and von Willebrand factor (vWF). It is used to replace fibrinogen.

Coagulation factor concentrates factor VIII and IX: Used for the treatment of conditions such as haemophilia and von Willebrand disease. Recombinant substitutes are preferred as they avoid infection risk.

I.V. immunoglobulin: Used to prevent infection in patients with hypogammaglobulinaemia. It is also used in idiopathic thrombocytopenic purpura and Guillain–Barré syndrome.

RED CELL COMPATIBILITY

There are four different ABO groups, determined by whether or not an individual's red cells express A or B antigens. Healthy individuals have antibodies directed against the A or B antigens that are not expressed on their own cells (Box 14.7). If red cells of an incompatible ABO group are transfused, the patient's antibodies bind to the transfused cells leading to red cell haemolysis. This is the main cause of an acute transfusion reaction, and can lead to disseminated intravascular coagulation (DIC), renal failure and death.

About 15% of Caucasians lack the Rhesus D (RhD) red cell antigen ('Rhesus-negative'). IgG antibodies to RhD-positive red cells are produced if such cells enter the circulation of an RhD-negative individual via fetomaternal haemorrhage during pregnancy. During a subsequent pregnancy with an RhD-positive fetus, these antibodies can cross the placenta and

14.7 THE ABO SYSTEM

Blood group	Red cell A or B antigens	Antibodies in plasma
O	None	Anti-A and anti-B
A	A	Anti-B
B	B	Anti-A
AB	A and B	None

cause haemolytic disease of the newborn and severe neurological damage. Administration of anti-RhD immunoglobulin (anti-D) after delivery blocks the immune response to the RhD antigen and prevents the development of Rhesus antibodies in RhD-negative women.

SAFE TRANSFUSION PROCEDURES

Red cells from the patient's blood sample are tested to determine the ABO and RhD type. The patient's plasma is tested to detect any red cell antibodies that could haemolyse transfused red cells. The transfusion laboratory will then perform either a 'type and screen' ('group and save') or a cross-match. In the type and screen procedure, the patient's sample is held in the laboratory and compatible blood can be prepared within 15 mins if required. Cross-matching involves allocating specific red cell units to a particular patient for transfusion.

It is essential to ensure that no ABO-incompatible red cell transfusion is ever given. Most incompatible transfusions result from:

• Mistakes in taking and labelling the blood sample for pre-transfusion testing. • Failure to perform standard checks before infusion to ensure the correct pack has been selected for the patient.

ADVERSE EFFECTS OF TRANSFUSION

• A temperature rise of <1.5°C in an otherwise well patient indicates a febrile non-haemolytic transfusion reaction. Paracetamol should be administered and the transfusion rate slowed. • A mild allergic reaction is characterised by urticaria; it is treated with an antihistamine (e.g. chlorphenamine 10 mg i.v.) and by slowing the transfusion rate. • In severe reactions (bronchospasm, angioedema, hypotension) the transfusion should be stopped and any unused units returned to the blood bank. The patient should be treated with oxygen, i.v. chlorphenamine, nebulised salbutamol and, in hypotensive patients, i.m. adrenaline (epinephrine, 0.5 ml of 1 in 1000). • ABO incompatibility causes red cell haemolysis leading to fever, rigors, tachycardia, hypotension, chest and abdominal pain, and shortness of breath. The transfusion must be stopped immediately and any unused blood returned to the blood bank. An i.v. saline infusion should be commenced to maintain an adequate urine output, and DIC should be treated with appropriate blood components. • Formerly, viral infections were transmitted by blood transfusion; however, testing of blood donations (see above) has dramatically reduced the incidence of such infections in the developed world. Transmission of malaria or Chagas disease by transfusion occasionally occurs in endemic areas. • Fluid overload is treated by stopping the transfusion and administering oxygen and i.v. furosemide.

ANAEMIAS

Around 30% of the world population is anaemic; iron deficiency is the cause in half of these.

IRON DEFICIENCY ANAEMIA

Causes of iron deficiency include:

Blood loss: The most common explanation in men and post-menopausal women is GI blood loss. This may result from gastric or colorectal malignancy, peptic ulceration, inflammatory bowel disease, diverticulitis and angiodysplasia. GI bleeding may be exacerbated by the use of aspirin or NSAIDs. In younger women, menstrual bleeding and pregnancy often contribute to iron deficiency.

Malabsorption: Gastric acid is required to release iron from food and helps keep it in the soluble ferrous (Fe^{2+}) state. Hypochlorhydria due to proton pump inhibitor (PPI) treatment or previous gastric surgery may contribute to deficiency. Iron is absorbed actively in the upper small intestine and absorption can be affected by coeliac disease.

Physiological demands: Increased demands for iron during puberty and pregnancy can lead to deficiency.

Investigations

• Blood film shows microcytic hypochromic red cells (low MCV, low mean cell Hb—MCH). • Iron deficiency is confirmed by a low plasma ferritin level; however, ferritin levels may also be raised by liver disease and in the acute phase response, even in the presence of iron deficiency. • In these patients, measurement of transferrin saturation (<16%) and soluble transferrin receptor (raised) may be helpful.

The underlying cause of the iron deficiency should be established. Men >40 yrs and post-menopausal women should undergo investigation of the upper and lower GI tract by endoscopy or barium studies. If coeliac disease is suspected, serum antigliadin and anti-endomysium antibodies and duodenal biopsy are indicated.

Management

Unless the patient has angina, heart failure or evidence of cerebral hypoxia, transfusion is not necessary and oral iron supplementation (ferrous sulphate 200 mg 8-hourly for 3–6 mths) is appropriate, together with treatment of the underlying cause. The Hb should rise by 10 g/l every 7–10 days.

MEGALOBLASTIC ANAEMIA

This results from deficiency of vitamin B_{12} or folic acid, both of which are required for DNA synthesis. Deficiency leads to red cells with arrested nuclear maturation but normal cytoplasmic development within the bone marrow (megaloblasts). There is a macrocytic anaemia with an MCV often >120 fl, and mature red cells are commonly oval in shape. Involvement of white cells and platelets can lead to neutrophils with hypersegmented nuclei and, in severe cases, pancytopenia. Bone marrow examination reveals hypercellularity and megaloblastic changes.

VITAMIN B_{12}

The average diet contains well in excess of the 1 μg daily requirement of vitamin B_{12}, mainly in meat, eggs and milk. In the stomach, gastric enzymes release vitamin B_{12} from food and it binds to a carrier protein called R protein. The gastric parietal cells produce intrinsic factor, a vitamin B_{12}-binding protein. As gastric emptying occurs, vitamin B_{12} released from the diet switches from the R protein to intrinsic factor. B_{12} is absorbed in the terminal ileum and is transported in plasma bound to transcobalamin II, a transport protein produced by the liver. The liver stores enough B_{12} for 3 yrs, and deficiency therefore takes many years to become manifest even if all dietary intake is stopped.

Vitamin B_{12} deficiency can result in neurological disease including peripheral neuropathy and subacute combined degeneration of the cord. The latter involves the posterior columns (resulting in diminished vibration sense and proprioception leading to sensory ataxia) and corticospinal tracts (resulting in upper motor neuron signs). Dementia and optic atrophy can also occur.

Causes of vitamin B_{12} deficiency

Dietary deficiency: This only occurs in strict vegans.

Gastric factors: Gastric surgery (including gastrectomy) can result in B_{12} deficiency due to impaired secretion of gastric acid and intrinsic factor.

Pernicious anaemia: This is an autoimmune disorder characterised by atrophy of the gastric mucosa. Loss of the parietal cells causes intrinsic factor deficiency leading to B_{12} malabsorption. Pernicious anaemia has an average age of onset of 60 yrs, and is associated with other autoimmune conditions including Hashimoto's thyroiditis, Graves' disease, vitiligo and Addison's disease. Antiparietal cell antibodies are present in 90% of cases and antibodies to intrinsic factor in 60%.

Small bowel factors: Terminal ileal disease (e.g. Crohn's disease) and ileal resection result in vitamin B_{12} malabsorption. Motility disorders can result in bacterial overgrowth and the resulting competition for free vitamin B_{12} can result in deficiency.

It is possible to distinguish B_{12} deficiency due to pernicious anaemia from that due to intestinal problems with a two-part Schilling test, although this is rarely performed in practice (Fig. 14.2).

FOLATE

Leafy vegetables, liver and kidney provide rich sources of dietary folate. An average Western diet meets the daily requirement, but total body stores are small and deficiency can develop within weeks. Causes of folate deficiency include:

• Diet, e.g. poor intake of vegetables. • Malabsorption, e.g. coeliac disease.
• Increased demand, e.g. pregnancy, haemolysis. • Drugs, e.g. phenytoin, contraceptive pill, methotrexate.

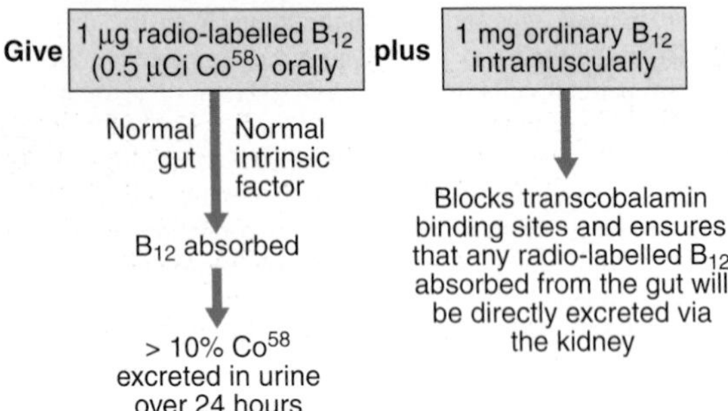

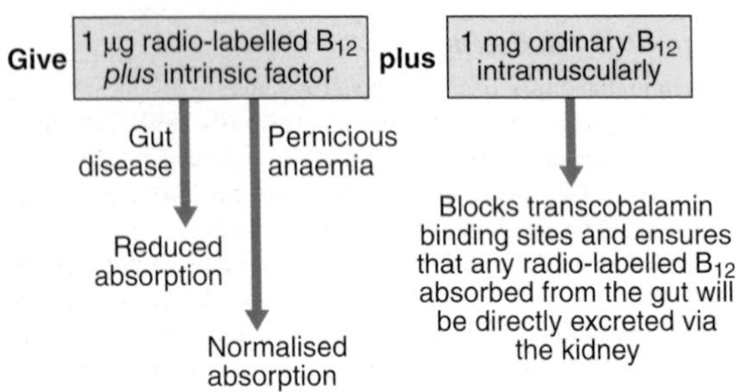

Fig. 14.2 The two-part Schilling test in the diagnosis of the cause of vitamin B12 deficiency.

Serum folate is very sensitive to dietary intake, and red cell folate is therefore a more accurate indicator of the body's folate stores.

MANAGEMENT OF MEGALOBLASTIC ANAEMIA

Vitamin B_{12} deficiency: Treated with i.m. hydroxycobalamin (1000 µg every 2 or 3 days for five doses followed by maintenance therapy of 1000 µg every 3 mths). Hb should rise by 10 g/l per wk, but neuropathy may take 6–12 mths to correct.

Folate deficiency: Treated with oral folic acid 5 mg daily. Folic acid supplementation in pregnancy may reduce the risk of neural tube defects. Prophylactic folic acid is also given in chronic haematological disease associated with reduced red cell lifespan (e.g. autoimmune haemolytic anaemia or haemoglobinopathies).

Where a patient with a severe megaloblastic anaemia requires treatment before vitamin B_{12} and red cell folate results are available, both folic acid and vitamin B_{12} are given. Folic acid therapy alone in the presence of vitamin B_{12} deficiency may result in worsening of neurological defects.

ANAEMIA OF CHRONIC DISEASE

This common type of anaemia occurs in the setting of chronic infections, chronic inflammation and neoplasia. The anaemia is mild and is usually associated with a normal MCV (normocytic, normochromic), though this may be reduced in long-standing inflammation. The pathogenesis of this type of anaemia is thought to involve abnormalities of iron metabolism and erythropoiesis. Raised ferritin and reduced total iron binding capacity (TIBC) and soluble transferrin receptor help to distinguish anaemia of chronic disease from iron deficiency. Measures which reduce the severity of the underlying disorder generally help to improve the anaemia.

HAEMOLYSIS

Normal red cells have a lifespan of 120 days. Increased red cell destruction (haemolysis) leads to increased LDH, a modest increase in serum unconjugated bilirubin and mild jaundice. Compensatory expansion of the active bone marrow results in increased reticulocytes (large red cell precursors) and immature granulocytes in peripheral blood, and blood films may also show the reason for haemolysis (e.g. spherocytosis). The erythroid hyperplasia may also cause folate deficiency, leading to megaloblastosis. When destruction exceeds production, haemolytic anaemia results.

Intravascular haemolysis: Releases free Hb into the plasma, where it binds to haptoglobin (an α_2 globulin produced by the liver), resulting in a fall in haptoglobin levels. Once haptoglobins are saturated, free Hb is oxidised to form methaemoglobin. Excess free Hb may also be absorbed by renal tubular cells, where it is degraded and the iron stored as haemosiderin. When the tubular cells are subsequently sloughed into the urine they give rise to haemosiderinuria.

Extravascular haemolysis: Occurs in the reticulo-endothelial cells of the liver and spleen, so avoiding free Hb in the plasma. In most haemolytic states, haemolysis is predominantly extravascular.

CONGENITAL HAEMOLYSIS

Inherited red cell defects may result in chronic haemolysis. The principal pathologies are:

• Red cell membrane defects. • Red cell enzymopathies. • Haemoglobinopathies.

RED CELL MEMBRANE DEFECTS

Hereditary spherocytosis

This is usually inherited as an autosomal dominant condition and has an incidence of 1 : 5000. The most common abnormalities are deficiencies of the red cell membrane proteins beta spectrin or ankyrin. The cells lose their normal elasticity and undergo destruction when they pass through the spleen. The severity of spontaneous haemolysis varies. Most cases are associated with an asymptomatic compensated chronic haemolytic state with spherocytes on the blood film and a reticulocytosis. The clinical course may be complicated by crises:

• A haemolytic crisis occurs when the severity of haemolysis increases. • A megaloblastic crisis follows the development of folate deficiency. • An aplastic crisis occurs in association with erythrovirus infection; the virus directly invades red cell precursors and switches off red cell production.

Pigment gallstones occur in up to 50% of patients and may cause cholecystitis.

Investigations are as follows:

• Hb levels are variable depending on the degree of compensation. • Reticulocyte count is raised. • The blood film shows spherocytes and reticulocytes. • The direct Coombs test is negative, excluding immune haemolysis. • Bilirubin is raised. • LDH is also raised.

Management is as follows:

• Family members should be screened. • Folic acid prophylaxis (5 mg weekly) should be given for life. • Splenectomy should be considered in moderate to severe cases but only after the age of 6 yrs because of the risk of sepsis. Splenectomised patients should receive pre-operative vaccination against pneumococcus, *Haemophilus influenzae* type B, meningococcus group C and influenza. They should undergo regular immunisation against pneumococcus and influenza, and should receive life-long penicillin V. • Acute severe haemolytic crises require transfusion.

Hereditary elliptocytosis

This is less common than hereditary spherocytosis and runs a milder clinical course. The blood film shows elliptocytic red cells and there is a variable degree of haemolysis. Most cases are asymptomatic and do not require specific treatment; more severe cases are managed in a similar way to hereditary spherocytosis.

GLUCOSE-6-PHOSPHATE DEHYDROGENASE DEFICIENCY (G6PD)

This is the most common inherited enzymopathy, affecting 10% of the world's population. G6PD is pivotal in the hexose monophosphate shunt and produces NADPH to protect the red cell against oxidative stress. G6PD deficiency is an X-linked condition principally affecting males. It results in acute intravascular haemolysis secondary to infection, drugs (e.g. antimalarials, sulphonamides, nitrofurantoin) and ingestion of fava beans. It can also cause chronic haemolysis and neonatal jaundice. Management involves stopping any precipitant drugs. Transfusion may be required in severe cases.

ACQUIRED HAEMOLYTIC ANAEMIA

AUTOIMMUNE HAEMOLYTIC ANAEMIA

This results from increased red cell destruction due to red cell autoantibodies. If an antibody avidly fixes complement, it will result in intravascular haemolysis, but if complement activation is weak, the haemolysis will be extravascular. Immune haemolysis is classified according to whether the antibodies bind best at 37°C (warm antibodies, 80% of cases) or 4°C (cold antibodies).

Warm autoimmune haemolysis

Warm autoimmune haemolysis occurs at all ages but is more common in middle age. Antibodies are usually IgG. No underlying cause is identified in up to 50% of cases. Secondary causes include:

• Lymphoid neoplasms, e.g. lymphoma. • Solid tumours, e.g. lung, colon. • Connective tissue disease, e.g. SLE, rheumatoid arthritis. • Drugs, e.g. methyldopa.

Investigations are as follows:

• Blood tests show evidence of haemolysis. • The diagnosis is confirmed by the direct Coombs or antiglobulin test, in which red cells are mixed with Coombs reagent containing antibodies against human IgG and IgM (Fig. 14.3). If the red cells have been coated by antibody in vivo, agglutination occurs. The test will miss IgA and IgE antibodies.

Management involves the following:

• Any underlying cause must be treated and any offending drugs stopped. • Corticosteroids (prednisolone 1 mg/kg) form the mainstay of treatment. They work by decreasing macrophage destruction of antibody-coated red cells and reducing antibody production. • Transfusion may be required for severe anaemia. • Splenectomy should be considered in refractory cases; this removes a main site of red cell destruction and antibody production. • Alternative immunosuppressive therapy (e.g. azathioprine, cyclophosphamide) may be required in some patients.

Cold agglutinin disease

This is due to antibodies ('cold agglutinins'), usually IgM, which bind to the red cells at 4°C and cause them to agglutinate. Causes include:

• Lymphoma. • Infections, e.g. *Mycoplasma pneumoniae*, infectious mononucleosis. • Paroxysmal cold haemoglobinuria.

Cold antibodies optimally bind red cells at lower temperatures. Red cell agglutination therefore occurs in small vessels in exposed areas, and patients may experience cold, painful and blue fingers and toes (acrocyanosis). Agglutination may cause intravascular haemolysis if complement fixation occurs.

Management involves the following:

• Any underlying cause must be treated. • Patients must keep extremities warm, especially in winter. • Corticosteroid therapy and blood transfusion may be required in some patients.

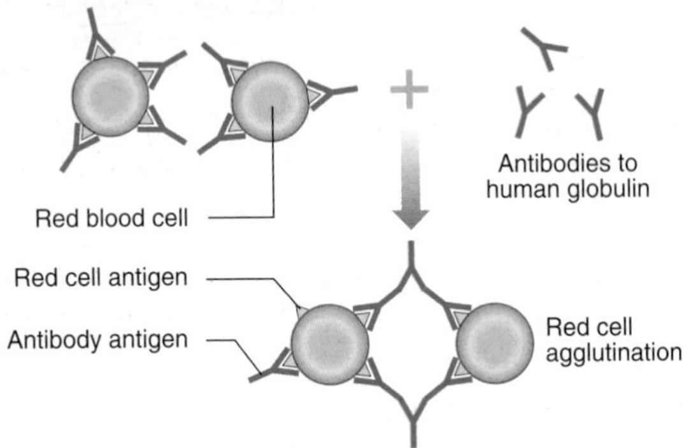

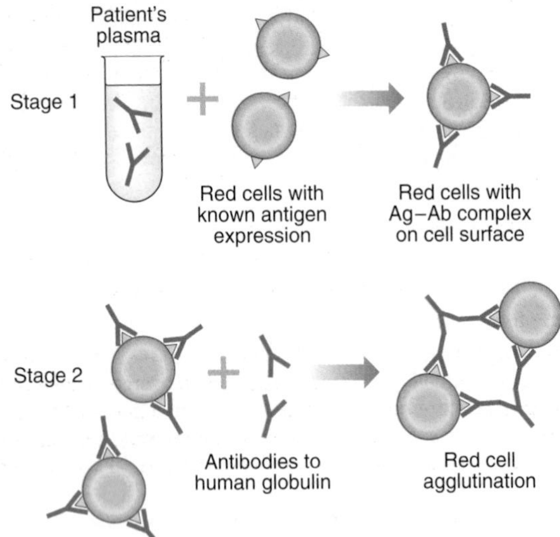

Fig. 14.3 Direct and indirect antiglobulin tests.

NON-IMMUNE HAEMOLYTIC ANAEMIA

Physical trauma

Physical disruption of red cells may occur in a number of conditions and is characterised by the presence of red cell fragments on the blood film and markers of intravascular haemolysis.

Mechanical heart valves: High flow through incompetent valves results in shear stress damage.

March haemoglobinuria: Prolonged marching or marathon running can cause red cell damage in the capillaries in the feet.

Microangiopathic haemolytic anaemia: Fibrin deposition in capillaries can cause severe red cell disruption. Causes include malignant hypertension, haemolytic uraemic syndrome and DIC.

Infection

Plasmodium falciparum malaria may be associated with intravascular haemolysis; when severe, this is termed blackwater fever due to the associated haemoglobinuria.

HAEMOGLOBINOPATHIES

SICKLE-CELL ANAEMIA

The normal Hb molecule is comprised of two alpha and two non-alpha globin polypeptide chains, each containing a haemoglobin group. Haemoglobin A (HbA-$\alpha_2\beta_2$) is the predominant form in adults. Sickle-cell disease results from a single glutamic acid to valine substitution at position 6 of the beta globin chain. It is inherited as an autosomal recessive trait.

Homozygotes: Only produce abnormal beta chains that make haemoglobin S (HbS, termed SS), resulting in the clinical syndrome of sickle-cell disease.

Heterozygotes: Produce a mixture of normal and abnormal beta chains that make normal HbA and HbS (termed AS), and this results in the clinically asymptomatic sickle trait.

Individuals with sickle-cell trait are relatively resistant to the lethal effects of *falciparum* malaria, which explains the high incidence of the sickle gene in equatorial Africa where *falciparum* malaria is endemic.

Clinical features

When HbS is deoxygenated, the Hb molecules polymerise and the red cell membrane becomes distorted, producing characteristic sickle-shaped cells. Sickling is precipitated by hypoxia, dehydration and infection. Sickled cells have a shortened survival and plug vessels in the microcirculation. This results in a number of acute syndromes termed 'crises' and chronic organ damage.

Vaso-occlusive crisis: Plugging of small vessels in the bone results in avascular necrosis, producing acute severe bone pain. Commonly affected sites include the femur, humerus, ribs, pelvis and vertebrae. Vaso-occlusion in the spleen can give rise to recurrent splenic infarction and adults may have no functional spleen. Occlusion at other sites can result in cerebrovascular accidents and proliferative retinopathy.

Sickle chest syndrome: This may follow on from a vaso-occlusive crisis and is the most common cause of death in adult sickle disease. Bone marrow infarction results in fat emboli to the lungs, which cause sickling and infarction, leading to ventilatory failure.

Sequestration crisis: Thrombosis of the venous outflow from an organ causes loss of function and acute painful enlargement. Massive splenic enlargement may result in severe anaemia and circulatory collapse. Sequestration in the liver leads to severe pain due to capsular stretching.

Aplastic crisis: Infection with human erythrovirus 19 results in severe red cell aplasia, producing a very low Hb.

Investigations

• Patients with sickle-cell disease have a compensated anaemia (usually 60–80 g/l) with a reticulocytosis. • Blood film shows sickle cells. • Hb electrophoresis demonstrates a predominance of HbS with absent HbA.

Management and prognosis

• Patients with sickle disease should receive prophylaxis with folic acid. • Pneumococcal infection may be lethal in the presence of hyposplenism; patients should therefore receive prophylaxis with daily penicillin V and should be vaccinated against pneumococcus. • Patients should also be vaccinated against *Haemophilus influenzae* B and hepatitis B. • Vaso-occlusive crises are managed by aggressive rehydration, oxygen therapy and adequate analgesia (which often requires opiates). • Top-up transfusion may be used in sequestration or aplastic crises. Exchange transfusion, where a patient is simultaneously venesected and transfused to replace HbS with HbA, may be used in life-threatening crises. • The oral cytotoxic agent hydroxycarbamide induces increased synthesis of fetal Hb (HbF-$\alpha_2\gamma_2$), which in turn inhibits polymerisation of HbS and reduces sickling; this may be helpful in individuals with recurrent severe crises. • Bone marrow transplantation is rarely performed but may be potentially curative. • Sickle-cell anaemia has mortality of 15% by the age of 20 yrs and 50% by the age of 40 yrs.

THE THALASSAEMIAS

The thalassaemias are a group of inherited disorders of Hb production in which there is impaired synthesis of a particular type of globin chain.

• In alpha-thalassaemia, there is impaired production of alpha chains. • In beta-thalassaemia there is impaired production of beta chains.

The resultant imbalance in the ratio of alpha to beta chains leads to precipitation of the excess chains, causing red cell membrane damage and reduced red cell survival.

Beta-thalassaemia

Failure to synthesise beta chains is the most common type of thalassaemia and most frequently occurs in the Mediterranean area.

Heterozygotes: Have beta-thalassaemia minor, a condition in which there is usually mild anaemia and little or no clinical disability. The anaemia has a microcytic hypochromic pattern, but individuals are not iron-deficient.

Homozygotes: Have beta-thalassaemia major and either are unable to synthesise HbA or at best produce very little. After the first 4 mths of life, they develop a profound hypochromic anaemia. Levels of HbF ($\alpha_2\gamma_2$) are raised.

Intermediate grades of severity also occur.

Management of beta-thalassaemia major is as follows:

• Blood transfusions to maintain the Hb level >100 g/l. • Daily folic acid should be prescribed. • Repeated transfusions can lead to iron overload, which is treated with the iron-chelating drug desferrioxamine. • Splenectomy is indicated for splenomegaly. • Cure is now a possibility for selected children, with allogeneic bone marrow transplantation.

Alpha-thalassaemia

Reduced or absent alpha-chain synthesis is common in Southeast Asia. There are two alpha gene loci on chromosome 16 and therefore four alpha genes.

• If one is deleted, there is no clinical effect. • If two are deleted, there may be a mild microcytic hypochromic anaemia. • If three are deleted, the patient has haemoglobin H disease; treatment is similar to that for beta-thalassaemia of intermediate severity. • If all four alpha genes are deleted, the baby is stillborn (hydrops fetalis).

HAEMATOLOGICAL MALIGNANCIES

Haematological malignancies arise when the processes of proliferation or apoptosis are corrupted in blood cells.

• If mature differentiated cells are involved, the cells produce indolent neoplasms such as low-grade lymphomas and chronic leukaemias, where patients have an expected survival of many years. • If more primitive stem cells are involved, the cells produce rapidly progressive life-threatening illnesses such as acute leukaemias and high-grade lymphomas.

LEUKAEMIAS

Leukaemias are malignant disorders of haematopoietic stem cells, associated with increased numbers of white cells in the bone marrow and/or peripheral blood. The aetiology is unknown in most patients, but several factors are associated with the development of leukaemia:

Ionising radiation: Both wartime exposure and iatrogenic exposure are known to increase risk.

Cytotoxic chemicals: Alkylating drugs can induce myeloid leukaemia after a latent period of several years. Industrial benzene exposure is associated with leukaemia.

Retroviruses: One rare form of T-cell leukaemia is associated with retroviral infection.

Genetic factors: Males are affected more than females. There is a greatly increased incidence in identical twins of affected individuals. Incidence is also increased in Down's syndrome. Racial variation also occurs; chronic lymphocytic leukaemia is rare in Chinese populations.

Immunological factors: Immune deficiency states (e.g. hypogammaglobulinaemia) are associated with an increase in haematological malignancy.

Leukaemias are traditionally classified into four main groups:

• Acute lymphoblastic leukaemia (ALL). • Acute myeloid leukaemia (AML). • Chronic lymphocytic leukaemia (CLL). • Chronic myeloid leukaemia (CML).

ACUTE LEUKAEMIA

Acute leukaemias occur at all ages, but ALL has a peak incidence in childhood. AML occurs mainly in middle and old age. In acute leukaemia there is proliferation of primitive stem cells leading to an accumulation of blast cells in the bone marrow, taking up marrow space at the expense of the normal haematopoietic elements. Eventually, this proliferation spills into the blood. The clinical features are usually those of bone marrow failure (anaemia, bleeding or infection).

Investigations

• FBC usually shows anaemia and thrombocytopenia. The leucocyte count varies from as low as $1 \times 10^9/l$ to as high as $500 \times 10^9/l$ or more. • The appearance of blast cells on the blood film is usually diagnostic. • Bone marrow aspiration is the most valuable investigation and provides material for cytology, cytogenetics and immunological phenotyping. The marrow is typically hypercellular, with replacement of normal elements by leukaemic blast cells in varying degrees. The presence of Auer rods in the cytoplasm of blast cells indicates myeloblastic leukaemia.

Management

Specific treatment for acute leukaemia is aggressive, has a number of side-effects, and may not be appropriate for very elderly patients or for those with significant comorbidity. In these patients supportive treatment only should be considered.

Specific therapy

Before embarking on specific therapy, any underlying infection should be treated. Anaemia and thrombocytopenia should be corrected with red cell and platelet transfusions. The aim of treatment is to destroy the leukaemic clone of cells without destroying the residual normal stem cell compartment. There are three phases:

Remission induction: The bulk of the tumour is destroyed by combination chemotherapy. The patient goes through a period of severe bone marrow hypoplasia, requiring intensive support and inpatient care.

Remission consolidation: Residual disease is attacked by several courses of chemotherapy during the consolidation phase. This again results in periods of marrow hypoplasia. In some patients this phase may include a stem cell transplant.

Remission maintenance: If the patient is still in remission after the consolidation phase for ALL, a period of maintenance therapy is given, consisting of a repeating cycle of drug administration. This is usually given on an outpatient basis. This maintenance phase is not of benefit in most patients with AML. In ALL, prophylactic cranial irradiation and intrathecal chemotherapy are used to ensure therapy penetrates the CNS.

Supportive therapy

Aggressive chemotherapy involves periods of bone marrow failure and requires adequate supportive care. The following problems are common:

Anaemia: This is treated with red cell transfusion to maintain Hb >100 g/l.

Bleeding: Thrombocytopenic bleeding requires platelet transfusions. Prophylactic platelet transfusion should be given to maintain the platelet count $>10 \times 10^9$/l. Coagulation abnormalities should be treated appropriately, usually with fresh frozen plasma.

Infection: Fever (>38°C) lasting over 1 hr in a significantly neutropenic patient (neutrophil count $<1.0 \times 10^9$/l) indicates possible septicaemia and constitutes a medical emergency. I.V. broad-spectrum antibiotic therapy is essential. Empirical therapy is given with a combination of an aminoglycoside (e.g. gentamicin) and a broad-spectrum penicillin (e.g. piperacillin/tazobactam). This combination is synergistic and bactericidal. The organisms most commonly associated with severe neutropenia are skin-based Gram-positive bacteria such as *Staphylococcus aureus* and *Staph. epidermidis* which gain entry via cannulae and central lines, and Gram-negative bacteria from the gut.

Patients with ALL are susceptible to infection with *Pneumocystis jirovecii*, which causes severe pneumonia. Diagnosis may require sputum induction, and if negative, bronchoalveolar lavage. Treatment is with high-dose i.v. co-trimoxazole. Susceptible patients should be given prophylactic oral co-trimoxazole.

Patients receiving intensive chemotherapy receive prophylaxis against fungal infections with fluconazole or itraconazole. Systemic fungal infection with *Candida* or aspergillosis is treated with i.v. amphotericin.

Herpes simplex infection frequently occurs around the lips and nose during chemotherapy and is treated with aciclovir. Herpes zoster should be treated early with high-dose aciclovir, as it can be fatal in immunocompromised patients.

Metabolic problems: Continuous monitoring of renal and hepatic function is necessary. Renal toxicity occurs with some antibiotics (e.g. aminoglycosides) and antifungal agents (amphotericin). Cellular breakdown during induction therapy increases uric acid production, which may cause renal failure; allopurinol and i.v. hydration are given as prophylaxis; renal failure; allopurinol and i.v. hydration are given as prophylaxis against this.

Prognosis

• Without treatment the median survival of patients with acute leukaemia is about 5 wks. • Around 80% of adult patients <60 yrs of age achieve remission with specific therapy. Remission rates are lower for older patients. However, the relapse rate continues to be high. • The introduction of the drug ATRA (all transretinoic acid) for acute promyelocytic leukaemia has greatly reduced the death rate from bleeding.

Bone marrow and peripheral blood stem cell transplantation

Haematological indications for bone marrow transplantation (BMT) include:

• Leukaemias (AML, ALL, CML). • Myeloma. • Myelodysplastic syndrome. • Non-Hodgkin lymphoma. • Severe aplastic anaemia. • Myelofibrosis. • Severe immune deficiency syndromes.

Allogeneic BMT

Healthy marrow or blood stem cells from a donor (usually an HLA-identical sibling) are infused intravenously into a recipient who has been suitably 'conditioned'. The conditioning treatment (chemotherapy with or without radiotherapy) destroys malignant cells and immunosuppresses the recipient as well as ablating the recipient's haematopoietic tissues. The injected donor cells 'home' to the marrow and produce enough erythrocytes, granulocytes and platelets for the patient's needs after 3–4 wks. During this period of aplasia patients are at risk of infection and bleeding. An advantage of receiving donor stem cells is that the donor's immunological system can recognise residual malignant recipient cells and destroy them ('graft versus disease' effect).

There is considerable morbidity and mortality associated with BMT. The best results are obtained in young patients with minimal residual disease. Around 25% die from complications such as graft-versus-host disease (see below), and there remains a significant risk of disease relapse. The long-term survival for patients undergoing allogeneic BMT in acute leukaemia is ~50%.

Graft-versus-host disease (GVHD)

GVHD is due to the cytotoxic activity of donor T lymphocytes which become sensitised to their new host, regarding it as foreign.

Acute GVHD: This occurs in the first 100 days after transplant in about one-third of patients. It varies from mild to lethal, causing skin rashes, jaundice and diarrhoea. Prevention includes HLA-matching of the donor and immunosuppressant drugs.

Chronic GVHD: This may follow acute GVHD or arise independently. It often resembles a connective tissue disorder, and is usually treated with corticosteroids and prolonged immunosuppression (e.g. ciclosporin).

Autologous BMT

In this procedure the patient's own stem cells are first harvested, usually from peripheral blood or alternatively from bone marrow, and frozen. After conditioning therapy, the autologous stem cells are reinfused. These stem cells engraft more quickly, marrow recovery occurring within 2–3 wks. There is no risk of GVHD and no immunosuppression is required.

CHRONIC MYELOID LEUKAEMIA (CML)

CML is a myeloproliferative stem cell disorder resulting in proliferation of all haematopoietic lineages but predominantly the granulocytic series. Cell maturation proceeds fairly normally. The peak incidence is at the age of 55 yrs. Around 95% of patients with CML have a chromosome abnormality (Philadelphia chromosome, Ph), a shortened chromosome 22 formed by reciprocal translocation with chromosome 9. A resulting chimeric gene (*BCR ABL*) codes for a protein with tyrosine kinase activity, which plays a causative role in the disease, influencing cellular proliferation and differentiation.

Clinical features

The disease has three phases:

• A chronic phase, in which the disease is responsive to treatment and is easily controlled, typically lasting 3–5 yrs. • An accelerated phase, in which disease control becomes more difficult. • Blast crisis, in which the disease transforms into an acute leukaemia (usually AML), which is relatively refractory to treatment.

Common symptoms include tiredness, weight loss, breathlessness and abdominal pain. About 25% of patients are asymptomatic at diagnosis. Splenomegaly is characteristic and may be massive; hepatomegaly occurs in 50% of cases.

Investigations

• FBC usually shows a normocytic, normochromic anaemia. • Leucocyte count is usually raised (average 220×10^9), but the range of values is wide. • Platelets may be low, normal or elevated. • Neutrophils are the predominant cell type on the blood film, although the full range of granulocyte precursors is seen. • The number of circulating blasts increases dramatically as the disease enters blast transformation. • Chromosome analysis of bone marrow reveals the Ph chromosome.

Management

Imatinib: This specifically inhibits *BCR ABL* tyrosine kinase activity and reduces white cell proliferation. It is first-line therapy in chronic phase CML, producing a complete response in almost 80% of patients. It is also useful for patients presenting in accelerated phase or blast crisis. Alternative agents such as hydroxycarbamide and alpha interferon are less effective.

Allogeneic BMT: This can provide a cure for younger patients in the chronic phase who are Imatinib resistant.

Treatment of blast crisis: Blast crisis is the main cause of death in patients with CML. It is treated as acute leukaemia but responds poorly, and supportive therapy alone may be appropriate in elderly patients.

CHRONIC LYMPHOCYTIC LEUKAEMIA (CLL)

This is the most common variety of leukaemia, typically presenting between the ages of 65 and 70 yrs. There is uncontrolled proliferation of immuno-incompetent B lymphocytes, leading to impaired immunity and haematopoiesis.

Clinical features

The onset is very insidious. In ~70% of patients the diagnosis is made incidentally on a routine FBC. Presenting problems include:

• Anaemia. • Infections. • Lymphadenopathy. • Systemic symptoms, such as night sweats and weight loss.

Investigations

• Peripheral blood shows a mature lymphocytosis ($>5 \times 10^9$/l). • Immunophenotyping confirms the monoclonal origin of the B cells. • Serum immunoglobulins indicate the degree of immunosuppression. • Direct Coombs test may show autoimmune haemolytic anaemia. • Bone marrow examination may be helpful in difficult cases.

Management and prognosis

• Many patients do not require specific treatment, particularly older individuals with less advanced disease. • Treatment is indicated if there is bone marrow failure, massive lymphadenopathy or splenomegaly, systemic symptoms or a rapidly increasing lymphocyte count. • Initial therapy comprises oral chemotherapy with the alkylating agent chlorambucil or the purine analogue fludarabine. • Supportive care is required in progressive disease, e.g. transfusions for symptomatic anaemia or thrombocytopenia and prompt treatment of infections. • The main prognostic factor is stage of disease. Older patients with early-stage disease usually have a normal life expectancy. • The overall median survival is about 6 yrs. • Approximately 50% of patients die of infection and 30% of causes unrelated to CLL.

MYELODYSPLASTIC SYNDROME (MDS)

MDS predominantly affects elderly patients, and is characterised by peripheral blood cytopenias and abnormal-looking (dysplastic) blood cells. It inevitably progresses to AML.

• Bone marrow failure results in symptoms of anaemia, recurrent infections or bleeding. • Bone marrow aspiration reveals hypercellular marrow with evidence of dysplasia. • MDS is usually incurable. Supportive care with red cell and platelet transfusions forms the mainstay of treatment. • Erythropoietin and granulocyte–colony stimulating factor (G–CSF) may improve Hb and white cell counts in selected individuals. • Allogeneic stem cell transplants may afford a cure in younger patients. • Survival ranges from months to years depending on subtype; >10% blasts in marrow indicates poor prognosis.

LYMPHOMAS

These neoplasms arise from lymphoid tissues, and are classified according to biopsy findings into Hodgkin and non-Hodgkin lymphoma. The majority are of B-cell origin.

HODGKIN LYMPHOMA (HL)

This typically affects young adults, although there is a second peak at 50–70 yrs of age. The condition is more common in individuals with a previous history of infectious mononucleosis, although no causal link has been proved. Reed–Sternberg cells, large malignant lymphoid cells of B-cell origin, are the histological hallmark of HL. Four histological patterns of classical HL are recognised according to the WHO classification:

• Nodular sclerosing (common in young patients and women). • Mixed cellularity. • Lymphocyte-rich. • Lymphocyte-depleted.

A nodular lymphocyte-predominant form of HL is also recognised, and carries a good prognosis.

Clinical features

• There is painless rubbery lymphadenopathy, usually in the neck or supraclavicular fossae. • Some patients have no systemic 'B' symptoms; others have weight loss and drenching sweats. • Hepatosplenomegaly may be present.

Investigations

• Lymph node biopsy is required to confirm the diagnosis.• FBC may be normal or show normocytic, normochromic anaemia. Lymphopenia may be present. • ESR may be raised. • Liver function may be abnormal with or without hepatic infiltration. • Raised LDH levels indicate adverse prognosis. • CXR may show a mediastinal mass. • CT of the chest and abdomen must be performed to permit staging, as this guides management (Box 14.8).

14.8 CLINICAL STAGES OF HODGKIN LYMPHOMA (ANN ARBOR CLASSIFICATION)

Stage	Definition
I	Involvement of a single lymph node region or extralymphatic site
II	Involvement of two or more lymph node regions or an extralymphatic site and lymph node regions on the same side of the diaphragm
III	Involvement of lymph node regions on both sides of the diaphragm with or without localised extralymphatic involvement or involvement of the spleen or both
IV	Diffuse involvement of one or more extralymphatic tissues, e.g. liver or bone marrow
A	No systemic symptoms
B	Weight loss, drenching sweats

Management and prognosis

Treatment options include radiotherapy, chemotherapy or a combination of the two.

• Radiotherapy is used for localised stage IA or IIA disease. • All other patients are initially treated with combination chemotherapy (chlorambucil, vinblastine, procarbazine and prednisolone); this is associated with an increased risk of infertility, especially in men. • Radiotherapy may be given to the original sites of bulky disease after chemotherapy to reduce the risk of relapse. • Stage IA disease has a 90% cure rate from radiotherapy alone. • Approximately 70% of those receiving chemotherapy are cured.

NON-HODGKIN LYMPHOMA (NHL)

NHL represents a monoclonal proliferation of lymphoid cells and may be of B-cell (70%) or T-cell (30%) origin. It has a peak incidence between 65 and 70 yrs of age. The most important factor influencing treatment and prognosis is grade.

High-grade NHL: Has high proliferation rates, rapidly produces symptoms and is fatal if untreated, but is potentially curable.

Low-grade NHL: Has low proliferation rates, may be asymptomatic for many months and runs an indolent course, but is not curable by conventional therapy.

Clinical features

The same staging system (Box 14.7) is used for both HL and NHL, but NHL is more likely to be stage III or IV at presentation. Features include: • Lymph node enlargement. • Systemic upset, e.g. weight loss, sweats and fever. • Hepatosplenomegaly. • Extranodal disease: more common in NHL, with involvement of the bone marrow, gut, thyroid, lung and skin. • Bone marrow involvement: more common in low-grade than high-grade disease.

Investigations

• In addition to the investigations listed for HL, patients should undergo bone marrow aspiration and trephine biopsy to identify marrow involvement. • Immunophenotyping of surface antigens allows T- and B-cell tumours to be distinguished.

Management and prognosis

Low-grade NHL: Asymptomatic patients may not require therapy. Indications for treatment include systemic symptoms, lymphadenopathy causing discomfort and bone marrow failure. Chemotherapy in combination with the monoclonal antibody Rituximab, which binds to the CD20 surface antigen in tumour cells and induces apoptosis, is first line therapy. This increases survival but is not curative. Radiotherapy can be used for localised disease. Autologous stem cell transplantation improves survival in relapsed disease.

High-grade NHL: Over 90% need combination chemotherapy with cyclophosphamide, doxorubicin, vincristine, prednisolone, and rituximab. Radiotherapy may be used for debulking, treating cord compression or in localised disease. Autologous stem-cell transplantation is used in relapsed disease.

Prognosis: Low-grade NHL runs an indolent remitting and relapsing course, with a median survival of 10 yrs. In high-grade NHL, 80% of patients initially respond to therapy but only 35% are disease-free at 5 yrs.

PARAPROTEINAEMIAS

A monoclonal increase in a single immunoglobulin class may occur in association with normal or reduced levels of the other immunoglobulins. Such monoclonal proteins are called paraproteins or M-proteins.

MONOCLONAL GAMMOPATHY OF UNCERTAIN SIGNIFICANCE (MGUS)

In this condition, a paraprotein is present in the blood but there are no other features of myeloma or related disease. It predominantly affects elderly patients, who are usually asymptomatic, and blood tests are otherwise normal. No specific treatment is required, but patients should receive annual monitoring to identify progression to myeloma.

WALDENSTRÖM MACROGLOBULINAEMIA

This rare low-grade lymphoma occurs in the elderly and is associated with the production of an IgM paraprotein. Patients present with features of hyperviscosity such as visual disturbance and confusion. Other features include anaemia, systemic symptoms, splenomegaly and lymphadenopathy. Plasma electrophoresis demonstrates an IgM paraprotein, and bone marrow aspiration shows infiltration of lymphoid cells. Severe hyperviscosity may require plasmapheresis to remove IgM. Treatment with chlorambucil or fludarabine may give effective control.

MULTIPLE MYELOMA

This is a malignant proliferation of plasma cells and has a peak incidence between the ages of 60 and 70 yrs. Normal plasma cells are derived from B cells and produce immunoglobulins containing heavy and light chains. In myeloma, plasma cells produce a monoclonal immunoglobulin (paraprotein). Light chains (kappa or lambda) may appear in the urine as Bence Jones proteinuria. IgG is the most common paraprotein type in myeloma.

Clinical features

• The malignant plasma cells stimulate osteoclastic bone resorption leading to lytic lesions, bone pain, fractures and hypercalcaemia. • Marrow involvement can result in anaemia or pancytopenia. • Renal failure can result from paraprotein deposition in the kidneys, hypercalcaemia, dehydration and amyloidosis. • Hyperviscosity due to paraproteinaemia can lead to retinal bleeds, bruising and cerebral ischaemia.

Investigations

The diagnosis of myeloma requires two of the following:

• Increased malignant plasma cells on bone marrow aspiration. • Paraprotein on plasma and/or urinary protein electrophoresis. • Lytic lesions on skeletal survey.

Other investigations include FBC, U&E and serum calcium. ESR is usually elevated. Alkaline phosphatase and bone scans are normal in the absence of fractures.

Management and prognosis

Supportive therapy: High fluid intake is necessary to treat renal impairment and hypercalcaemia. Analgesia is given for bone pain. Bisphosphonates are required for hypercalcaemia and to reduce the incidence of fractures. Plasmapheresis is given, as necessary, for hyperviscosity.

Specific therapy: Chemotherapy with melphalan is effective. Radiotherapy is useful for bone pain not responding to simple analgesia and for pathological fractures. Stem cell or bone marrow transplantation may prolong survival in selected patients. Thalidomide has anti-angiogenic effects against tumour blood vessels and is effective in myeloma, but is teratogenic.

Prognosis: The median survival of patients receiving standard treatment is 40 mths. Autologous BMT improves survival to around 54 mths.

APLASTIC ANAEMIA

PRIMARY IDIOPATHIC ACQUIRED APLASTIC ANAEMIA

This is a rare disorder in developed countries. It is characterised by failure of the pluripotent stem cells, resulting in hypoplasia of the bone marrow with pancytopenia. Usually no cause is found but enquiry should be made into causes of secondary aplasia.

Clinical features and investigations

• Patients present with symptoms of bone marrow failure, including anaemia, bleeding and infection. • FBC demonstrates pancytopenia with low reticulocytes. • Bone marrow aspiration reveals hypocellularity.

Management

• Patients require supportive treatment with red cell and platelet transfusions and aggressive management of infection. • The curative treatment for patients <30 yrs of age is allogeneic BMT, which offers a 75–90% chance of long-term cure. • Immunosuppressive therapy with ciclosporin and antithymocyte globulin is used in older patients.

14.9 CAUSES OF ACQUIRED APLASTIC ANAEMIA	
Drugs	Cytotoxic drugs Antibiotics: chloramphenicol, sulphonamides Antirheumatic agents: penicillamine, gold Antithyroid drugs Anticonvulsants Immunosuppressives: azathioprine
Chemicals	Benzene toluene solvent misuse: glue-sniffing Insecticides: organophosphates
Radiation	
Viral hepatitis	
Pregnancy	
Paroxysmal nocturnal haemoglobinuria	

SECONDARY APLASIA

Causes of secondary aplasia are listed in Box 14.9. In some instances the cytopenia is more selective and affects only one cell line, most often the neutrophils. Clinical features and investigations are the same as for primary aplastic anaemia. Any underlying cause should be addressed.

MYELOPROLIFERATIVE DISORDERS

This is a group of chronic conditions characterised by clonal proliferation of marrow erythroid precursors (polycythaemia rubra vera, PRV), megakaryocytes (primary thrombocythaemia and myelofibrosis) or myeloid cells (chronic myeloid leukaemia).

MYELOFIBROSIS

Myelofibrosis is characterised by bone marrow fibrosis with extramedullary haematopoiesis (blood cell formation outside the bone marrow). The marrow is initially hypercellular, with an excess of abnormal megakaryocytes which release growth factors, resulting in fibroblast proliferation. As the disease progresses, the marrow becomes fibrosed.

Clinical features

• Most patients present over the age of 50 yrs with fatigue, weight loss and night sweats. • The spleen may be massively enlarged due to extramedullary haematopoiesis, and painful splenic infarcts may occur.

Investigations

• There is anaemia with a leucoerythroblastic blood picture (circulating immature red cells and granulocyte precursors). • White count and platelet count may be high, normal or low. • Increased cell turnover commonly leads to high urate levels and folate deficiency. • Bone marrow is often difficult to aspirate; trephine biopsy shows replacement by fibrous tissue.

Management

• Supportive treatment includes red cell transfusions for anaemia. • Folic acid should be given to prevent deficiency. • Cytotoxic therapy with hydroxycarbamide may help reduce the WCC. • Splenectomy may be required for massive splenomegaly. • BMT may be considered in younger patients. • Survival is variable with a median of 4 yrs.

PRIMARY THROMBOCYTHAEMIA

This is characterised by a raised level of circulating platelets that are often dysfunctional. Reactive causes of increased platelets must be excluded before making the diagnosis. Patients present at a median age of 60 yrs with vascular occlusion or bleeding events. A small percentage may transform to acute leukaemia or myelofibrosis.

Hydroxycarbamide may be used to control platelet numbers. Aspirin should be considered for all patients to reduce the risk of thrombosis.

POLYCYTHAEMIA RUBRA VERA (PRV)

PRV occurs mainly in patients over the age of 40 yrs. It is characterised by increased erythropoiesis due to a primary increase in marrow activity.

Clinical features

• Patients present with an incidental finding of a high Hb, or with symptoms of hyperviscosity such as fatigue, headaches, dizziness and pruritus. • Some present with manifestations of peripheral arterial disease or a cerebrovascular accident. • Patients are often plethoric and have splenomegaly. • There is an increased risk of thrombosis and bleeding. • Thrombotic complications may occur and peptic ulceration is common, sometimes complicated by bleeding.

Investigations

• The diagnosis of PRV requires a raised Hb with an increased red cell mass, in the absence of causes of secondary polycythaemia (Box 14.1). • Neutrophil and platelet counts are often raised. • Bone marrow examination shows evidence of increased erythropoiesis and the presence of a JAK2 mutation.

Management and prognosis

• Venesection should be performed to maintain the haematocrit <45%. • Hydroxycarbamide or interferon can be used to suppress the underlying myeloproliferation. • Radioactive phosphorus (^{32}P) is reserved for older patients, as it greatly increases the risk of transformation to acute leukaemia. • Aspirin reduces the risk of thrombosis. • Median survival exceeds 10 yrs. • 15% develop myelofibrosis and a small percentage develop acute leukaemia.

BLEEDING DISORDERS

DISORDERS OF PRIMARY HAEMOSTASIS

Platelet functional disorders, thrombocytopenia, von Willebrand disease and diseases affecting the vessel wall may all result in failure of platelet plug formation in primary haemostasis.

VESSEL WALL ABNORMALITIES

Hereditary haemorrhagic telangiectasia (HHT)

HHT is a dominantly inherited condition characterised by abnormalities of vascular modelling.

Telangiectasia and small aneurysms occur on the fingertips, on the face, in the nasal passages, on the tongue, in the lung and in the GI tract. Many patients develop larger pulmonary arteriovenous malformations that cause arterial hypoxaemia and are associated with stroke and cerebral abscess due to paradoxical embolism; these should be treated by percutaneous embolisation. Patients present with recurrent bleeds (particularly epistaxis) or with iron deficiency due to occult GI bleeding.

Treatment includes iron therapy and local cautery or laser therapy to prevent lesions from bleeding.

THROMBOCYTOPENIA

Causes of thrombocytopenia are listed in Box 14.4. Treatment should be directed at the underlying condition. Indications for platelet transfusion include:

• A platelet count $<10 \times 10^9$/l. • Troublesome bleeding such as persistent epistaxis. • Life-threatening bleeding such as GI haemorrhage.

Transfusions provide only temporary relief because the survival of the platelets in the circulation is a few days at most.

IDIOPATHIC THROMBOCYTOPENIC PURPURA (ITP)

The presence of autoantibodies directed against platelets results in platelet destruction. ITP in children typically presents 2–3 wks after a viral illness with sudden onset of purpura and sometimes oral and nasal bleeding. Adult ITP usually has a more insidious onset. Some cases may be associated with connective tissue disease. The condition is likely to become chronic, with remissions and relapses. The peripheral blood film is normal, apart from a greatly reduced platelet number, whilst the bone marrow reveals increased megakaryocytes.

Management

• Most cases of childhood ITP are self-limiting and resolve within a few weeks. • Indications for oral prednisolone include severe purpura, bruising or epistaxis, and a platelet count $<10 \times 10^9$/l. • Adults are also treated with prednisolone, although this is often less effective than in children. • Persistent or potentially life-threatening bleeding should be treated with platelet transfusion. • Intravenous IgG (IVIgG) raises the platelet count and is indicated if the bleeding is immediately life-threatening. • Splenectomy should be considered in patients with relapsing disease.

THROMBOTIC THROMBOCYTOPENIC PURPURA

This is a rare cause of thrombocytopenia requiring urgent management. Platelet thrombi form in the microvasculature, and affect the renal and cerebral circulation in particular. Excessive platelet aggregation occurs because of the lack of a protease enzyme, which results in the presence of extra-large von Willebrand factor molecules. The condition may be associated with infection (e.g. *E. coli* O157).

Clinically there are five features:

• Thrombocytopenia. • Microangiopathic haemolytic anaemia. • Neurological signs. • Renal impairment. • Fever.

Untreated mortality rates are 90%. Management includes plasma exchange.

COAGULATION DISORDERS

Coagulation factor disorders can arise from deficiency of a single factor (usually congenital, e.g. haemophilia A) or of multiple factors (often acquired, e.g. liver disease).

CONGENITAL BLEEDING DISORDERS

HAEMOPHILIA A

Haemophilia A is the most common congenital coagulation disorder. It affects 1 : 10 000 individuals and is characterised by a reduction in factor VIII. The factor VIII gene is located on the X chromosome. Haemophilia A is inherited as an X-linked recessive disorder and patients are therefore male. All daughters of haemophiliacs are carriers. If a carrier has a son, he will have a 50% chance of having haemophilia, and a daughter will have a 50% chance of being a carrier.

Clinical features and investigations

The diagnosis is normally made after the age of 6 mths, when babies become more mobile and first experience bruising or haemarthrosis. The features of haemophilia A are related to the plasma factor VIII level (Box 14.10). Individuals with severe haemophilia experience recurrent haemarthroses in large joints, which over time lead to secondary osteoarthrosis. Although joints and muscles are the most common sites for haemorrhage, bleeding can occur at almost any site. Intracranial haemorrhage is often fatal.

Management

• Bleeding episodes should be treated early with i.v. factor VIII concentrate. • Freeze-dried factor VIII concentrates can be stored at 4°C in domestic

14.10 SEVERITY OF HAEMOPHILIA		
Degree of severity	**Factor VIII or IX level**	**Clinical presentation**
Severe	<2%	Spontaneous haemarthroses and muscle haematomas
Moderate	2–10%	Mild trauma or surgery causes haematomas
Mild	10–50%	Major injury or surgery results in excess bleeding

refrigerators, and many patients are therefore able to treat themselves at home. • The concentrates are prepared from blood donor plasma which has been screened for hepatitis B, C and HIV, and has undergone a viral inactivation process during manufacture. • Factor VIII concentrates prepared by recombinant technology are also now widely available and, although more expensive, are perceived as being safer than those derived from plasma. • In individuals with mild haemophilia A, i.v. or intranasal desmopressin can be used to increase factor VIII levels. This is often sufficient to treat a mild bleed or cover minor surgery such as dental extraction.

Complications of therapy

Before 1985 concentrates were not virally inactivated. As a result, many patients treated became infected with hepatitis B, hepatitis C and HIV. All potential recipients of pooled blood products should therefore be offered hepatitis A and B immunisation. There is also now concern that the infectious agent which causes variant CJD might be transmissible via blood and blood products.

The other serious consequence of factor VIII infusion is the development of anti-factor VIII antibodies, which arise in about 20–30% of severe haemophiliacs. Such antibodies rapidly neutralise therapeutic infusions, making treatment relatively ineffective. Infusion of factor VIIa may stop bleeding.

HAEMOPHILIA B (CHRISTMAS DISEASE)

This is caused by deficiency of factor IX and is also an X-linked condition. The disorder is clinically indistinguishable from haemophilia A but is less common. Treatment is with factor IX concentrate.

VON WILLEBRAND DISEASE

Von Willebrand disease is a common but usually mild bleeding disorder with autosomal dominant inheritance. Von Willebrand factor (vWF) is a protein that performs two principal functions:

• It acts as a carrier protein for factor VIII; deficiency of vWF therefore results in a secondary reduction in the plasma factor VIII level. • Its other role is in platelet binding to subendothelial collagen; deficiency therefore also leads to prolonged primary haemorrhage after trauma.

Clinical features

Patients present with haemorrhagic manifestations similar to those in individuals with reduced platelet function. Superficial bruising, epistaxis, and menorrhagic and GI haemorrhage are common. Bleeding episodes are usually far less common and severe than in severe haemophilia.

Investigations

• Reduced level of vWF, with secondary reduction in factor VIII. • Prolonged bleeding time.

Management

• Mild haemorrhage can be treated with desmopressin, which raises the vWF level. • Factor VIII concentrates can be used for more severe bleeds.

ACQUIRED BLEEDING DISORDERS

DISSEMINATED INTRAVASCULAR COAGULATION (DIC)

DIC can be initiated by a number of mechanisms. Examples include infection (particularly endotoxaemia due to Gram-negative septicaemia), cancer and obstetric problems (e.g. placental abruption, amniotic fluid embolism). Expression of tissue factor leads to activation of the coagulation cascade through the extrinsic pathway. Intravascular coagulation takes place with consumption of platelets, coagulation factors and fibrinogen. This results in depletion of haemostatic components and therefore a potential haemorrhagic state. This may be exacerbated by activation of the fibrinolytic system secondary to the deposition of fibrin.

Investigations

• Thrombocytopenia. • Prolonged PT and APTT due to coagulation factor deficiency. • Low fibrinogen. • Increased levels of D-dimer (a fibrin degradation product).

Management

• Therapy should be aimed at treating the underlying condition causing DIC (e.g. i.v. antibiotics for septicaemia). • Blood products such as platelets and/or fresh frozen plasma should be given to correct identified abnormalities.

LIVER DISEASE

In severe parenchymal liver disease, bleeding may arise from many different causes. These include reduced synthesis of coagulation factors, DIC and thrombocytopenia secondary to hypersplenism. Cholestatic jaundice reduces vitamin K absorption and leads to deficiency of factors II, VII, IX and X. This deficiency can be treated with parenteral vitamin K.

VENOUS THROMBOSIS

Venous thrombosis may arise either because of damage to or pressure on veins (e.g. varicose veins, pelvic tumour) or as a result of changes in the blood. Predisposing conditions for venous thromboembolism are listed in Box 14.11. Clinical features and investigations are described on page 532.

HAEMATOLOGICAL DISORDERS PREDISPOSING TO VENOUS THROMBOEMBOLISM

When a thrombotic event arises in an individual under the age of 40 yrs, investigations for a predisposing blood abnormality (thrombophilia) should be undertaken. This is particularly relevant if there is a family history of thrombosis.

14.11 FACTORS PREDISPOSING TO VENOUS THROMBOSIS	
Patient factors	
• Age > 40 yrs • Obesity • Varicose veins • Previous DVT	• Oral contraceptive • Pregnancy/puerperium • Dehydration • Immobility
Surgical conditions	
• Surgery, especially if >30 mins' duration • Abdominal or pelvic	• Orthopaedic to lower limb
Medical conditions	
• MI/heart failure • Inflammatory bowel disease • Malignancy	• Nephrotic syndrome • Pneumonia • Homocystinaemia
Haematological disorders	
• PRV (primary proliferative polycythaemia) • Essential thrombocythaemia	• Paroxysmal nocturnal haemoglobinuria • Myelofibrosis
Deficiency of anticoagulants	
• Antithrombin • Protein C	• Protein S • Factor V Leiden
Antiphospholipid antibody	
• Lupus anticoagulant	• Anticardiolipin antibody

14.12 CLINICAL ASSOCIATIONS WITH ANTIPHOSPHOLIPID SYNDROME	
Primary antiphospholipid syndrome	
• Venous thromboembolic disease • Arterial thromboembolic disease	• Sterile (Liebmann–Sachs) endocarditis with embolism • Recurrent pregnancy failure
Secondary antiphospholipid syndrome	
• SLE • Rheumatoid arthritis	• Systemic sclerosis • Sjögren's syndrome

Antithrombin deficiency: Antithrombin is a protein which inactivates factors IIa (thrombin), IXa, Xa and XIa. Its activity is greatly potentiated by heparin. Familial deficiency of antithrombin is a dominantly inherited disorder and is associated with a marked predisposition to venous thromboembolism.

Protein C and S deficiencies: Protein C inactivates factors Va and VIIIa; protein S acts as a co-factor for protein C. Inherited deficiency of either protein C or S therefore results in a prothrombotic state.

Factor V Leiden: This condition is caused by an amino acid substitution in factor Va which prevents its inactivation. Factor Va therefore persists, resulting in a tendency to venous thrombosis.

Antiphospholipid antibody syndrome: In this syndrome, antiphospholipid antibodies (which include lupus anticoagulant and anticardiolipin antibodies) interact with the coagulation cascade, causing arterial and venous thromboembolism. The exact mechanism of thrombosis is unclear. The syndrome sometimes occurs in patients with SLE (secondary antiphospholipid syndrome); when it occurs in the absence of features of SLE, it is known as the primary antiphospholipid syndrome (Box 14.12). The antibody is also associated with recurrent spontaneous abortions.

MANAGEMENT OF VENOUS THROMBOEMBOLISM

ANTICOAGULANT THERAPY

Heparin

Standard (unfractionated) heparin produces its anticoagulant effect by potentiating the activity of antithrombin. This results in prolongation of the APTT. The low molecular weight heparins (LMWHs) augment antithrombin activity preferentially against factor Xa. LMWH does not affect the APTT. It is given as a subcutaneous injection in a weight-related dose. Normally, therefore, the plasma LMWH level does not need to be measured. Indications for heparin are given in Box 14.12.

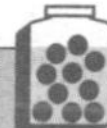

14.13 INDICATIONS FOR ANTICOAGULATION

Heparin

- Treatment and prevention of DVT
- Pulmonary embolism
- Post-thrombolysis for MI, to prevent coronary re-occlusion
- Unstable angina pectoris
- Acute peripheral arterial occlusion

Warfarin

Indication	Target
• Prophylaxis against DVT • Treatment of DVT and pulmonary embolism • Arterial embolism • Atrial fibrillation with specific stroke risk factors • Mobile mural thrombus on echo post-MI • Extensive anterior MI	Therapeutic corrected prothrombin ratio (INR) 2.5
• Recurrent DVT whilst on warfarin • Mechanical prosthetic cardiac valves	INR 3.5

LMWHs are now widely used for the treatment of both DVT and pulmonary embolism, and have replaced standard heparin as the initial treatment of choice. As LMWH injections need only be given once daily subcutaneously and no monitoring is required, many patients can be treated at home. Standard heparin is started with a loading dose of 5000 U i.v., followed by a continuous infusion adjusted to maintain the patient's APTT at 1.5–2.5 times the control time. The half-life of i.v. heparin is about 1 hr, and if a patient bleeds, it is usually sufficient just to discontinue the infusion; however, if bleeding is severe, the excess can be neutralised with i.v. protamine. The short half-life of standard heparin makes it useful for those with a predisposition to bleeding (e.g. patients with a peptic ulcer). It is usually appropriate to start warfarin therapy at the same time as heparin, as it takes several days to decrease the concentration of the vitamin K-dependent clotting factors. Heparin should be continued until the INR is >2.0 for 2 consecutive days.

Heparin-induced thrombocytopenia (HIT): In a small proportion of patients treated with heparin the platelet count declines after 5–7 days due to the development of an antibody directed against a factor on the platelet surface. Heparin should be discontinued immediately and the direct thrombin inhibitor, hirudin, given instead.

Warfarin

Warfarin inhibits the vitamin K-dependent carboxylation of factors II, VII, IX and X in the liver (Fig. 14.4). Indications for warfarin and appropriate target INRs are listed in Box 14.13. Warfarin therapy must be initiated with a loading dose (e.g. 10 mg orally) on the first day; subsequent daily doses

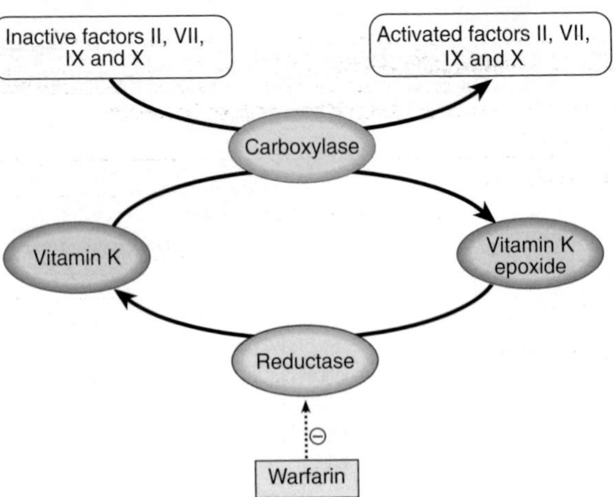

Fig. 14.4 The role of vitamin K in clotting and the mechanism of action of warfarin.

depend on the INR and can be predicted using an algorithm. Following a single episode of venous thromboembolism, oral anticoagulation is usually continued for 3 mths if the cause is known and reversed, or 6 mths if idiopathic. After two thromboembolic episodes, life-long warfarin is often considered appropriate.

Bleeding is the most common serious side-effect of warfarin. If the INR is above the desired therapeutic level, the warfarin dose should be reduced or withheld. The anticoagulant effect of warfarin may be reversed by administering vitamin K, but this takes about 6 hrs. If the patient has a serious haemorrhage, reversal can be effected quickly by giving coagulation factor concentrate or fresh frozen plasma.

PREVENTION OF VENOUS THROMBOSIS

All patients admitted to hospital should be assessed for their risk of developing venous thromboembolism (Box 14.14). Early mobilisation of all patients is important to prevent DVTs. Patients at medium or high risk may require additional antithrombotic measures such as graduated compression stockings and standard heparin or LMWH.

14.14 ANTITHROMBOTIC PROPHYLAXIS 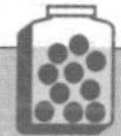
Patients in the following categories should be considered for specific antithrombotic prophylaxis:
Moderate risk of DVT
• Major surgery in patients >40 yrs or with other risk factor • Major medical illness, e.g. heart failure, chest infection, malignancy, inflammatory bowel disease
High risk of DVT
• Hip or knee surgery • Major abdominal or pelvic surgery for malignancy or with history of DVT or known thrombophilia

15 Musculoskeletal disorders

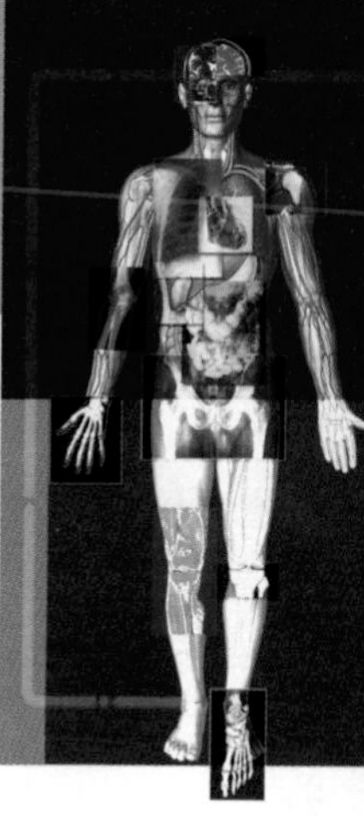

Disorders of the musculoskeletal (MSK) system are extremely common, accounting for up to a quarter of new consultations in general practice. They are the single most frequent cause of physical disability in the elderly. The principal manifestations are pain and impairment of locomotor function. Non-inflammatory conditions are far more prevalent than inflammatory disease. Osteoarthritis is the most common joint disorder, with knee involvement a major cause of disability. Osteoporosis is the most prevalent bone disorder, with 1 in 3 women sustaining an osteoporotic fracture at some point during their lifetime.

PRESENTING PROBLEMS

JOINT PAIN

ACUTE MONOARTHRITIS

Causes of acute inflammation in a single joint are listed in Box 15.1. The site affected rarely helps to identify the cause except in the case of gout, which typically affects the first metatarsophalangeal joint.

Joint aspiration is normally required to exclude sepsis and to look for crystals.

OLIGOARTHRITIS

Oligoarthritis is arthritis affecting two, three or four joints. By far the most common cause is osteoarthritis (OA), which is a non-inflammatory condition characterised by degenerative joint change. Inflammatory oligoarthritis mainly targets lower limb joints and is usually asymmetrical; it is a common

CLINICAL EXAMINATION OF THE MUSCULOSKELETAL SYSTEM

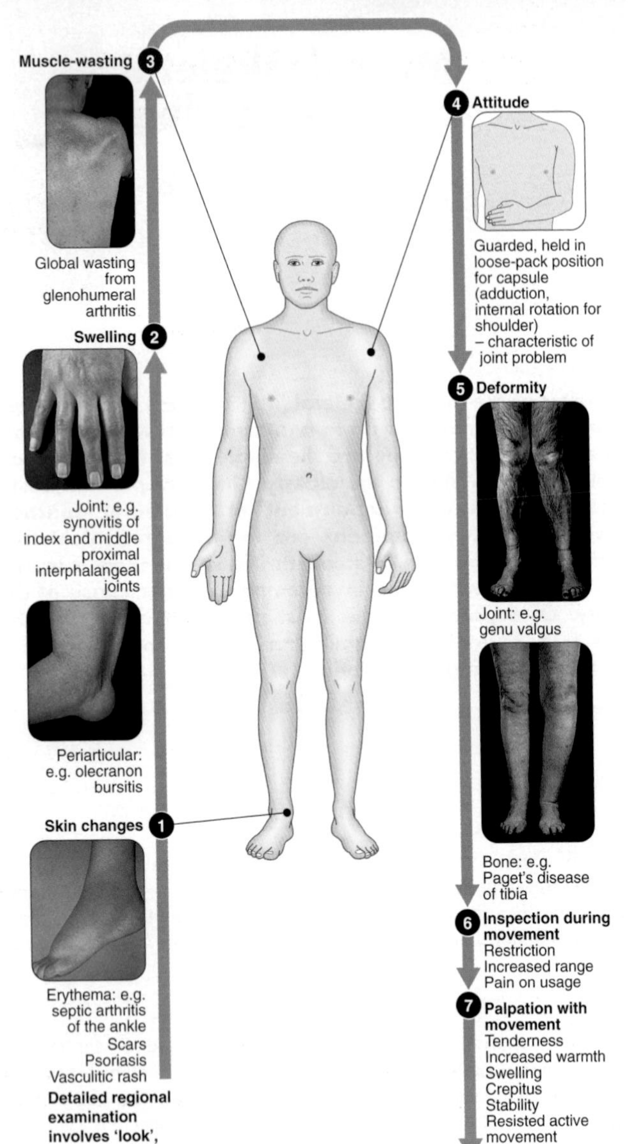

Detailed regional examination involves 'look', 'feel' and 'move'

15.1 CAUSES OF ACUTE MONOARTHRITIS

- Septic arthritis
- Crystal synovitis: gout, pseudogout
- Monoarticular presentation of oligo- or polyarthritis (e.g. rheumatoid arthritis, seronegative spondarthritis)
- Haemarthrosis associated with clotting abnormality or trauma

15.2 CAUSES OF POLYARTHRITIS

Cause	Characteristics
Non-inflammatory	
Generalised osteoarthritis	Small and large joints, only a few joints symptomatic at any one time
Inflammatory	
Rheumatoid arthritis, juvenile idiopathic arthritis	Symmetrical, small and large joints, upper and lower limbs
Seronegative spondarthritis (psoriasis, reactive, ankylosing spondylitis, enteropathic arthropathy)	Asymmetrical, large > small joints, lower > upper limbs, spondylitis
Lupus	Symmetrical, small > large joints, joint damage uncommon
Chronic gout	Distal > proximal joints preceded by acute attacks
Viral arthritis	Very acute, self-limiting (<6 wks)
Chronic sarcoidosis	Symmetrical, small and large joints

presentation of seronegative spondarthritis (e.g. reactive arthritis, psoriatic arthritis, ankylosing spondylitis, enteropathic arthritis). Sequential joint involvement ascending a limb suggests sepsis.

POLYARTHRITIS

Polyarthritis is inflammation affecting five or more joints. The symmetry and pattern of involved joints are important in determining the cause (Box 15.2). Accompanying periarticular or extra-articular features may aid diagnosis.

Many viral infections can cause the rapid onset of an acute symmetrical inflammatory polyarthritis affecting small and large joints of the upper and lower limbs. The arthritis is usually self-limiting within 6 wks. Typical viruses include hepatitis B and C, mumps, rubella and infectious mononucleosis. The rapidity of onset, the presence of fever and the characteristic 'viral' rash suggest the diagnosis.

REGIONAL PERIARTICULAR PAIN

SINGLE REGIONAL PAIN

This usually results from over-usage strain or injury affecting a periarticular structure. Certain movements reproduce the pain. Examination reveals localised periarticular tenderness but minimal signs of inflammation. The pain may be reproduced by resisted active movement or by stressing the involved structure. Diagnosis is usually clinical. Management is aimed towards avoiding predisposing mechanical factors, pain relief and appropriate exercise to restore function.

Shoulder pain

Rotator cuff syndrome: In this common condition, tendinitis or bursitis around the glenohumeral joint causes pain which is reproduced by resisted movement. Treatment is by physiotherapy, analgesia and steroid injections.

Adhesive capsulitis ('frozen shoulder'): This presents with upper arm pain that progresses over 4–10 wks before receding over a similar time course. Glenohumeral restriction is present from the outset, but progresses and reaches its maximum as the pain is receding. In the early phase there is marked anterior joint tenderness and pain at extremes of movement; later there is painless restriction, often affecting all movements. Treatment comprises analgesia, local corticosteroid injection and regular 'pendulum' exercises of the arm. The natural history is for slow but complete recovery.

Elbow pain

Lateral epicondylitis ('tennis elbow'): The most common periarticular lesion (Box 15.3).

Olecranon bursitis: Can follow local repetitive trauma but may also be secondary to infection, gout or RA.

15.3 PERIARTICULAR LESIONS PRESENTING AS ELBOW PAIN

Lesion	Pain	Examination findings, tests
'Tennis elbow'	Lateral epicondyle Radiation to extensor forearm	Tender over epicondyle Pain reproduced by resisted active wrist extension
'Golfer's elbow'	Medial epicondyle Radiation to flexor forearm	Tender over epicondyle Pain reproduced by resisted active wrist flexion
Olecranon bursitis	Olecranon	Fluctuant tender swelling over olecranon

15.4 PERIARTICULAR LESIONS IN THE LOWER LIMB		
Lesion	**Pain**	**Examination findings, tests**
Trochanteric bursitis	Upper lateral thigh, worse on lying on that side at night	Tender over greater trochanter
Pre-patellar bursitis	Anterior patella	Tender fluctuant swelling in front of patella
Popliteal cyst ('Baker's cyst')	Popliteal fossa	Tender swelling of popliteal fossa, usually reducible by massage with knee in mid-flexion
Plantar fasciitis	Under heel, worse on standing and walking	Tender under distal calcaneus/ plantar fascia insertion site
Achilles tendinitis	Localised to tendon	Tender on squeezing tendon Pain reproduced by standing on toes or resisted plantar flexion

Disorders of the hand and wrist

Trigger finger: This tenosynovitis in the flexor tendon sheath causes intermittent locking of the finger in flexion. Local corticosteroid injection often relieves the problem and surgery is rarely required.

De Quervain's tenosynovitis: Inflammation of the tendon sheaths of abductor pollicis longus and extensor pollicis brevis leads to pain over the radial aspect of the distal forearm and wrist. Examination reveals distal radial tenderness, sometimes with associated crepitus. The condition is usually caused by repetitive over-usage.

Dupuytren's contracture: Results from fibrosis and contracture of the superficial palmar fascia. Inability to extend the fingers fully is associated with puckering of the skin. The ring and little fingers are generally the worst affected but the condition is usually painless. Dupuytren's contracture is age-related, more common in men and often familial. It is also associated with alcohol misuse.

Lower limb pain

Causes of periarticular pain affecting the lower limb are listed in Box 15.4.

BACK AND NECK PAIN

LOW BACK PAIN

Back pain is extremely common. In the UK, 7% of the adult population consult their GP each year with back pain, at a cost of 80 million lost working days.

Clinical assessment

The vast majority of cases are due to simple mechanical back pain and are managed conservatively. The aim of history and examination is to identify the small number of patients with serious spinal pathology who require specific investigation and treatment.

Mechanical pain: Accounts for >90% of back pain episodes, usually affecting patients aged 20–55 yrs. It is more common in heavy manual workers. The pain is often sudden in onset, and is associated with lifting or bending. Symptoms are worsened by activity and relieved by rest. Pain is typically asymmetrical and is confined to the lumbosacral region, buttock or thigh, but there is no clear-cut nerve root distribution (unlike radicular pain). Examination may reveal local paraspinal muscle spasm with painful restriction of movement. Mechanical pain has a good prognosis, with 90% recovery at 6 wks. Psychological factors (e.g. job dissatisfaction, depression) increase the risk of progression to chronic disability.

Non-mechanical pain: Causes of non-mechanical pain include bony destruction due to malignancy, fracture or infection. The pain is constant and progressive, and shows little variation with activity. 'Red flag' features suggesting serious spinal pathology include:
• Age <20 or >50 yrs. • Constant, progressive pain unrelieved by rest. • Thoracic pain. • Past medical history or symptoms of malignancy or TB. • Systemic corticosteroid use. • Constitutional symptoms: sweats, malaise, weight loss.

Examination may reveal painful spinal deformity with signs at multiple nerve root levels. In all cases it is important to exclude signs of cauda equina syndrome (see below).

Inflammatory pain: Pain due to spondylitis is gradual in onset and often occurs before the age of 30 yrs. It is usually axial, symmetrical and spread over many segments. Sacroiliitis causes maximal pain in the buttock, with radiation down the posterior thigh. Patients often experience morning stiffness which improves with activity.

Radicular (nerve root) pain: This is commonly caused by a prolapsed intervertebral disc in young adults, most commonly at L4 or L5. Patients experience severe, sharp pain radiating down the back of the leg beyond the knee ('sciatica'). The unilateral leg pain is worse than the low back pain, and is aggravated by coughing and straining. Straight leg raising reproduces the pain, and examination may reveal motor weakness and/or sensory loss limited to one nerve root with loss of the corresponding reflex. Around 50% of patients recover by 6 wks with conservative management only. Compression of multiple nerve roots in the cauda equina constitutes a medical emergency (Box 15.5).

Investigations

• Plain X-rays are rarely helpful in acute mechanical low back pain, unless 'red flag' features are present. They can also be useful in cases of ankylosing spondylitis and osteoporotic crush fractures. • A low Hb and raised CRP

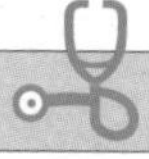

15.5 FEATURES OF CAUDA EQUINA SYNDROME

- Difficulty with micturition
- Loss of anal sphincter tone or faecal incontinence
- Saddle anaesthesia
- Progressive motor weakness/gait disturbance
- Sensory level

15.6 CAUSES OF NECK PAIN	
Mechanical	e.g. Postural, 'whiplash', disc prolapse, cervical spondylosis
Inflammatory	e.g. Infection, spondylitis, RA, polymyalgia rheumatica
Neoplasia	e.g. Bony metastases, myeloma
Fibromyalgia	
Referred pain	e.g. Pharynx, teeth, angina, Pancoast tumour

or ESR may suggest inflammation or malignancy. • Raised alkaline phosphatase is associated with bony metastases and Paget's disease. • Raised prostate-specific antigen (PSA) is associated with metastatic prostate cancer. • A monoclonal band on serum immunophoresis and Bence Jones proteinuria suggest myeloma. • MRI is useful in assessing soft tissue structures including nerve roots in patients with 'red flag' features or signs of cauda equina syndrome.

Management

• Treatment of mechanical back pain involves reassurance, education, simple analgesia and early mobilisation. • ~90% of patients will have recovered by 6 wks, although recurrent back pain is common. • Bed rest is not helpful and increases the risk of chronic disability. • Physiotherapy may be required in individuals not settling with the above measures. • <1% of patients require surgery. • The management of serious spinal pathology is dictated by the cause.

NECK PAIN

Neck pain is less common than back pain but is a particular problem in elderly patients. It is usually due to mechanical or degenerative problems (Box 15.6). Nerve roots and/or the cervical cord may be compromised by osteophytes or disc prolapse (usually C6 disc compressing the C7 root). Surgery is occasionally required for severe radiculopathy or cervical myelopathy. The principles of investigation and management are similar to those for back pain.

15.7 CAUSES OF BONE PAIN

Cause	Characteristics
Fracture (high-energy fractures, osteoporotic fractures, pathological fractures, e.g. secondary to bony metastases)	Acute pain, tenderness and deformity
Metastatic bone disease or primary bone tumour	Progressive, localised, associated weight loss and fatigue
Paget's disease	Localised to affected sites +/– deformity
Osteomalacia	Bone tenderness and associated limb girdle weakness
Chronic infection (osteomyelitis)	
Renal bone disease	

15.8 CAUSES OF PROXIMAL MUSCLE PAIN AND WEAKNESS

Inflammatory	e.g. Polymyositis, dermatomyositis
Endocrine	e.g. Hypothyroidism, hyperthyroidism, Cushing's syndrome, Addison's disease
Metabolic	e.g. Glycogen storage disorders, hypokalaemia, osteomalacia
Drugs/toxins	e.g. Alcohol, fibrates, statins
Infections	e.g. HIV, cytomegalovirus, Epstein–Barr, schistosomiasis
Genetic	e.g. Muscular dystrophies

BONE PAIN

Causes of bone pain are listed in Box 15.7.

MUSCLE PAIN AND WEAKNESS

It is important to distinguish between a subjective feeling of generalised weakness or fatigue, and 'true' weakness with objective loss of muscle power. The former is a non-specific manifestation of many organic diseases and also of psychological distress. The latter, however, may indicate intrinsic muscle disease. Proximal muscle weakness causes difficulty in standing from a seated position, squatting and lifting overhead. Distal power (e.g. grip) is usually preserved. Causes of proximal myopathy are listed in Box 15.8. Distal muscle weakness normally has a neurological cause.

The most sensitive biochemical test of muscle injury is creatine kinase (CK). However, although a raised level confirms the suspicion of muscle inflammation or necrosis, it does not establish the cause. Muscle biopsy and electromyography (EMG) may therefore be required to reach a precise diagnosis.

PRINCIPLES OF MANAGEMENT OF MUSCULOSKELETAL DISORDERS

Key aims of management of MSK conditions are:

• Patient education. • Pain control. • Optimising function. • Beneficially modifying the disease process.

These therapeutic objectives are achieved most effectively via a multidisciplinary team approach.

NON-PHARMACOLOGICAL INTERVENTIONS

Patient education has been shown to reduce pain and disability. Regular exercise helps strengthen muscles acting over compromised joints and improves function. Adverse mechanical factors should be addressed; examples include shock-absorbing footwear, walking aids, and weight loss in obese patients. Physical treatments such as local heat and ice packs can help induce muscle relaxation and symptom relief. Splints and orthoses help provide rest and support, and reduce joint instability. For those with severe disabilities, a variety of aids and appliances can be used to modify the environment and promote independence. Examples include raised toilet seats, high chairs, extended tap handles and devices to help pull on socks. Occupational therapy input is crucial for these individuals. Tuition in coping strategies (e.g. yoga, relaxation, avoiding maladaptive pain behaviour) can assist patients with incurable disease to deal with their chronic pain and disability.

PHARMACOLOGICAL OPTIONS FOR DIRECT SYMPTOM CONTROL

SIMPLE ANALGESIA

Paracetamol is effective for the treatment of mild to moderate pain. It acts by inhibiting central prostaglandin synthesis but has little effect on peripheral prostaglandin production. It is safe, has few contraindications and drug interactions, and is low in cost. It is therefore an appropriate first-line analgesic in most patients.

NON-STEROIDAL ANTI-INFLAMMATORY DRUGS (NSAIDS)

NSAIDs (e.g. ibuprofen, diclofenac) are effective in combating pain and stiffness associated with inflammatory disease. They also help reduce bone pain due to metastatic deposits. They act by inhibiting cyclo-oxygenase (COX) and thereby reducing prostaglandin synthesis (Fig. 15.1). There are two isoforms of COX, encoded by distinct genes.

Details of the usage, dose and side-effects of NSAIDs are given on page 776.

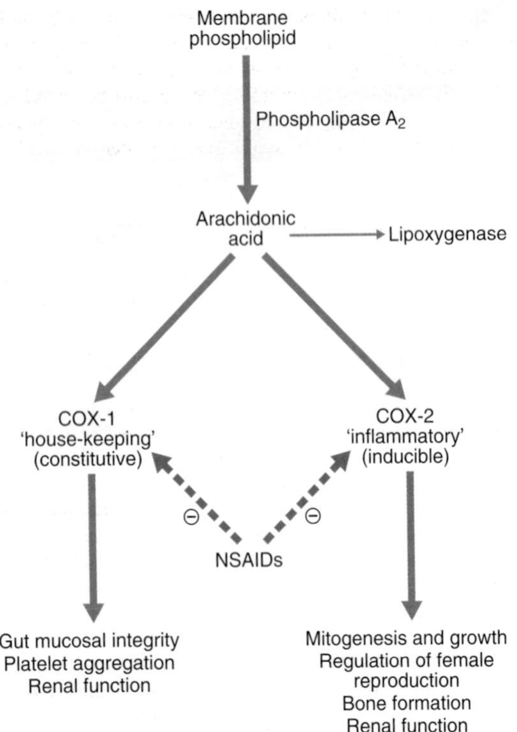

Fig. 15.1 COX-1 and COX-2 pathways.

NUTRIPHARMACEUTICALS

A wide variety of nutritional supplements are available for the relief of MSK symptoms. There are some data that glucosamine and chondroitin may provide modest pain relief in knee OA.

TOPICAL AGENTS

NSAID and capsaicin (chilli extract) creams provide safe and effective pain relief from arthritis (especially OA) and periarticular lesions. They may be used as monotherapy or as an adjunct to oral analgesics. Topical capsaicin causes pain fibres to discharge substance P. Initial application results in a burning sensation, but continued use reduces substance P activity with consequent pain reduction.

OTHER ANALGESICS

Stronger analgesics are sometimes required for moderate to severe pain. The weak opioids codeine and dihydrocodeine are relatively mild analgesics, but may be effective when combined with paracetamol. Their use is often limited by side-effects such as constipation and confusion, particularly in the elderly. Continuous opioid use can give rise to dependence and tolerance. The centrally acting analgesic tramadol can also be useful for severe pain, but can cause nausea, constipation, dizziness, somnolence and confusion. Patients with refractory symptoms may merit referral to a specialist pain team.

SLOW-ACTING ANTIRHEUMATIC DRUGS

These drugs suppress chronic inflammatory disease, but can take several months to exert a beneficial effect. They may reduce target tissue damage and are therefore also called 'disease-modifying antirheumatic drugs' (DMARDs). They are used in the management of RA, seronegative spondarthritis and connective tissue diseases. All DMARDs carry potentially toxic side-effects, and regular monitoring is therefore required. Some of these drugs increase the risk of infection due to their immunosuppressant effect, and patients should therefore receive annual influenza vaccination, and pneumococcal vaccination every 5–10 yrs. The drugs may also compromise immunosurveillance, increasing the risk of solid tumours and lymphomas. Further details of individual DMARDs are given in Box 15.9.

OTHER TREATMENTS

ANTICYTOKINES

The pro-inflammatory cytokine tumour necrosis factor alpha (TNF-α) plays an important role in the pathogenesis of RA and is therefore a prime therapeutic target. Infliximab is an anti-TNF-α monoclonal antibody which is administered by i.v. infusion. Etanercept is a synthetic anti-TNF biological agent. Although these drugs are more effective than standard DMARDs, they are costly. They also have potential side-effects including the risk of serious infection and of immunosuppression-related malignancy, particularly lymphoma. They are therefore recommended in the UK for active RA when treatment with at least two other DMARDs has failed. Rituximab may be used with methotrexate in patients who have not responded to anti-TNF therapy.

CORTICOSTEROIDS

Glucocorticoids have a rapid and dramatic anti-inflammatory action. However, prolonged use is accompanied by an unacceptable level of side-effects, including the risk of iatrogenic Cushing's syndrome, steroid-induced diabetes and osteoporosis. Their use in MSK disorders is therefore generally reserved for rapid and short-term control of severe synovitis or systemic inflammation. They are also useful for control of inflammatory disease during pregnancy (when DMARDs are contraindicated) and for the treatment of polymyalgia rheumatica. Prednisolone is the oral steroid of

15.9 EXAMPLES OF SLOW-ACTING ANTIRHEUMATIC DRUGS*

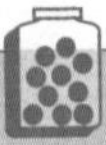

Drug	Disease indications	Side-effects	Monitoring requirement
Methotrexate	RA, seroneg, lupus, CTD, vasculitis, PMR	GI upset, mouth ulcers, alopecia, hepatotoxicity, hepatic fibrosis, acute pneumonitis	FBC, LFTs: monthly
Sulfasalazine	RA, seroneg	GI upset, hepatitis	FBC, LFTs: monthly for 3 mths, then 3-monthly
Hydroxychloroquine	RA, lupus	Diarrhoea, headache, corneal deposits, retinopathy	Visual acuity, fundoscopy: 6–12-monthly
Leflunomide	RA	GI upset, alopecia, hepatitis, hypertension	FBC, LFTs, BP: 2–4-weekly
Gold	RA	Mouth ulcers, alopecia, proteinuria	FBC, urine (protein): at each monthly injection
Penicillamine	RA	Mouth ulcers, metallic taste, proteinuria	FBC, urine (protein): initially 1–2-weekly, later 4–6-weekly
Azathioprine	RA, seroneg, lupus, CTD, vasculitis, PMR	GI upset, mouth ulcers, hepatitis	FBC, LFTs: initially weekly, then monthly
Cyclophosphamide	Vasculitis, lupus, myositis	GI upset, alopecia, cystitis, azoospermia, anovulation	FBC, urine (blood): each i.v. injection

*Most DMARDs can cause a rash, nausea and myelosuppression as well as the individual side-effects listed above.
DMARD = disease-modifying antirheumatic drug; RA = rheumatoid arthritis; PMR = polymyalgia rheumatica; seroneg = peripheral arthritis due to seronegative spondarthritis; CTD = connective tissue disease; FBC = full blood count; LFTs = liver function tests.

choice. The aim is to use the lowest effective dose for the shortest possible time to avoid unnecessary side-effects.

LOCAL INJECTIONS

Intra-articular injection of a long-acting corticosteroid (e.g. triamcinolone) can be a useful adjunctive therapy for controlling synovitis affecting one or a few joints. Symptom relief typically lasts for 2–8 wks. Iatrogenic infection is the most important adverse effect, which can be avoided by proper aseptic technique. Other side-effects include local skin atrophy and temporary symptom exacerbation. Periarticular steroid injections can be used to provide rapid, effective pain relief for conditions such as bursitis, tenosynovitis and lateral epicondylitis. The steroid is sometimes combined with local anaesthetic to provide more rapid analgesia.

SURGERY

A variety of surgical interventions may help relieve pain and improve function in patients with MSK disorders. Knee and hip replacement are commonly done and highly successful. Other examples include carpal tunnel release for median nerve compression, tendon repairs and synovectomy. In some cases, joint fusion (arthrodesis) may be appropriate. Each operation should be considered as part of an integrated programme of management, and this is often best achieved via a multidisciplinary team approach.

OSTEOARTHRITIS (OA)

OA is by far the most common form of arthritis. It is strongly associated with ageing, with 80% of people over the age of 65 showing radiographic evidence of OA, although only 25–30% are symptomatic. It is characterised by focal loss of articular cartilage with new bone proliferation and remodelling of the joint contour. Inflammation is not a prominent feature. OA preferentially targets certain small and large joints (Fig. 15.2); the knee and hip are the principal large joints involved.

Family history is a major risk factor for OA. The condition is more common in Caucasians, and women are more commonly symptomatic. Most cases of OA are 'primary', meaning the cause of joint damage remains unclear; 'secondary' OA affects joints which have been subject to trauma or adverse loading over prolonged periods (e.g. knee OA in miners and footballers).

The pathogenesis of OA involves enzymatic degradation of aggrecan and collagen within the articular cartilage, with fissuring and thinning of the cartilage surface (Fig. 15.3). Cysts develop within the subchondral bone, possibly due to osteonecrosis resulting from increased pressure on the bone as the cartilage fails. At the joint margins there is new fibrocartilage production which then ossifies, forming osteophytes. Bone remodelling and cartilage thinning gradually alter the shape of the OA joint. This is commonly accompanied by wasting of the muscles acting across the joint, synovial hyperplasia and thickening of the joint capsule.

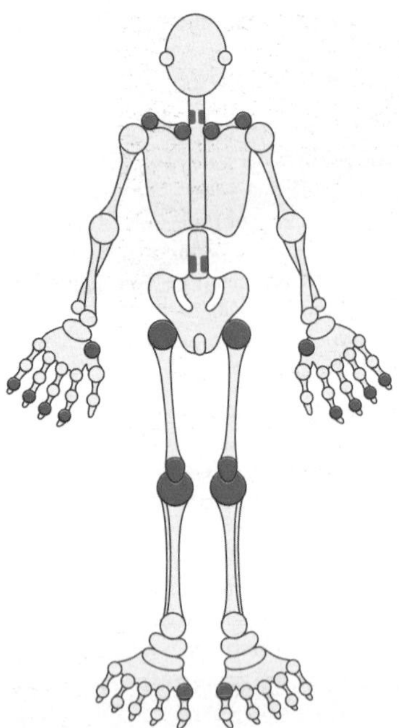

Fig. 15.2 The distribution of osteoarthritis. Although OA can affect any synovial joint, those shown in red are the most commonly targeted.

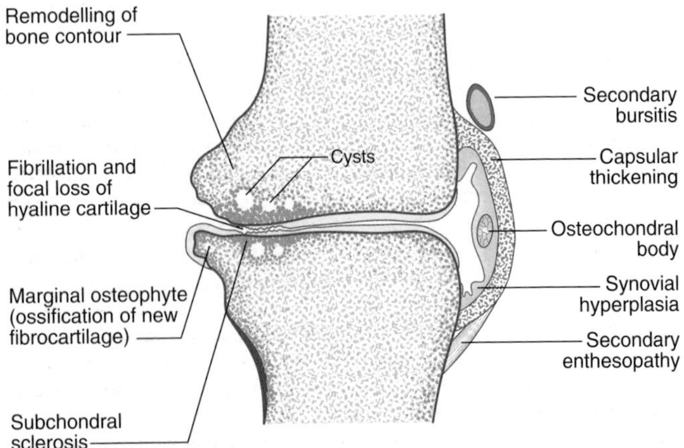

Fig. 15.3 Pathological changes in OA.

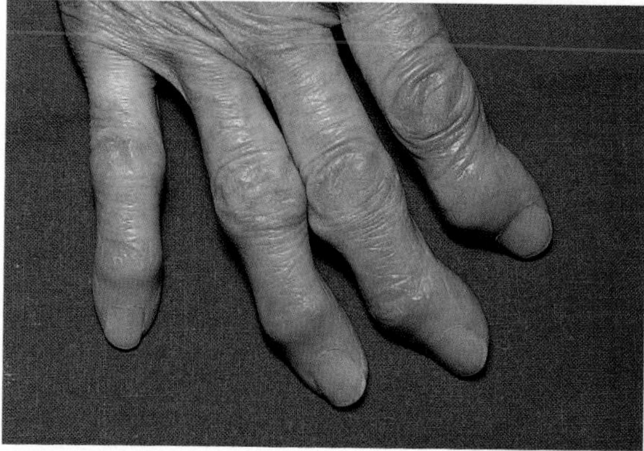

Fig. 15.4 Nodal osteoarthritis. Heberden's nodes and lateral deviation of distal interphalangeal joints, with mild Bouchard's nodes at the proximal interphalangeal joints.

Clinical features

• Main symptoms: pain and functional restriction. • Insidious onset of symptoms over months or years. • Pain worsened by movement and relieved by rest. • Only brief (<15 mins) morning stiffness and brief 'gelling' after rest (in contrast to inflammatory arthritis). • Usually only one or a few painful joints.

Physical examination reveals:

• Bony swelling and deformity around joint margins. • Joint-line or periarticular tenderness. • Restricted range of movement. • Palpable coarse crepitus. • Muscle-wasting. • No or only mild synovitis (effusion, increased warmth).

Nodal generalised OA: This common form of OA has a strong genetic predisposition and is more common in middle-aged women. Patients develop pain, stiffness and swelling affecting the finger interphalangeal joints (IPJs) (distal > proximal). Affected joints develop swellings which harden to become Heberden's (distal IPJ) and Bouchard's (proximal IPJ) nodes (Fig. 15.4). Involvement of the first carpometacarpal joint is also common. The condition is associated with a good functional prognosis. There is, however, an increased risk of OA at other sites ('generalised OA'), especially the knee.

Knee OA: May be primary or may be secondary to trauma; the latter is more common in men and is typically unilateral. Pain is usually localised to the anterior and medial aspects of the knee. Functional difficulties include prolonged walking, rising from a chair and bending to put on shoes. Examination findings may include:

• A jerky, asymmetric 'antalgic' gait (less time weightbearing on the painful side). • A varus (bow-legged) or less commonly valgus (knock-kneed) deformity. • A fixed flexion deformity. • Bony swelling around the joint line. • Wasting of the quadriceps muscle. • Joint line and/or periarticular tenderness. • Restricted range of movement. • Coarse crepitus.

Hip OA: Pain due to hip OA is usually maximal deep in the anterior groin, with variable radiation to the buttock, thigh or knee. Lateral hip pain, worse on lying on that side with tenderness over the greater trochanter, suggests secondary trochanteric bursitis. Functional difficulties are similar to those for knee OA. Examination may reveal:

• An antalgic gait. • Wasting of quadriceps and gluteal muscles. • Pain and restriction of internal rotation with the hip flexed (the earliest sign of hip OA); other movements may subsequently be affected. • Anterior groin tenderness. • Fixed flexion, external rotation deformity of the hip.

Investigations

• Plain X-rays may reveal joint space narrowing, subchondral sclerosis, osteophytes and bone cysts. However, the correlation between the presence of radiographic changes and the level of pain and disability is variable. • OA does not trigger an acute inflammatory response and therefore has no impact on the FBC, ESR or CRP.

Management

Treatment follows the principles set out on page 577 and includes:

• Full explanation of the nature of OA. • Local strengthening and aerobic exercises. • Reducing adverse mechanical factors (e.g. weight loss if obese, shock-absorbing footwear, walking aids). • Local physical therapies such as heat or cold. • Analgesia (initially paracetamol, then consider topical NSAID or capsaicin, then paracetamol plus oral NSAIDs, then opioid analgesics). • Intra-articular corticosteroid injection: may provide temporary relief of moderate to severe pain. • Surgery: should be considered for patients with uncontrolled pain and progressive functional impairment despite medical treatment; options include osteotomy and joint replacement.

INFLAMMATORY JOINT DISEASE

RHEUMATOID ARTHRITIS (RA)

RA is the most common form of inflammatory arthritis in women. The typical clinical phenotype of RA is a symmetrical, deforming, small and large joint polyarthritis, often associated with systemic disturbance and extra-articular disease. The clinical course is usually life-long, with intermittent exacerbations and remissions and highly variable severity. RA occurs throughout the world and in all ethnic groups. The prevalence is lowest in black Africans and Chinese; in Caucasians it is around 1.0–1.5% with a female : male ratio of 3 : 1. Prevalence increases with age, with 5% of women and 2% of men >55 yrs being affected. Concordance rates are higher in monozygotic twins (12–15%) than in dizygotic twins (3%). Up to 50% of the genetic contribution to susceptibility is due to genes in the HLA region, particularly HLA-DR4.

RA is an autoimmune condition characterised by chronic inflammation, granuloma formation and joint destruction. The earliest change is swelling and congestion of the synovial membrane and the underlying connective tissues, which become infiltrated with lymphocytes, plasma cells and macrophages. Effusion of synovial fluid into the joint space takes place during active phases of the disease. Hypertrophy of the synovial membrane occurs, and inflammatory granulation tissue (pannus) spreads over the articular cartilage, causing progressive cartilage destruction. Muscles adjacent to inflamed joints atrophy and there may be focal infiltration with lymphocytes. Subcutaneous rheumatoid nodules are granulomatous lesions consisting of a central area of fibrinoid material surrounded by proliferating mononuclear cells. Similar nodules may occur in the pleura, lung and pericardium.

Clinical features

The diagnosis of RA is made clinically, and is supported by a raised ESR or CRP and, in the majority, a positive rheumatoid factor. The clinical hallmark of inflammatory joint disease is persistent synovitis. Diagnostic criteria for RA are listed in Box 15.10.

• The most common presentation is with a gradual onset of symmetrical arthralgia and synovitis of small joints of the hands, feet and wrists. • Morning and inactivity stiffness is a characteristic feature. • Involvement of other synovial structures (tenosynovium, bursae) is also common.

Other patterns of presentation also exist:

• A dramatic acute onset of synovitis, sometimes over just a few days, with florid morning stiffness and polyarthritis, occurs more commonly in the elderly. • Some elderly patients present acutely with an initial polymyalgic illness with marked proximal muscle stiffness, the synovitis appearing only after several months as initial corticosteroid therapy is withdrawn. • Occasionally the onset is palindromic, with recurrent symmetrical acute episodes of joint pain and swelling which last for only a few hours or days before settling.

Specific joints: The hand is crucial to patient function and provides a good reflection of overall disease activity. The typical features are sym-

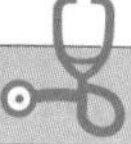

15.10 CRITERIA FOR DIAGNOSIS OF RHEUMATOID ARTHRITIS*

Diagnosis of RA is made with four or more of the following:

- Morning stiffness (>1 hr)
- Arthritis of three or more joint areas
- Arthritis of hand joints
- Symmetrical arthritis
- Rheumatoid nodules
- Rheumatoid factor
- Radiological changes
- Duration of 6 wks or more

*American Rheumatism Association 1988 revision.

A

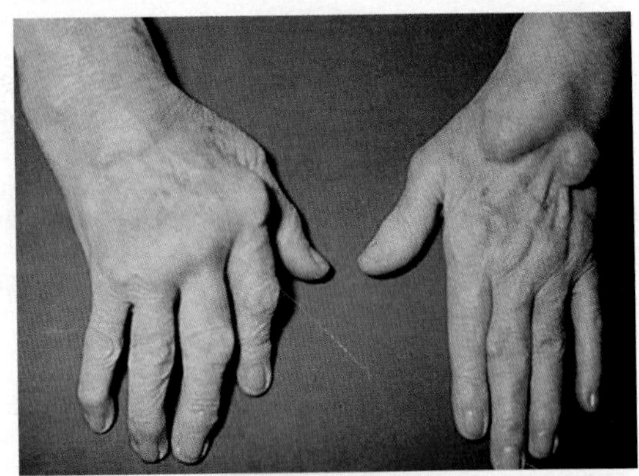

B

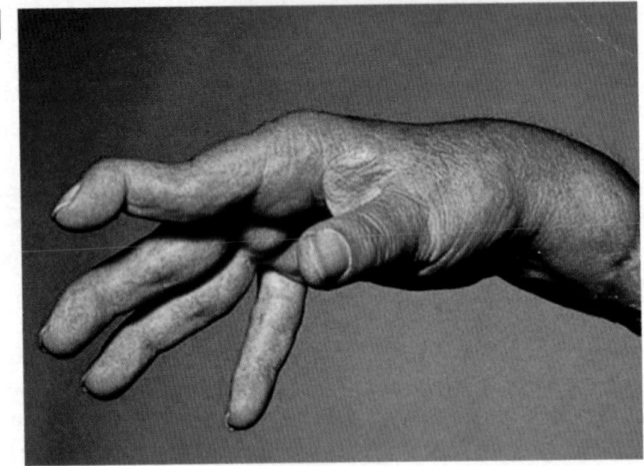

Fig. 15.5 The hand in rheumatoid arthritis. **A** Ulnar deviation of the fingers with wasting of the small muscles of the hands and synovial swelling at the wrists, the extensor tendon sheaths, the metacarpophalangeal and proximal interphalangeal joints. **B** 'Swan neck' deformity of the fingers.

metrical swelling of the metacarpophalangeal (MCP) and proximal interphalangeal (PIP) joints. Actively inflamed joints are tender on pressure and have stress pain on passive movement or non-bony swelling/effusion. Erythema is not a feature of RA and usually implies coexistent sepsis. Specific hand abnormalities, usually seen with long-standing active disease (Fig. 15.5), include:

• 'Swan neck' deformity. • Boutonnière deformity. • Z deformity of the thumb. • Dorsal subluxation of the ulnar styloid of the wrist, which may contribute to rupture of the fourth and fifth extensor tendons. • Triggering of fingers due to nodules in the flexor tendon sheath.

15.11 EXTRA-ARTICULAR MANIFESTATIONS OF RHEUMATOID DISEASE	
Systemic	Fever, fatigue, weight loss, susceptibility to infection
MSK	Muscle-wasting, tenosynovitis, bursitis, osteoporosis
Haematological	Microcytic anaemia (NSAID-induced GI blood loss), normocytic normochromic anaemia (chronic disease), thrombocytosis
Lymphatic	Splenomegaly, Felty's syndrome (RA, splenomegaly and neutropenia)
Nodules	Sinuses, fistulae
Ocular	Episcleritis, scleritis, scleromalacia, keratoconjunctivitis sicca (Sjögren's syndrome)
Vasculitis	Digital arteritis causing nailfold infarcts, skin ulcers, pyoderma gangrenosum, mononeuritis multiplex, visceral arteritis
Cardiac	Pericarditis, myocarditis
Pulmonary	Nodules, pleural effusions, pulmonary fibrosis, Caplan's syndrome (RA plus pneumoconiosis), bronchiolitis, bronchiectasis
Neurological	Cervical cord compression due to atlantoaxial subluxation, compression neuropathies (e.g. carpal tunnel syndrome), peripheral neuropathy, mononeuritis multiplex
Amyloidosis	

Popliteal ('Baker's') cysts usually occur in combination with knee synovitis. Cyst rupture, often induced by knee flexion in the presence of a large effusion, leads to calf pain and swelling. Deep venous thrombosis (DVT) is an important differential, and Doppler USS is required to establish the correct diagnosis.

Extra-articular features: RA is a systemic disease. Anorexia, weight loss and fatigue are common and may occur throughout the disease course. Extra-articular features (Box 15.11) are more common in patients with long-standing erosive disease and positive rheumatoid factor (RF), but may occasionally occur at presentation, especially in men.

Subcutaneous rheumatoid nodules occur almost exclusively in seropositive patients, usually at sites of pressure such as the extensor surfaces of the forearm, Achilles tendon and toes.

The most common ocular symptom is dry eyes (keratoconjunctivitis sicca) due to secondary Sjögren's syndrome. Painless episcleritis may cause intense redness but is not usually associated with visual disturbance. Scleritis is more serious and potentially sight-threatening; the eye is red and painful, and the pupil may appear irregular due to adhesions (synechiae). Scleromalacia is painless thinning of the sclera, with the affected area appearing blue or grey (the colour of the underlying choroid). No specific treatment is required.

Investigations

• Diagnosis should be confirmed according to clinical criteria. • CRP and ESR are usually elevated in patients with active disease. • Rheumatoid factor (an antibody directed against a specific region of human IgG) is positive in about 70% of patients, but has low diagnostic specificity and sensitivity; a high titre at presentation is, however, associated with a poorer prognosis. • Typical X-ray appearances of RA are periarticular osteopenia and marginal erosions. These changes may take several months to develop, so it is not appropriate to await radiographic changes before making the diagnosis. It is not always necessary to X-ray all symptomatic joints; erosions appear first in the wrists, hands and feet, even if they are asymptomatic.

Management

This follows the principles outlined on pages 577–581 and includes:

Non-pharmacological interventions: Physical rest, joint splinting, hydrotherapy, physiotherapy and patient education may all be beneficial.

Drug therapy: Oral analgesics and NSAIDs provide symptomatic relief. Intra-articular corticosteroids may be useful for acute RA. DMARDs are crucial in the modern management of RA. They do not have immediate anti-inflammatory effects but improve symptoms and the acute phase response, and reduce radiographic progression. They are most useful when started early in disease before irreversible damage has occurred. Methotrexate and sulfasalazine are currently first-choice DMARDs for RA. Anti-TNF therapy should be considered in disease resistant to DMARDs.

Surgery: Synovectomy of wrist or finger tendon sheaths may provide pain relief when medical interventions have failed. Osteotomy, arthrodesis or arthroplasties may be beneficial in later stages of disease.

Prognosis

Prognosis is variable; 40% of patients will be registered disabled within 3 yrs, and 80% will be moderately to severely disabled within 20 yrs. Factors at presentation associated with a poor prognosis include:

• A higher level of baseline disability. • Female gender. • Positive RF.

SERONEGATIVE SPONDARTHRITIS

This term is applied to a group of inflammatory joint diseases distinct from RA:

• Ankylosing spondylitis. • Reactive arthritis, including Reiter's syndrome. • Psoriatic arthropathy. • Arthritis associated with inflammatory bowel disease (Crohn's disease, ulcerative colitis).

They share a number of clinical features (Box 15.12). An association with HLA-B27 occurs in all seronegative spondarthritides but is particularly strong for ankylosing spondylitis (>95%) and Reiter's disease (90%). The suggested pathogenesis is an aberrant response to infection in genetically predisposed individuals. In some situations a triggering organism can

15.12 CLINICAL FEATURES COMMON TO SERONEGATIVE SPONDARTHRITIS

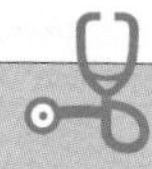

- Asymmetrical inflammatory oligoarthritis (lower > upper limb)
- Sacroiliitis and inflammatory spondylitis
- Inflammatory enthesitis (e.g. tendons, ligaments)
- Tendency for familial aggregation
- No association with seropositivity for RF
- Absence of nodules and other extra-articular features of RA
- Strong association with HLA-B27

be identified, as in Reiter's disease following bacterial dysentery or chlamydial urethritis, but in others the environmental trigger remains obscure.

ANKYLOSING SPONDYLITIS

Ankylosing spondylitis is a chronic inflammatory arthritis with a predilection for the sacroiliac joints and spine. The condition typically presents in the teens or twenties, with a male : female ratio of 3 : 1. It is characterised by progressive stiffening and fusion of the axial skeleton. Periarticular inflammation tends to resolve with extensive fibrosis which in turn calcifies and ossifies, ultimately leading to spinal fusion (ankylosis).

Clinical features

Spinal features are as follows:

• Insidious onset over months or years. • Recurrent episodes of low back pain and marked stiffness. • Symptoms worst in early morning and after inactivity, and relieved by movement. • Possible involvement of the entire spine as disease progresses. • Restriction of lumbar spinal movements: revealed by examination. • Progressive spinal fusion: results in loss of lumbar lordosis, marked thoracic kyphosis and reduced chest expansion. • Spinal rigidity and secondary osteoporosis: predispose to spinal fracture.

Extraspinal features are as follows:

• Plantar fasciitis and Achilles tendinitis: result from enthesitis (inflammation of the attachment of tendons or ligaments to bone). • Extraspinal joint involvement (up to 40% of patients): typically causes asymmetrical inflammatory arthritis affecting hips, knees, ankles or shoulders and can precede spinal involvement. • Anterior uveitis (25%). • Aortic incompetence. • Cardiac conduction defects. • Upper lobe pulmonary fibrosis.

Investigations

• ESR and CRP are usually raised. • Serum RF is negative or present in low titre. • X-ray changes may take years to develop. Erosions occur at the margins of the sacroiliac joints with subsequent sclerosis, joint space narrowing and fusion. Thoracolumbar spine X-rays may show 'squaring' of the vertebrae due to erosion and sclerosis of the corners. The formation of syndesmophytes (bony spurs bridging adjacent vertebral bodies), coupled with ossification of the spinal ligaments, gives rise to the typical 'bamboo' spine.

Management and prognosis

• Education in good posture and regular back exercises are essential to maintain mobility and avoid deformity. • NSAIDs are effective in relieving symptoms but do not alter the course of the disease. Long-acting NSAIDs at night are particularly helpful for morning stiffness. • Sulfasalazine, methotrexate or azathioprine may control peripheral arthritis but have little impact on axial disease. • Anti-TNF therapy is indicated in active disease resistant to standard therapy, and may improve symptoms including spinal mobility. • Local corticosteroid injections may help persistent plantar fasciitis and other forms of enthesitis. • Severe hip, knee, ankle or shoulder symptoms may require surgery. • ~75% of patients with ankylosing spondylitis are able to remain in employment and enjoy a good quality of life. Severe hip, knee or shoulder disease carries a worse prognosis.

REACTIVE ARTHRITIS

Reactive arthritis classically affects young men. It follows an episode of bacterial dysentery (due to *Salmonella, Shigella, Campylobacter* or *Yersinia*) or non-specific urethritis (due to *Chlamydia*). The classic triad of urethritis, conjunctivitis and reactive arthritis constitutes Reiter's disease.

Clinical features

Patients present with acute-onset, inflammatory oligoarthritis affecting the large and small joints of the lower limbs 1–3 wks following sexual exposure or an attack of dysentery. Symptoms of urethritis and conjunctivitis may be present. Less classical attacks are common, with insidious onset of single joint involvement, minimal features of urethritis and conjunctivitis, and no clear history of 'trigger' illness. Achilles tendinitis or plantar fasciitis may occur.

Extra-articular features are as follows:

• Circinate balanitis: causes vesicles (often painless) on the prepuce and glans. • Buccal erosions on the tongue, palate and buccal mucosa. • Keratoderma blennorrhagica: waxy yellow-brown skin lesions, particularly affecting the palms and soles. • Nail dystrophy with subungual hyperkeratosis, identical to psoriatic nail dystrophy.

The first attack of reactive arthritis is usually self-limiting, with spontaneous remission within 2–4 mths. Recurrent arthritis develops in >60% of patients. Uveitis is rare with the first attack but occurs in 30% of patients with recurring arthritis.

Investigations

• Raised ESR and CRP. • Aspirated synovial fluid: inflammatory and often contains macrophages. • High vaginal swab culture in female patients: may reveal *Chlamydia*. • Stool cultures: usually negative by the time the arthritis presents. • Serum RF and antinuclear antibody (ANA): negative. • X-ray changes: usually absent during the acute attack, other than soft tissue swelling. Joint space narrowing and marginal erosions may develop with recurrent disease.

Management

• NSAIDs provide symptomatic relief during the acute phase. • Joint aspiration and intra-articular corticosteroid injections may be helpful. • Systemic steroids are rarely required. • DMARDs (azathioprine, methotrexate) are occasionally used for severe progressive arthritis and keratoderma blennorrhagica. • Non-specific chlamydial urethritis is treated with a short course of tetracycline. • Anterior uveitis is a medical emergency requiring topical or systemic corticosteroids.

PSORIATIC ARTHROPATHY

Psoriatic arthritis affects 7% of patients with psoriasis. It typically presents between the ages of 25 and 40 yrs. The seronegative arthritis usually occurs in individuals with pre-existing skin disease but can predate the onset of psoriasis.

Clinical features

Five major presentations of joint disease are recognised:

Asymmetrical inflammatory oligoarthritis (40%): May affect lower and upper limb joints. Involvement of a finger or toe by synovitis, together with enthesitis and inflammation of intervening tissue, can give rise to a 'sausage digit' or dactylitis. Usually only one or two large joints are involved, mainly knees.

Symmetrical polyarthritis (25%): May strongly resemble RA, with symmetrical involvement of small and large joints in both upper and lower limbs. However, nodules and other extra-articular features of RA are absent.

Predominant distal interphalangeal joint (DIPJ) arthritis (15%): Predominantly affects men, almost invariably with accompanying nail dystrophy.

Psoriatic spondylitis (15%): Presents a similar clinical picture to ankylosing spondylitis but tends to be less severe.

Arthritis mutilans (5%): This deforming erosive arthritis targets fingers and toes. Marked cartilage and bone attrition results in loss of the joint and instability.

The general pattern of psoriatic arthritis is one of intermittent exacerbation followed by periods of remission. Residual damage and disability are relatively mild, except in arthritis mutilans.

Extra-articular features include:

• Skin lesions. • Nail changes: pitting, onycholysis (separation of the nail from the nail bed) and subungual hyperkeratosis. • Uveitis.

Investigations

• ESR and CRP: may be raised but are often normal. • Serum RF and ANA: negative. • X-rays: may be normal or show erosive change with joint space narrowing.

Management and prognosis

• Regular exercise is important in maintaining mobility. • Simple analgesics and NSAIDs provide symptomatic relief. • Intra-articular corticosteroids may help control florid synovitis. • Sulfasalazine, methotrexate or azathioprine may be required for peripheral arthritis, but have little effect on axial disease. Methotrexate is the treatment of choice as it may also help severe skin psoriasis. • The retinoid acitretin is effective in treating both the arthritis and the skin lesions but is teratogenic. • Excepting arthritis mutilans, the prognosis is better than for RA.

ARTHRITIS ASSOCIATED WITH INFLAMMATORY BOWEL DISEASE

Two patterns of inflammatory arthritis are associated with ulcerative colitis and Crohn's disease:

• Enteropathic arthritis is an acute oligoarthritis with a predilection for large lower limb joints. The arthritis coincides with exacerbations of the underlying bowel disease. • Sacroiliitis and ankylosing spondylitis: not correlated with the activity of the bowel disease. Such axial disease is indistinguishable from classic ankylosing spondylitis.

CRYSTAL-ASSOCIATED DISEASE

Crystal deposition in and around joints can result in acute and chronic inflammatory arthritis.

GOUT

Gout is caused by the deposition of monosodium urate monohydrate (MSUM) crystals in and around synovial joints. It has a prevalence of ~1%, and is more common in men, in certain ethnic groups and with increasing age. Uric acid is derived from the metabolism of purines, which are largely synthesised in the body but are also to a lesser extent obtained from food. Prolonged hyperuricaemia is necessary, but not sufficient, for the development of gout. Causes of hyperuricaemia are shown in Box 15.13.

Clinical features

Acute gout: First attacks usually affect a single distal joint, commonly the first metatarsophalangeal joint—'podagra' (Fig. 15.6A). Other common sites include the ankle, midfoot, knee, hand, wrist and elbow. Patients present with rapid onset of severe pain. Examination reveals marked synovitis with swelling, red shiny skin and extreme tenderness. Periarticular swelling and fever may also be present. Symptoms are usually self-limiting

15.13 FACTORS PREDISPOSING TO CHRONIC HYPERURICAEMIA AND GOUT
Diminished renal excretion (>90% of cases)
• Inherited isolated renal tubular defect ('under-excretors') • Renal failure • Chronic drug therapy (e.g. thiazide and loop diuretics, low-dose aspirin, ciclosporin) • Lead toxicity (e.g. in 'moonshine' drinkers) • Lactic acidosis (alcohol)
Increased production of uric acid (uncommon)
• Increased purine turnover: chronic myeloproliferative or lymphoproliferative disorders, chemotherapy for leukaemias • Increased de novo synthesis ('over-producers'): cause unknown in most, rarely specific enzyme defects, e.g. glucose-6-phosphatase deficiency

over 5–14 days. The differential diagnosis includes septic arthritis, cellulitis and other crystal diseases.

Recurrent and chronic gout: Following an acute attack, most patients go on to experience a second attack within a year. The frequency of attacks increases with time. Involvement of several joints with continued MSUM deposition eventually leads to joint damage and chronic pain.

Chronic tophaceous gout: MSUM crystal deposits produce irregular firm nodules ('tophi') around extensor surfaces of fingers, forearms, elbows, Achilles tendons and ears (Fig. 15.6B). Tophi are usually a late feature of gout.

Renal and urinary tract manifestations: Uric acid stones form within the urinary tract and cause renal colic in ~10% of gout patients. The deposition of MSUM crystals within the renal medulla in untreated chronic tophaceous gout can lead to chronic inflammation and progressive renal impairment.

Investigations

• Joint fluid aspiration reveals long, needle-shaped MSUM crystals which are negatively birefringent under polarised light. Synovial fluid in acute gout shows increased turbidity due to the greatly elevated cell count (>90% neutrophils). • Serum uric acid is usually elevated, but hyperuricaemia itself does not confirm gout. Equally, acute inflammation reduces levels, so a normal uric acid level does not exclude gout. • Serum creatinine should be checked to screen for renal impairment. • FBC, CRP and ESR: neutrophilia with a raised CRP occurs in acute gout; FBC and ESR may detect myeloproliferative disorders during remission of the acute episode. • Joint X-rays are usually normal in early gout. Changes of secondary OA and gouty erosions may develop with chronic disease.

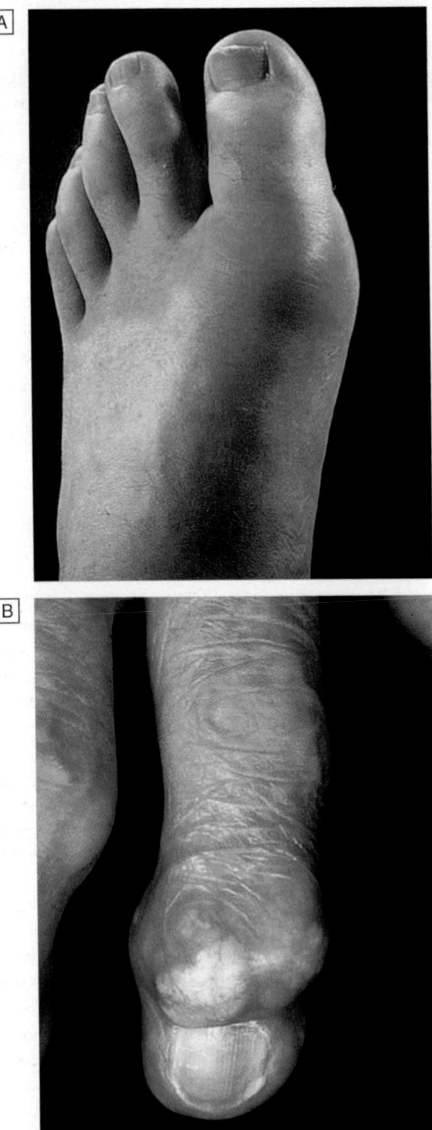

Fig. 15.6 Gout. A Acute gout causing inflammation of the first metatarsophalangeal joint (podagra). B Tophus.

Management

For the acute attack:

• Oral NSAIDs (e.g. naproxen) provide effective pain relief. • Oral colchicine (an inhibitor of neutrophil microtubular assembly) is an alternative when NSAIDs are contraindicated. Vomiting and diarrhoea are common side-effects. • Joint aspiration and intra-articular corticosteroid injection are effective in more severe cases.

As regards long-term management:

• Predisposing factors should be addressed. • Weight loss is advised in obese patients. • Excess beer consumption should be reduced. • Stop diuretics if possible. • Avoid a very high purine diet (seafood, red meat and offal).

Allopurinol inhibits xanthine oxidase and reduces the conversion of hypoxanthine and xanthine to uric acid, thereby lowering serum uric acid levels. It is indicated in patients with recurrent attacks of acute gout, tophi, joint damage or renal impairment. Allopurinol initiation can trigger an acute attack; it should therefore be initiated after the acute attack has settled, following which it should be co-prescribed with an NSAID or colchicine for the first few weeks.

CALCIUM PYROPHOSPHATE DIHYDRATE (CPPD) CRYSTAL DEPOSITION

CPPD crystal deposition within articular cartilage causes chondrocalcinosis. The condition is usually sporadic and occurs in the elderly. In rare cases it is associated with metabolic disease (e.g. haemochromatosis, hyperparathyroidism, hypomagnesaemia and Wilson's disease). It is often clinically silent, but can cause episodes of acute synovitis ('pseudogout') or occur as a chronic arthritis which is associated with OA.

Clinical features

Acute synovitis ('pseudogout'): The most common cause of acute monoarthritis in the elderly. The knee is by far the most common site, followed by the wrist, shoulder and ankle. The typical attack resembles acute gout with rapid onset of pain, stiffness and swelling. Examination reveals erythema, marked joint tenderness and signs of synovitis (large effusion, warmth and restricted movement). Fever may be present. Septic arthritis and gout are the main differential diagnoses.

Chronic ('pyrophosphate') arthritis: Chronic symptoms usually occur in elderly women. The distribution is similar to that of pseudogout. Symptoms are chronic pain with variable early morning stiffness. Affected joints show features of OA (bony swelling, crepitus, restriction) with varying degrees of synovitis.

Investigations

• Joint fluid aspiration in acute pseudogout reveals small, rhomboid-shaped CPPD crystals which are positively birefringent under polarised light. Gram stain and culture of the fluid will exclude sepsis. • X-rays may show chondrocalcinosis within the articular cartilage. • Blood tests should be performed to exclude metabolic causes of CPPD crystal deposition in younger patients and in individuals with recurrent attacks.

Management

• Oral NSAIDs and colchicine are effective for acute pseudogout. • Joint aspiration with intra-articular corticosteroid injection provides rapid pain relief.

BONE AND JOINT INFECTION

SEPTIC ARTHRITIS

Septic arthritis is a medical emergency. It usually arises from haematogenous spread of bacterial infection from another site, commonly the skin or upper respiratory tract. Infection from direct puncture wounds or secondary to joint aspiration is uncommon. Risk factors for septic arthritis include increasing age, pre-existing joint disease, diabetes mellitus and immunosuppression. Lyme disease (p. 85) may present with monoarthritis.

Clinical features

• The usual presentation is with acute or subacute monoarthritis. The joint is usually swollen, hot and red, with rest pain and stress pain on movement. The knee and hip are the most common sites. • The usual culprit organism is *Staphylococcus aureus*. Disseminated gonococcal infection is another cause in young, sexually active adults. This presents with migratory arthralgia and low-grade fever followed by the development of oligo- or monoarthritis. Painful pustular skin lesions may also be present.

Investigations

• Joint fluid aspiration for Gram stain and culture is essential, under image guidance if deep; aspirated fluid often looks turbid or blood-stained. • Blood cultures may be positive due to bacteraemia. • Blood tests may reveal leucocytosis with raised ESR, although these may be absent in elderly or immunocompromised patients. • Concurrent cultures from the genital tract are indicated if gonococcal infection is likely.

Management

• Pain relief. • I.V. antibiotics: the recommended first-line agent is i.v. flucloxacillin, until identification of the organism and its sensitivities is possible. I.V. treatment is usually continued for 2–3 wks, followed by oral treatment for a total duration of 6 wks. • Daily joint aspiration: should be performed in the initial stages to minimise the effusion. If this is unsuccessful, surgical drainage may be required. • Early mobilisation: should be encouraged.

VIRAL ARTHRITIS

Erythrovirus is the most common cause of viral arthritis; other causes include hepatitis B and C, rubella and HIV. The usual presentation is with acute polyarthritis, fever and rash. Symptoms are usually self-limiting. Diagnosis is confirmed by viral serology.

OSTEOMYELITIS

Infection of the bone usually arises from haematogenous spread, although directly introduced infection may complicate a compound fracture, penetrating injury or orthopaedic surgery. Organisms most frequently implicated are staphylococci, *Pseudomonas* and *Mycobacterium tuberculosis*. Risk factors include young age, diabetes, immunodeficiency and sickle-cell disease. Infection often results in a florid inflammatory response and localised areas of osteonecrosis.

Clinical features and investigations

• Presentation is with localised bone pain and tenderness, fever and night sweats. • X-rays may be normal for the first few weeks, but bone technetium scans, labelled white cell scans and MRI are much more sensitive. • Confirmation of the diagnosis may be obtained by blood culture and/or culture of a bone aspirate or biopsy.

Management

• Pain relief. • I.V. followed by oral antibiotics. • Surgical decompression and removal of any dead bone. • Rehabilitation.

TUBERCULOSIS OF BONE AND JOINTS

This is usually secondary to an established focus in the lung or kidney. The hip, knee and vertebrae are key target sites. Patients develop chronic pain, swelling and eventual deformity. Definitive diagnosis requires synovial or bone biopsy for PCR and culture. Management is with antituberculous combination chemotherapy, as for pulmonary TB (see p. 300). Surgical débridement may be required for extensive disease.

FIBROMYALGIA

This is a common cause of multiple regional MSK pain. It has a prevalence of 2–3% and increases in frequency with age. There is a strong female predominance of around 10 : 1. The condition is associated with stressful life events including divorce, marital disharmony, low income and childhood abuse. The condition is poorly understood and is associated with other medically unexplained symptoms. No structural, inflammatory or metabolic abnormality has been identified, although abnormalities of non-REM sleep and of central pain processing have been postulated as potential aetiological factors.

Clinical features and investigations

• The main presenting feature is multiple regional pain. At various times this affects the neck, back, both arms and both legs. The pain is characteristically unresponsive to analgesics and NSAIDs. • Patients commonly report fatigability, particularly in the morning, and reported disability is often marked. Although people can usually dress and groom themselves, they may struggle with daily tasks such as shopping and housework, and may have given up work because of pain and fatigue. • Additional non-locomotor features include tension headache, irritable bowel syndrome and irritable bladder.

Examination usually reveals hyperalgesia at multiple specific tender sites. Moderate pressure at each site may be uncomfortable in a normal subject but in fibromyalgia it produces a wince/withdrawal response. Although there are no abnormal investigations associated with fibromyalgia, it is important to screen for alternative MSK conditions.

Management

• Patient education about the nature of the condition is crucial. • NSAID therapy is ineffective. • Low-dose amitriptyline with or without fluoxetine may be useful. • Graded exercise may improve well-being. • Relaxation techniques and coping strategies employing a cognitive behavioural approach should be encouraged. • Patient organisations can provide valuable support.

DISEASES OF BONE

OSTEOPOROSIS

Osteoporosis is by far the most common bone disease. It is characterised by reduced bone mineral density (BMD) with an increased risk of fracture, and increases markedly with age. The condition affects up to 30% of women and 12% of men at some time during their life.

In normal individuals, bone mass increases to reach a peak between the ages of 20 and 40 yrs but falls thereafter. Bone turnover throughout life depends on the balance between bone formation by osteoblasts and bone resorption by osteoclasts. There is an accelerated phase of bone loss in women after the menopause as a result of oestrogen deficiency which alters this balance in favour of increased bone resorption. This leads to an increased risk of osteoporosis and fractures, particularly in women who have attained a low peak bone mass or who have other risk factors (Box 15.14).

Corticosteroid therapy is an important cause of osteoporosis, the risk of which is directly related to the dose and duration of therapy. Steroids result in reduced intestinal calcium absorption, increased renal calcium excretion, secondary hyperparathyroidism and direct inhibition of osteoblast activity. The risk is minimised by prescribing systemic steroids at the lowest effective dose for the shortest possible duration. Osteoporosis may also occur in patients taking inhaled glucocorticoids, especially with high doses.

Clinical features

Osteoporosis is asymptomatic unless it causes fragility fractures. The most common sites are the forearm (Colles fracture), spine (vertebral fractures

15.14 RISK FACTORS FOR OSTEOPOROSIS	
Early menopause	
Endocrine disease	e.g. Hypogonadism, hyperthyroidism, hyperparathyroidism, Cushing's syndrome
Inflammatory disease	e.g. Inflammatory bowel disease
Drugs	e.g. Corticosteroids, anticonvulsants, heparin, alcohol excess
GI disease	e.g. Malabsorption, chronic liver disease
Miscellaneous	e.g. Myeloma, anorexia nervosa, lack of exercise, immobilisation, poor diet/low body weight, smoking

causing back pain, height loss and kyphosis), and femur (hip fracture).

Investigations

BMD is measured using dual energy X-ray absorptiometry (DEXA), usually of the lumbar spine and hip. Bone densitometry should be performed in patients sustaining low trauma fractures, those with clinical features of osteoporosis, and individuals with significant osteoporotic risk factors. In addition to providing absolute BMD values, DEXA machines give results as 'T-scores' and 'Z-scores'.

The T-score measures by how many standard deviations the patient's BMD value differs from that of a young healthy control. The Z-score measures by how many standard deviations the BMD deviates from that of an age-matched control. Osteoporosis is diagnosed when the T-score value falls to –2.5 or below, whereas T-score values between –1.0 and –2.5 indicate osteopenia. BMD values above –1.0 are regarded as normal.

If the diagnosis of osteoporosis is confirmed by bone densitometry, any predisposing factors should be identified. Relevant blood tests include:

• Serum calcium and phosphate. • TFTs. • Immunoglobulins (for myeloma). • ESR. • Anti-TTG (for coeliac disease).

In some cases it may be appropriate to check serum vitamin D, parathyroid hormone (PTH), sex hormone and gonadotrophin levels.

Management

Patients with osteopenia should be given lifestyle advice such as:

• Stopping smoking. • Limiting alcohol intake. • Maintaining an adequate dietary calcium intake (1500 mg daily). • Taking regular exercise.

Osteopenic patients should be offered a repeat BMD measurement in 2–3 yrs. Pharmacological treatment should be reserved for those patients with BMD values in the osteoporotic range.

Bisphosphonates: Bisphosphonates are first-line drugs in the treatment of osteoporosis (see p. 778).

Calcium and vitamin D supplements: Calcium (500–1000 mg daily) and vitamin D supplements (400–800 U daily) are generally used as an adjunct to other treatments. They do not reduce the risk of fractures in patients with osteoporosis when given as monotherapy.

Raloxifene: Raloxifene is a selective oestrogen receptor modulator, which useful in post-menopausal patients with vertebral osteoporosis who are intolerant of bisphosphonates.

Strontium ranelate: Strontium ranelate inhibits bone resorption and increases BMD. It is effective in secondary prevention of vertebral and non-vertebral fractures in post-menopausal women but can cause GI upset and thrombosis.

Hormone replacement therapy (HRT): HRT with oestrogen and progestogens prevents post-menopausal bone loss and reduces the risk of vertebral and non-vertebral osteoporotic fractures. However, the use of HRT as a treatment for osteoporosis has diminished following publication of data showing that long-term HRT increases the risk of breast cancer, thromboembolic disease, stroke and cardiovascular disease. HRT is therefore regarded as second-line treatment for post-menopausal osteoporosis.

OSTEOMALACIA AND RICKETS

Defective bone mineralisation leads to rickets in children, and to osteomalacia following epiphyseal fusion in adults. Osteomalacia is characterised by bone pain, increased bone fragility and fractures; patients with rickets also develop bone deformity. Full-blown osteomalacia is now rare in developed countries, but subclinical disease remains quite common in people with a poor diet or limited sunlight exposure such as elderly housebound individuals and Muslim women living in northern latitudes. Causes of osteomalacia and rickets include:

• Deficiency of vitamin D or defects in vitamin D metabolism. • Hypophosphataemia. • Drug-induced inhibition of bone mineralisation.

The role of vitamin D in calcium metabolism is described on p. 357. Vitamin D occurs in only small quantities in most foods, so dietary intake is generally insufficient to meet requirements. Maintenance of normal vitamin D levels depends on ultraviolet sunlight exposure which permits formation of cholecalciferol (D) in the skin from 7-dehydrocholesterol. Lack of cholecalciferol due to inadequate sunlight exposure, dietary deficiency or malabsorption is accompanied by a reduction in 25(OH)D3 synthesis in the liver. This causes reduced production of the active metabolite 1,25$(OH)_2$D3 in the kidneys, reduced intestinal calcium absorption and low serum calcium. The low serum calcium level stimulates PTH secretion, resulting in secondary hyperparathyroidism and subsequent increased osteoclastic bone resorption, reduced renal calcium excretion and increased renal phosphate excretion. This sequence represents an attempt by the parathyroid glands to restore serum calcium levels to normal; however, this cannot be achieved with continuing vitamin D deficiency so there is progressive loss of both calcium and phosphate from bone and defective mineralisation.

Osteomalacia also occurs in association with defects of vitamin D metabolism and function. Patients with chronic renal failure cannot synthesise the active metabolite of vitamin D (1,25$(OH)_2$D3) due to renal damage.

• Vitamin D-resistant rickets (VDRR) type I is caused by inactivating mutations in the renal α-hydroxylase enzyme, rendering it unable to convert 25(OH)D3 to 1,25$(OH)_2$D3. • In VDRR type II, mutations occur in the vitamin D receptor, rendering it resistant to activation by 1,25$(OH)_2$D3.

Clinical features

• Manifestations of rickets in children include enlargement of epiphyses at the lower end of the radius and swelling of the costochondral junctions ('rickety rosary'). • Osteomalacia in adults presents more insidiously and may be asymptomatic. Further progression leads to bone pain and pathological fractures. Proximal muscle weakness is prominent and may result in a waddling gait and difficulty climbing stairs or rising from a chair.

Investigations

• Renal function, serum calcium, phosphate, albumin, alkaline phosphatase, serum 25(OH)D3 and PTH levels should be measured. Vitamin D-deficient osteomalacia is suggested by low or low–normal calcium and phosphate, raised alkaline phosphatase, low 25(OH)D3 and raised PTH. • X-rays are of limited value in diagnosis, but may show focal radiolucent areas (Looser's zones) in advanced cases. Osteopenia is a common finding. • Bone biopsy can be used to confirm the diagnosis.

Management

• Rickets and osteomalacia caused by vitamin D deficiency respond rapidly to treatment with oral vitamin D and calcium supplementation. Higher doses may be required in patients with malabsorption. • Osteomalacia due to renal failure and VDRR type I requires treatment with active vitamin D metabolites (1-α-(OH)D3 or 1,25$(OH)_2$D3) since these bypass the metabolic defect in 1-α-hydroxylation of 25(OH)D3. Serum calcium and alkaline phosphatase should be monitored to assess response to treatment.

PAGET'S DISEASE

Paget's disease of bone (PDB) is a common condition characterised by focal areas of increased and disorganised bone remodelling. The condition increases in frequency with age, affecting 10% of the UK population by the age of 85. Genetic factors are implicated in the aetiology of PDB; 15–40% have a positive family history. The presence of inclusion bodies within osteoclasts has led to speculation that a slow virus infection may also play a role. The primary abnormality in PDB is increased osteoclastic bone resorption accompanied by increased osteoblast activity. The resultant bone is architecturally abnormal and has reduced mechanical strength. Other features of PDB are marrow fibrosis and increased bone vascularity.

Clinical features

PDB most commonly affects the pelvis, femur, tibia, lumbar spine and skull. Patients classically present with bone pain, deformity and pathological fractures, although many cases are asymptomatic. Clinical signs include bone deformity and expansion with increased warmth over affected bones. Bone deformity is most evident in the femur, tibia and skull. Neurological complications include deafness and spinal cord compression. The deafness is often conductive in nature due to osteosclerosis of the temporal bone. Other rare complications include high-output cardiac failure (due to increased bone vascularity) and osteosarcoma.

Investigations

• Serum biochemistry shows an isolated elevation in alkaline phosphatase with normal calcium and phosphate levels. • X-rays show areas of osteosclerosis alternating with areas of osteolysis, together with bone expansion and deformity. • Radionuclide bone scanning is useful in confirming PDB and documenting its extent. • Bone biopsy is not usually required to make the diagnosis, but can be helpful in differentiating PDB from sclerotic bony metastases.

Management

Treatment of PDB is primarily indicated for control of bone pain.

• If paracetamol and NSAIDs are ineffective then bisphosphonates (e.g. oral risedronate, i.v. pamidronate, i.v. zoledronic acid) are helpful in suppressing bone turnover, reducing serum alkaline phosphatase and controlling pain. • Subcutaneous calcitonin can be used as an alternative to bisphosphonates, but is less convenient to administer and significantly more expensive. • The long-term effects of therapy with bisphosphonates and calcitonin on complications such as deafness, bone deformity and fracture are unknown. • Currently, there is no evidence to show that prophylactic therapy with bisphosphonates in asymptomatic patients is effective in preventing complications.

PRIMARY BONE TUMOURS

Primary bone tumours are less common than secondary bone metastases. They have a peak incidence in childhood and adolescence, although osteosarcoma secondary to PDB develops in later adulthood.

• Primary bone tumours present with local pain and swelling. • Plain X-rays show expansion of the bone and diagnosis is confirmed by biopsy. • Treatment usually involves surgical removal followed by chemotherapy and radiotherapy. • The prognosis is generally good in cases presenting in childhood and adolescence, but poor in elderly patients with osteosarcomas related to PDB.

OSTEOGENESIS IMPERFECTA (OI)

OI is a rare disease characterised by bone fragility presenting with multiple fractures in infancy and childhood. The condition is caused by reduced or abnormal collagen production. Other common features include blue sclerae and abnormal dentition. Treatment is multidisciplinary in nature, involving orthopaedic surgery for the management of fractures and limb deformities, physiotherapy and occupational therapy.

SYSTEMIC CONNECTIVE TISSUE DISEASE

The connective tissue diseases are a group of chronic inflammatory disorders that involve multiple body systems and therefore exhibit a wide spectrum of clinical manifestations. Their aetiology is multifactorial and involves genetic, immunological (especially autoantibody production) and environmental factors.

SYSTEMIC LUPUS ERYTHEMATOSUS (SLE)

SLE is the most common multisystem connective tissue disease. It predominantly affects women, has a peak onset in the second and third decades, and is more common in individuals of Afro-Caribbean origin.

Several autoantibodies are associated with SLE. Many of the target autoantigens are intracellular and intranuclear components. It is likely that the wide spectrum of autoantibody production results from polyclonal B- and T-cell activation. Although the triggers that lead to autoantibody production in SLE are unknown, one mechanism may be exposure of intracellular antigens on the cell surface during apoptosis.

Clinical features

Raynaud's phenomenon: Arthralgia or arthritis in combination with Raynaud's phenomenon is the most common presentation of SLE. Raynaud's phenomenon in a teenage girl with no other associated symptoms is likely to be idiopathic 'primary' Raynaud's. By contrast, onset in a male, or in a woman over the age of 30 yrs, suggests underlying connective tissue disease.

MSK features: A variety of joint problems may occur, including migratory arthralgia with mild morning stiffness, and small-joint synovitis that may mimic RA. In contrast to RA, joint deformities are rare.

Mucocutaneous features: Painful oral ulcers are common. Certain types of rash are characteristic of SLE:

• The classic butterfly (malar) facial rash is raised and painful or pruritic and occurs in a photosensitive distribution (Fig. 15.7). • Discoid lupus lesions are characterised by hyperkeratosis and follicular plugging, and may cause scarring alopecia if present on the scalp.

Other skin manifestations include diffuse non-scarring alopecia, vasculitis and livedo reticularis, the latter also being a common feature of the antiphospholipid syndrome.

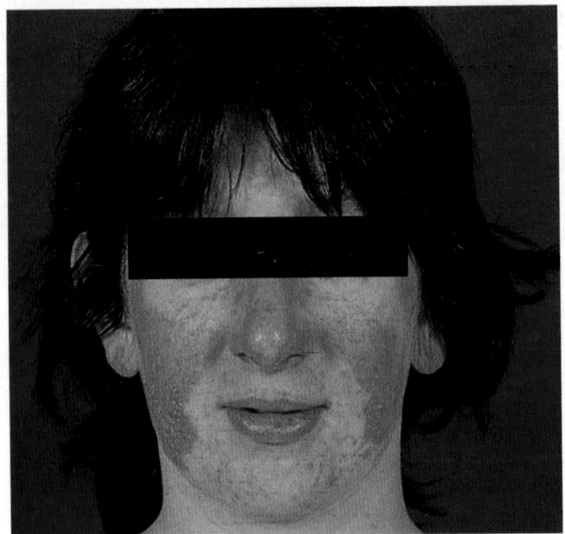

Fig. 15.7 Butterfly (malar) rash of systemic lupus erythematosus.

Renal features: The typical renal lesion is a proliferative glomerulonephritis, characterised by haematuria, proteinuria and casts on urine microscopy.

Cardiopulmonary features: Pleurisy can cause pleuritic chest pain, a rub or a pleural effusion. Alveolitis, lung fibrosis and diaphragmatic paralysis can also occur. Cardiac involvement can lead to pericarditis, myocarditis and Libman–Sacks endocarditis (due to non-infectious vegetations). The antiphospholipid syndrome (APS) is characterised by recurrent arterial and venous thromboses, recurrent fetal losses and thrombocytopenia. It is associated with antiphospholipid antibodies and may occur in lupus (secondary APS) or in isolation (primary APS; see p. 564).

CNS features: Features of cerebral lupus include visual hallucinations, chorea, organic psychosis, seizures, lymphocytic meningitis, hemiparesis and transverse myelitis.

Other manifestations: Non-specific features of SLE include fever, weight loss, mild lymphadenopathy and fatigue.

Investigations

FBC: Antibody-mediated destruction of peripheral blood cells may cause neutropenia, lymphopenia, thrombocytopenia or haemolytic anaemia. The degree of lymphopenia is often a good guide to disease activity.

ESR and CRP: ESR is usually elevated in active disease; CRP is often normal unless serositis or infection is present.

U&Es, urine dip test, urine microscopy: To assess renal function and to detect haematuria, proteinuria and casts suggestive of glomerulonephritis.

Autoantibodies: ANA are autoantibodies directed against components of the nucleus. There are many causes of a positive ANA. For SLE, ANA has high sensitivity (negative ANA virtually excludes SLE) but low specificity (a positive result does not make the diagnosis). Anti-double-stranded DNA antibodies (anti-dsDNA) are specific for SLE but are only present in 30–50% of patients. Anti-extractable nuclear antigen antibodies (anti-ENA) associated with SLE include anti-Smith (anti-Sm) and anti-Ro. The presence of antiphospholipid antibodies directed against components of the coagulation cascade is associated with the antiphospholipid syndrome.

Management and prognosis

• Patients should avoid sun exposure and should apply high-factor sun blocks. • Mild disease may require only intermittent analgesics or NSAIDs. • Hydroxychloroquine is used for more troublesome skin and joint symptoms. • Short courses of oral corticosteroids may be required for mild to moderate disease (e.g. rashes, synovitis, pleuro-pericarditis). • Acute or life-threatening disease (e.g. renal, cerebral) requires high-dose corticosteroids (oral prednisolone 40–60 mg daily or i.v. methylprednisolone) in combination with pulse i.v. cyclophosphamide. • Other immunosuppressive drugs (e.g. azathioprine, ciclosporin) may also be useful for severe disease. • Lupus patients with the antiphospholipid syndrome who have had previous thrombosis require life-long warfarin. • Overall 5-yr survival is >90%. Organ failure is associated with early mortality, and renal involvement is a major adverse prognostic factor.

SYSTEMIC SCLEROSIS

Systemic sclerosis (scleroderma) is a generalised multisystem connective tissue disorder. The peak age of onset is in the fourth and fifth decades, and it has a 4 : 1 female : male ratio. It is subdivided into diffuse cutaneous systemic sclerosis (DCSS) and limited cutaneous systemic sclerosis (LCSS). Many patients with LCSS have features which are grouped into the 'CREST' syndrome (**c**alcinosis, **R**aynaud's, o**e**sophageal involvement, **s**clerodactyly, **t**elangiectasia).

The aetiology of systemic sclerosis is unknown. Early in the disease there is skin infiltration by T lymphocytes and abnormal fibroblast activation leading to increased production of collagen in the dermis. This results in symmetrical thickening, tightening and induration of the skin, leading to sclerodactyly in the fingers. In addition to skin changes there is arterial and arteriolar narrowing due to intimal proliferation and vessel wall inflammation. Endothelial injury causes release of vasoconstrictors and platelet activation, resulting in further ischaemia.

Clinical features

Cutaneous changes: Raynaud's phenomenon occurs early in the disease. The skin of the fingers becomes tight, shiny and thickened (sclerodactyly) (Fig. 15.8). Subcutaneous deposition of calcium can lead to nodules on the fingers (calcinosis). Involvement of the face causes thinning and radial

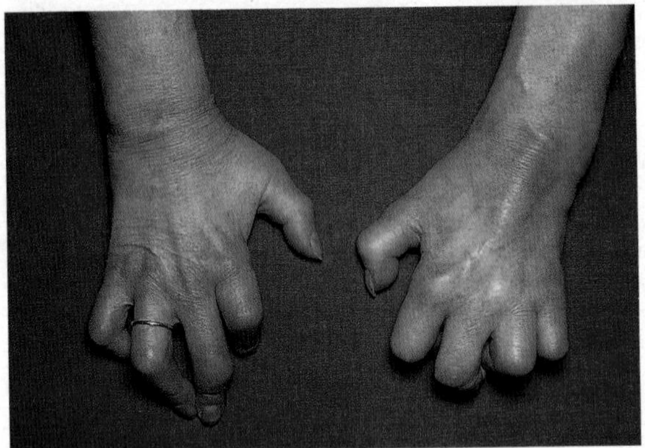

Fig. 15.8 Systemic sclerosis. Hands showing tight shiny skin, sclerodactyly and flexion contractures of the fingers.

furrowing of the lips. Telangiectasia may be present. Skin involvement restricted to sites distal to the elbow or knee (apart from the face) is classified as LCSS or CREST syndrome. Involvement proximal to the knee and elbow and on the trunk is classified as DCSS. In the distal extremities, the combination of intimal fibrosis and vessel wall inflammation may cause tissue ischaemia, leading to skin ulceration and localised areas of infarction.

MSK features: Arthralgia, morning stiffness and flexor tenosynovitis are common. Restricted hand function is usually due to skin rather than joint disease.

GI features: Smooth muscle atrophy and fibrosis in the lower oesophagus lead to acid reflux with erosive oesophagitis; this may in turn progress to further fibrosis. Dysphagia may also occur. Involvement of the stomach causes early satiety and occasionally outlet obstruction. Small intestine involvement may lead to malabsorption due to bacterial overgrowth and intermittent bloating or pain. Dilatation of the large or small bowel due to autonomic neuropathy may cause pseudo-obstruction.

Cardiorespiratory features: Pulmonary involvement is a major cause of morbidity and mortality. Pulmonary fibrosis mainly affects patients with diffuse disease. Pulmonary hypertension is a complication of long-standing limited disease, characterised by rapidly progressive dyspnoea and right heart failure.

Renal features: One of the main causes of death is hypertensive renal crisis characterised by rapidly developing malignant hypertension and renal failure. It is much more likely to occur in patients with diffuse disease.

Investigations

ANA is usually positive. Anti-topoisomerase I (anti-Scl-70) antibodies are specific for diffuse systemic sclerosis, and anti-centromere antibodies are relatively specific for limited systemic sclerosis. However, autoantibodies are not present in all patients, and the diagnosis is predominantly a clinical one.

Management and prognosis

• Patients should avoid peripheral cold exposure; conventional or heated gloves can be effective. • Prompt treatment with antibiotics is required for infected skin ulcers. • Vasodilators such as calcium antagonists (e.g. nifedipine, amlodipine) and angiotensin II receptor antagonists (e.g. valsartan) may be effective for Raynaud's symptoms. • Intermittent infusions of epoprostenol may be helpful for severe digital ischaemia. • PPIs are used to treat reflux oesophagitis. • Corticosteroids are indicated for alveolitis. • Treatment strategies for pulmonary hypertension include vasodilators, continuous infusions of epoprostenol, the oral endothelin 1 antagonist bosentan and heart-lung transplantation. • Hypertensive renal crises are treated with ACE inhibitors. • 5-yr survival is ~70%. Diffuse skin disease, pulmonary hypertension and renal involvement are associated with a poor prognosis.

POLYMYOSITIS AND DERMATOMYOSITIS

These are rare connective tissue disorders characterised by muscle weakness and inflammation. The onset is usually between 40 and 60 yrs of age. There is an increased risk of malignancy in patients with dermatomyositis (about a threefold increase) and polymyositis (an increase of ~30%).

Clinical features

Polymyositis: Presents with symmetrical proximal muscle weakness, usually affecting the lower extremities first. Patients report difficulty rising from a chair, climbing stairs and lifting, sometimes in combination with muscle pain. The onset is typically gradual, over a few weeks. Systemic features of fever, weight loss and fatigue are common. Respiratory or pharyngeal muscle involvement leading to ventilatory failure/aspiration is ominous and requires urgent treatment.

Dermatomyositis: Has identical muscle manifestations to polymyositis but these occur in combination with characteristic cutaneous manifestations. Gottron's papules are scaly erythematous/violaceous plaques or papules occurring over the extensor surfaces of the fingers (Fig 17.4, p. 712). The heliotrope rash is a violaceous discoloration of the eyelid associated with periorbital oedema.

Investigations

• CK is usually raised and tracks disease activity. • ANA and anti-Jo1 antibodies may be positive. • EMG may confirm the presence of myopathy and exclude neuropathy. • Muscle biopsy shows typical features of fibre necrosis and inflammatory cell infiltration. • MRI can help identify areas of abnormal muscle.

Management

• Oral corticosteroids (e.g. prednisolone) are the mainstay of initial treatment. • Patients with severe weakness or respiratory or pharyngeal involvement may require i.v. methylprednisolone. • Additional immunosuppressive therapy with azathioprine or methotrexate is often required.

MIXED CONNECTIVE TISSUE DISEASE

This is an overlap connective tissue disease with features of SLE, systemic sclerosis and polymyositis. Most patients have anti-ribonucleoprotein (anti-RNP) antibodies, although these can also occur in SLE without overlap features.

SJÖGREN'S SYNDROME

This is an idiopathic autoimmune disorder characterised by lymphocytic infiltration of salivary and lachrymal glands, leading to glandular fibrosis and exocrine failure. It predominantly affects women and has a peak onset between the ages of 40 and 60 yrs. There is an association with HLA-B8 and DR3. The disease may be primary or secondary in association with other autoimmune diseases such as RA, SLE or primary biliary cirrhosis.

Clinical features

• Dry eyes (keratoconjunctivitis sicca) due to a lack of tears. • Dry mouth (xerostomia). • Vaginal dryness. • Other features: fatigue, non-erosive arthritis and Raynaud's phenomenon. • The condition is associated with a 40-fold lifetime increased risk of lymphoma.

Investigations

• ESR is usually elevated. • Autoantibodies frequently detected include RF, ANA, anti-Ro (SS-A) and anti-La (SS-B). • Sicca can be established by the Schirmer test, which measures the flow of tears using an absorbent paper strip placed in the lower eyelid; a normal result is >6 mm of wetting over 5 mins. • In cases of diagnostic doubt, lip biopsy can be performed to identify lymphocytic infiltration of the minor salivary glands.

Management

Treatment is largely symptomatic:

• Artificial tears and lubricants for dry eyes. • Artificial saliva for xerostomia. • Lubricants such as K-Y jelly for vaginal dryness.

INHERITED DISEASES OF CONNECTIVE TISSUE

Marfan's syndrome: Characterised by skeletal disproportion (arm span greater than height), arachnodactyly (long, thin, 'spider' fingers), hypermobility of joints, lens dislocation and a high arched palate. It results from mutations of the fibrillin gene, a component of the extracellular matrix. The most serious complications are mitral valve prolapse, aortic incompetence and aortic dissection.

Ehlers–Danlos syndrome: Characterised by generalised hypermobility, skin laxity and easy bruising. It may result from mutations in several genes including elastin.

SYSTEMIC VASCULITIS

The primary systemic vasculitides are a heterogeneous group of diseases characterised by inflammation and necrosis of blood vessel walls (Box 15.15). Vasculitis may also occur in many types of inflammatory or infectious diseases, such as SLE, RA and endocarditis. Clinical features are due to a combination of local tissue ischaemia and systemic effects of widespread inflammation. Multisystem involvement is a typical feature.

Antineutrophil cytoplasmic antibodies (ANCA) are directed against enzymes present in neutrophil granules. Two main patterns of immunofluorescence are distinguished: cytoplasmic (c-ANCA) and perinuclear (p-ANCA).

• c-ANCA are directed against proteinase 3 and are particularly associated with Wegener's granulomatosis and Churg–Strauss syndrome. • p-ANCA are directed against myeloperoxidase and are associated with microscopic polyangiitis.

POLYMYALGIA RHEUMATICA (PMR)

PMR is not a true vasculitis but is closely associated with giant cell arteritis. The mean age of onset is 70 and the condition is more common in women.

Clinical features

• The cardinal features are muscle stiffness and pain, symmetrically affecting the proximal muscles of the neck, upper arms and, less commonly, buttocks and thighs. There is marked early morning stiffness. • Constitutional features including weight loss and fatigue also occur. • Examination may reveal stiffness and painful restriction of active shoulder movement. Muscles may be tender to palpation but wasting is not a feature.

15.15 SIZE OF VESSEL INVOLVEMENT IN VASCULITIS

Large vessel	Giant cell arteritis, Takayasu's arteritis
Medium vessel	Classical polyarteritis nodosa, Kawasaki disease (in childhood)
Small vessel	ANCA-positive: microscopic polyangiitis, Wegener's granulomatosis, Churg–Strauss syndrome ANCA-negative: Henoch–Schönlein purpura, mixed essential cryoglobulinaemia

Investigations

• ESR is usually elevated >40 mm/hr. • A normochromic, normocytic anaemia may be present.

Management

• Treatment is with oral corticosteroids (prednisolone 15 mg daily). The dose is gradually reduced after 1 mth. • Most patients require steroids for an average of 12–18 mths, and osteoporosis prophylaxis with bisphosphonates should be considered. • Between 15 and 20% of patients develop symptoms of giant cell arteritis at some point.

GIANT CELL ARTERITIS (GCA)

GCA is a large-vessel vasculitis affecting branches of the temporal and ophthalmic arteries. The mean age of onset is 70, with a 4 : 1 female : male ratio.

Clinical features

The onset of symptoms may be insidious or abrupt. Features include:

Headache: Usually the first symptom and often localised to the temporal or occipital region, with scalp tenderness.

Jaw pain: Brought on by chewing or talking and due to ischaemia of the masseters.

Visual disturbance: The optic nerve head is supplied by the posterior ciliary artery, vasculitis of which leads to occlusion and acute anterior ischaemic optic neuropathy. Sudden visual symptoms in one eye, leading rapidly to blindness, constitute the most common pattern.

Constitutional symptoms: Anorexia, fatigue, weight loss and fever may occur.

Investigations

• ESR and CRP are elevated. • A temporal artery biopsy should be obtained, but corticosteroid treatment should not be delayed whilst this is organised. 'Skip' lesions (i.e. sections of unaffected vessel) are common and a negative biopsy does not exclude the diagnosis.

Management

If GCA is suspected, systemic corticosteroid therapy (prednisolone 60 mg daily) should be started immediately to prevent visual loss. Steroid reduction should be guided by symptoms and ESR. Maintenance therapy is required for at least 1 yr but relapse occurs in 30%.

TAKAYASU'S ARTERITIS

This is a granulomatous large-vessel vasculitis affecting the aorta and the carotid, brachial, radial and axillary arteries.

• The usual presentation is with claudication and systemic symptoms of fever and weight loss. • Diagnosis is based on angiographic findings of coarctation, vessel occlusion and aneurysmal dilatation. • Treatment is with oral prednisolone combined with methotrexate or cyclophosphamide.

CLASSICAL POLYARTERITIS NODOSA (PAN)

PAN is a rare necrotising vasculitis affecting medium-sized and small arteries which predominantly affects middle-aged men. Hepatitis B is a risk factor for PAN.

• Clinical presentation is with myalgia, arthralgia, fever and weight loss together with manifestations of multisystem disease. • Skin involvement can cause a palpable purpuric rash, ulceration, infarction and livedo reticularis. • Arteritis of the vasa nervorum leads to a symmetrical sensory and motor neuropathy. • Severe hypertension and renal impairment may occur due to multiple renal infarctions. • Diagnosis is confirmed by finding multiple aneurysms and narrowing of the mesenteric, hepatic or renal vessels on angiography. • Tissue biopsy may be definitive. • Treatment is with corticosteroids and cyclophosphamide.

ANCA-ASSOCIATED VASCULITIS

Microscopic polyangiitis, Wegener's granulomatosis and Churg–Strauss syndrome are rare conditions which can be grouped together as 'ANCA-associated vasculitis'.

Microscopic polyangiitis (MPA)

This classically presents with rapidly progressive glomerulonephritis, often associated with pulmonary alveolar haemorrhage. Cutaneous involvement similar to PAN is common. Patients are usually p-ANCA-positive.

Wegener's granulomatosis (WG)

Airway involvement may lead to epistaxis, nasal crusting, sinusitis, mucosal ulceration and subglottic airway stenosis. Lung involvement results in haemoptysis with migratory pulmonary infiltrates and cavitating nodules. Glomerulonephritis may also occur. Patients are usually c-ANCA-positive.

Churg–Strauss syndrome (CSS)

CSS classically presents as a triad comprising skin lesions (purpura or nodules), mononeuritis multiplex and eosinophilia on a background of resistant asthma. Pulmonary infiltrates may be present. Mesenteric vasculitis can cause abdominal symptoms. Either c-ANCA or p-ANCA is present in ~40% of cases.

Investigation and management of MPA, WG and CSS

• The diagnosis should ideally be confirmed by tissue biopsy (e.g. skin, nasal septal tissue). • Urine dip testing for protein and blood should be performed. • Renal biopsy must be considered in patients with abnormal renal function. • Treatment of ANCA-associated vasculitis should be instituted as early as possible to prevent irreversible organ damage. • Remission can be induced with oral or i.v. corticosteroids together with cyclophosphamide. The cyclophosphamide is usually replaced with azathioprine once remission has occurred.

OTHER FORMS OF VASCULITIS

Henoch–Schönlein purpura

This small-vessel vasculitis usually occurs in children and young adults, and has a good prognosis. Typical presentation is with purpura over the buttocks and lower legs, abdominal symptoms (pain and bleeding) and arthritis (knee or ankle) following an upper respiratory tract infection. Nephritis may occur and can result in renal impairment. The diagnosis is confirmed by demonstrating IgA deposition within blood vessel walls. Treatment is with corticosteroids; additional immunosuppressive drugs are required in patients with nephritis.

Behçet's syndrome

This is a rare vasculitis which characteristically targets venules. The diagnosis is clinical, and is based on the presence of recurrent oral ulceration together with two of the following:

• Recurrent oral and genital ulceration. • Eye lesions: anterior or posterior uveitis, retinal vasculitis. • Skin lesions: erythema nodosum, papulopustular lesions, acneiform nodules. • Positive pathergy test: skin pricking with a needle results in pustule development within 48 hrs.

Other features include meningitis, encephalitis and recurrent thromboses.

• Treatment of oral ulceration is with topical corticosteroids. • Thalidomide is effective for resistant oral and genital ulceration but is teratogenic. • Systemic disease requires oral corticosteroids in combination with other immunosuppressive drugs.

16

Neurological disease

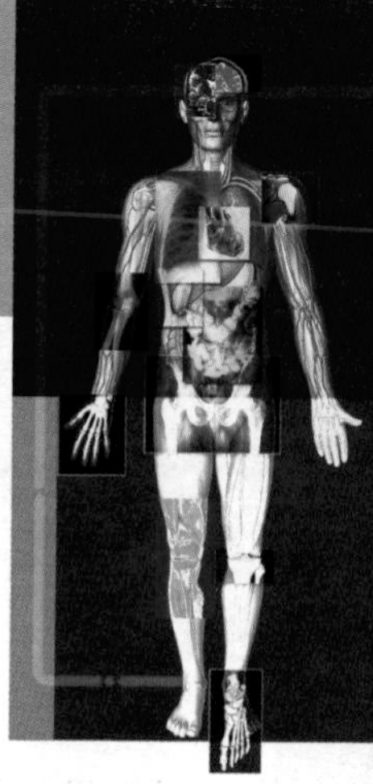

The brain, spinal cord and peripheral nerves constitute an organ responsible for perception of the environment, a person's behaviour within it, and the maintenance of the body's internal milieu in readiness for this behaviour. In the UK some 10% of the population consult their GP each year with a neurological symptom, and neurological disorders account for about one-fifth of acute medical admissions and a large proportion of chronic physical disability.

PRESENTING PROBLEMS

HEADACHE

Headache is a frequently encountered neurological symptom but is seldom associated with significant neurological disease unless accompanied by other symptoms or neurological signs.

ACUTE HEADACHE

Serious acute neurological disease should always be considered in patients with headaches of very sudden onset. Subarachnoid haemorrhage causes a very sudden headache, followed by vomiting and neck stiffness which may take hours to develop. The main differential diagnosis is between subarachnoid haemorrhage and a migraine variant.

SUBACUTE HEADACHE

Headache coming on over the course of hours is likely to be migraine, unless accompanied by other symptoms or signs. Migraine headaches may be accompanied or preceded by vomiting and focal neurological symptoms.

CLINICAL EXAMINATION OF THE NERVOUS SYSTEM

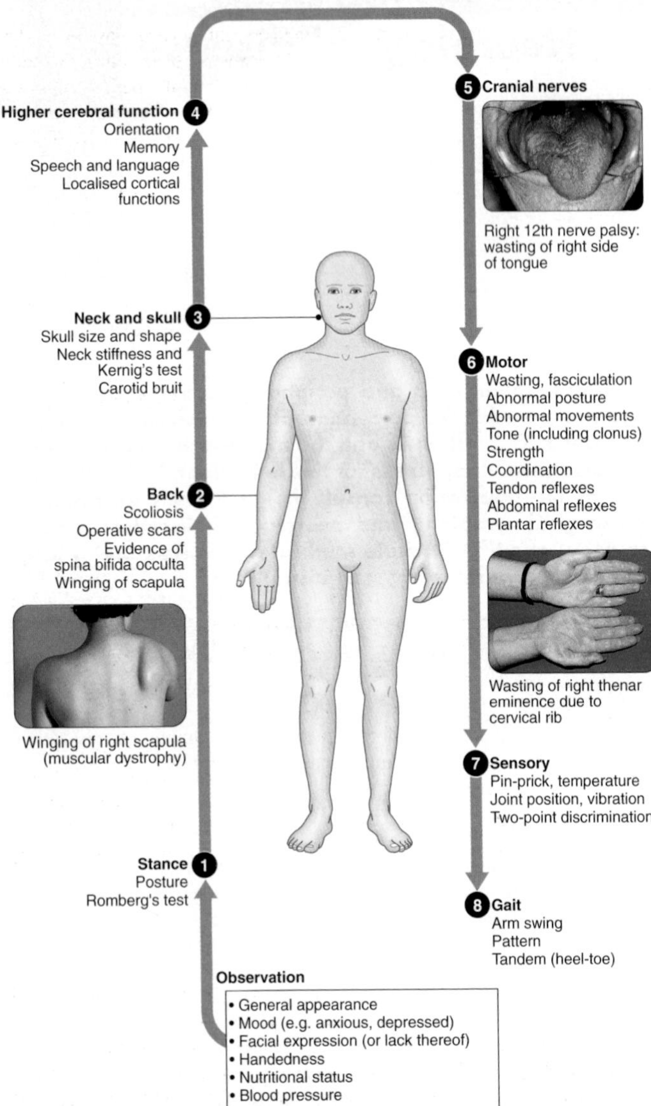

Patients with bacterial meningitis are usually pyrexial and exhibit meningism (p. 664). Patients with viral meningitis may present with a pyrexia and quite sudden and severe headache, but may not have meningism.

INTERMITTENT HEADACHE

When headaches are intermittent rather than continuous over days or weeks, they are most likely to be migrainous. The headache of raised intracranial pressure is present on waking and often improves as the patient becomes upright or takes simple analgesia. It is unusual for a patient with an intracranial mass to present with such a headache alone since it is usually not sufficiently severe to cause alarm; seizure or other focal signs are more common presenting features. The exceptions to this are patients with acute hydrocephalus who present with a more severe headache.

CHRONIC HEADACHE

Headaches that persist for weeks, are present all day and are poorly responsive to simple analgesia are very likely to be tension-type headaches. Headaches so well localised by the patient that a finger is used to locate the exact spot on the skull are never associated with significant disease. In a patient >60 yrs with head pain localised to one or both temples, giant cell arteritis should be considered.

TENSION-TYPE HEADACHE

Clinical assessment

This is the most common type of headache.

• The pain is constant and generalised but often radiates forward from the occipital region. • It is described as 'dull', 'tight' or like a 'pressure'. • The pain may continue for weeks without interruption, although the severity may vary. • There is no vomiting or photophobia. • The pain is characteristically more troublesome as the day goes on.

Management

• Discussion of likely precipitants and explanation that the symptoms are not due to sinister pathology are more likely to help than analgesics. • Excessive use of analgesics, particularly codeine, may worsen the headache (analgesic headache). • Physiotherapy (with muscle relaxation and stress management). • Low-dose amitriptyline (10 mg at night increased gradually to 30–50 mg) may be necessary.

MIGRAINE

Clinical assessment

Migraine is a triad of paroxysmal headache, nausea and/or vomiting, and an 'aura' of focal neurological events. Patients with all three features have migraine with aura ('classical' migraine). Migraine without aura, with or without vomiting, is called 'common' migraine. A classical migraine attack starts with a prodrome of malaise and irritability followed by the 'aura' of a focal neurological event, and then a severe, throbbing, hemicranial headache with photophobia and vomiting. The headache may persist for several days.

The 'aura' typically lasts 20–30 mins, and usually takes the form of 'fortification spectra': shimmering zigzag lines which march across the visual fields. Some patients experience a sensory aura: tingling then numbness moving from one part of the body to another. Patients may also experience transient aphasia. True weakness is distinctly unusual, so 'hemiplegic migraine' should be diagnosed with caution.

The aetiology of migraine is largely unknown.

• The headache may be caused by vasodilatation of extracranial vessels. • There is often a family history, suggesting a genetic predisposition. • The female preponderance hints at hormonal influences. The contraceptive pill appears to exacerbate migraine in many patients. • In some patients there are identifiable dietary precipitants such as cheese, chocolate or red wine. • When psychological stress is involved, the migraine attack often occurs after the period of stress.

Management

Acute attack: Simple analgesia with aspirin or paracetamol, often with an antiemetic. Severe attacks can be treated with one of the 'triptans' (e.g. sumatriptan), 5-HT agonists that are potent vasoconstrictors of the extracranial arteries.

Prevention: Identification and avoidance of precipitants or exacerbating factors. If frequent, try propranolol (80–160 mg daily, sustained-release), amitriptyline (10–50 mg at night), sodium valproate (300–600 mg/day) or pizotifen (1.5–3.0 mg daily). Women should be warned that the small risk of ischaemic stroke attributable to taking oral contraception is increased if they have migraine, especially if they also smoke.

CLUSTER HEADACHE (MIGRAINOUS NEURALGIA)

Clinical assessment

This is much less common than migraine. There is a predominance of males and onset is usually in the third decade. The syndrome comprises periodic, severe, unilateral periorbital pain accompanied by unilateral lacrimation, nasal congestion and conjunctival injection. The pain is characteristically brief (30–90 mins). The syndrome may occur repeatedly for a number of weeks, followed by months of respite before another cluster occurs.

Management

• Acute attacks are usually halted by subcutaneous injections of sumatriptan or by inhalation of 100% oxygen. • Attacks can be prevented by verapamil (80–120 mg 8-hourly), methysergide (4–10 mg daily, for a maximum of 3 mths only) or short courses of corticosteroids. • Severe and debilitating clusters can be helped with lithium therapy.

FACIAL PAIN

Pain in and around the eye not caused by ocular disease should be considered as a headache. Most patients with persisting pain in the face have trigeminal neuralgia (see below), atypical facial pain or post-herpetic neuralgia. Atypical facial pain is continuous and unremitting, and is centred over the maxilla, usually on the left side. Post-herpetic neuralgia is a continuous burning pain throughout the affected territory, often very sensitive to light touch. The cause is usually obvious from a history of 'shingles' in the ophthalmic division of the trigeminal nerve.

TRIGEMINAL NEURALGIA

Clinical assessment

• Trigeminal neuralgia causes lancinating pains ('like lightning') in the second and third divisions of the trigeminal nerve territory. The pain is severe and very brief but repetitive, causing the patient to flinch as if with a motor tic. • It may be precipitated by touching trigger zones within the trigeminal territory or by eating. • There is a tendency for the condition to remit and relapse over years.

Management

The pain usually responds to carbamazepine (up to 1200 mg daily). If patients cannot tolerate carbamazepine, gabapentin or phenytoin may help.

Various surgical treatments are available:

• Alcohol or phenol injection into a peripheral branch of nerve. • Percutaneous placing of a radiofrequency lesion in the nerve. • Posterior craniotomy to relieve vascular compression of nerve. This latter approach is favoured in younger patients in whom injection treatments may have to be repeated and become less effective.

DIZZINESS, BLACKOUTS AND 'FUNNY TURNS'

Episodes of lost or altered consciousness are frequent. After a careful history from the patient, supplemented by a witness account, it should be clear whether the patient is describing loss of consciousness, altered consciousness, vertigo, transient amnesia or something else. The diagnostic approach is shown in Figure 16.1.

VERTIGO

Abnormal perception of movement of the environment occurs as a result of a mismatch between the information about a person's position reaching the brain from the eyes, limb proprioception and the vestibular system. Vertigo arising from inappropriate input from the labyrinthine apparatus is usually short-lived, though it may recur, whilst vertigo arising from central (brain-stem) disorders is often persistent and accompanied by other signs of brain-stem dysfunction.

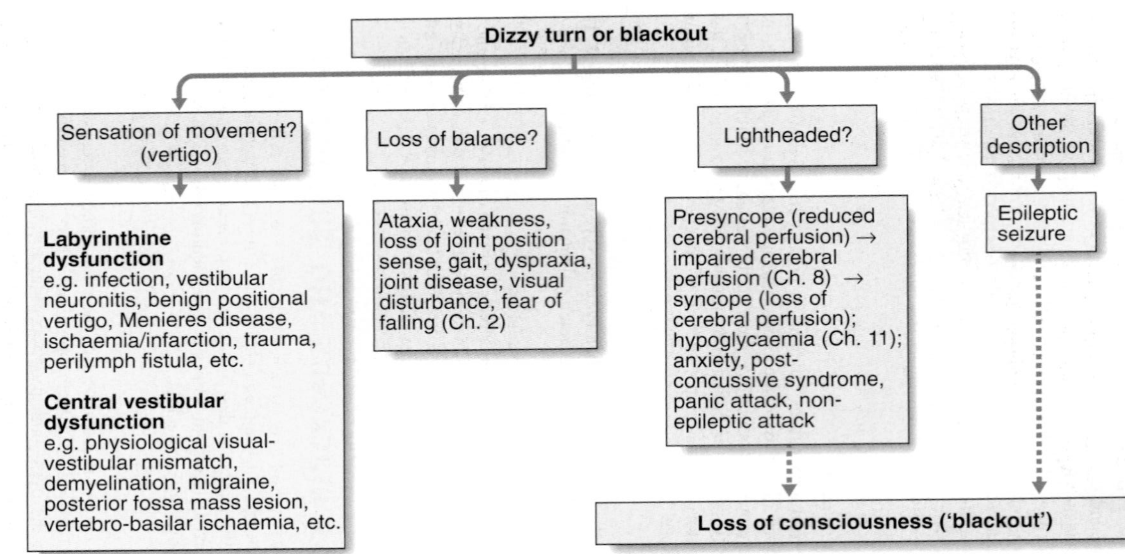

Fig. 16.1 A diagnostic approach to the patient with dizziness, funny turns or blackouts.

VERTIGO CAUSED BY LABYRINTHINE DISTURBANCES

Labyrinthitis ('vestibular neuronitis'): Usually presents in the 3rd or 4th decade as severe vertigo, with vomiting and ataxia but no tinnitus or deafness. The vertigo is most severe at onset and settles down over the next few days. Nystagmus is present during the attack but does not persist for long.

Benign paroxysmal positional vertigo: Paroxysms of vertigo occurring with certain head movements may be due to degenerative material affecting endolymph flow in the labyrinth. Each attack lasts seconds but patients may become reluctant to move their head, producing a muscle tension-type headache. The diagnosis can be confirmed by using the 'Hallpike manoeuvre' in which the head is swung briskly back to demonstrate positional nystagmus. The vertigo fatigues with repetitive positioning of the head and can be treated with vestibular exercises.

Ménière's disease: Patients usually present with tinnitus and distorted hearing, and then develop paroxysmal vertigo preceded by a sense of fullness in the ear. Examination shows sensorineural hearing loss on the affected side.

Drug treatment of labyrinthine vertigo: Symptomatic relief can be achieved with 'vestibular sedatives' (e.g. cinnarizine, prochlorperazine, betahistine). Patients with intractable symptoms should be referred to an ENT specialist for assessment.

CENTRAL CAUSES OF VERTIGO

Any disease that affects the vestibular nucleus in the brain stem or its connections can cause vertigo. Positionally induced central vertigo persists for as long as the position is maintained, unlike peripheral positional vertigo that fatigues if the inducing position is maintained. Causes such as brainstem ischaemia may be associated with dysarthria or diplopia. If deafness is present, consider compression of the 8th cranial nerve.

EPISODIC LOSS OF CONSCIOUSNESS

Transient loss of consciousness occurs because of a recoverable loss of adequate blood supply to the brain (syncope), or from sudden electrical dysfunction of the brain during a seizure (epileptic fit). Many patients have psychogenic blackouts or non-epileptic seizures which may confuse this distinction. No amount of investigation can replace a clear history in these circumstances. Features in the history useful in distinguishing a seizure from a faint are shown in Box 16.1.

SYNCOPE

A brief feeling of 'lightheadedness' often precedes a faint; vision then darkens and there may be a ringing in the ears. Vasovagal syncope (p. 211) may be provoked by some emotionally charged event (e.g. venepuncture) and usually occurs while standing. Cardiac syncope, caused by a sudden decline in cardiac output and hence cerebral perfusion, may be exertional

16.1 FEATURES HELPFUL IN DISTINGUISHING SEIZURES FROM FAINTS		
	Seizure	**Faint**
Aura (e.g. olfactory)	+	–
Cyanosis	+	–
Tongue-biting	+	–
Post-ictal confusion	+	–
Post-ictal amnesia	+	–
Post-ictal headache	+	–
Rapid recovery	–	+

(e.g. with severe aortic stenosis) or may occur completely 'out of the blue' (as in heart block). During a syncopal attack, incontinence of urine can occur and there is often stiffening and brief twitching of the limbs, but tongue-biting never occurs. Recovery is rapid and without confusion.

SEIZURES

A seizure is any clinical event caused by an abnormal electrical discharge in the brain, whilst epilepsy is the tendency to have recurrent seizures. The division of seizure types on physiological grounds is between partial (focal) seizures in which paroxysmal neuronal activity is limited to one part of the cortex, and generalised seizures where the electrophysiological abnormality involves both hemispheres simultaneously.

Clinical assessment

Tonic clonic seizures: These may be preceded by a partial seizure (the 'aura'). The patient then goes rigid, stops breathing, becomes unconscious and cyanosed, and may fall. After a few moments, the rigidity is periodically relaxed, producing clonic jerks. Urinary incontinence or tongue-biting may occur. The patient then gradually regains consciousness, but is drowsy or confused for some hours.

Complex partial seizures: Partial seizures cause episodes of altered consciousness without the patient collapsing to the ground. The patient stares blankly, often making rhythmic smacking movements of the lips or other automatisms. After a few minutes the patient returns to consciousness but may be muddled or drowsy. Immediately before the attack there may be alterations of mood, memory and perception. If these occur without subsequent alteration in awareness, the seizure is a simple partial seizure.

Absence seizures: These are generalised seizures which always start in childhood. The child goes blank and stares for a few seconds only. The attacks resemble complex partial seizures but are usually shorter, more frequent and not associated with post-ictal confusion.

Partial motor seizures: Epileptic activity in the pre-central gyrus causes partial motor seizures affecting the contralateral face, arm, trunk or leg.

There is rhythmical jerking or sustained spasm of the affected parts. They may remain localised to one part, or may spread to involve the whole side. Some attacks begin in one part and spread gradually ('Jacksonian epilepsy'). Prolonged episodes may leave paresis of the involved limb lasting for several hours (Todd's palsy).

Partial sensory seizures: Seizures arising in the sensory cortex cause unpleasant tingling or 'electric' sensations in the contralateral face and limbs. A spreading pattern like a Jacksonian seizure may occur, but is much faster (in seconds) than the 'march' of a migrainous focal sensory attack (10–15 mins).

Factors precipitating seizures

Sometimes specific trigger factors can be identified, such as sleep deprivation, alcohol excess or withdrawal, flickering lights or intercurrent illness.

EPILEPSY

Epilepsy is a tendency to have seizures and is a symptom of brain disease rather than a disease itself. A single seizure is not epilepsy but is an indication for investigation. The recurrence rate after a first seizure approaches 70% during the first year. The lifetime risk of having a single seizure is ~5%, whilst the prevalence of epilepsy is ~0.5%.

Types of epilepsy

Primary generalised epilepsy: This makes up 10% of all epilepsies, including 40% of those with tonic clonic seizures. Onset is usually in childhood or adolescence. No structural abnormality is present and there is often a substantial genetic predisposition. Some varieties, like childhood absence epilepsy, are relatively uncommon, whilst others, like juvenile myoclonic epilepsy, are common (5–10% of all patients with epilepsy).

Secondary generalised epilepsy: Generalised epilepsy may arise from spread of partial seizures due to structural disease, or may be secondary to drugs or metabolic disorders. Epilepsy presenting in adult life is almost always secondary generalised, even if there is no clear history of a partial seizure before the onset of a major attack.

Partial epilepsy: Partial seizures may arise from any disease of the cerebral cortex, congenital or acquired, and frequently generalise. With the exception of a few idiopathic partial epilepsies of benign outcome in childhood, the presence of partial seizures signifies the presence of focal cerebral pathology.

Investigations

No cause is found in most patients. However, investigations are necessary to confirm the diagnosis, characterise the type of epilepsy, and identify any underlying cause.

Cerebral imaging: After a single seizure, head CT or MRI is advisable, although the yield of structural lesions is low unless there are focal features.

EEG: May be more helpful in showing focal features if performed very soon after a seizure than after an interval. It can also help establish the type of epilepsy and guide therapy.

Other investigations: These should identify any metabolic, infective, inflammatory or toxic causes. They include FBC, ESR, CRP, U&Es, glucose, LFTs, CXR, syphilis serology, HIV, collagen disease, CSF examination.

Management

• Explain the nature and cause of seizures to patients and their relatives. • Instruct relatives in the first aid management of major seizures. • Emphasise that epilepsy is a common disorder and that good control can be expected in >80% of patients.

Immediate care of seizures: Little can or need be done for a person whilst a major seizure is occurring except first aid and common-sense manoeuvres (Box 16.2).

Restrictions: Patients should be made aware of the riskiness of activities where loss of awareness would be dangerous, until good control of seizures has been established. This includes work or recreational activities involving exposure to heights, dangerous machinery, open fires or water. In the UK and many other countries, legal restrictions regarding vehicle driving apply to patients with epilepsy.

Anticonvulsant drug therapy (see also p. 781)***:*** Drug treatment should be considered after more than one seizure has occurred. Of patients whose epilepsy is controllable, only a single drug is necessary in 80%. Dose regi-

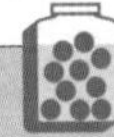

16.2 IMMEDIATE CARE OF SEIZURES
First aid (by relatives and witnesses)
• Move person away from danger (fire, water, machinery, furniture) • After convulsions cease, turn into 'recovery' position (semi-prone) • Ensure airway is clear • Do **NOT** insert anything in mouth (tongue-biting occurs at onset and cannot be prevented) • If convulsions continue for >5 mins or recur without person regaining consciousness, summon urgent medical attention • Person may be drowsy/confused for 30–60 mins and should not be left alone until recovered
Immediate medical attention
• Ensure airway is patent • Give oxygen to offset cerebral hypoxia • Give i.v. anticonvulsant (e.g. diazepam 10 mg) **ONLY IF** convulsions are continuous or repeated (if so, manage as for status epilepticus: Box 16.4) • Consider taking blood for anticonvulsant levels (if known epileptic) • Investigate cause

16.3 GUIDELINES FOR CHOICE OF ANTI-EPILEPTIC DRUGS 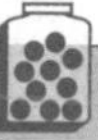		
Epilepsy type	**First-line**	**Second-line**
Partial and/or secondary GTCS	Carbamazepine	Lamotrigine Sodium valproate Topiramate Gabapentin Levetiracetam
Primary GTCS	Sodium valproate	Lamotrigine Topiramate
Absence	Ethosuximide	Sodium valproate
Myoclonic	Sodium valproate	Clonazepam
N.B. Preferably one and no more than two drugs should be used at one time. (GTCS = generalised tonic clonic seizure.)		

mens should be kept as simple as possible to promote compliance. The first line of treatment should be one of the established drugs (Box 16.3), with more recently introduced drugs as second choice. Try up to three agents singly before resorting to combinations; beware drug interactions. Phenytoin and carbamazepine induce liver enzymes and therefore are not ideal for women wishing to use oral contraception. Occasional phenytoin and carbamazepine blood levels can be checked to confirm appropriate dose and to check compliance. There is no relationship between drug levels of sodium valproate and anticonvulsant efficacy.

Prognosis

Generalised seizures are more readily controlled than partial seizures. A structural lesion makes complete control less likely. After 20 yrs:

• 50% have been seizure-free for the last 5 yrs without medication. • 20% are seizure-free with medication. • Seizures continue in 30% despite medication.

There is a 40-fold increased risk of sudden unexplained death in epilepsy and patients may need to be made aware of this to help them rearrange their lifestyle and comply with treatment.

Withdrawal of anticonvulsant therapy: After complete control of seizures for 2–4 yrs, withdrawal of medication may be considered. Childhood-onset epilepsy carries the best prognosis for successful drug withdrawal. Overall, the recurrence rate of seizures after drug withdrawal is ~40%. Withdrawal should be undertaken slowly, reducing the drug dose gradually over 6–12 mths.

STATUS EPILEPTICUS

Status epilepticus exists when a series of seizures occurs over 30 mins without the patient regaining awareness between attacks. This usually refers

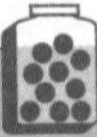

16.4 MANAGEMENT OF STATUS EPILEPTICUS

General

- Immediate care (Box 16.2)
- Secure i.v. access
- Blood for glucose, U&Es, Ca, Mg, LFTs and sample for future analysis (e.g. drug misuse)
- Diazepam 10 mg i.v. (or rectally)—repeat *once only* after 15 mins; *or* lorazepam 4 mg i.v.
- Transfer to intensive care area, monitoring neurological condition, BP, respiration and ABG

Pharmacological

If seizures continue after 30 mins

- I.V. infusion (with cardiac monitoring) with one of:
  Phenytoin: i.v. infusion of 15 mg/kg at 50 mg/min
  Fosphenytoin: i.v. infusion of 15 mg/kg at 100 mg/min
  Phenobarbital: i.v. infusion of 10 mg/kg at 100 mg/min

If seizures still continue after 30–60 mins

- Start treatment for refractory status with intubation and ventilation, and general anaesthesia using propofol or thiopental

Once status controlled

- Commence longer-term anticonvulsant medication with one of:
  Sodium valproate 10 mg/kg i.v. over 3–5 mins, then 800–2000 mg/day
  Phenytoin: give loading dose (if not already used) of 15 mg/kg, infuse at <50 mg/min, then 300 mg/day
  Carbamazepine 400 mg by nasogastric (NG) tube, then 400–1200 mg/day
- Investigate cause

to recurrent tonic clonic seizures and is a medical emergency. Status is never the presenting feature of idiopathic epilepsy but may be precipitated by abrupt withdrawal of anticonvulsant drugs, a major structural lesion or acute metabolic disturbance. Management is summarised in Box 16.4.

NON-EPILEPTIC ATTACK DISORDER ('PSYCHOGENIC ATTACKS', 'PSEUDO-SEIZURES')

Patients may present with attacks that superficially resemble epileptic seizures but which are caused by psychological phenomena and not associated with abnormal epileptic discharges in the brain. Clues pointing towards non-epileptic attacks include elaborate arching of the back, pelvic thrusting and/or wild flailing of limbs. Cyanosis and severe biting of the tongue are rare, but urinary incontinence can occur. Treatment is often difficult and usually requires psychotherapy and/or counselling rather than drug therapy.

SLEEP DISORDERS

Disturbances of sleep are common. Apart from insomnia, patients may complain of:

• Excessive daytime sleepiness, often a sign of upper airway obstruction (see p. 277). • Disturbed behaviour during night-time sleep. • The parasomnias (sleep walking and talking, night terrors). • Disturbing subjective experiences during sleep and/or its onset (nightmares, hypnagogic hallucinations (frightening hallucinations during sleep or waking), sleep paralysis).

NARCOLEPSY

In this disorder recurrent bouts of irresistible sleep are experienced. Patients will report at least one other of the 'narcolepsy tetrad':

• Sleep attacks. • Cataplexy (sudden loss of muscle tone triggered by surprise, laughter, emotion). • Hypnagogic hallucinations. • Sleep paralysis.

Narcoleptic attacks can be treated with modafinil (200–400 mg per day). Cataplexy responds to clomipramine (25–50 mg 8-hourly) or fluoxetine (20 mg per day).

RESTLESS LEG SYNDROME

This is a common disorder, also known as Ekbom's syndrome. Unpleasant sensations in the legs that are ameliorated by moving the legs occur when the patient is tired and at the onset of sleep. Restless legs can also be symptomatic of an underlying peripheral neuropathy or iron deficiency, or of general medical conditions (e.g. uraemia). Treatment is with clonazepam (0.5–2.0 mg), levodopa (100–200 mg) or dopamine agonists at night.

DISORDERS OF MOVEMENT

Lesions in various parts of the motor system produce distinctive patterns of motor deficit. These can be 'negative' symptoms (weakness, lack of coordination, lack of stability and stiffness) or 'positive' symptoms (tremor, dystonia, chorea, athetosis, hemiballismus, tics and myoclonus). When the lower limbs are affected, characteristic patterns of gait disorder may result.

THE MOTOR SYSTEM

A programme of movement formulated by the pre-motor cortex is converted into a series of muscle movements in the motor cortex and then transmitted to the spinal cord in the pyramidal tract (Fig. 16.2).

Lower motor neuron lesions: Loss of function of lower motor neurons causes loss of contraction in their units' muscle fibres and the muscle will be weak and flaccid. Denervated muscle fibres atrophy, causing wasting. Re-innervation from neighbouring motor neurons occurs but the neuromuscular junctions are unstable, causing fasciculations (visible to the naked eye because the motor units are larger than normal).

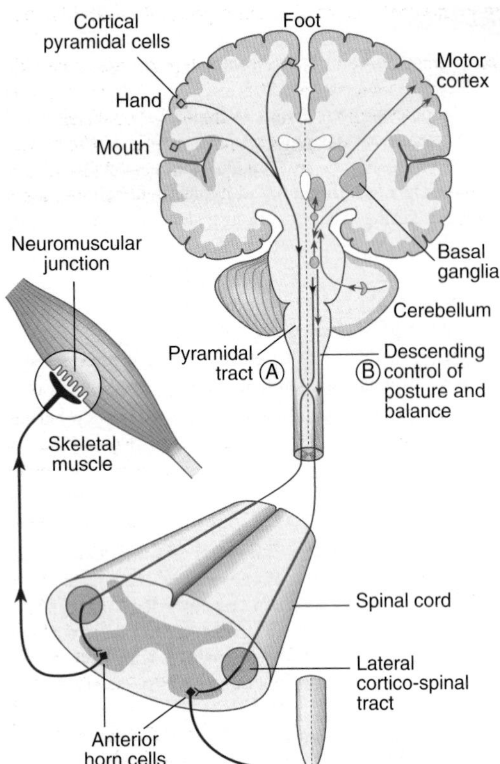

Fig. 16.2 The motor system. Neurons from the motor cortex descend as the pyramidal tract in the internal capsule and cerebral peduncle to the ventral brain stem, where most cross low in the medulla (A). In the spinal cord the upper motor neurons form the cortico-spinal tract in the lateral column before synapsing with the lower motor neurons in the anterior horns. The activity in the motor cortex is modulated by influences from the basal ganglia and cerebellum. Pathways descending from these structures control posture and balance (B).

Upper motor neuron (pyramidal) lesions: When the spinal cord is disconnected from the higher motor hierarchies, the anterior horn motor neurons are under the uninhibited influence of the spinal reflex mechanisms. An upper motor neuron lesion therefore manifests clinically with brisk tendon stretch reflexes, 'spastic' increase in tone, and extensor plantar responses. Spasticity takes time to develop and may not be present for weeks.

Extrapyramidal lesions: There is an increase in tone, which is continuous throughout the range of movement at any speed of stretch ('lead-pipe' rigidity). Involuntary movements are present, and a tremor combined with rigidity produces typical 'cogwheel' rigidity. Rapid movements are slowed (bradykinesia). Extrapyramidal lesions also cause postural instability, precipitating falls.

Cerebellar lesions: These cause lack of coordination on the same side of the body. The initial movement is normal but accuracy deteriorates as the target is approached, producing an 'intention tremor'. The distances of targets are misjudged (dysmetria), resulting in 'past-pointing'. The ability to produce rapid, regularly alternating movements is impaired (dysdiadochokinesis). Disorders of the central vermis of the cerebellum produce a characteristic ataxic gait.

A DIAGNOSTIC APPROACH TO LIMB WEAKNESS (Box 16.5, Fig. 16.3)

• Weakness in only some muscles in a limb suggests a problem in the peripheral nerve(s) or motor root(s). • Weakness of the whole limb may be due to problems in the brachial or lumbosacral plexuses, or to a central lesion. • Weakness in both lower limbs (paraparesis) or all four limbs (tetraparesis) suggests either a spinal cord lesion or a diffuse peripheral nerve problem such as Guillain–Barré syndrome. • The reflexes are absent in Guillain–Barré syndrome (or other lower motor nerve lesions) and brisk in spinal cord (upper motor neuron) lesions. • Patients with a bradykinetic limb often complain of weakness. • Patients with Parkinson's disease usually present with symptoms in one limb that may be described as weak and clumsy, especially for fine manipulations. Often the typical rest tremor is a clue to the diagnosis. • Weakness down one side of the body (hemiparesis) is almost always due to a cerebral hemisphere lesion, although it can be caused by spinal cord or brain-stem lesions. The lesion is of upper motor neuron type and the site can be deduced by other signs, such as higher cerebral abnormalities or sensory change. • The evolution of a motor deficit over time suggests the likely underlying pathology (Box 16.6).

GAIT DISORDERS

Patterns of weakness, loss of coordination and proprioceptive sensory loss produce a range of abnormal gaits. Neurogenic disorders need to be distinguished from skeletal abnormalities, usually characterised by pain producing an antalgic gait, or limp.

Pyramidal gait: Upper motor neuron (pyramidal) lesions cause a gait in which the upper limb is held in flexion and the lower limb is kept relatively extended. In a hemiplegia, the asymmetry between the affected and normal sides is obvious. In a paraparesis, both lower limbs move slowly, swung from the hips and dragged on the ground in extension.

Foot drop: Weakness of ankle dorsiflexion disrupts the normal gait cycle. Descent of the foot is less controlled, making a slapping noise, and the foot may be lifted higher, producing a high-stepping gait.

Waddling gait of proximal muscle weakness: In proximal muscle weakness, usually caused by muscle disease, the hips are not properly fixed and trunk movements are exaggerated, producing a rolling or waddling gait.

16.5 PHYSICAL SIGNS IN DIFFERENT TYPES OF MOTOR DEFICIT

Clinical sign	Upper motor (pyramidal) lesion	Lower motor lesion	Extrapyramidal lesion	Cerebellar lesion	Functional
Power	Weak Upper limbs: extensors weaker Lower limbs: flexors weaker	Weak	No weakness	No weakness	Give-way weakness
Wasting	None	Yes, after interval	None	None	None
Fasciculation	None	Yes, after interval	None	None	None
Tone	Spastic increase (after interval)	Flaccid from onset	Rigidity (cogwheel)	Normal/reduced	Normal
Reflexes	Increased	Reduced/absent	Normal	Normal	Normal
Plantar response	Extensor	Flexor	Flexor	Flexor	Normal
Coordination	Reduced by weakness	Reduced by weakness	Normal (but slowed)	Impaired	Normal (may be elaborated)

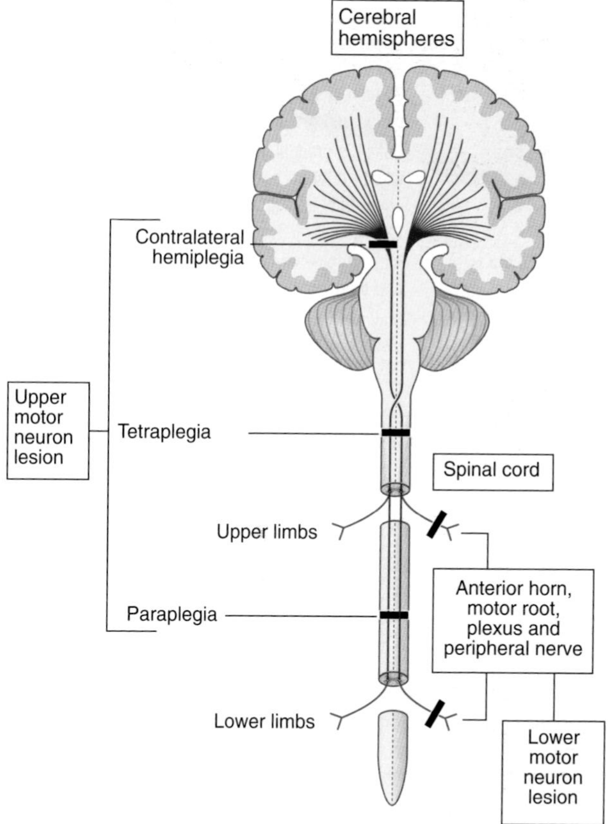

Fig. 16.3 Patterns of motor loss according to the anatomical site of the lesion.

Cerebellar ataxia: Patients with lesions of the central parts of the cerebellum (the vermis) walk with a characteristic broad-based gait, 'like a drunken sailor'.

Gait apraxia: There is normal power in the legs and no abnormal cerebellar signs or proprioception loss, yet the patient cannot formulate the motor act of walking. This higher cerebral dysfunction occurs in bilateral hemisphere disease, such as normal pressure hydrocephalus and diffuse frontal lobe disease.

Sensory ataxia: Loss of joint position sense makes walking unreliable. The feet tend to be placed on the ground with greater emphasis, resulting in a 'stamping' gait.

16.6 LIMB WEAKNESS: ASSESSING THE CAUSE	
Vascular (stroke) lesions	Sudden onset (over mins) followed by a stable period and gradual recovery
Neoplastic lesions	Deficit is gradual in onset and progressive over wks or mths There may be signs caused by the mass effect of the lesion
Inflammatory lesions	May be fairly acute (over days), persist for a time and then improve (e.g. MS)
Degenerative disorders	May evolve over mths/yrs (e.g. motor neuron disease or cervical myelopathy)

Extrapyramidal gait: Patients have difficulty initiating walking and controlling the pace of their gait. This produces the festinant gait: initial stuttering steps that quickly increase in frequency while decreasing in length.

INVOLUNTARY MOVEMENTS

Abnormal movements usually imply a disorder in the basal ganglia, in which there is disinhibition of intrinsic rhythm generators or a disorder of postural control.

Rest tremor: A tremor is a rhythmic oscillating movement of a limb or part of a limb, or of the head. Rest tremor is pathognomonic of Parkinson's disease. It is characteristically 'pill-rolling' and asymmetrical. Tremor of the head in the upright position ('titubation') is not a rest tremor since this is a postural tremor, disappearing when the head is supported.

Action tremor: More common than rest tremor. The potential causes are numerous:

• Physiological tremor: may be exaggerated by anxiety, fatigue, thyrotoxicosis, drugs, or alcohol withdrawal. • Essential tremor: slower than physiological tremor, often familial and responds to propranolol. • Parkinson's disease (resting tremor more usual). • Wilson's disease. • Postural tremor (e.g. MS, cerebellar outflow lesions). • Intention tremor (cerebellar hemisphere disease). • Asterixis: a 'flapping' tremor seen in metabolic disturbances (renal failure, liver failure, hypercapnia) or acute parietal lesions (usually vascular).

Chorea: Jerky, small-amplitude, purposeless involuntary movements. There are numerous potential causes:

• Hereditary (Huntington's disease, Wilson's disease). • Drugs (dopaminergic, phenothiazines, tricyclics, oral contraceptive). • Infective/inflammatory (e.g. Sydenham's post-streptococcal chorea, CJD, SLE). • Endocrine (pregnancy, thyrotoxicosis, hypoparathyroidism, hypoglycaemia). • Vascular (lacunar infarction, AV malformation).

Ballism: More dramatic than chorea, ballistic movements of the limbs usually occur unilaterally (hemiballismus) in vascular lesions of the subthalamic nucleus.

Athetosis: Slower writhing movements of the limbs. These are often combined with chorea and are then termed 'choreo-athetoid' movements.

Dystonia: A movement disorder in which a limb (or the head) involuntarily takes up an abnormal posture. This may be generalised in basal ganglia disease, or may be focal or segmental, as in spasmodic torticollis when the head involuntarily turns to one side. Other segmental dystonias may cause abnormal disabling postures during specific actions (e.g. writer's cramp) and can be treated with botulinum toxin to the responsible muscles.

Myoclonus: Brief, isolated, random, non-purposeful jerks of muscle groups in the limbs. They occur normally at the onset of sleep (hypnic jerks). Myoclonus can occur in epilepsy, from subcortical structures or from diseased segments of the spinal cord.

Tics: Repetitive semi-purposeful movements such as blinking, winking, grinning or screwing up of the eyes. Unlike with other involuntary movements, patients can suppress tics, at least for a short time.

SENSORY DISTURBANCE

Sensory symptoms are very common but do not always denote nervous system disorder. For example, tingling in the fingers of both hands and around the mouth commonly suggests hyperventilation. Damage to the afferent nervous pathways conveying touch and pain produces either the negative sensation of numbness, or positive symptoms such as paraesthesia and pain.

A DIAGNOSTIC APPROACH TO SENSORY SYMPTOMS

In the history, the most useful features are:

• Anatomical distribution. • Mode of onset of numbness. • Paraesthesia or pain.

Certain patterns can be recognised. For example, in migraine the aura may consist of a front of paraesthesia followed by numbness which takes 20–30 mins to spread over one half of the body. Sensory loss due to a vascular lesion, on the other hand, will occur more or less instantaneously. The numbness and paraesthesia of spinal cord lesions often ascend one or both lower limbs to a level on the trunk over hours or days.

PATTERNS OF SENSORY DISTURBANCE (Fig. 16.4)

Peripheral nerve lesions

In peripheral nerve lesions, the symptoms are usually of sensory loss and simple paraesthesia (pins and needles). Single peripheral nerve lesions will cause disturbance in the sensory distribution of that nerve. In diffuse

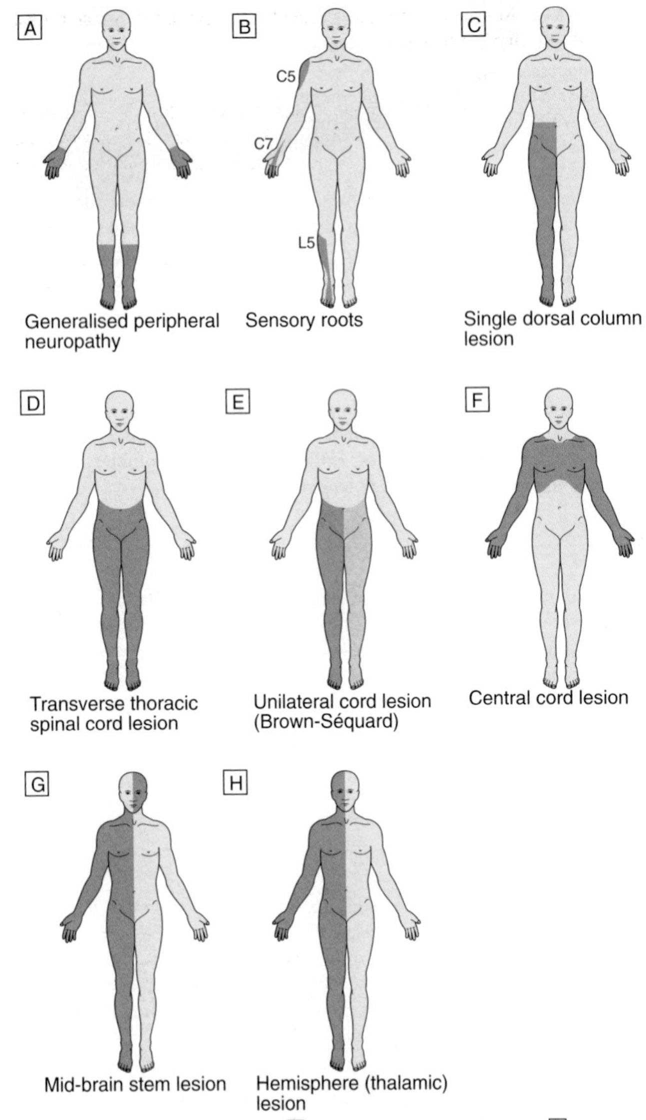

Fig. 16.4 Patterns of sensory loss. **A** Generalised peripheral neuropathy. **B** Sensory roots. **C** Single dorsal column lesion (proprioception and some touch loss). **D** Transverse thoracic spinal cord lesion. **E** Unilateral cord lesion (Brown-Séquard): ipsilateral dorsal column (and motor) deficit and contralateral spinothalamic deficit. **F** Central cord lesion: 'cape' distribution of spinothalamic loss. **G** Mid brain stem lesion: ipsilateral facial sensory loss and contralateral loss on body. **H** Hemisphere (thalamic) lesion: contralateral loss on one side of face and body.

neuropathies the longest neurons are affected first, giving the characteristic 'glove and stocking' distribution.

Nerve root lesions

Pain is more often a feature of lesions of nerve roots within the spine or of the limb plexuses. It is often felt in the muscles innervated by a root. The site of nerve root lesions may be deduced from the dermatomal pattern of sensory loss.

Spinal cord lesions

Sensory information ascends the nervous system in two anatomically discrete systems, differential involvement of which is often of diagnostic assistance (Fig. 16.5).

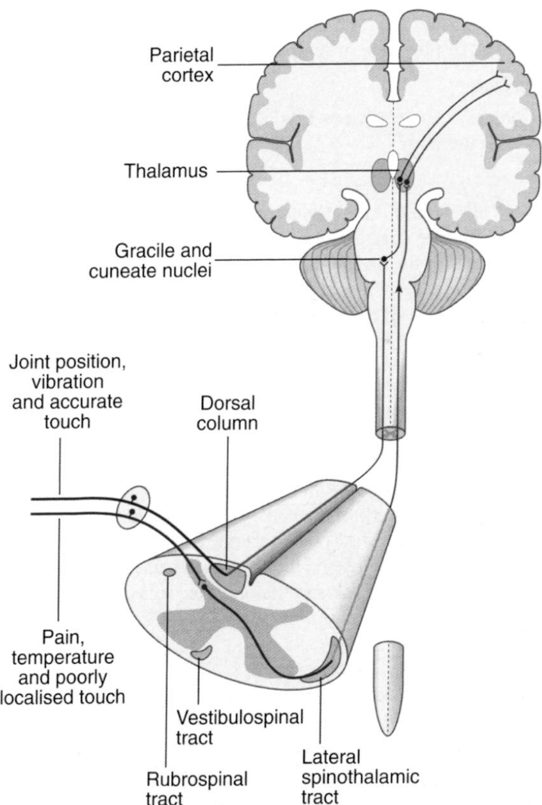

Fig. 16.5 The main somatic sensory pathways.

Transverse spinal cord lesions: There is loss of all modalities below that segmental level. Often a band of paraesthesia or hyperaesthesia is found at the top of the area of loss. If vascular in origin (e.g. due to anterior spinal artery thrombosis), the posterior one-third of the spinal cord (dorsal column modalities) may be spared.

Unilateral spinal cord lesions: There is loss for spinothalamic modalities (pain and temperature) on the opposite side of the lesion. There is also loss for dorsal column modalities (joint position and vibration) on the same side as the lesion (e.g. Brown-Séquard syndrome).

Central spinal cord lesions (e.g. syringomyelia): These spare the dorsal columns but affect spinothalamic fibres from both sides over the length of the lesion. The sensory loss is therefore dissociated (in terms of the modalities affected) and suspended (segments above and below the lesion are spared).

Single dorsal column lesion (e.g. MS): The patient experiences an unpleasant tight feeling over the limb involved. There is loss of proprioception without any loss of pin-prick or temperature sensation.

Brain-stem lesions

Brain-stem lesions can cause sensory loss affecting all modalities on the contralateral side of the body.

Hemisphere lesions

These may affect all modalities of sensation. In the thalamus, discrete lesions (e.g. small lacunar strokes) can cause loss of sensation over the whole contralateral half of the body. With substantial lesions of the parietal cortex (as with large strokes) there is severe loss of proprioception and even loss of conscious awareness of the existence of the affected limb(s).

Neuropathic pain

Pain is of two main types: nociceptive pain, arising from a pathological process in a body part, and neuropathic pain, caused by dysfunction of the pain perception apparatus itself. Neuropathic pain is a very unpleasant persistent burning sensation, often with increased sensitivity to touch. The most common syndromes include partial damage to peripheral nerves ('causalgia'), the trigeminal nerve (post-herpetic neuralgia) or the thalamus. Drugs (carbamazepine, tricyclics or phenothiazines) may help but usually only partially. Neurosurgical attempts to interrupt pain pathways sometimes succeed. Implantation of electrical stimulators has occasionally proved successful.

COMA AND BRAIN DEATH

COMA

Persistent loss of consciousness or coma indicates disorder of the arousal mechanisms in the brain stem and diencephalon. There are many causes of coma (Box 16.7). The history is crucial to establishing the cause and should be obtained from any witnesses. Neurological examination may reveal

16.7 CAUSES OF COMA	
Metabolic disturbance	Drug overdose, diabetes mellitus (hypoglycaemia, ketoacidosis, hyperosmolar coma), hyponatraemia, uraemia, liver failure, respiratory failure, hypothermia, hypothyroidism
Trauma	Cerebral contusion, extradural haematoma, subdural haematoma
Cerebrovascular disease	Subarachnoid haemorrhage, intracerebral haemorrhage, brain-stem infarction/haemorrhage, cerebral venous sinus thrombosis
Infections	Meningitis, encephalitis, cerebral abscess, general sepsis
Others	Epilepsy, brain tumour, thiamine deficiency

important findings, e.g. evidence of head injury, papilloedema, meningism or eye movement disorder.

Assessment of conscious level

Systematic assessment using the Glasgow Coma Scale provides a grading of coma which allows serial comparison and may provide prognostic information, particularly in traumatic coma (Box 16.8).

BRAIN DEATH

The availability of mechanical ventilators has resulted in the survival of patients with severe irreversible brain damage but functioning cardiovascular systems. Diagnostic criteria for brain death have been established in order that those patients without functioning brains who have no chance of recovery may be identified, organ donation options considered, and ventilation discontinued.

ACUTE CONFUSIONAL STATE (DELIRIUM)

This is much more common than dementia. Unlike in dementia, there is a disturbance of arousal that accompanies the global impairment of mental function. There is drowsiness with disorientation, perceptual disturbances and muddled thinking. Patients typically fluctuate, confusion being worse at night, and there may be associated emotional disturbance or psychomotor changes. There are many possible causes (Box 16.9).

Diagnosis

It is vital to take a history from a witness. Examination may yield other clues. It is important to distinguish confusion from a fluent aphasia. Often, however, the cause is not immediately obvious and a wide screen of tests must be performed (Box 16.10).

16.8 GLASGOW COMA SCALE	
Eye-opening (E)	
• Spontaneous	4
• To speech	3
• To pain	2
• Nil	1
Best motor response (M)	
• Obeys	6
• Localises	5
• Withdraws	4
• Abnormal flexion	3
• Extensor response	2
• Nil	1
Verbal response (V)	
• Orientated	5
• Confused conversation	4
• Inappropriate words	3
• Incomprehensible sounds	2
• Nil	1
Coma score = E + M + V	
• Minimum	3
• Maximum	15

Management

• Identify the cause and correct it if possible. • Nurse in a well-lit room. • Avoid sedative drugs which may exacerbate the confusion. • Occasionally drugs such as haloperidol (1–10 mg 8-hourly) may be required. • In delirium tremens (alcohol withdrawal) the treatment is a tapered course of diazepam with i.v. thiamine.

DISTURBANCE OF MEMORY

It is important to determine for how long the problem has existed, and exactly which aspects of memory are affected. Disturbance of episodic memory ('short-term memory') must be distinguished from semantic memory. The former can be selectively impaired in Korsakoff's syndrome (often secondary to alcohol) or bilateral temporal lobe damage.

TRANSIENT AMNESIA

Loss of memory for a period of time may be due to:

16.9 CAUSES OF ACUTE CONFUSIONAL STATE		
Type	**Common**	**Unusual**
Infective	Chest infection Urinary infection Septicaemia Viral illness Meningitis, encephalitis	Cerebral abscess Subdural empyema AIDS
Metabolic/ endocrine	Hypoxia (cardiac/respiratory failure) Acute haemorrhage Hyper-/hypoglycaemia Hyper-/hypocalcaemia Hyponatraemia Liver failure, renal failure	Hypo-/hyperthyroidism Adrenal disease Porphyria
Vascular	Acute cerebral haemorrhage/ infarction Subarachnoid haemorrhage	Vasculitis (e.g. SLE) Cerebral venous thrombosis
Toxic	Alcohol intoxication/withdrawal Drugs (therapeutic/illicit)	Carbon monoxide poisoning Industrial exposure (e.g. heavy metals)
Neoplastic	Secondary deposits	Primary cerebral tumour Paraneoplastic syndrome
Trauma	Cerebral contusion, subdural haematoma	
Other	Post-ictal state Perioperative Acute decompensation of dementia	Acute hydrocephalus Complex partial status epilepticus Hashimoto's encephalopathy

16.10 INVESTIGATION OF ACUTE CONFUSIONAL STATE		
	First-line	**Other useful tests**
Blood tests	FBC, ESR U&Es, Ca, Mg Glucose LFTs TFTs	Cardiac enzymes Protein electrophoresis, tumour markers Vitamin B_{12}, copper studies Syphilis serology Autoantibodies
CNS tests	Head imaging (CT and/or MRI)	Lumbar puncture, EEG
Other	ABGs, ECG Infection screen (blood cultures, CXR, urine culture)	Viral screen, as appropriate (e.g. HIV) Urinary porphyrins

• Transient toxic confusional state. • Psychological fugue state. • Post-ictal period after seizure. • Transient global amnesia.

These are usually distinguished from the history. Transient global amnesia is a syndrome affecting middle-aged patients in which there is an abrupt, discrete and reversible loss of short-term memory function. After 4–6 hrs, memory functions and behaviour return to normal. There are none of the phenomena associated with seizures, and transient global amnesia tends not to recur. The patient has no physical signs and further investigation may not be needed if epilepsy can be excluded.

DEMENTIA

Progressive memory deterioration over months suggests an underlying dementia, which is characterised by a loss of previously acquired intellectual function in the absence of impairment of arousal. There are many causes but Alzheimer's disease and diffuse vascular disease are the most common. Rarer causes should be sought in younger patients and those with short histories. Many primary degenerative diseases have characteristic features that may help diagnosis:

• CJD is rapidly progressive (over months), associated with myoclonus, and may have characteristic EEG abnormalities. • Pick's disease presents with focal dysfunction often affecting language early. • Lewy body dementia may present with visual hallucinations.

Investigations

The aim is to discover a treatable cause, if present, and to try to give an idea of prognosis. Standard investigations include:

• CT and/or MRI brain imaging. • CXR. • FBC, ESR. • U&Es, glucose. • Calcium, LFTs. • TFTs. • Vitamin B_{12}. • ANA, anti-dsDNA. • VDRL. • EEG. • In selected patients: HIV testing, lumbar puncture (LP) or brain biopsy may be indicated.

Management

• Remove correctable causes. • Provide support for patient and carers if no specific treatment exists. • Anticholinesterases (donepezil, rivastigmine and galantamine) or memantine appear to improve cognitive function to some extent in Alzheimer's disease.

CHANGES IN PERSONALITY AND BEHAVIOUR

Organic conditions can result in altered personality and behaviour. This particularly applies to disorders affecting the frontal lobes, which control executive function, movement and behaviour. The frontal lobes may be damaged structurally (e.g. trauma, strokes, hydrocephalus or tumour) or functionally (e.g. metabolic disturbances). Personality can be affected in three broad directions:

• Patients with mesial frontal lesions become withdrawn, unresponsive and mute, often with associated urinary incontinence, gait apraxia and increased tone. • Patients with dorsolateral pre-frontal cortical lesions develop difficulties with speech and motor planning and organisation. • Patients with orbitofrontal lesions become disinhibited or exhibit irresponsible behaviour. Memory is substantially intact, and there may be focal physical signs such as a grasp reflex, palmo-mental response or pout.

SPEECH AND LANGUAGE DISTURBANCE

Speech is the process whereby vocal sounds are used to convey meaning between individuals. A large volume of the cerebral cortex is involved in this complex process, mostly in the dominant hemisphere. The temporal speech comprehension region is referred to as Wernicke's area. The language information then passes to Broca's area. The motor commands generated here pass to the lips, tongue, palate, pharynx, larynx and respiratory muscles via the facial nerve and cranial nerves 9, 10 and 12, resulting in speech.

DYSPHONIA AND DYSARTHRIA

The vocal cords may fail to generate sounds properly in speech, resulting in hoarse or whispered speech (dysphonia). This may be due to a local problem affecting the cords or a higher-level problem (dystonia) of vocal cord operation. If the muscles or nerves controlling the mouth, tongue, pharynx and lips are not functioning correctly, poorly articulated speech will result (dysarthria). Cerebellar or brain-stem disease, lower cranial nerve lesions, myasthenia or muscle disease may all result in dysarthria.

APHASIA

Aphasia (or dysphasia) is a disorder of the language content of speech. It can occur with lesions over a wide area of the dominant hemisphere. Aphasia is detected by the patient's inability to produce the correct word. If a patient has difficulty with speech comprehension there is likely to be a lesion in Wernicke's area. Patients with large lesions over much of the speech area have no language production and have 'global aphasia'.

DISORDERS OF PERCEPTION

The temporal, parietal and occipital lobes receive sensory information including touch, vision, hearing and balance. Damage to any of these areas will result in loss of the ability to perceive that particular modality. Abnormal excitation (e.g. epilepsy, migraine) results in an apparent perception not based in physical reality. This can be visual (flashing lights), somatosensory (tingling, burning or pain), auditory (noises) or vestibular (vertigo).

The parietal lobes are also involved in the higher processing and integration of primary sensory information. Damage here gives rise to sensory (including visual) inattention and apraxia. Apraxia is the inability to perform complex, organised activity in the presence of a normal basic motor, sensory and cerebellar system (e.g. dressing, using cutlery and finding one's way around geographically).

PROBLEMS WITH BRAIN-STEM FUNCTION

Many different functional areas are tightly packed into the brain stem. Damage to even a small area potentially causes major disturbance of several systems. An example would be upper motor neuron features affecting the right face, arm and leg in association with a left 3rd nerve palsy. The lesion would have to be in the left cerebral peduncle in the brain stem ('Weber's syndrome'). The lower cranial nerves, 9, 10, 11 and 12, are frequently affected bilaterally (by vascular, degenerative, infective/inflammatory or neoplastic conditions), producing dysphagia and dysarthria:

• The term 'bulbar palsy' is used if this results from lower motor neuron lesions. The tongue is wasted and fasciculating, and the palate moves very little. • A 'pseudobulbar palsy' arises from an upper motor neuron lesion of the bulbar muscles. Here the tongue is small and contracted, and moves slowly; the jaw jerk is brisk.

SWALLOWING DIFFICULTIES

Swallowing is a complex activity involving the coordinated action of lips, tongue, soft palate, pharynx and larynx, which are innervated by the facial nerve and cranial nerves 9, 10, 11 and 12.

• Acute dysphagia may result from a brain-stem stroke, a rapidly developing neuropathy (e.g. Guillain–Barré syndrome) or diphtheria. • Dysphagia developing subacutely may be seen in myasthenia gravis, motor neuron disease, polymyositis, basal meningitis and inflammatory brain-stem disease. • More slowly developing dysphagia suggests a myopathy or possibly a brain-stem or skull-base tumour.

DISORDERS OF BALANCE

Disorders of balance can arise from a number of different abnormalities affecting:

• Input (loss of vision, vestibular disorders or lack of joint position sense). • Processing (damage to vestibular nuclei or cerebellum). • Motor function (spinal cord lesions, leg weakness of any cause).

Loss of joint position sense or cerebellar function may result in a sensation of 'unsteadiness', while damage to the vestibular nuclei or labyrinth may cause an illusory sensation of movement, i.e. 'vertigo'. Sensory abnormalities may be manifest as altered visual acuities or visual fields, altered eye movements, impaired vestibular function or lack of joint position sense. Disturbance of cerebellar function may be manifest as nystagmus, dysarthria or ataxia.

VISUAL DISTURBANCE

VISUAL LOSS

The visual pathway from the retina to the occipital cortex is topographically organised, so the pattern of visual field loss allows localisation of the site of the lesion (Fig. 16.6, Box 16.11). Patients often present with transient visual loss.

• Visual loss lasting from 1 min to 15 mins is likely to have a vascular cause. This can affect one eye (amaurosis fugax) or one visual field. The field loss may be monocular (carotid circulation) or a homonymous hemianopia (vertebro-basilar circulation). • Transient visual loss lasting 20–30 mins suggests migraine, especially if accompanied by headache and/or positive visual phenomena.

EYE MOVEMENT DISORDERS

The control of eye movements begins in the cerebral hemispheres, and the pathway then descends to the brain stem with input from the visual cortex and cerebellum. Horizontal and vertical gaze centres in the pons and midbrain coordinate output to the ocular motor nerve nuclei (3, 4 and 6). These are connected to each other by the medial longitudinal fasciculus (MLF). The extraocular muscles are then supplied by the oculomotor (3rd), trochlear (4th) and abducens (6th) nerves.

Diplopia ('double vision')

The pattern of double vision and associated features allow localisation of the lesion, whilst the mode of onset and subsequent behaviour suggest the aetiology. The trochlear (4th) nerve innervates the superior oblique muscle, and the abducens (6th) nerve innervates the lateral rectus. The oculomotor (3rd) nerve innervates the remainder of the extraocular muscles along with the levator palpebrae superioris and the ciliary body (pupil constriction and accommodation). Causes of ocular motor nerve palsies are given in Box 16.12.

Complete oculomotor (3rd) nerve lesions: There is ptosis and a dilated pupil. The eye rests in a 'down and out' position (due to unaffected lateral rectus and superior oblique muscles). The pupil is often spared in ischaemic lesions (e.g. in diabetes). Pupillary involvement requires that compressive lesions (e.g. aneurysm) be excluded.

Trochlear (4th) nerve palsy: There is vertical diplopia and head tilt to the contralateral side, with double vision when looking down to the side opposite the lesion.

Abducens (6th) nerve palsy: There is horizontal double vision when looking towards the side of the lesion.

Myasthenia gravis: Can cause diplopia by affecting any or all of the extraocular muscles. It is often associated with ptosis. The hallmark is fatigability.

Extraocular muscle disease: Thyroid eye disease, myopathies and orbital myositis.

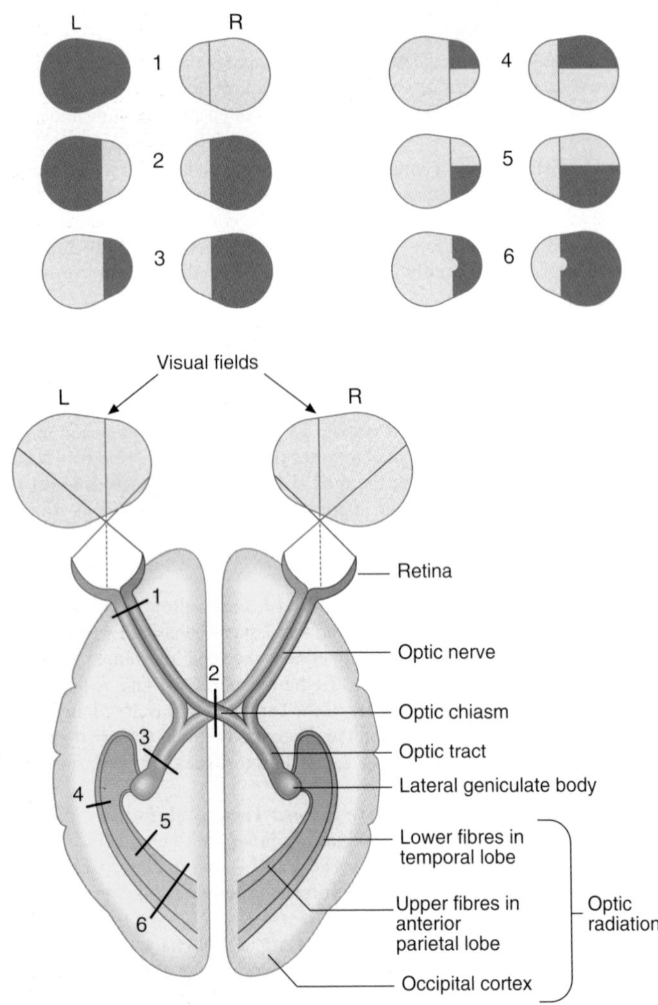

Fig. 16.6 Visual pathways and visual field defects. Schematic representation of eyes and brain in transverse section.

16.11 CLINICAL MANIFESTATIONS OF VISUAL FIELD LOSS

Site	Common causes	Complaint	Visual field loss	Associated physical signs
Retina/ optic disc	Vascular disease (including vasculitis) Glaucoma Inflammation	Partial/complete visual loss depending on site	Altitudinal field defect Arcuate scotoma	Reduced acuity Visual distortion (macula) Abnormal retinal appearance
Optic nerve	Optic neuritis Sarcoidosis Tumour Leber's hereditary optic neuropathy	Partial/complete loss of vision in one eye Often painful Central vision particularly affected	Central scotoma Paracentral scotoma Monocular blindness	Reduced acuity Reduced colour vision Relative afferent pupillary defect Optic atrophy (late)
Optic chiasm	Pituitary tumours Craniopharyngioma Sarcoidosis	May be none Rarely diplopia ('hemifield slide')	Bitemporal hemianopia	Pituitary function abnormalities
Optic tract	Tumour Inflammatory disease	Disturbed vision to one side of midline	Incongruous contralateral homonymous hemianopia	
Temporal lobe	Stroke Tumour Inflammatory disease	Disturbed vision to one side of midline	Contralateral homonymous upper quadrantanopia	Memory/language disorders
Parietal lobe	Stroke Tumour	Disturbed vision to one side of midline Bumping into things	Contralateral homonymous lower quadrantanopia	Contralateral sensory disturbance Asymmetry of optokinetic nystagmus
Occipital lobe	Stroke Tumour Inflammatory disease	Disturbed vision to one side of midline Difficulty reading Bumping into things	Homonymous hemianopia (may be macula-sparing)	Damage to other structures supplied by posterior cerebral circulation

Central lesions: Brain-stem lesions affecting the 3rd, 4th or 6th nerves or nuclei. In lesions of the MLF the hallmark is an internuclear ophthalmoplegia (e.g. in MS). The ipsilateral eye will either fail to adduct past midline or adduct very slowly.

Nystagmus

If the eye movement control systems are defective, the eyes may drift off target, resulting in a repetitive to-and-fro movement (drift-correction-drift) known as nystagmus. The direction of the fast phase is designated as the direction of the nystagmus because it is easier to see, although the abnormality is the slower drift of the eyes off target.

Vestibular system lesions: Damage to the horizontal canal allows output from the healthy, contralateral side to cause the eyes to drift towards the side of the lesion. Recurrent compensatory fast movements away from the lesion cause unidirectional horizontal nystagmus to the opposite side. Nystagmus of peripheral labyrinthine lesions fatigues quickly and is always accompanied by vertigo and/or nausea and vomiting. Central vestibular nystagmus is more persistent.

Brain-stem/cerebellar lesions: Lesions allow the eyes to drift back in towards their primary position, producing nystagmus whose fast component beats in the direction of gaze. They are bi-directional and not accompanied by vertigo. Brain-stem disease may also cause vertical nystagmus. Unilateral cerebellar lesions may cause nystagmus in the direction of the lesion (fast phases are directed towards the side of the lesion).

Other causes: These include physiological (in response to vestibular stimulation), toxicity (especially drugs), nutritional (thiamine) deficiency, and congenital ('pendular' rather than 'jerking') causes.

EYELID, GLOBE AND PUPIL DISORDERS

Ptosis may result from a 3rd nerve palsy (Box 16.12), sympathetic nerve damage (Horner's syndrome) or muscle disorders (e.g. myasthenia gravis or myotonic dystrophy).

When the globe is pushed forward in the orbit, either unilaterally (proptosis) or bilaterally (exophthalmos), the causes include:

• Thyroid eye disease (most common). • Orbital tumours or granulomas. • Cavernous sinus disease. • Inflammatory orbital disease ('pseudotumour').

Disorders of the pupil

Pupillary response to light is due to a combination of parasympathetic and sympathetic activity.

• Third nerve lesions cause pupillary dilatation with complete ptosis and extraocular muscle palsy. • Sympathetic lesions cause partial ptosis and pupillary constriction. • Holmes–Adie pupils are dilated and constrict to accommodation but not to light. • Afferent pupillary disorders occur when the direct light reflex is impaired because of optic nerve damage (consensual response from stimulation of the normal eye remains intact).

16.12 COMMON CAUSES OF DAMAGE TO CRANIAL NERVES 3, 4 AND 6

Site	Common pathology	Nerve(s) involved	Associated features
Brain stem	Infarction Haemorrhage Demyelination Intrinsic tumour	3 (mid-brain) 6 (ponto-medullary junction)	Contralateral pyramidal signs Ipsilateral lower motor neuron 7 palsy Other brain-stem/cerebellar signs
Intrameningeal	Meningitis	3, 4 and/or 6	Meningism
	Raised intracranial pressure	6 3 (uncal herniation)	Papilloedema Features of space-occupying lesion
	Aneurysms	3 (posterior communicating artery) 6 (basilar artery)	Pain Features of subarachnoid haemorrhage
	Cerebello-pontine angle tumour	6	8, 7, 5 lesions Ipsilateral cerebellar signs
	Trauma	3, 4 and/or 6	Other features of trauma
Cavernous sinus	Infection/thrombosis Carotid artery aneurysm Caroticocavernous fistula	3, 4 and/or 6	May be 5th nerve involvement also Pupil may be fixed, mid-position
Superior orbital fissure	Tumour (e.g. sphenoid wing meningioma) Granuloma	3, 4 and/or 6	May be proptosis, chemosis
Orbit	Vascular, infections, tumour, granuloma, trauma	3, 4 and/or 6	Pain Pupil often spared in vascular 3 palsy

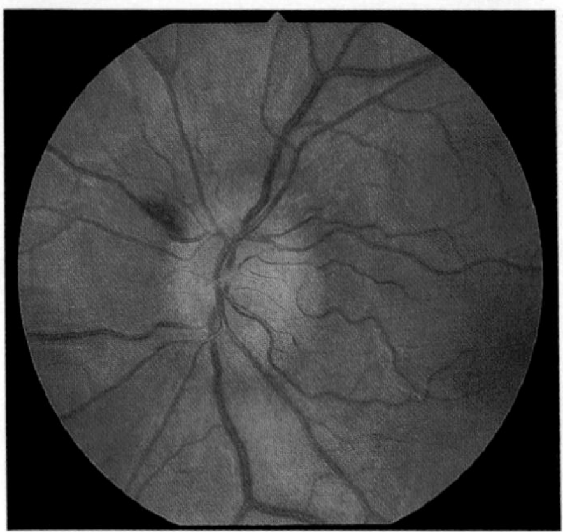

Fig. 16.7 Optic disc oedema (papilloedema). Fundus photograph of the left eye showing optic disc oedema with a small haemorrhage on the nasal side of the disc. (Courtesy of Dr B. Cullen.)

Optic disc disorders

Optic disc swelling: This occurs with:

• Raised intracranial pressure ('papilloedema'). • Venous obstruction. • Systemic disorders affecting retinal vessels (hypertension, hypercapnia, vasculitis). • Optic nerve damage (e.g. with demyelination, ischaemia, sarcoid, glioma).

There is the cessation of normal venous pulsation at the disc, and the disc margins then become red. The margins become indistinct and the whole disc is raised up, often with haemorrhages in the retina (Fig. 16.7).

Optic atrophy: Optic nerve damage makes the optic disc appear pale (Fig. 16.8). Causes include:

• Previous optic neuritis. • Ischaemic damage. • Chronic papilloedema. • Optic nerve compression. • Trauma. • Degenerative conditions.

SPHINCTER DISTURBANCE DUE TO NEUROLOGICAL DISEASE

BLADDER

The bladder is analogous to skeletal muscle in that neural control can be divided into upper and lower motor neuron components.

• An atonic (lower motor neuron) bladder is distended with overflow, and occurs in disease affecting the sacral cord or roots. • A hypertonic (upper motor neuron) bladder occurs in spinal cord or brain stem disease and presents with urgency with urge incontinence. • In cortical disease there may be a loss of awareness of bladder fullness and inappropriate micturition.

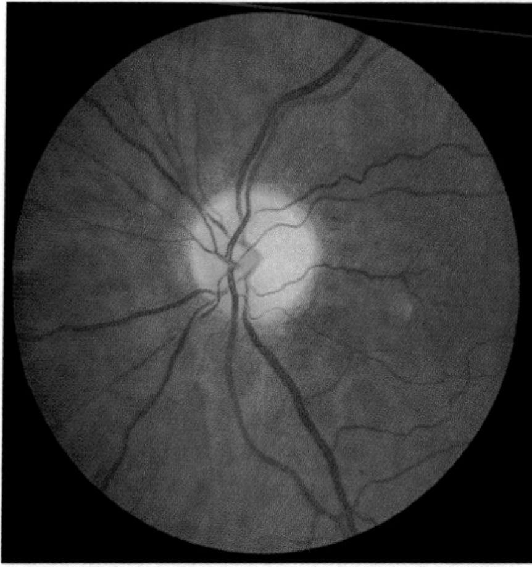

Fig. 16.8 Fundus photograph of the left eye of a patient with familial optic atrophy. Note marked pallor of optic disc.

RECTUM

The rectum has an excitatory cholinergic input from the parasympathetic sacral outflow, and inhibitory sympathetic supply similar to the bladder. Continence depends on skeletal muscle contraction in the pelvic floor muscles supplied by the pudendal nerves, as well as the internal and external anal sphincters.

• Damage to the autonomic components usually causes constipation. • Lesions affecting the conus medullaris, the somatic S2–4 roots and the pudendal nerves cause faecal incontinence.

PENILE ERECTION AND EJACULATION

These related functions are under autonomic control via the pelvic (parasympathetic, S2–4) and hypogastric nerves (sympathetic, L1–2).

• Erection is largely parasympathetic and is impaired by anticholinergic drugs and also by some antihypertensive and antidepressant agents. • Sympathetic activity is important for ejaculation, and may be inhibited by α-adrenoceptor antagonists.

CEREBROVASCULAR DISEASE

Stroke is a common medical emergency with an annual incidence of between 180 and 300 per 100 000. The incidence rises with age. One-fifth of patients with an acute stroke will die within a month of the event, and at least half of those who survive will be left with physical disability.

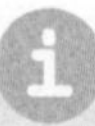

16.13 DIFFERENTIAL DIAGNOSIS OF STROKE AND TIA

- Space-occupying lesions (cerebral tumours, subdural haematoma, cerebral abscess)
- Peripheral nerve lesions (vascular or compressive)
- Todd's paresis (after epileptic seizure)
- Demyelination
- Hypoglycaemia
- Encephalitis
- Conversion disorder
- Migrainous aura (with or without headache)
- Focal seizures

ACUTE STROKE

Acute stroke is characterised by the rapid appearance (over minutes) of a focal deficit of brain function, most commonly a hemiplegia with or without signs of focal higher cerebral dysfunction (such as aphasia), hemisensory loss, visual field defect or brain-stem deficit.

Clinical classification of stroke

Transient ischaemic attack (TIA): Symptoms resolve completely within 24 hrs. This includes transient monocular blindness (amaurosis fugax), usually due to vascular occlusion in the retina.

Stroke: Symptoms last more than 24 hrs. With a clear history of rapid-onset transient or sustained focal deficit, the alternative diagnoses (Box 16.13) account for only 5% of cases.

Progressing stroke ('stroke in evolution'): Focal neurological deficit worsens after the patient first presents. It may be due to increasing volume of infarction, haemorrhage or related oedema.

Completed stroke: Focal deficit persists but is not progressing.

Clinical features

• A unilateral motor deficit, higher cerebral function deficit (e.g. aphasia or neglect) or a visual field defect usually places the lesion in the cerebral hemisphere. • Ataxia, diplopia, vertigo and/or bilateral weakness usually indicates a lesion in the brain stem or cerebellum. • Different combinations of these deficits result in distinct stroke syndromes (Box 16.14). • Clinical examination may provide clues to the cause of the stroke and should include the fundus (diabetic or hypertensive change), the heart (atrial fibrillation or valve lesions), the peripheral pulses (arteriopathy) and the skin (xanthelasma, arteritis, splinter haemorrhages, livedo reticularis).

CEREBRAL INFARCTION (85%)

Cerebral infarction is mostly due to thromboembolic disease secondary to atherosclerosis in the major extracranial arteries (carotid artery and aortic arch). About 20% are due to embolism from the heart, and a further 20% are due to intrinsic disease of small perforating vessels, producing so-called

16.14 SYNDROMES OF ACUTE STROKE	
Total anterior circulation syndrome (TACS)	Higher cerebral function deficit + hemiplegia + hemianopia
Partial anterior circulation syndrome (PACS)	Higher cerebral function deficit alone Combination of any 2 of higher cerebral function deficit, hemiplegia, hemianopia
Lacunar syndrome (pure motor stroke) (LACS)	Hemiplegia alone
Posterior circulation syndrome (POCS)	Brain-stem symptoms ± hemianopia ± hemiplegia Hemianopia alone

'lacunar' infarctions. Perhaps 5% are due to rare causes, including vasculitis, endocarditis and cerebral venous disease. Risk factors for ischaemic stroke are similar to those for coronary artery disease (p. 229).

INTRACEREBRAL HAEMORRHAGE (15%)

This usually results from rupture of a blood vessel within the brain parenchyma: a primary intracerebral haemorrhage. It may also occur in a patient with a subarachnoid haemorrhage if the artery ruptures into the brain substance as well as the subarachnoid space. Haemorrhage frequently occurs into an area of brain infarction; if large, it may be difficult to distinguish from primary intracerebral haemorrhage. Risk factors for intracerebral haemorrhage include:

• Age. • Hypertension. • Anticoagulant therapy. • Intracranial vascular malformations. • Substance abuse.

INVESTIGATION OF ACUTE STROKE

Investigation aims to confirm the vascular nature of the lesion, distinguish cerebral infarction from haemorrhage and identify the underlying vascular disease and risk factors (Box 16.15). Further investigations are indicated if the nature of the stroke is uncertain, especially for younger patients who are less likely to have atherosclerotic disease.

Imaging the brain

Brain imaging should be performed in all patients. CT is the most practical and widely available (Fig. 16.9). It will usually exclude non-stroke lesions (subdural haematomas and brain tumours) and demonstrate intracerebral haemorrhage. CT changes in cerebral infarction may be absent within the first few hours after symptom onset. For most purposes, a CT scan within the first day or so is adequate. However, an immediate CT scan is essential if the patient has abnormal coagulation, a progressing deficit or suspected cerebellar haematoma, or if thrombolysis is planned.

16.15 INVESTIGATION OF A PATIENT WITH AN ACUTE STROKE	
Is it a vascular lesion?	CT/MRI
Is it ischaemic or haemorrhagic?	CT/MRI
Is it a subarachnoid haemorrhage?	CT, lumbar puncture
Is there any cardiac source of embolism?	ECG, echocardiogram
What is the underlying vascular disease?	Duplex USS of carotids Magnetic resonance angiography (MRA) CT angiography (CTA) Contrast angiography
What are the risk factors?	FBC, cholesterol, glucose
Is there an unusual cause?	ESR, clotting/thrombophilia screen

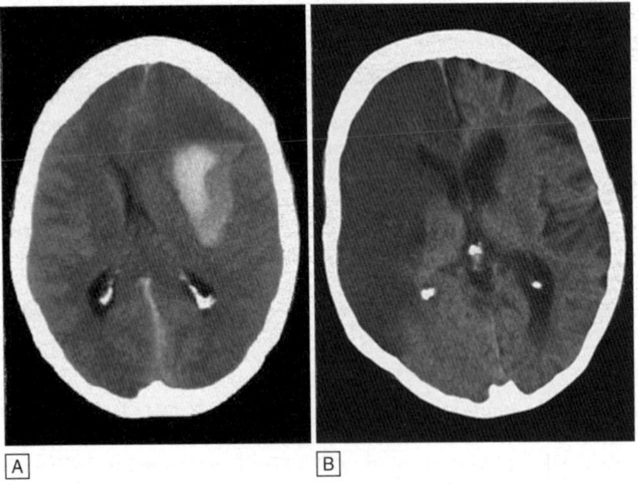

Fig. 16.9 CT scans in stroke. A Large intracerebral haemorrhage with mass effects. B Large middle and anterior cerebral artery territory infarct with mass effect. (Courtesy of Dr A. Farrell and Professor J. Wardlaw.)

Imaging blood vessels

Detection of extracranial vascular disease can help establish why the patient has had an ischaemic stroke and may lead on to specific treatments including carotid endarterectomy to reduce the risk of further stroke. A carotid bruit is not a reliable indicator of the degree of carotid stenosis. Extracranial arterial disease can be non-invasively identified with duplex USS, MR angiography or CT angiography.

Detecting a cardiac source of embolism

The most common causes of cardiac embolism are atrial fibrillation, prosthetic heart valves, other valvular abnormalities and recent myocardial infarction. A transthoracic or transoesophageal echocardiogram can identify an unsuspected source such as endocarditis, atrial myxoma, intracardiac thrombus or patent foramen ovale.

GENERAL MANAGEMENT OF PATIENTS WITH ACUTE STROKE

Management is aimed at minimising the volume of brain that is irreversibly damaged, preventing complications, reducing disability and handicap through rehabilitation, and reducing the risk of recurrent episodes. Early admission to a specialised stroke unit facilitates coordinated care from a multidisciplinary team and reduces mortality and residual disability amongst survivors. In the acute phase it may be useful to refer to a checklist (Box 16.16) to ensure that all the factors which might influence outcome have been addressed.

The deteriorating stroke patient

Neurological deficits may worsen during the hours or days after their onset. This is most common with lacunar infarction but may occur in other patients, due to extension of the area of infarction, haemorrhage into it or the development of oedema with consequent mass effect. It is important to distinguish this from deterioration caused by complications (hypoxia, sepsis, seizures, metabolic abnormalities), which may be more easily reversed. Patients with cerebellar haematomas or infarcts with mass effect may develop obstructive hydrocephalus and might benefit from insertion of a ventricular drain and/or decompressive surgery. Patients with massive cerebral oedema may benefit from anti-oedema agents (mannitol), artificial ventilation and/or surgical decompression to reduce intracranial pressure, although evidence for these interventions is still incomplete.

Specific medical treatment for ischaemic stroke

Thrombolysis and other revascularisation treatments: I.V. thrombolysis with recombinant tissue plasminogen activator (rt-PA) increases the risk of haemorrhagic transformation of the cerebral infarct with potentially fatal results. However, if given within 3 hrs of symptom onset to highly selected patients, the haemorrhagic risk may be offset by an improvement in overall outcome.

Aspirin: Aspirin (300 mg daily) should be started immediately after an ischaemic stroke unless rt-PA has been given, in which case it should be withheld for at least 24 hrs. Aspirin reduces the risk of early recurrence and improves long-term outcome.

Specific treatment for haemorrhagic stroke

Coagulation abnormalities, most commonly due to oral anticoagulants, should be reversed immediately to reduce the likelihood of the haematoma enlarging.

16.16 ACUTE STROKE MANAGEMENT: ADMISSION CHECKLIST	
Airway	Can patient protect airway? Can he/she swallow without evidence of aspiration? Perform a swallow screen and keep patient nil by mouth if swallowing unsafe
Breathing	Check oxygen saturation Give supplementary oxygen if oxygen saturation <95%
Circulation	Are peripheral perfusion, pulse and BP adequate? Treat as appropriate
Hydration	Is patient dehydrated or unable to swallow? I.V. or NG fluids if swallow is unsafe
Nutrition	Consider nutritional supplements If dysphagia persists, start feeding via NG tube
Medication	If patient is dysphagic, consider alternative routes for essential medications
BP	Unless there is heart failure/renal failure/hypertensive encephalopathy/aortic dissection, do not lower BP in 1st wk, as it will often return towards patient's normal level within a few days Early BP reduction may decrease cerebral perfusion and increase infarction
Blood glucose	Is blood glucose ≥11.1 mmol/l? Hyperglycaemia may increase infarct volume; therefore use insulin (via infusion or glucose/potassium/insulin (GKI)) to normalise levels
Temperature	Is patient pyrexial? Investigate and treat any cause but give antipyretics early
Pressure areas	Formally assess and reduce risk Treat infection, maintain nutrition, provide a pressure-relieving mattress and turn immobile patients regularly
Incontinence	Ensure patient is not constipated or in urinary retention Avoid catheterisation unless acute retention or incontinence threatening pressure areas

Reducing the risk of further strokes and other vascular problems

The average risk of a further stroke is 5–10% within the first week of a stroke or TIA, 15% in the first year and 5%/yr thereafter. Patients with ischaemic events should be put on long-term antiplatelet drugs and statins to lower cholesterol. For patients in atrial fibrillation the risk can be reduced by ~60% by oral anticoagulation to achieve an INR of 2–3. The risk of recurrence after both ischaemic and haemorrhagic strokes can be reduced by BP reduction.

Carotid endarterectomy and angioplasty: Patients with a carotid territory ischaemic event and >70% carotid artery stenosis on the side of the brain lesion have a higher risk of stroke recurrence. For those without major residual disability, removal of the stenosis reduces the overall risk of recurrence, although the operation itself carries a 5% risk of stroke. Carotid angioplasty and stenting are technically feasible but the long-term effects are unclear.

SUBARACHNOID HAEMORRHAGE

About 85% of cases of spontaneous arterial bleeding into the subarachnoid space are caused by rupture of saccular ('berry') aneurysms at bifurcations of the cerebral arteries; 10% are non-aneurysmal haemorrhages; and 5% are due to rarities (arteriovenous malformations, vertebral artery dissection). Subarachnoid haemorrhage is rare (incidence 6/100 000); about three-quarters are <65 yrs and women are more frequently affected.

Clinical features

• There is typically a sudden, severe 'thunderclap' headache (often occipital) which lasts for hours or even days, often accompanied by vomiting. • Physical exertion, straining and sexual excitement are common antecedents. • Usually the patient is distressed and irritable, with photophobia, but there may be loss of consciousness. • Neck stiffness, focal hemisphere signs and subhyaloid haemorrhage on fundoscopy may be found.

Investigations

• All patients with a sudden severe headache require urgent CT to exclude a subarachnoid haemorrhage. • If the CT scan is negative (up to 15% of subarachnoid haemorrhages), then CSF should be obtained by LP at least 12 hrs after symptom onset to detect blood and xanthochromia. • If the CT scan and CSF at 12 hrs are negative, then subarachnoid haemorrhage can be excluded.

Management and prognosis

• The immediate mortality is ~30%. • Endovascular insertion of coils into an aneurysm or surgical clipping of the aneurysm neck reduces recurrence. • Nimodipine (60 mg) is given to prevent vasospasm in the acute phase. • Survivors have a re-bleed rate of 40% in the first 4 wks and 3% annually thereafter.

CEREBRAL VENOUS DISEASE

Thrombosis of cerebral veins and venous sinuses is relatively uncommon. Predisposing systemic causes include:

• Dehydration. • Pregnancy. • Thrombophilia. • Oral contraceptives. • Hypotension.

Local causes include:

• Paranasal sinusitis. • Meningitis. • Facial skin infection. • Otitis media, mastoiditis. • Penetrating head/eye wounds. • Skull fracture.

Anticoagulation is usually given, and management of underlying causes and complications is important.

CORTICAL VEIN THROMBOSIS

This may present with focal cortical deficits (aphasia, hemiparesis) or epilepsy, according to the area involved.

CEREBRAL VENOUS SINUS THROMBOSIS

• Cavernous sinus thrombosis causes proptosis, ptosis, headache, ophthalmoplegias, papilloedema and numbness in the trigeminal first division dermatome. • Superior sagittal sinus thrombosis causes headache, papilloedema and seizures. • Transverse sinus thrombosis causes hemiparesis, seizures and papilloedema.

About 10% of cases are associated with infection and require antibiotics; otherwise treatment is by anticoagulation.

SUBDURAL HAEMATOMA

This is a collection of blood between the dura and the surface of the brain, due to rupture of veins on the brain surface. It usually follows trauma but may occur spontaneously, particularly with anticoagulants. It is common in the elderly and in patients who misuse alcohol. Patients present with subacute impairment of brain function, both globally (obtundation, coma) and focally (hemiparesis, seizures). CT is the investigation of choice, and management entails surgical drainage, usually via a burr hole.

INFLAMMATORY DISEASES

MULTIPLE SCLEROSIS (MS)

In MS the myelin-producing oligodendrocytes of the CNS are the target of recurrent cell-mediated autoimmune attack. In the UK the prevalence is 120/100 000, with an annual incidence of 7/100 000. The incidence is higher at temperate than equatorial latitudes, and the disease is twice as common in women as men. Although the exact cause is uncertain, an interplay of genetic and environmental factors probably occurs. The risk of familial recurrence is 15%. Histologically, the characteristic lesion is a plaque of demyelination in the periventricular regions of the brain, the optic nerves or the subpial regions of the spinal cord.

Clinical features

Diagnosis requires the demonstration of lesions in more than one anatomical site at more than one time for which there is no other explanation. There are several recognisable clinical courses:

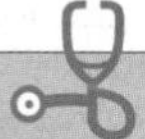

16.17 CLINICAL FEATURES OF MS
Common presentations of MS
• Optic neuritis • Relapsing and remitting sensory symptoms • Subacute painless spinal cord lesion • Acute brain-stem syndrome • Subacute loss of function of upper limb (dorsal column deficit) • 6th cranial nerve palsy
Other symptoms and syndromes suggestive of CNS demyelination
• Afferent pupillary defect and optic atrophy (previous optic neuritis) • Lhermitte's symptom (tingling in spine or limbs on neck flexion) • Progressive non-compressive paraparesis • Partial Brown-Séquard syndrome • Internuclear ophthalmoplegia with ataxia • Postural ('rubral', 'Holmes') tremor • Trigeminal neuralgia under the age of 50 • Recurrent facial palsy

• Relapsing and remitting clinical course (80%) with variable recovery. • Primary progressive clinical course (10–20%). • Secondary progressive disease (supersedes relapse and remission phase). • Fulminant disease (<10%), leading to early death.

There are a number of clinical syndromes suggestive of multiple sclerosis (Box 16.17).

Demyelinating lesions cause symptoms and signs that come on over days or weeks and resolve over weeks or months. Frequent relapses with incomplete recovery indicate a poor prognosis. In a minority, there is an interval of years between attacks, and in some there is no recurrence. The physical signs depend on the anatomical site of demyelination. Combinations of spinal cord and brain-stem signs are common, maybe with evidence of previous optic neuritis. Significant intellectual impairment is unusual until late in the disease.

Investigations

There is no specific test for MS, and the clinical diagnosis should be supported by investigations to:

• Exclude other conditions. • Provide evidence for an inflammatory disorder. • Identify multiple sites of neurological involvement.

Visual evoked potentials: Detect clinically silent lesions in up to 70% of patients.

CSF examination: Lymphocytic pleocytosis in acute phase and oligoclonal bands of IgG in 70–90% of patients between attacks. Oligoclonal bands denote intrathecal inflammation and occur in a range of other disorders.

MRI: Provides images of lesions in both brain and spinal cord, and excludes other causes of the neurological deficit (Fig. 16.10). However, appearances may be confused with cerebrovascular disease or cerebral vasculitis.

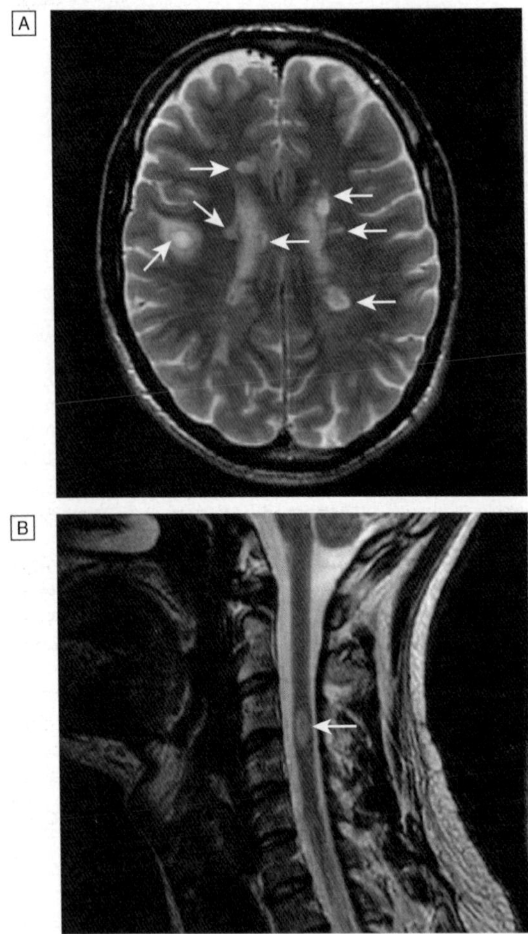

Fig. 16.10 Multiple sclerosis. A Brain MRI in MS: multiple high-signal lesions (arrows) are seen particularly in the paraventricular region on T2 image. B Demyelinating lesion in cervical spinal cord: high-signal T2 images (sagittal plane).

16.18 TREATMENT OF COMPLICATIONS OF MS	
Spasticity	Physiotherapy Baclofen 15–100 mg*, tizanidine 18–32 mg Local injection of botulinum toxin, chemical neuronectomy
Ataxia	Isoniazid 600–1200 mg*, clonazepam 2–8 mg*
Dysaesthesia	Carbamazepine 200–1800 mg*, gabapentin 900–2400 mg, phenytoin 200–400 mg, amitriptyline 10–100 mg
Bladder symptoms	Anticholinergics for hypertonic bladder, intermittent catheterisation
Fatigue	Amantadine 100–300 mg, modafinil 100–400 mg, amitriptyline 10–50 mg
Impotence	Sildenafil 50–100 mg/24 hrs
*In divided doses.	

Management

This involves:

• Treatment of the acute relapse. • Prevention of future relapses. • Treatment of complications. • Management of disability.

Acute relapse: Pulses of high-dose methylprednisolone, either i.v. (1 g daily for 3 days) or orally (500 mg daily for 5 days), shorten the duration of relapse but do not affect long-term outcome. Pulses of steroids can be given up to three times in a year but should be restricted to significant function-threatening deficits.

Preventing relapses: Immunosuppressive agents, including azathioprine, have some effect in reducing relapses and improving long-term outcome. In relapsing and remitting MS, interferon beta-1a/b reduces relapses by some 30%, with a small effect on long-term disability; glatiramer acetate has similar effects.

Complications: Treatment of complications is summarised in Box 16.18. Specialist nurses are of great value in managing the chronic phase of the disease. Physiotherapy and occupational therapy may improve functional capacity in patients who become disabled. Bladder care is particularly important. Urgency and frequency may be treated pharmacologically, but this may lead to retention and infection. Retention can be managed initially by intermittent urinary catheterisation but an indwelling catheter may become necessary.

Prognosis

This is difficult to predict, especially early in the disease:

• ~15% of those having one attack of demyelination do not suffer further events. • Those with relapsing and remitting symptoms have about 1–2 relapses every 2 yrs. • After 10 yrs about one-third of patients are sufficiently disabled to need help with walking.

ACUTE DISSEMINATED ENCEPHALOMYELITIS

This is an acute monophasic condition with areas of perivenous demyelination throughout the brain and spinal cord. The illness often occurs a week or so after a viral infection (e.g. measles, chickenpox, recent vaccination), suggesting that it is immunologically mediated.

Clinical features

• Headache, vomiting, pyrexia, confusion and meningism, often with focal brain and spinal cord signs. • Possibly, seizures or coma.

Investigations

• MRI shows multiple high-signal areas in a pattern similar to that of MS. • CSF may be normal or show an increase in protein and lymphocytes; oligoclonal bands may be found acutely but do not persist on recovery (unlike in MS).

Management

• The disease may be fatal in the acute stages but is otherwise self-limiting. • A minority have recurrent episodes. • Treatment is with high-dose i.v. methylprednisolone.

ACUTE TRANSVERSE MYELITIS

Transverse myelitis is an acute, monophasic, inflammatory demyelinating disorder affecting the spinal cord. Patients present with a subacute paraparesis with a sensory level, often with severe neck or back pain at onset. MRI is needed to distinguish this from a compressive spinal cord lesion. CSF examination shows cellular pleocytosis and oligoclonal bands are usually absent. Treatment is with high-dose i.v. methylprednisolone. The outcome is variable; in some cases, near-complete recovery occurs despite a severe initial deficit. Some patients go on to develop MS in later years.

DEGENERATIVE DISEASES

• Degeneration of the cerebral cortex causes dementia. • Degeneration of the basal ganglia results in movement disorder. • Cerebellar degeneration usually causes ataxia. • Degeneration can also occur in the spinal cord or peripheral nerves, giving rise to motor, sensory or autonomic disturbance.

DEGENERATIVE CAUSES OF DEMENTIA

As many as 5% of the population >65 yrs of age suffer from a dementing illness. Over the age of 80, this rises to >20%.

ALZHEIMER'S DISEASE

This is the most common cause of dementia. About 15% of cases are familial. The brain is atrophic, with senile plaques and neurofibrillary tangles in the cerebral cortex. Many different neurotransmitter abnormalities have been described, in particular impairment of cholinergic transmission.

Clinical features

• Patients present with gradual impairment of memory, usually in association with disorders of other cortical functions. Both short-term and long-term memory are affected. • Later in the disease, patients commonly deny their disabilities, and typical features are apraxia, visuo-spatial impairment, depression and aphasia.

Investigations and management

• Investigation is aimed at excluding other treatable causes of dementia, such as chronic subdural haematoma, infections (syphilis, HIV), thiamine or B_{12} deficiency, or hydrocephalus. • Anticholinesterases (donepezil, rivastigmine, galantamine) and the NMDA receptor antagonist memantine may be of modest benefit in mild to moderate disease. • Depression should be treated with antidepressants. • Support for carers is crucial.

OTHER DEGENERATIVE CAUSES OF DEMENTIA

WERNICKE–KORSAKOFF DISEASE

Thiamine (vitamin B_1) deficiency presents with an acute confusional state (Wernicke's encephalopathy) and brain-stem abnormalities (ataxia, nystagmus, extraocular muscle weakness). If this is inadequately treated, it results in a profound disturbance of short-term memory with a tendency to confabulate (Korsakoff's syndrome). The deficiency can arise as a result of malnutrition (particularly in chronic alcohol misuse). It must be considered in any confused patient; if in doubt, treat anyway. Treatment consists of i.v. thiamine (Pabrinex, 2 vials 8-hourly for 48 hrs), followed by oral thiamine (100 mg 8-hourly), in addition to treating the underlying cause.

PICK'S DISEASE

In this rare condition degeneration affects frontal and temporal lobes. Patients present with personality change or progressive aphasia. Memory is relatively preserved in the early stages. There is no specific treatment.

LEWY BODY DEMENTIA

Pathology similar to Parkinson's disease is found in the cerebral cortex. This condition presents as cognitive impairment in the context of an extrapyramidal syndrome. Patients' cognitive state often fluctuates and there may be visual hallucinations. They are particularly sensitive to the side-effects of anti-parkinsonian medication. There may be clinical benefit with anticholinesterase agents.

PARKINSON'S DISEASE AND AKINETIC-RIGID SYNDROMES

Several degenerative diseases affect the basal ganglia, presenting with differing combinations of bradykinesia, rigidity, tremor and loss of postural reflexes. The most common cause of these parkinsonian or akinetic-rigid syndromes is idiopathic Parkinson's disease.

IDIOPATHIC PARKINSON'S DISEASE

The incidence and prevalence increase with age, the latter rising to >1% in those >60 yrs. Sex incidence is equal. It is less common in cigarette smokers. Depletion of the dopaminergic neurons in the substantia nigra leads to reduced inhibition of the subthalamic nucleus. This becomes more active in inhibiting cortical activation, resulting in bradykinesia.

Clinical features

The presentation is usually unilateral: e.g. a resting tremor in an upper limb. Typical features of an established case include:

• Resting tremor (4–6 Hz), diminished on action: starts in fingers/thumb, may affect arms, legs, feet, jaw, tongue. • Rigidity: cogwheel type mostly affects upper limbs; plastic (lead-pipe) type mostly affects legs. • Bradykinesia: slowness in initiating or repeating movements, impaired fine movements, expressionless face. • Gait: slow to start walking, reduced arm swing, rapid small steps, tendency to run (festination).

The classical features may be absent initially, but non-specific tiredness, mental slowness, depression and small handwriting (micrographia) may be noticed. One-third of patients develop cognitive impairment as the disease progresses.

Investigations

• Diagnosis is made clinically. • Patients <50 yrs are usually tested for Wilson's disease. • Brain imaging may be needed if any features suggest pyramidal, cerebellar or autonomic involvement, or if the diagnosis is in doubt.

Management: drug therapy (see also p. 783)

Levodopa: This provides the mainstay of treatment together with a peripheral-acting dopa-decarboxylase inhibitor. Therapy should be delayed until there is significant disability. Decarboxylase inhibitors (carbidopa and benserazide) reduce peripheral side-effects and are available as combination preparations with levodopa (Sinemet and Madopar). Levodopa is particularly effective at improving bradykinesia and rigidity. Side-effects are: • Postural hypotension. • Nausea and vomiting. • Involuntary movements (orofacial dyskinesias, limb and axial dystonias). • Occasionally depression, hallucinations and delusions.

Late deterioration despite levodopa occurs after 3–5 yrs in up to 50% of patients. The simplest form is end-of-dose deterioration; this may be improved by using smaller, more frequent doses or a slow-release preparation. More complex fluctuations present as periods of severe parkinsonism alternating with dyskinesia and agitation (the 'on-off' phenomenon).

Anticholinergic agents (e.g. trihexyphenidyl, orphenadrine): These help tremor and rigidity, but not bradykinesia. Side-effects are:

• Confusion and hallucinations in the elderly. • Dry mouth. • Blurred vision. • Difficulty with micturition. • Constipation.

Amantadine: This has a mild, short-lived effect on bradykinesia, but may be useful early in the disease. It can help control the dyskinesias produced by dopaminergic treatment later in the disease. Side-effects are:

• Livedo reticularis. • Peripheral oedema. • Confusion and seizures.

Selegiline: Has a mild therapeutic effect in its own right. Evidence that it slows the progression of the disease is highly controversial.

COMT (catechol-O-methyl-transferase) inhibitors: When used with levodopa, entacapone prolongs the effects of each dose and reduces motor fluctuations. This allows the levodopa dose to be reduced.

Dopamine receptor agonists: Apomorphine alone causes marked vomiting and has to be administered parenterally with concomitant antiemetic medication (e.g. domperidone). More easily administered oral drugs include bromocriptine, pergolide, cabergoline, ropinirole and pramipexole. These are less powerful than levodopa but cause fewer dose fluctuations or dyskinesia. Side-effects are:

• Nausea. • Vomiting. • Confusion. • Hallucinations.

Management: non-pharmacological

Surgery: Stereotactic thalamotomy can treat tremor (rarely needed). Other stereotactic lesions are currently undergoing evaluation.

Physiotherapy and speech therapy: Physiotherapy reduces rigidity and corrects abnormal posture. Speech therapy may help dysarthria and dysphonia.

Prognosis

If symptoms start in middle life, the disease is usually slowly progressive and likely to shorten lifespan. Onset after 70 is unlikely to shorten life or become severe.

OTHER AKINETIC-RIGID SYNDROMES

Many conditions can manifest as parkinsonian syndromes:

• Other degenerative diseases (e.g. Huntington's disease, Wilson's disease (p. 509)). • Infective diseases (e.g. syphilis). • Drug-induced parkinsonism (neuroleptic agents, antiemetics).

Several specific degenerative conditions mimic idiopathic Parkinson's disease, particularly in the early stages. About 10% of those thought to have idiopathic Parkinson's disease have one of these variants, which cause rapid clinical deterioration and are more resistant to dopaminergic medication.

Multiple systems atrophy (previously Shy–Drager syndrome)

Features of parkinsonism are combined with degrees of autonomic failure, cerebellar involvement and pyramidal tract dysfunction. Diagnosis is assisted by autonomic function tests. Falls are more common than in idiopathic Parkinson's disease, and life expectancy is reduced.

Progressive supranuclear palsy

Clinical features include parkinsonism (rigidity in extension rather than flexion) with supranuclear paralysis of eye movements. Other features are pyramidal signs and cognitive impairment.

HUNTINGTON'S DISEASE

This is an autosomal dominant inherited disorder usually starting in adult life. It is due to expansion of a trinucleotide repeat on chromosome 4 and frequently demonstrates anticipation (younger age of onset in subsequent generations).

Clinical features

• Gradually progressive chorea is the earliest symptom. • This is accompanied by cognitive impairment which later becomes frank dementia. • Seizures may occur late in the disease.

Investigations

• The diagnosis is made clinically, supported by atrophy of the caudate nucleus on CT/MRI. • DNA analysis can confirm the diagnosis and provide pre-symptomatic testing for family members after counselling.

Management

• Chorea may respond to tetrabenazine or dopamine antagonists. • Long-term psychological support and eventually institutional care are often needed. • Depressive symptoms are common and may be helped by antidepressant medication. • Genetic counselling is needed for relatives.

HEREDITARY ATAXIAS

This is a group of inherited disorders in which degenerative changes occur to varying extents in the cerebellum, brain stem, pyramidal tracts, spinocerebellar tracts, and optic and peripheral nerves. They present in childhood with ataxia and a variety of associated neurological symptoms and signs. Genetic testing facilitates diagnosis and counselling in some.

MOTOR NEURON DISEASE

In this disease there is progressive degeneration of motor neurons in the spinal cord and cranial nerve nuclei, and of pyramidal neurons in the motor cortex. About 5% of cases are familial (autosomal dominant); for the remaining 95% the cause is unknown. The prevalence is 5/100 000. Onset

16.19 PATTERNS OF INVOLVEMENT OF MOTOR NEURON DISEASE 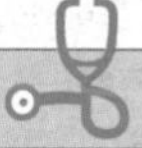
Progressive muscular atrophy
• Predominantly spinal motor neurons affected • Weakness and wasting of distal limb muscles at first • Fasciculation in muscles; tendon reflexes may be absent
Progressive bulbar palsy
• Early involvement of tongue, palate and pharyngeal muscles (dysarthria/dysphagia) • Wasting and fasciculation of tongue (there may be pyramidal signs as well)
Amyotrophic lateral sclerosis
• Combination of distal and proximal muscle-wasting and weakness, fasciculation • Spasticity, ↑ reflexes, extensor plantars; bulbar/pseudobulbar palsy follow eventually • Pyramidal tract features may predominate

is usually after the age of 50 yrs and is very uncommon before the age of 30 yrs. Males are more commonly affected.

Clinical features

• Patients present with a combination of lower and upper motor neuron signs without sensory involvement. • The presence of brisk reflexes in wasted fasciculating limb muscles is typical. • There may also be dysarthria or dysphagia, but there is usually no intellectual impairment. • Symptoms often begin focally, then spread gradually but relentlessly to become widespread. • Three common patterns of involvement are described in Box 16.19.

Investigations

• The diagnosis is clinical. • Exclude potentially treatable disorders (diabetic amyotrophy, spinal disorders, multifocal motor neuronopathy). • EMG helps confirm fasciculation and denervation. • Spinal and brain imaging exclude focal spinal or cerebral disease.

Management and prognosis

• The glutamate antagonist, riluzole, may prolong life expectancy by ~2 mths. • Psychological and physical support (occupational therapy, speech therapy, physiotherapy) is essential. • Feeding by percutaneous gastrostomy may be necessary if bulbar palsy is marked. • Non-invasive ventilatory support may help distress from weak respiratory muscles. • The mean time from diagnosis to death is 1 yr, with most patients dying within 3–5 yrs of the onset of symptoms. • Death is usually from respiratory infection and failure.

INFECTIONS OF THE NERVOUS SYSTEM

MENINGITIS

Acute infection of the meninges presents with pyrexia, headache and meningism. Meningism, which can occur in other situations (e.g. subarachnoid haemorrhage), consists of stiffness of the neck. Abnormalities in the CSF (Box 16.20) are helpful in distinguishing the cause of meningitis. Causes are listed in Box 16.21.

VIRAL MENINGITIS

Viral infection is the most common cause of meningitis.

Clinical features

The condition occurs mainly in children or young adults, with acute headache, irritability and meningism. In viral meningitis, the headache is usually the most severe feature.

Investigations

• CSF contains an excess of lymphocytes, but glucose and protein are commonly normal or the protein may be raised. • This picture can also be found in partially treated bacterial meningitis.

Management

• No specific treatment. • Usually benign and self-limiting. • Treat symptomatically in a quiet environment. • Recovery usually occurs within days.

Meningitis may also occur as a complication of viral infection in other organs (e.g. mumps, measles, infectious mononucleosis, herpes zoster and hepatitis). Complete recovery without specific therapy is the rule.

PYOGENIC BACTERIAL MENINGITIS

Many bacteria can cause meningitis and certain organisms are particularly common at different ages (see Box 16.22 below). Bacterial meningitis is usually secondary to a bacteraemic illness, although infection may result from a focus of infection in the ear, skull fracture or sinus. Bacterial meningitis has become less common but the mortality and morbidity remain significant. The meningococcus *(Neisseria meningitidis)* is second to *Streptococcus pneumoniae* as the most common cause in Western Europe.

Epidemics of meningococcal meningitis occur, particularly in cramped living conditions or where the climate is hot and dry. In pneumococcal and *Haemophilus* infections there may be associated otitis media. Pneumococcal meningitis may be associated with pneumonia and occurs especially in older patients and alcoholics. *Listeria monocytogenes* has emerged as an increasing cause of meningitis and brain-stem encephalitis in the immunosuppressed, people with diabetes, alcoholics and pregnant women.

16.20 CSF INDICES IN MENINGITIS*

Condition	Cell type	Cell count	Glucose	Protein	Gram stain
Normal	Lymphocytes	$0–4 \times 10^6$/l	>60% of blood glc	Up to 0.45 g/l	–
Viral	Lymphocytes	10–2000	Normal	Normal	–
Bacterial	Polymorphs	1000–5000	Low	Normal/elevated	+
Tuberculous	Mixed	50–5000	Low	Elevated	Often –
Fungal	Lymphocytes	50–500	Low	Elevated	±
Malignant	Lymphocytes	0–100	Low	Normal/elevated	–

16.21 CAUSES OF MENINGITIS

Infective	Bacteria	Adults: *Streptococcus pneumoniae, Neisseria meningitidis, Mycobacterium tuberculosis* Young children: *H. influenzae, Strep. pneumoniae, N. meningitidis* Neonates: Gram –ve bacilli, group B streptococci, *Listeria monocytogenes*
	Viruses	Enteroviruses (echo, Coxsackie, polio), mumps, influenza Herpes simplex, varicella zoster, Epstein–Barr, HIV
	Protozoa and parasites	*Toxoplasma, Amoeba, Cysticercus*
	Fungi	*Cryptococcus, Candida, Histoplasma*
Non-infective ('sterile')	Malignant disease	Breast cancer, bronchial cancer, leukaemia, lymphoma
	Inflammatory disease (may be recurrent)	Sarcoidosis, SLE, Behçet's disease

16.22 CHEMOTHERAPY OF BACTERIAL MENINGITIS WHEN CAUSE IS KNOWN

Pathogen	Regimen of choice	Alternative agent(s)
N. meningitidis	Benzylpenicillin 2.4 g i.v. 4-hourly for 5–7 days	Cefuroxime, ampicillin Chloramphenicol*
Strep. pneumoniae (sensitive to β-lactams)	Cefotaxime 2 g i.v. 6-hourly or ceftriaxone 2 g i.v. 12-hourly for 10–14 days	Chloramphenicol*
Strep. pneumoniae (resistant to β-lactams)	Add vancomycin 1 g i.v. 12-hourly or rifampicin 600 mg i.v. 12-hourly	Vancomycin + rifampicin*
H. influenzae	Cefotaxime 2 g i.v. 6-hourly or ceftriaxone 2 g i.v. 12-hourly for 10–14 days	Chloramphenicol*
L. monocytogenes	Ampicillin 2 g i.v. 4-hourly plus gentamicin 5 mg/kg i.v. daily	Ampicillin + co-trimoxazole 50 mg/kg daily

*For patients with a history of anaphylaxis to β-lactam antibiotics.

Clinical features

• Headache, drowsiness, fever and neck stiffness are the usual presenting features. • Meningococcal meningitis is associated with a purpuric rash in 70% of cases. • When accompanied by septicaemia, it may present very rapidly, with abrupt obtundation due to cerebral oedema and circulatory collapse.

Investigations

CT head: If there is drowsiness, focal neurological signs or seizures, CT is required prior to LP to exclude a mass lesion (there is a risk of coning if LP is performed in the presence of raised intracranial pressure).

LP: CSF is cloudy due to neutrophils. Protein is significantly elevated and glucose is reduced. A Gram film and culture may identify the organism.

Other: Blood cultures may be positive. PCR of blood and CSF can identify bacterial DNA.

Management

• If bacterial meningitis is suspected, the patient should be given parenteral antibiotics immediately and admitted to hospital. • Before the cause of meningitis is known, patients with a typical meningococcal rash should receive benzylpenicillin (2.4 g i.v. 4-hourly); those without a typical rash should be given cefotaxime (2 g i.v. 6-hourly) or ceftriaxone (2 g i.v. 12-hourly). • The antibiotic regimen may be modified after CSF examination, depending on the infecting organism (Box 16.22). • Adjunctive corticosteroid therapy is useful in both children and adults.

Prevention of meningococcal infection

• Close contacts of patients with meningococcal infections (especially children) should be given 2 days of oral rifampicin. • In adults, a single dose of ciprofloxacin is an alternative. • If not treated with ceftriaxone, patients should be given similar treatment to clear nasopharyngeal carriage. • Vaccines are available for the prevention of disease caused by meningococci of groups A and C.

TUBERCULOUS MENINGITIS

Tuberculous meningitis remains common in developing countries and is seen more frequently as a secondary infection in AIDS. It occurs most frequently shortly after a primary infection in childhood or as part of miliary TB. The usual source of infection is a caseous focus in the meninges or brain.

Clinical features

• Symptoms include headache, low-grade fever, vomiting, lassitude, depression, confusion and behavioural changes. • Signs include meningism, oculomotor palsies, papilloedema, reduced conscious level and focal hemisphere signs.

Investigations

• CSF is under increased pressure and contains up to 5×10^8 cells/litre, predominantly lymphocytes. • There is elevated protein and markedly reduced glucose. • CSF culture takes up to 6 wks so treatment must be started empirically. • Brain imaging may show hydrocephalus, brisk meningeal enhancement on enhanced CT, and/or an intracranial tuberculoma.

Management and prognosis

• Chemotherapy should be started with a regimen including pyrazinamide. • Corticosteroids are controversial; they may improve mortality but not focal neurological damage. • Surgical ventricular drainage may be needed if obstructive hydrocephalus develops. • Untreated tuberculous meningitis is fatal. • Complete recovery is the rule if treatment is started before focal signs or stupor. • When treatment is started later, the recovery rate is <60% and survivors show permanent neurological deficit.

PARENCHYMAL VIRAL INFECTIONS

VIRAL ENCEPHALITIS

Only a minority of patients have a history of recent viral infection. In Europe, the most serious cause is herpes simplex. In some parts of the world, viruses transmitted by mosquitoes and ticks (arboviruses) are an important cause. Acute encephalitis may occur in HIV infection.

Clinical features

• Viral encephalitis presents with acute onset of headache, fever, focal neurological signs (aphasia and/or hemiplegia) and seizures. • Disturbance of consciousness ranging from drowsiness to deep coma supervenes early. • Meningism is common.

Investigations

• CT of the head (should precede LP) may show low-density lesions in the temporal lobes. • CSF usually contains excess lymphocytes but is occasionally normal. The protein may be elevated but the glucose is normal. • The EEG is usually abnormal in the early stages, especially in herpes simplex encephalitis. • Virological investigations of the CSF may reveal the causative organism but treatment should not await this.

Management

• Raised intracranial pressure is treated with dexamethasone (8 mg 12-hourly). • Herpes simplex encephalitis responds to aciclovir (10 mg/kg i.v. 8-hourly for 2–3 wks). This should be given early to all patients with suspected viral encephalitis. • Mortality is 10–30% and significant proportions of survivors have residual epilepsy or cognitive impairment.

BRAIN-STEM ENCEPHALITIS

This presents with ataxia, dysarthria, diplopia or other cranial nerve palsies. The CSF is lymphocytic, with a normal glucose. The causative agent is presumed to be viral. However, *L. monocytogenes* may cause a similar syndrome and requires specific treatment with ampicillin (500 mg 6-hourly).

RABIES

Rabies is caused by a rhabdovirus which infects the central nervous tissue and salivary glands of mammals, and is usually conveyed by saliva through bites. Humans are most frequently infected from dogs. The incubation period varies but is usually between 4 and 8 wks.

Clinical features

• A prodromal period of 1–10 days leads to 'hydrophobia'; although the patient is thirsty, drinking provokes violent contractions of the diaphragm and inspiratory muscles. • Delusions and hallucinations may develop, with lucid intervals. • Cranial nerve lesions and terminal hyperpyrexia are common. • Death ensues, usually within a week of symptoms.

Investigations

• The diagnosis is made on clinical grounds. • Rapid immunofluorescent techniques can detect antigen in corneal smears or skin biopsies.

Management

• A few patients have survived; all received post-exposure prophylaxis and needed intensive care facilities. • Only palliative treatment is possible once symptoms have appeared. • The patient should be heavily sedated with diazepam, supplemented by chlorpromazine if necessary.

Prevention

Pre-exposure prophylaxis: This is required by those who professionally handle potentially infected animals, work with rabies virus in laboratories or live at special risk in rabies-endemic areas. Protection is afforded by two injections of human diploid cell strain vaccine given 4 wks apart, followed by yearly boosters.

Post-exposure prophylaxis: The wounds should be cleaned, damaged tissues excised and the wound left unsutured. Rabies can usually be prevented if treatment is started within a day or two of biting. For maximum protection, hyperimmune serum (human rabies immune globulin) and vaccine (human diploid cell strain vaccine) are required.

POLIOMYELITIS

The disease is caused by one of three polioviruses. It is much less common in developed countries following the use of oral vaccines. Infection occurs through the nasopharynx, causing a lymphocytic meningitis and infecting the grey matter of the nervous system. There is a propensity to damage anterior horn cells.

Clinical features

• The incubation period is 7–14 days. • Many patients recover fully after a few days of mild fever and headache. • In others, there is recurrence of pyrexia, headache and meningism. • Weakness may start later and can progress to widespread paresis. • Respiratory failure may supervene if intercostal muscles or the medullary motor nuclei are involved.

Investigations

• CSF shows a lymphocytic pleocytosis, raised protein and normal glucose. • Poliomyelitis virus may be cultured from CSF and stool.

Management and prognosis

• Bed rest is imperative, as exercise appears to worsen or precipitate the paralysis. • A tracheostomy and ventilation are required for respiratory difficulties. • Subsequent treatment is by physiotherapy and orthopaedic measures. • Epidemics vary widely in mortality rate. • Death occurs from respiratory paralysis. • Gradual recovery may take place over several months. • Muscles showing no signs of recovery after 1 mth will probably not regain function. • Prevention is by immunisation with live (Sabin) vaccine.

SUBACUTE SCLEROSING PANENCEPHALITIS

This is a rare, chronic and progressive neurological disease caused by the measles virus. It occurs in children and adolescents, usually many years after the primary virus infection. The onset is insidious, with intellectual deterioration, apathy and clumsiness followed by myoclonic jerks, rigidity and dementia. The EEG is distinctive, with periodic bursts of triphasic waves. Antiviral therapy is ineffective and death ensues within years.

PROGRESSIVE MULTIFOCAL LEUCOENCEPHALOPATHY

This is an infection of oligodendrocytes by human polyomavirus JC, which causes widespread demyelination of the white matter of the cerebral hemispheres. It occurs most frequently as a feature of AIDS. Clinical signs include dementia, hemiparesis and aphasia, which progress rapidly, leading to death within weeks or months. MRI reveals diffuse high signal in the cerebral white matter.

PARENCHYMAL BACTERIAL INFECTIONS

CEREBRAL ABSCESS

The site of abscess formation and the causative organism are both related to the source of infection (Box 16.23).

Clinical features

• A cerebral abscess may present acutely with fever, headache, meningism and drowsiness, but more commonly presents over days or weeks as a cerebral mass lesion with little or no evidence of infection. • Seizures, raised intracranial pressure and focal hemisphere signs occur alone or in combination.

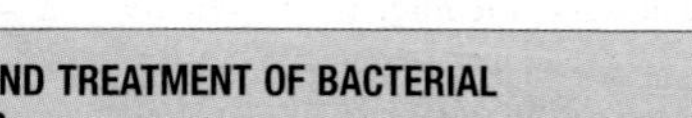
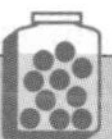

16.23 AETIOLOGY AND TREATMENT OF BACTERIAL CEREBRAL ABSCESS

Site of abscess	Source of infection	Likely organisms	Recommended treatment
Frontal lobe	Paranasal sinuses Teeth	Streptococci Anaerobes	Cefuroxime 1.5 g i.v. 8-hourly *plus* metronidazole 500 mg i.v. 8-hourly
Temporal lobe	Middle ear	Streptococci Enterobacteriaceae	Ampicillin 2–3 g i.v. 8-hourly *plus* metronidazole 500 mg i.v. 8-hourly *plus* either ceftazidime 2 g i.v. 8-hourly *or* gentamicin* 5 mg/kg i.v. daily
Cerebellum	Sphenoid sinus Mastoid/middle ear	*Pseudomonas* spp. Anaerobes	As for temporal lobe
Any site	Penetrating trauma	Staphylococci	Flucloxacillin 2–3 g i.v. 6-hourly *or* cefuroxime 1.5 g i.v. 8-hourly
Multiple	Metastatic and cryptogenic	Streptococci Anaerobes	Benzylpenicillin 1.8–2.4 g i.v. 6-hourly if endocarditis or cyanotic heart disease Otherwise cefuroxime 1.5 g i.v. 8-hourly *plus* metronidazole 500 mg i.v. 8-hourly

*Monitor gentamicin levels.

Investigations

• LP is potentially hazardous in the presence of raised intracranial pressure and CT should always precede it. • CT reveals single or multiple low-density areas, which show ring enhancement and surrounding cerebral oedema. • There may be an elevated WBC and ESR with active infection. • Cerebral toxoplasmosis or tuberculous disease secondary to HIV infection should always be considered.

Management and prognosis

• Antimicrobial therapy is indicated once the diagnosis is made. • Surgical treatment by burr-hole aspiration or excision may be necessary. • Anticonvulsants are often necessary, as epilepsy frequently develops. • The mortality rate remains high at 10–20%.

SPINAL EPIDURAL ABSCESS

The characteristic clinical features are pain in a root distribution and progressive transverse spinal cord syndrome with paraparesis, sensory impairment and sphincter dysfunction. Infection is usually haematogenous. Staphylococcal infection, often linked to i.v. drug misuse, has contributed to a marked rise in incidence. MRI or myelography should precede urgent neurosurgical intervention. Decompressive laminectomy with draining of the abscess relieves the pressure on the dura. This, together with appropriate antibiotics, may prevent complete and irreversible paraplegia.

TETANUS

This results from infection with *Clostridium tetani*, a commensal in the gut of humans and domestic animals, which is found in soil. Infection enters the body through wounds. It is rare in the UK but is a major killer in developing countries. Spores germinate and bacilli multiply in areas of tissue necrosis. The bacilli remain localised but produce an exotoxin with an affinity for motor nerve endings and cells. The anterior horn cells are affected, resulting in rigidity and convulsions. Symptoms appear from 2 days to several weeks after injury—the shorter the incubation period, the worse the prognosis.

Clinical features

• The most important early symptom is trismus—painless spasm of the masseter muscles ('lockjaw'). • The tonic rigidity spreads to the muscles of the face, neck and trunk. Contraction of facial muscles leads to the so-called 'risus sardonicus'. The back is usually slightly arched ('opisthotonus') and there is a board-like abdominal wall. • In more severe cases, painful violent spasms or convulsions can occur which may lead to exhaustion, asphyxia or aspiration pneumonia. • Autonomic involvement may cause cardiovascular complications such as hypertension.

Investigations and management

The diagnosis is made on clinical grounds. Treatment of an established case involves:

• Human tetanus antitoxin (3000 U i.v.) to neutralise absorbed toxin. • Débridement of wounds. • I.V. metronidazole or benzylpenicillin. • Nursing in a quiet room and avoidance of unnecessary stimuli. • Diazepam i.v. to control spasms; if ineffective, paralyse and ventilate the patient. • Fluid and nutritional support.

Prevention

• Active immunisation: must be given. • Débridement of contaminated injuries. • Penicillin (1.2 g injection followed by a 7-day oral course). • I.M. injection of 250 U of human tetanus antitoxin, along with toxoid (repeated at 1 and 6 mths). • If already immunised: only a booster of toxoid is required.

16.24 CLINICAL AND PATHOLOGICAL FEATURES OF NEUROSYPHILIS		
Type (interval from primary)	**Pathology**	**Clinical features**
Meningovascular (5 yrs)	Endarteritis obliterans Meningeal exudate Granuloma (gumma)	Stroke Cranial nerve palsies Seizures/mass lesion
General paralysis of the insane (5–15 yrs)	Degeneration in cerebral cortex/cerebral atrophy Thickened meninges	Dementia Tremor Bilateral upper motor signs
Tabes dorsalis (5–20 yrs)	Degeneration of sensory neurons Wasting of dorsal columns Optic atrophy	Lightning pains Sensory ataxia Visual failure Abdominal crises Incontinence Trophic changes

NEUROSYPHILIS

Neurosyphilis may involve the meninges, blood vessels and/or the brain and spinal cord. In developed countries syphilis is now most commonly seen in AIDS. Although rare, early diagnosis and treatment remain important.

Clinical features

The three most common presentations are summarised in Box 16.24. The 'Argyll Robertson' pupillary abnormality may accompany any neurosyphilitic syndrome; the pupils are small and react to convergence but not directly to light.

Investigations

• Routine screening is warranted in many neurological patients. • Serological tests are positive in most patients. • CSF examination is essential; active disease is suggested by an elevated cell count, and protein may be elevated.

Management

• Procaine benzylpenicillin and probenecid are given for 17 days. • Further courses must be given if symptoms persist/recur or if the CSF continues to show signs of active disease.

PRION DISEASES: TRANSMISSIBLE SPONGIFORM ENCEPHALOPATHIES

Transmissible spongiform encephalopathies are characterised by the histopathological triad of spongiform change, neuronal cell loss and brain gliosis. There is also deposition of an abnormal prion protein. These diseases can be transmitted by inoculation; they may also occur spontaneously or as an inherited disorder. Diseases affecting animals include bovine spongiform encephalopathies (BSE). In humans, the most common condition is Creutzfeldt–Jakob disease (CJD). Some 10% of cases arise due to a mutation in the gene coding for the prion protein. A variant form of CJD is probably due to the same agent which causes BSE.

CREUTZFELDT–JAKOB DISEASE (CJD)

Sporadic CJD usually occurs in middle-aged to elderly patients. Clinical features usually involve a rapidly progressive dementia, myoclonus and a characteristic EEG pattern (repetitive slow wave complexes). Death occurs after a mean of 4–6 mths. There is no known treatment.

Variant CJD

A variant of CJD has been described in a few patients, mostly in the UK. The causative agent appears identical to that causing BSE in cows, and the disease may have appeared as a result of the BSE epidemic in the UK in the 1980s. Affected patients are typically younger than those with sporadic CJD and present with neuropsychiatric changes and sensory symptoms in the limbs, followed by ataxia, dementia and death (mean time to death is over a year). Characteristic EEG changes are not present but MRI scans show typical changes.

INTRACRANIAL MASS LESIONS AND RAISED INTRACRANIAL PRESSURE

Intracranial mass lesions may be:

• Traumatic: subdural or extradural haematoma. • Vascular: intracranial haemorrhage. • Infective: e.g. abscess, tuberculoma, cysticercosis. • Inflammatory: sarcoid. • Neoplastic: benign or malignant.

Symptoms and signs are produced by three distinct mechanisms:

• Direct effects on adjacent tissue. • Raised intracranial pressure. • False localising signs.

RAISED INTRACRANIAL PRESSURE

Raised intracranial pressure may be caused by:

• Mass lesions. • Cerebral oedema. • Obstruction to CSF circulation (causing hydrocephalus). • Impaired CSF absorption (idiopathic intracranial hypertension, cerebral venous obstruction).

Clinical features

• Headache, papilloedema, impaired consciousness and vomiting are typical features. • Impairment of conscious level is related to the level of intracranial pressure. • Cerebral mass lesions increase intracerebral pressure, but the amount by which the pressure is raised depends on the rate of growth of the mass. • Rapid growth does not allow compensatory mechanisms to take place, and so raised intracranial pressure develops early.

Management

This is largely dictated by the cause.

'CONING' AND FALSE LOCALISING SIGNS

The rise in intracranial pressure from a mass lesion may not be uniform; alterations in pressure relationships may displace the brain between its compartments.

• Downward displacement of the temporal lobes through the tentorium may cause 'temporal coning'. This may stretch the 3rd and/or 6th cranial nerves, or cause pressure on the contralateral cerebral peduncle (causing ipsilateral upper motor neuron signs). • Downward movement of the cerebellar tonsils through the foramen magnum may compress the medulla—'tonsillar coning'. • As coning progresses, the patient may adopt a decerebrate posture and, unless rapidly treated, death almost invariably ensues. • The process may be accelerated if pressure dynamics are suddenly disturbed by LP.

INTRACRANIAL NEOPLASMS

In the developed world, cerebral tumours account for 2% of deaths at all ages. The majority are metastatic from malignancies outside the nervous system.

PRIMARY AND SECONDARY BRAIN TUMOURS

Common sources of metastases from extracranial primary tumours are bronchus, breast and GI tract. Primary intracerebral tumours are classified by their cell of origin and degree of malignancy (Box 16.25). Even when malignant, they do not metastasise outside the nervous system.

Clinical features

• Headache is not invariable. • There may be symptoms of raised intracranial pressure. • Focal deficits are of slow onset and progressive. • The nature of the deficit depends on the site of the tumour. • Seizures are caused by tumour cells infiltrating an area of cerebral cortex which excites seizure activity.

Investigations

• CT or MRI allows localisation of the tumour and provides some guidance as to the likely histological type. • MRI is of particular value in posterior fossa/brain-stem tumours and in delineating tumours prior to surgery.

16.25 PRIMARY INTRACRANIAL TUMOURS

Histological type	Common site	Age
Malignant		
Glioma (astrocytoma)	Cerebral hemisphere	Adulthood
	Cerebellum	Childhood/adulthood
	Brain stem	Childhood/young adulthood
Oligodendroglioma	Cerebral hemisphere	Adulthood
Medulloblastoma	Posterior fossa	Childhood
Ependymoma	Posterior fossa	Childhood/adolescence
Cerebral lymphoma	Cerebral hemisphere	Adulthood
Benign		
Meningioma	Cortical dura, parasagittal, sphenoid ridge, suprasellar, olfactory groove	Adulthood
Neurofibroma	Acoustic neuroma	Adulthood
Craniopharyngioma	Suprasellar	Childhood/adolescence
Pituitary adenoma	Pituitary fossa	Adulthood
Colloid cyst	Third ventricle	Any age
Pineal tumours	Quadrigeminal cistern	Childhood (teratomas) Young adult (germ cell)

• Plain skull X-rays are rarely of value except in pituitary tumours. • CXR may reveal a primary tumour or other systemic malignancy.

Management

Medical: Dexamethasone (8 mg 12-hourly) lowers intracranial pressure by resolving the reactive oedema. In severely raised intracranial pressure, 16–20 mg of dexamethasone or 200 ml of 20% mannitol may be infused. Seizures may treated with anticonvulsants. Prolactin or growth hormone-secreting pituitary tumours may respond to dopamine agonists.

Surgical: Surgery is the mainstay of treatment. Only partial excision may be possible if tumour is inaccessible or if removal will cause unacceptable brain damage. Biopsy should be considered even if tumour cannot be removed (histology has implications for management). Meningiomas and acoustic neuromas offer the best prospects for complete removal. Pituitary adenomas may be removed by a trans-sphenoidal route, avoiding craniotomy.

Radiotherapy and chemotherapy: These have only a marginal effect on cerebral metastases and malignant gliomas in adults. Radiotherapy reduces recurrence of pituitary adenoma after surgery. Radiotherapy may be an adjunct to surgery for meningiomas which cannot be completely excised or whose histology suggests an increased tendency to recurrence.

Prognosis

• Gliomas are rarely completely excised and recurrence is therefore common. • Prognosis is related to histological grade; patients with better grades may survive many years, whilst only 20% of patients with high-grade gliomas survive 1 yr. • The prognosis for benign tumours is good, provided complete surgical excision can be achieved.

NEUROFIBROMATOSIS

This is a disorder of autosomal dominant inheritance due to an abnormal gene on chromosome 17 (type 1 neurofibromatosis, NF1) or 22 (type 2 neurofibromatosis, NF2). Multiple fibromatous tumours develop from the neurilemmal sheaths of peripheral and cranial nerves.

NF1 (von Recklinghausen's disease): Clinical features include: • multiple cutaneous neurofibromas, • café au lait spots in the skin, • plexiform and spinal neurofibroma, • scoliosis and • endocrine tumours. Investigation and treatment are only indicated if there are new symptoms or if malignant change is suspected.

NF2: Patients present with acoustic neuromas and/or spinal neurofibromas, meningiomas and other central neoplasms with few or no cutaneous neurofibromas. Relatives may require screening for acoustic neuromas.

ACOUSTIC NEUROMA

This is a benign tumour of Schwann cells of the 8th cranial nerve, which may arise in isolation or as part of NF2. As an isolated finding, it occurs after the third decade and is more frequent in females.

Clinical features

• Hearing loss is almost invariable. • Sensory symptoms in the face and vertigo are common. • Distortion of the brain stem or cerebellum may cause ataxia and/or cerebellar signs. • Distortion of the fourth ventricle and cerebral aqueduct may cause hydrocephalus.

Investigations and management

• MRI is the investigation of choice. • Management involves surgical removal. If this is complete, the prognosis is excellent. • Deafness and facial weakness may result from the operation.

VON HIPPEL–LINDAU DISEASE

This is a dominantly inherited disease characterised by the combination of retinal and intracranial (typically cerebellar) haemangiomas and haemangioblastomas. There may be associated extracranial hamartomatous lesions.

PARANEOPLASTIC NEUROLOGICAL DISEASE

Mild degrees of myopathy and neuropathy are quite frequent with systemic malignant tumours in the absence of metastases. Much rarer are certain disabling paraneoplastic syndromes, with associated autoantibodies cross-reacting with neural and tumour antigens.

Clinical features

These are summarised in Box 16.26. The neurological disease often precedes clinical presentation of the primary neoplasm.

Investigations

• Characteristic autoantibodies are present in many cases (e.g. anti Jo-1 in dermatomyositis). • CT of the chest or abdomen is often necessary to find

16.26 PARANEOPLASTIC SYNDROMES

Syndrome	Clinical features	Associated tumours
Sensory neuropathy	Limb pain, paraesthesia Distal numbness	Small-cell carcinoma of lung Hodgkin lymphoma
Limbic encephalitis	Memory loss, progressive dementia Seizures	Small-cell carcinoma of lung Hodgkin lymphoma
Myelitis	Progressive spinal cord lesion (usually cervical)	Small-cell carcinoma of lung
Cerebellar degeneration	Progressive ataxia, nystagmus, vertigo	Small-cell carcinoma of lung Ovarian, Hodgkin lymphoma
Subacute motor neuropathy	Subacute, patchy progressive, usually lower limb, weakness and wasting	Hodgkin lymphoma Small-cell carcinoma of lung
Sensorimotor peripheral neuropathy	Mild, non-disabling peripheral limb numbness and paraesthesia	Small-cell carcinoma of lung Breast, other carcinoma
Lambert–Eaton myasthenic syndrome	Weakness of proximal limb muscles, fatigue with exertion after initial improvement, areflexia	Small-cell carcinoma of lung
Dermatomyositis/ polymyositis	Proximal limb weakness and pain, heliotrope skin rash, Gottron's papules on knuckles	Lung, breast, ovary
Guillain–Barré	Ascending weakness, distal paraesthesia	Hodgkin lymphoma

the causative tumour. • CSF often shows increased protein and lymphocytes with oligoclonal bands.

Management

• This is directed at the primary tumour. • Some improvement may occur following administration of i.v. immunoglobulin.

HYDROCEPHALUS

COMMUNICATING AND OBSTRUCTIVE HYDROCEPHALUS

Hydrocephalus (dilatation of the ventricular system) may be due to obstruction of CSF circulation. Causes are given in Box 16.27. Diversion of the CSF by a shunt procedure between the ventricular system and peritoneal cavity or right atrium may relieve symptoms.

NORMAL PRESSURE HYDROCEPHALUS

Dilatation of the ventricular system is caused by intermittent rises in CSF pressure. It occurs in old age and is suggested by gait apraxia and dementia, often with urinary incontinence. The result of shunting procedures is unpredictable.

IDIOPATHIC (BENIGN) INTRACRANIAL HYPERTENSION

This usually occurs in obese young women. Raised intracranial pressure develops without a space-occupying lesion, ventricular dilatation or impairment of consciousness. The aetiology is uncertain. It can be precipitated by drugs (tetracycline, vitamin A, retinoids), Addison's disease and withdrawal of corticosteroids.

Clinical features

• Headache is present, sometimes with transient diplopia and visual obscurations. • There are usually no signs other than papilloedema.

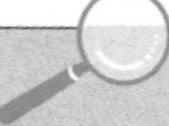

16.27 CAUSES OF HYDROCEPHALUS	
Communicating (obstruction outside ventricular system)	
• Bacterial meningitis (especially tuberculous) • Sarcoidosis	• Subarachnoid haemorrhage • Head injury • Idiopathic ('normal pressure')
Non-communicating (obstruction within ventricular system)	
• Tumours • Colloid cyst • Arnold–Chiari malformation	• Aqueduct stenosis • Cerebellar abscess • Cerebellar or brain-stem haematoma

Investigations

• CT is normal. • LP (after CT) confirms raised CSF pressure and forms part of treatment. • MR angiography will exclude cerebral venous sinus thrombosis or stenosis of other cause.

Management

• Avoid precipitants; reduce weight if obese. • Acetazolamide may lower intracranial pressure. • Repeated LP helps but is often unacceptable to the patient. • Patients failing to respond, in whom chronic papilloedema threatens vision, may require optic nerve sheath fenestration or a lumbo-peritoneal shunt.

DISORDERS OF THE SPINE AND SPINAL CORD

CERVICAL SPONDYLOSIS

Degeneration of the intervertebral discs and secondary osteoarthrosis (cervical spondylosis) is often asymptomatic but may cause neurological dysfunction. The C5/6, C6/7 and C4/5 vertebral levels and C6, C7 and C5 roots, respectively, are most commonly affected.

CERVICAL SPONDYLOTIC RADICULOPATHY

Compression of a nerve root occurs when a disc prolapses laterally, which may develop acutely or more gradually due to osteophytic encroachment of the intervertebral foramina.

Clinical features

• Neck pain may radiate in the distribution of the affected nerve root. • Neck movements may exacerbate pain. • Paraesthesia and sensory loss may be found in the affected segment and there may be lower motor neuron signs (Box 16.28).

Investigations

• Plain X-rays: confirm degenerative changes. • MRI: if surgery is contemplated. • Electrophysiological studies: if in doubt about the differential diagnosis.

16.28 PHYSICAL SIGNS IN CERVICAL ROOT COMPRESSION

Root	Muscle weakness	Sensory loss	Reflex loss
C5	Biceps, deltoid, spinati	Upper lateral arm	Biceps
C6	Brachioradialis	Lower lateral arm, thumb, index finger	Supinator
C7	Triceps, finger and wrist extensors	Middle finger	Triceps

Management

• Analgesia and physiotherapy usually help. • A minority require surgery (foraminotomy or disc excision).

CERVICAL SPONDYLOTIC MYELOPATHY

Dorsomedial herniation of a disc may cause pressure on the spinal cord or the anterior spinal artery (which supplies the anterior two-thirds of the cord).

Clinical features

• The onset is usually insidious and painless, but acute deterioration may occur after trauma. • Upper motor neuron signs develop in the limbs. • Sensory loss in the upper limbs is common. • Disturbance of micturition is a very late feature.

Investigations

• Plain X-rays: confirm degenerative changes. • MRI or myelography: if surgery is considered.

Management and prognosis

• Often stabilises or improves without intervention. • Surgery may arrest progression but may not result in improvement. • Cervical spine manipulation is of no proven benefit. • If progressive disability develops, surgical decompression should be considered.

LUMBO-SACRAL SPONDYLOSIS

Low back pain is usually due to abnormalities of joints and ligaments in the lumbar spine. Pain in the distribution of the lumbar or sacral roots ('sciatica') is often due to disc protrusion but can be a feature of rare disorders (e.g. spinal tumour, pelvic malignancy or vertebral TB).

LUMBAR DISC HERNIATION

Acute lumbar disc herniation is often precipitated by lifting heavy weights while the spine is flexed.

Clinical features

• The onset may be sudden or gradual. • Constant aching pain in the lumbar region may radiate to the buttock, thigh, calf and foot. • Pain is exacerbated by straining but may be relieved by lying flat. • Root pressure is suggested by limited hip flexion on the affected side if the straight leg is raised (Lasègue's sign). • If the L3 or L4 is involved, back pain may be induced by hyperextension of the hip (femoral nerve stretch test). • The roots most frequently affected are L4, L5 and S1 (Box 16.29).

Investigations

• MRI is the investigation of choice. • Plain X-rays of the lumbar spine are of little value.

16.29 PHYSICAL SIGNS IN LUMBAR ROOT COMPRESSION				
Disc level	**Root**	**Sensory loss**	**Weakness**	**Reflex loss**
L3/L4	L4	Inner calf	Inversion of foot	Knee
L4/L5	L5	Outer calf and dorsum of foot	Dorsiflexion of hallux/toes	Hamstring
L5/S1	S1	Sole and lateral foot	Plantar flexion	Ankle

Management

• 90% of patients recover with analgesia and early mobilisation. • Avoid physical manoeuvres likely to strain the lumbar spine. • Local anaesthetic or corticosteroid injections may help in ligamentous injury or joint dysfunction. • Consider surgery if there is no response to conservative treatment or if there is a progressive neurological deficit. • Central disc prolapse with bilateral symptoms and sphincter dysfunction requires urgent surgical decompression.

LUMBAR CANAL STENOSIS

This is congenital narrowing of the lumbar spinal canal, exacerbated by age-related degenerative change. Patients are usually elderly. There is exercise-induced weakness and paraesthesia in the legs, which is quickly relieved by rest (cauda equina claudication). Peripheral pulses are preserved and ankle reflexes are absent. Myelography, CT or MRI will demonstrate narrowing of the lumbar canal. Lumbar laminectomy often results in complete relief of symptoms.

COMPRESSION OF THE SPINAL CORD

Acute spinal cord compression is a common neurological emergency most commonly caused by trauma or metastatic tumours. Rarer causes include intervertebral disc prolapse, extradural abscess, tuberculoma, and tumours of the meninges or spinal cord. The early stages of damage are reversible but severely damaged neurons do not recover; therefore, patients with a short history should be investigated urgently.

Clinical features (Box 16.30)

• The onset of symptoms is usually slow (over weeks), but can be acute as a result of trauma or metastases. • Pain and sensory symptoms occur early, while weakness and sphincter dysfunction are late manifestations. • Root involvement causes dermatomal sensory impairment and corresponding lower motor signs. • Spinal cord interruption causes sensory loss, upper motor neuron signs below the lesion, and sphincter dysfunction. • The Brown-Séquard syndrome (p. 632) results if damage is confined to one side of the cord.

16.30 SIGNS OF SPINAL CORD COMPRESSION	
Cervical, above C5	Upper motor neuron signs and sensory loss in all four limbs Diaphragm weakness (phrenic nerve)
Cervical, C5–T1	Lower motor neuron signs and segmental sensory loss in the arms; upper motor neuron signs in the legs Respiratory (intercostal) muscle weakness
Thoracic cord	Spastic paraplegia with a sensory level on the trunk
Conus medullaris	Sacral loss of sensation and extensor plantar responses
Cauda equina	Spinal cord ends at approximately the T12/L1 spinal level; lesions below this can only cause lower motor neuron signs by affecting the cauda equina

Investigations

• Plain X-rays may show bony destruction and soft-tissue abnormalities. • Routine investigations, including CXR, may reveal systemic disease. • MRI of the spine is the investigation of choice. • Needle biopsy is required prior to radiotherapy to establish tumour histology.

Management

Benign tumours: Should be surgically excised. Recovery is good unless there is a marked neurological deficit before diagnosis.

Extradural compression due to malignancy: Prognosis is poor; useful function may be regained if treatment is initiated within 24 hrs of severe weakness or sphincter dysfunction. Surgical decompression may be appropriate in some; outcome is similar to radiotherapy.

Spinal cord compression due to TB: Surgical treatment is performed if the patient is seen early. Appropriate anti-tuberculous chemotherapy should be given.

Traumatic lesions of the vertebral column: Require specialised neurosurgical treatment.

INTRINSIC DISEASES OF THE SPINAL CORD

There are many disorders which interfere with spinal cord function due to non-compressive involvement of the spinal cord itself (Box 16.31). The symptoms and signs are similar to extrinsic compression, although a suspended sensory loss can only occur with intrinsic disease such as syringomyelia. Investigation starts with imaging, which is important for excluding a compressive lesion. MRI provides the most information about structural lesions (e.g. diastematomyelia, syringomyelia or intrinsic tumours) (Fig. 16.11). Non-specific signal change may be seen in inflammatory or infective conditions. Other investigations such as LP or blood tests are required to make a specific diagnosis.

16.31 INTRINSIC DISEASES OF THE SPINAL CORD

Type of disorder	Condition	Clinical features
Congenital	Diastematomyelia (spina bifida)	LMN features, deformity and sensory loss of legs, sphincter dysfunction Hairy patch or pit over low back Incidence ↓ by maternal intake of folic acid during pregnancy
	Hereditary spastic paraplegia	Autosomal dominant; onset usually in adult life. Slowly progressive UMN features (legs > arms), little sensory loss
Infective/ inflammatory	Transverse myelitis (viruses, e.g. HZV, HIV), schistosomiasis, MS, sarcoidosis	Weakness, sensory loss ± pain, developing over hours to days UMN features below lesion, impaired sphincter function
Vascular	Anterior spinal artery infarct Intervertebral disc embolus	Abrupt onset LMN signs at level of lesion, UMN features below it Spinothalamic sensory loss below lesion (spared dorsal column sensation)
	Spinal AVM/dural fistula	Onset variable (acute to slowly progressive) Variable LMN, UMN, sensory and sphincter disturbance
Neoplastic	Glioma, ependymoma	Weakness, sensory loss ± pain, developing over months/years UMN features below lesion; LMN features in conus; sphincter dysfunction
Metabolic	Vitamin B_{12} deficiency (subacute combined degeneration)	Progressive spastic paraparesis with proprioception loss, absent reflexes due to peripheral neuropathy ± optic nerve and cerebral involvement
Degenerative	Motor neuron disease	Progressive LMN and UMN features, bulbar weakness, no sensory loss
	Syringomyelia	Gradual onset over months or years, pain in cervical segments LMN signs at level of lesion, UMN features below it Suspended spinothalamic sensory loss at lesion, dorsal columns preserved

(AVM = arteriovenous malformation; HZV = herpes zoster virus; LMN = lower motor neuron; UMN = upper motor neuron)

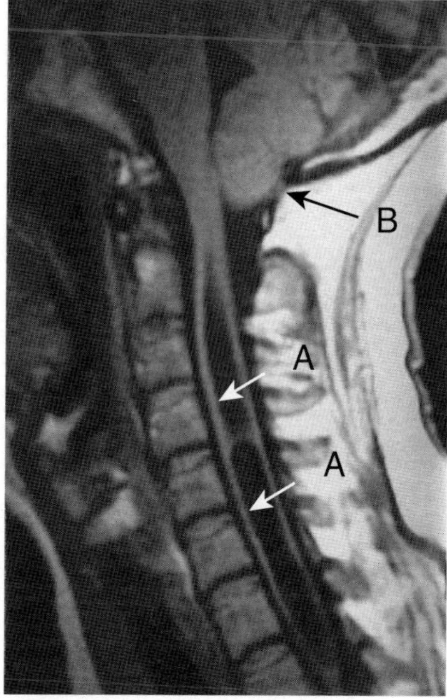

Fig. 16.11 MRI scan showing syrinx (arrows A), with herniation of cerebellar tonsils (arrow B).

DISEASES OF NERVE AND MUSCLE

DISEASES OF THE PERIPHERAL NERVOUS SYSTEM

Pathological processes may affect the nerve roots (radiculopathy), the nerve plexuses (plexopathy) and/or the individual nerves (neuropathy). Nerve fibres of different types (motor, sensory or autonomic) may be involved. Disorders may be primarily directed at the axon, the myelin sheath (Schwann cells) or both. An acute or chronic peripheral nerve disorder may be focal (affecting a single nerve: mononeuropathy), multifocal (several nerves: mononeuropathy multiplex) or generalised (polyneuropathy). Neurophysiological tests, and sometimes nerve biopsy, will help determine whether the pathology is primarily affecting the nerve axon (axonal neuropathy) or the myelin sheath (demyelinating neuropathy).

16.32 INVESTIGATION OF PERIPHERAL NEUROPATHY

	First-line tests	Second-line tests
Haematology	FBC, ESR, B_{12} and folate	
Biochemistry	U&Es, calcium Creatinine LFTs Blood glucose ± tolerance test/HbA_{1c} TFTs Plasma protein electrophoresis	Serum lipids Cryoglobulins Toxic metal and drug screen Prostate-specific antigen Urinary porphyrins Urinary Bence Jones protein Faecal occult blood Vitamin assay
Immunology	VDRL test Serum autoantibodies (ANF, dsDNA, RF, ENA)	Antiganglioside antibodies Antineuronal antibodies
Other	Nerve conduction/EMG	Genetic tests, nerve biopsy CXR/CT, mammogram Abdominal imaging

Causes of peripheral neuropathy include:

• Metabolic disease: diabetes, chronic kidney disease. • Toxins: alcohol, lead, thallium, many drugs. • Inflammatory conditions: e.g. polyarteritis, SLE, rheumatoid arthritis. • Infections: e.g. HIV. • Neoplasms: lymphoma, carcinoma, myeloma. • Vitamin deficiencies: especially B_{12}, thiamine, folic acid, E.

Investigations required in peripheral neuropathy reflect this spectrum of causes (Box 16.32).

FOCAL NEUROPATHY (MONONEUROPATHY)

Entrapment is the usual cause of a mononeuropathy (Box 16.33). Certain conditions increase the propensity to develop entrapment neuropathies, including acromegaly, hypothyroidism, pregnancy, any pre-existing generalised axonal neuropathy (e.g. diabetes), and bone damage near the nerve. Unless axonal loss has occurred, entrapment neuropathies will recover, provided the pressure on the nerve is relieved, either by avoiding precipitating activities or by surgical decompression.

CRANIAL NEUROPATHIES

• Lesions of ocular motor nerves (3rd, 4th and 6th) are reviewed on page 641. • An isolated lesion of an 8th cranial nerve may be caused by compression (e.g. by acoustic neuroma) near the cerebellopontine angle. • Isolated lesions of the 9th, 10th, 11th or 12th cranial nerves are uncommon, since they are usually caused by structural pathology.

16.33 SYMPTOMS AND SIGNS IN COMMON ENTRAPMENT NEUROPATHIES

Nerve	Symptoms	Muscle weakness/muscle-wasting	Area of sensory loss
Median (at wrist) (carpal tunnel syndrome)	Pain and paraesthesia on palmar aspect of hands. Pain may extend to arm and shoulder	Abductor pollicis brevis	Lateral palm and thumb, index, middle and lateral half 4th finger
Ulnar (at elbow)	Paraesthesia on medial border of hand, wasting and weakness of hand muscles	All small hand muscles, excluding abductor pollicis brevis	Medial palm and little finger, and medial half 4th finger
Radial	Weakness of extension of wrist and fingers, often precipitated by sleeping in abnormal posture, e.g. arm over back of chair	Wrist and finger extensors, supinator	Dorsum of thumb
Peroneal	Foot drop, trauma to head of fibula	Dorsiflexion and eversion of foot	Nil or dorsum of foot
Lateral cutaneous nerve of the thigh	Tingling and dysaesthesia on lateral border of the thigh	Nil	Lateral border of thigh

Trigeminal neuropathy

Isolated trigeminal sensory neuropathy is rare. It causes unilateral facial sensory loss and is sometimes associated with connective tissue disorders. Patients with trigeminal neuralgia do not have sensory loss unless there has been previous nerve surgery. Reactivation of varicella virus in the trigeminal nerve causes herpes zoster and is followed in one-third of patients by post-herpetic neuralgia.

Idiopathic isolated facial nerve palsy (Bell's palsy)

This is a common condition affecting all ages and both sexes. The lesion may be due to reactivation of latent herpes simplex virus 1 infection. Symptoms develop over hours, with pain around the ear preceding unilateral facial weakness. There is no sensory loss, hyperacusis can occur, and there may be diminished salivation and tear secretion. Examination reveals an ipsilateral lower motor neuron facial nerve palsy. Vesicles in the ear or palate indicate herpes zoster rather than Bell's palsy.

Management involves:

• Prednisolone 40–60 mg daily for a week: may speed recovery if started within 72 hrs. • Artificial tears prevent exposure keratitis. The eye should be taped shut overnight.

About 80% recover spontaneously within 12 wks. Poor recovery is predicted by complete paralysis, older age and reduced facial motor action potential amplitude after the first week. Recurrences should prompt further investigation.

Hemifacial spasm

This presents after middle age with intermittent twitching around one eye, spreading ipsilaterally over months to affect other facial muscles. The spasms are exacerbated by talking, eating or stress. The facial nerve should be imaged to exclude a structural lesion. Injections of botulinum toxin into affected muscles help, but have to be repeated every 3 mths.

MULTIFOCAL NEUROPATHY (MONONEURITIS MULTIPLEX)

When multiple nerve root, peripheral nerve or cranial nerve lesions occur serially or concurrently, the pathology is due either to involvement of the vasa nervorum or to malignant infiltration of the nerves. Investigation should be urgent since vasculitis is a common cause.

GENERALISED NEUROPATHY (POLYNEUROPATHY)

The clinical effects of a generalised pathological process occur in the longest peripheral nerves first, affecting the distal lower limbs before the upper limbs, with sensory symptoms and signs of an ascending 'glove and stocking' distribution. In inflammatory demyelinating neuropathies, the pathology may be patchier and variations from this ascending pattern occur.

ACUTE INFLAMMATORY DEMYELINATING POLYNEUROPATHY (GUILLAIN–BARRÉ SYNDROME)

This develops 1–4 wks after respiratory infection or diarrhoea (particularly that caused by *Campylobacter*) in 70% of patients. There is a cell-mediated inflammatory response directed at the myelin protein of spinal roots, and peripheral and extra-axial cranial nerves.

Clinical features

• Distal paraesthesia precedes a rapidly ascending muscle weakness. • Facial and bulbar weakness is common. • Respiratory weakness requiring ventilatory support occurs in 20% of cases. • Weakness usually progresses for 1–3 wks but respiratory failure can develop within hours. • Examination reveals diffuse weakness with widespread loss of reflexes. • An unusual variant (Miller Fisher) includes ophthalmoplegia, ataxia and areflexia.

Investigations

• CSF protein is elevated (may initially be normal) but there is no rise in CSF cell number. • Electrophysiology shows conduction block and motor slowing after a week. • Investigations may identify an underlying cause (CXR, stool culture, immunological blood tests).

Management and prognosis

• Regular monitoring of respiratory function (vital capacity and ABGs). • General management to protect the airway and prevent pressure sores and venous thrombosis. • Plasma exchange or i.v. immunoglobulin therapy: shorten the illness and improve prognosis if started within 14 days. • Steroids are ineffective. • Overall, 80% of patients recover completely within 3–6 mths, 4% die, and the remainder suffer residual neurological disability. • Adverse prognostic features include older age, rapid deterioration to ventilation and evidence of axonal loss on EMG.

CHRONIC POLYNEUROPATHY

A chronic symmetrical polyneuropathy is the most common neuropathy. In ~30% of patients no cause can be established. These patients usually have a mild axonal neuropathy which, whilst causing unpleasant symptoms, does not lead to motor disability.

Chronic demyelinating polyneuropathy

This is either hereditary or immune-mediated. Many genotypes cause hereditary demyelinating peripheral neuropathies, most characteristically Charcot–Marie–Tooth disease. This produces distal wasting ('inverted champagne bottle' legs), pes cavus and a predominantly motor involvement. Chronic inflammatory demyelinating peripheral neuropathy causes a generalised neuropathy which responds to immunosuppressive or immunomodulatory treatments.

16.34 PHYSICAL SIGNS IN BRACHIAL PLEXUS LESIONS			
Site	**Root**	**Affected muscles**	**Sensory loss**
Upper plexus (Erb–Duchenne)	C5/6	Biceps, deltoid, spinati, rhomboids, brachioradialis	Patch over deltoid
Lower plexus (Déjerine–Klumpke)	C8/T1	Small hand muscles, claw hand (ulnar wrist flexors)	Ulnar border hand/forearm
Thoracic outlet syndrome	C8/T1	Small hand muscles, ulnar forearm	Ulnar border hand/ forearm/upper arm

Chronic axonal polyneuropathy

This is the most common type of chronic polyneuropathy. It is usually an acquired (drugs and toxins) or genetic disorder affecting axonal metabolism and transport.

PLEXUS LESIONS

Brachial plexopathy

Trauma usually damages either the upper or the lower parts of the brachial plexus, according to the mechanics of the injury. The clinical features depend upon the anatomical site of damage (Box 16.34). The lower brachial plexus is vulnerable to breast or apical lung tumours, therapeutic irradiation, or compression by thoracic outlet anomalies such as a cervical rib.

Lumbosacral plexopathy

This may be caused by neoplastic infiltration or compression by retroperitoneal haematomas. A small vessel vasculopathy can produce a lumbar plexopathy, especially in elderly patients with type 2 diabetes mellitus ('diabetic amyotrophy') or a vasculitis. This presents with painful wasting of the quadriceps and an absent knee reflex.

SPINAL ROOT LESIONS (RADICULOPATHY)

These are caused by compression at or near spinal exit foramina by prolapsed intervertebral discs or degenerative spinal disease. Spinal roots may also be infiltrated by tumour masses and inflammatory or infective processes. Clinical features include muscle weakness and wasting and dermatomal sensory loss with reflex changes reflecting the roots involved (Box 16.29). Pain in the muscles whose innervating roots are involved is common.

DISORDERS OF THE NEUROMUSCULAR JUNCTION

MYASTHENIA GRAVIS

This is characterised by progressive fatigable weakness, particularly of the ocular, neck, facial and bulbar muscles. The disease is caused by autoantibodies to acetylcholine receptors in the neuromuscular junction. About 15% of patients have a thymoma, and a majority of the remainder have thymic follicular hyperplasia. Penicillamine can cause an antibody-mediated myasthenic syndrome and some drugs may exacerbate the neuromuscular blockade.

Clinical features

The disease usually presents between 15 and 50 yrs, with women affected more often than men in the younger age groups and the reverse at older ages. The cardinal symptom is abnormal fatigable weakness of the muscles; movement is initially strong but rapidly weakens. Worsening towards the end of the day or following exercise is characteristic. Intermittent ptosis or diplopia is common, but weakness of chewing, swallowing, speaking or limb movement also occurs. Sudden weakness from a cholinergic or myasthenic crisis may require ventilatory support.

Investigations

Tensilon test: I.V. injection of an anticholinesterase, edrophonium, causes improved muscle power within 30 secs which persists for 2–3 mins.

EMG: Repetitive stimulation may show a characteristic decremental response.

Autoantibodies: Anti-acetylcholine receptor antibody is found in >80% of cases. Screen for other autoimmune disorders.

Thoracic CT: Required to exclude thymoma (may not be visible on plain X-ray).

Management

Anticholinesterases: Maximise activity of acetylcholine at receptors in the neuromuscular junction. Pyridostigmine is given (30–120 mg 6-hourly). Muscarinic side-effects may be controlled by propantheline (15 mg as required). Anticholinesterase over-dosage may cause a cholinergic crisis (muscle fasciculation, paralysis, pallor, sweating, salivation and small pupils); this may be distinguished from a myasthenic crisis clinically and, if necessary, by a dose of edrophonium.

Immunological treatment: This limits the immunological attack on motor end plates. Thymectomy should be considered in antibody-positive patients under 45 yrs with symptoms outside extraocular muscles (unless disease has been established for >7 yrs). Plasma exchange or i.v. immunoglobulin is required for severe myasthenia or pre-operative preparation. Corticosteroids (can cause initial exacerbation) may need to continue for months or years. Azathioprine may allow steroids to be reduced or withdrawn.

Prognosis

Prognosis is variable; remissions sometimes occur spontaneously. When disease is confined to the eye muscles, the prognosis is excellent. Rapid progression >5 yrs after onset is uncommon.

OTHER MYASTHENIC SYNDROMES

In the Lambert–Eaton myasthenic syndrome transmitter release is impaired, often with antibodies to prejunctional calcium channels. The cardinal sign is absent tendon reflexes which return immediately after sustained contraction of the relevant muscle. The syndrome is often associated with underlying malignancy. It is diagnosed electrophysiologically and treatment is with 3,4-diaminopyridine.

DISEASES OF MUSCLE

Disease of voluntary muscle most commonly presents as symmetrical weakness of the large proximal muscles (proximal myopathy). Other presenting symptoms include myotonia (an abnormality of muscle relaxation) and muscle pain. Diagnosis depends upon the clinical picture along with EMG studies, muscle biopsy and sometimes genetic studies.

MUSCULAR DYSTROPHIES

These inherited disorders are characterised by progressive degeneration of muscle groups, sometimes with involvement of the heart muscle or conducting tissue (Box 16.35).

Clinical features

• Wasting and weakness are usually symmetrical. • There is no fasciculation and no sensory loss. • Tendon reflexes are preserved until a late stage, except in myotonic dystrophy.

Investigations

• Specific genetic testing, with EMG and muscle biopsy if necessary. • Creatine kinase is markedly elevated in Duchenne muscular dystrophy (normal or moderately elevated in other dystrophies). • Screening for cardiomyopathy or dysrhythmia.

Management and prognosis

• No specific therapy. • Physiotherapy and occupational therapy. • Treatment of cardiac failure, arrhythmia or respiratory complications. • Genetic counselling. • Patients with Duchenne dystrophy are now living into the third decade. • The lifespan in limb girdle and facioscapulohumeral dystrophies is normal. • In myotonic dystrophy, the prognosis is variable, limited by cardiac and respiratory complications.

ACQUIRED MYOPATHIES

Muscle weakness may be caused by a range of metabolic, endocrine, toxic or inflammatory disorders (Box 16.36). Disorders affecting the muscles' structural integrity can be distinguished by EMG from those caused by metabolic derangement. In metabolic disorders, weakness is often acute and generalised, while a proximal myopathy predominantly affecting the pelvic girdle is a feature of some endocrine disorders.

16.35 THE MUSCULAR DYSTROPHIES

Type	Genetics	Muscles affected	Other features
Myotonic dystrophy (Onset any age)	AD; expanded triplet repeat chromosome 19q	Face (incl. ptosis), sternomastoids, distal limb, generalised later	Myotonia, cognitive dulling, cardiac conduction abnormalities, lens opacities, frontal balding, hypogonadism
Proximal myotonic myopathy (Onset adulthood)	AD; quadruplet repeat in chromosome 3q	Proximal, especially thigh, muscle hypertrophy	As above but cognition not affected Muscle pain
Duchenne (Onset first 5 yrs)	X-linked; deletions in dystrophin gene	Proximal and limb girdle	Pseudohypertrophy of calves Cardiomyopathy
Becker (Onset childhood/early adult)	X-linked; deletions in dystrophin gene	Proximal and limb girdle	Pseudohypertrophy of calves Cardiomyopathy
Limb girdle (Onset childhood/early adult)	AD or AR	Limb girdle	Some have calf hypertrophy Some have cardiac conduction defects
Facioscapulohumeral (Onset 7–30 yrs)	AD; repeat deletion chromosome 4q	Face and upper limb girdle	Pain in shoulder girdle common

(AD = autosomal dominant; AR = autosomal recessive.)

16.36 CAUSES OF ACQUIRED PROXIMAL MYOPATHY	
Inflammatory	Polymyositis, dermatomyositis
Endocrine and metabolic	Hypothyroidism, hyperthyroidism, acromegaly, Cushing's syndrome, Addison's disease, Conn's syndrome, osteomalacia, hypokalaemia (liquorice, diuretic and purgative abuse), hypercalcaemia (disseminated bony metastases)
Toxic	Alcohol (chronic and acute syndromes), vitamin E, organophosphates, snake venoms
Drugs	Corticosteroids, chloroquine, amiodarone, β-blockers, statins, clofibrate, ciclosporin, vincristine, zidovudine, opiates, ε-aminocaproic acid
Paraneoplastic	Carcinomatous neuromyopathy, dermatomyositis

17

Skin disease

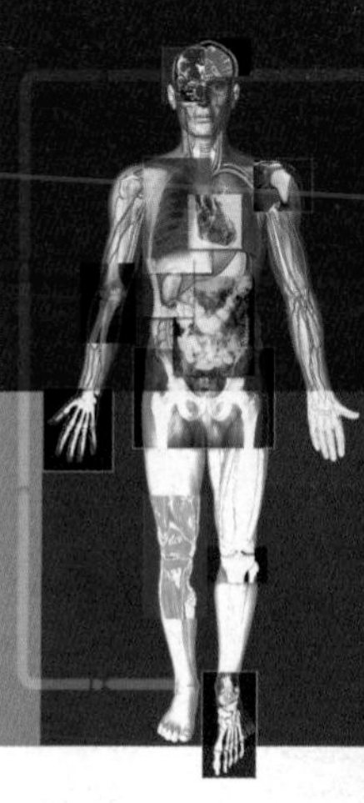

Skin disease is common. Surveys in Europe suggest that approximately 1 in 7–10 of all visits to a primary care physician is for a skin problem. Consultations for skin disease are becoming more common as the absolute incidence of many diseases (e.g. skin cancer, atopic dermatitis) has increased. In addition, the therapeutic options for diseases previously viewed as untreatable have increased and awareness of these therapies is spreading as patients take a greater interest in their health.

A glossary of dermatological words is shown in Box 17.1.

PRESENTING PROBLEMS

THE CHANGING MOLE

The challenge when assessing any pigmented lesion is distinguishing between common benign lesions such as seborrhoeic keratoses and melanocytic naevi, and the more serious diagnosis of melanoma. The history and examination may help to make this distinction, but where doubt exists, a biopsy should be taken. If the lesion does not appear malignant, it may be helpful to photograph it with a millimetre scale and review the patient for change in 6 mths.

History

• Change in size, shape or colour of lesion: over what time period? • Symptoms arising from the lesion: bleeding, tenderness, excessive itch. • Occupation: jobs involving outdoor work suggest a high lifetime actinic exposure.

CLINICAL EXAMINATION IN SKIN DISEASE

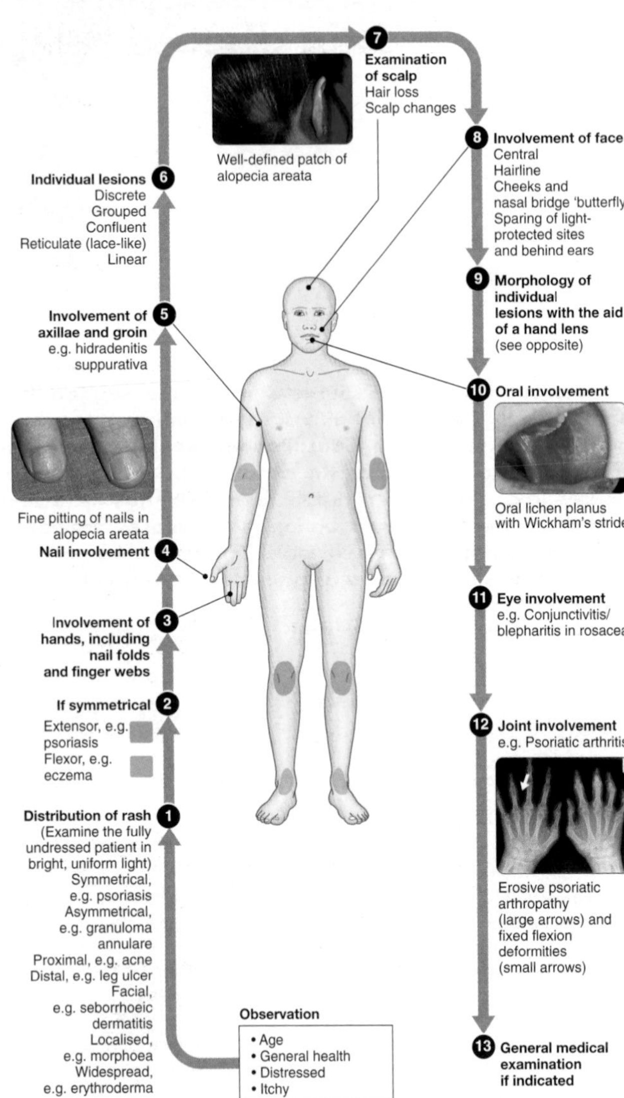

17.1 TERMS USED TO DESCRIBE SKIN LESIONS	
Primary lesions	
Macule	A small flat area of altered colour, e.g. freckle
Papule	A discrete raised lesion, which may be coloured; called a nodule if >1 cm
Plaque	A raised area of skin with a flat top, typically several cm across; often scaly
Vesicle, bulla	A small (~several mm)/larger (~several cm) blister, respectively
Pustule	A focal visible accumulation of pus in the skin; usually yellow or green
Abscess	A localised collection of pus in a cavity, >1 cm in diameter
Weal	An evanescent dermal collection of fluid; the fluid is diffuse, unlike in a blister
Papilloma	A projecting nipple-like mass, e.g. skin tag
Petechiae, purpura, ecchymosis	Petechiae are flat, pinhead-sized macules of extravascular blood in the dermis; larger ones (purpura) may be palpable; deeper bleeding causes an ecchymosis
Burrow	A linear or curvilinear papule, caused by a burrowing scabies mite
Comedone	A plug of keratin and sebum in a dilated pilosebaceous orifice
Telangiectasia	Visible dilatation of small cutaneous blood vessels
Secondary lesions (which evolve from primary lesions)	
Scale	A flake arising from the stratum corneum, e.g. psoriasis
Crust	Exudate of blood or serous fluid, e.g. eczema or tissue fluid
Ulcer	An area from which the epidermis and the upper part of the dermis have been lost
Excoriation	Damage resulting from scratching; usually a linear ulcer or erosion
Erosion	An area of skin denuded by complete or partial loss of the epidermis
Fissure	A deep, slit-shaped ulcer, e.g. irritant dermatitis of the hands
Sinus	A cavity or channel that permits the escape of pus or fluid
Scar	Permanent fibrous tissue resulting from healing
Atrophy	Loss of substance due to diminution of the epidermis, dermis or subcutaneous fat
Stria	A streak-like, atrophic, pink/purple/white lesion in the connective tissue

• Family history of melanoma. • Has the patient ever lived abroad in a sunny climate? • Skin type: pale/tending to burn easily or darker-skinned/tanning readily?

Examination

• Use both the naked eye and a magnifying glass or a dermatoscope. • Examine other pigmented lesions on the patient's body; a good degree of homogeneity between individual lesions in size and colour is reassuring. • Use the ABCDE rule (p. 729) to help determine the likelihood of melanoma.

ITCH (PRURITUS)

Pruritus is defined as an unpleasant sensation that provokes the desire to scratch, characteristic of many skin diseases and some medical conditions. The biological mechanisms governing itch are poorly understood.

History

Assessment of the itchy patient is one of the most difficult clinical problems in dermatology. Helpful hints from the history include:

Time course: Acute (as in urticaria, infestations) or chronic (eczema)?

Localisation: E.g. extensor surfaces of wrists are classically affected in lichen planus, limb flexures in childhood eczema.

Exacerbating factors: Most causes of itch are increased by heating and reduced by cooling. In cholinergic urticaria, exercise or heat dramatically induces itching.

Involvement of other family members: E.g. a scabietic infestation affecting more than one family member.

General health of the patient: A review of systems may uncover a medical cause of pruritus such as a malignancy, liver disease or anaemia.

Examination

The most important distinction is whether the itch is due to a primary skin condition or secondary to an underlying medical cause.

Generalised pruritus associated with skin disease: Eczema, urticaria, xeroderma (dry skin, often occurring in the elderly), scabies.

Local pruritus associated with skin disease: Lichen planus, psoriasis, dermatitis herpetiformis.

Pruritus with no evidence of skin disease: In the absence of clues pointing to a primary skin disease, detailed physical examination and investigations, including a careful search for lymphadenopathy, may be required. Investigations should include:

• FBC. • Iron status. • U&Es. • LFTs. • TFTs. • Possibly a CXR.

Examples of systemic diseases causing itch include:

• Renal failure, • Liver failure, • Anaemia, • Hyper- or hypothyroidism, • Malignancy.

Management

Management of the underlying primary skin condition or medical condition may alleviate the itch. For those who experience ongoing symptoms in spite of specific management, application of cooling emollients such as 1% menthol in aqueous cream may help. Alternatively, phototherapy with UVB may afford some relief. Although frequently the subject of ridicule, significant itch may incapacitate, cause embarrassment, disrupt sleep and ruin the patient's self-image. It is easily underestimated and trivialised as a symptom.

THE SCALY RASH (PAPULOSQUAMOUS ERUPTIONS)

A common presenting complaint in general practice is an eruptive scaly rash sometimes associated with itching. Causes are summarised in Box 17.2.

History

How long has the rash been present? Atopic eczema often starts in infancy or early childhood, pityriasis rosea and psoriasis between the ages of 15 and 40. Drug eruptions are acute in onset and a temporal relationship between starting the medicine and the onset of the rash should be sought.

Where on the body did it start? Localisation or distribution of the rash (see Box 17.2) may give clues to aetiology. The 'herald patch' of pityriasis rosea is a solitary erythematous lesion on the trunk, which enlarges rapidly.

Is it itchy? Atopic eczema is extremely itchy, psoriasis and pityriasis rosea less so. Drug eruptions and tinea corporis are usually pruritic.

Was there a preceding illness or systemic symptoms? Guttate psoriasis is often preceded by a β-haemolytic streptococcal sore throat. A small percentage of people with pityriasis rosea have a prodromal illness with malaise, headache and arthralgia.

Examination

The distribution of the rash can be very useful in discriminating between the various causes of a scaly rash. Morphological features noted on assessment with a magnifying lens may help to narrow down the diagnosis (see Box 17.2).

ERYTHRODERMA

Eczema, psoriasis, drug eruptions and lichen planus rarely progress to erythroderma, defined as erythema with or without scaling involving >90% of the body surface. It is associated with systemic symptoms due to excessive heat loss through extensively involved skin, and haemodynamic upset characterised by hypotension and tachycardia as a response to a large increase in insensible losses. Causes include:

17.2 CLINICAL FEATURES OF COMMON SCALY RASHES			
Type of rash	**Distribution**	**Morphology**	**Associated clinical signs**
Eczema	Face/flexures	Poorly defined erythema and scaling; lichenification	Shiny nails, infra-orbital crease, 'dirty neck'
Psoriasis	Extensor surfaces	Well-defined plaques with a silvery scale	Nail pitting and onycholysis; scalp involvement, axillae and genital areas often affected
Pityriasis rosea	Initial 'herald patch' precedes 'fir tree' pattern on torso	Well-defined erythematous papules and plaques with collarette of scale	
Pityriasis versicolor	Upper torso and upper shoulders	Hypo- and hyperpigmented scaly patches	
Drug eruption	Widespread	Maculo-papular erythematous scaly areas which merge and are followed by exfoliation	
Lichen planus	Distal limbs, esp. volar aspect of wrists; lower back	Shiny, flat-topped violaceous papules with Wickham's striae	White lacy network on buccal mucosa; rarely, nail changes
Tinea corporis	Asymmetrical, often isolated, red scaly lesions	Scaly plaques which expand with central healing	Nail involvement

• Severe eczema. • Severe psoriasis. • Cutaneous T-cell lymphoma (Sézary's syndrome). • Pityriasis rubra pilaris (a variant of psoriasis).

URTICARIA (NETTLE RASH, HIVES)

Urticaria refers to an area of focal dermal oedema secondary to a transient increase in capillary permeability, largely mediated by mast cell degranula-

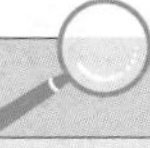

17.3 CAUSES OF URTICARIA	
Acute and chronic urticaria	
• Autoimmune due to production of antibodies that cross-link the IgE receptor on mast cells • Allergens (in foods, inhalants and injections) • Drugs (see Box 17.9) • Physical (e.g. heat, cold, pressure, sun, water)	• Contact (e.g. animal saliva, latex) • Infection (e.g. viral hepatitis, infectious mononucleosis, HIV during seroconversion) • Other conditions (e.g. SLE, pregnancy, intestinal parasites) • Idiopathic
Urticarial vasculitis	
• Hepatitis B • SLE	• Idiopathic

tion. The principal mediator released is histamine, which explains the efficacy of H_1-blocking drugs in the management of this condition. On certain body sites such as the lips or hands the oedema spreads and is traditionally referred to as angioedema. By definition the swelling lasts <24 hrs. Urticarial vasculitis has a similar clinical presentation but lesions last >24 hrs.

Most cases are idiopathic but physical, drug-induced, infection-related and autoimmune forms exist (Box 17.3).

Clinical assessment

Two important questions are:

• How long does the individual lesion last? (<24 hrs urticaria, >24 hrs urticarial vasculitis).

• How long has the condition been present? (<6 wks acute, >6 wks chronic urticaria).

A directed history is still the best way to elicit any causes or precipitants of urticaria. A record of possible allergens, including drugs (see Box 17.9), should be determined. A family history must be sought in cases of angioedema, in order to determine the likelihood of a C1 esterase inhibitor deficiency. Dermographism may be elicited on examination.

Investigations

These need to be directed at the possible underlying cause, as elicited from the clinical history. Some or all of the following may be appropriate:

• FBC, including eosinophil count in suspected parasitic infection. • ESR: elevated in vasculitis. • U&Es, LFTs and TFTs: to detect underlying disorders. • Total and specific IgE to possible allergens, e.g. shellfish and peanuts. • Antinuclear factor in chronic urticaria or urticarial vasculitis. • CH50 as a general guide to complement activation and C_3 and C_4 levels as evidence of complement consumption via both the classical and the alternative pathways. • Incisional biopsy: may be required for diagnosis of urticarial vasculitis.

Management

• Non-sedating antihistamines (e.g. loratadine) are the mainstay of management. • The patient should be advised to avoid medicines known to provoke urticaria, such as NSAIDs and codeine-containing preparations. • The addition of an H_2-blocking drug such as cimetidine may be helpful in cases refractory to H_1-blockers alone. • Those with features of angio-edema should carry a kit for self-administration of adrenaline (epinephrine) (p. 23).

BLISTERS

Loss of adhesion between adjacent keratinocytes, between keratinocytes and the basement membrane, or between the basement membrane and the dermis leads to a potential space which, because of negative extracellular pressure, fills with fluid: a blister. There is an artificial distinction made by some between small (vesicles, <0.5 cm) and large blisters (bullae, >0.5 cm). The site of blister formation within the skin therefore depends on the aetiology and underlying pathogenesis. The classification of blistering disorders may be considered as:

• Congenital or genetic. • Acquired (often infective in origin). • Autoimmune.

Clinical assessment

Genetic causes of blistering: These often present at birth or shortly after. They include epidermolysis bullosa, bullous ichthyosis and incontinentia pigmenti. Infection is a more common cause of blistering at birth, including herpes simplex acquired through vertical transmission, and impetigo.

Acquired forms of blistering: These are common in childhood and adulthood (Box 17.4), and may be infectious in origin (e.g. staphylococcal scalded skin syndrome), drug-related, metabolic (e.g. porphyria), or part of another primary skin complex such as acute eczema or pompholyx. Toxic epidermal necrolysis may be life-threatening, can occur at any age and is often due to drugs. Loss of skin compromises fluid balance and thermoregulation and leads to severe pain and risk of infection. Intensive care is often required.

Autoimmune blistering diseases (Box 17.5): These are more common in later life, with the exception of dermatitis herpetiformis and pemphigus gestationis which occur in younger patients. Diagnosis is based on clinical features and immunopathology of biopsies. Rarely, some of these conditions may be related to an underlying malignancy (e.g. paraneoplastic pemphigus, epidermolysis bullosa acquisita associated with lymphoma, multiple myeloma or inflammatory bowel disease). Patients with a suspected diagnosis of dermatitis herpetiformis should be investigated for coeliac disease.

17.4 CAUSES OF ACQUIRED BLISTERS			
	Localised	**Generalised**	
		With mucosal involvement	**With no mucosal involvement**
Vesicular	Herpes (simplex or zoster), impetigo, pompholyx	Eczema herpeticum	Eczema herpeticum, dermatitis herpetiformis, epidermolysis bullosa acquisita
Bullous	Impetigo, bullous cellulitis, bullous stasis oedema, acute eczema, insect bites, fixed drug eruptions	Pemphigus, bullous erythema multiforme/ Stevens–Johnson syndrome, toxic epidermal necrolysis, epidermolysis bullosa acquisita	Acute eczema, erythema multiforme, bullous pemphigoid, epidermolysis bullosa acquisita, bullous lupus erythematosus, pseudoporphyria, porphyria cutanea tarda, drug eruptions (e.g. barbiturates)

LEG ULCERS

Ulceration of the skin is the complete loss of the epidermis and part of the dermis. There are numerous aetiologies, summarised in Box 17.6, but when present on the lower limb, ulceration is usually due to arterial or venous insufficiency. The site of the ulceration gives clues as to its aetiology (Fig. 17.2).

Clinical assessment

• The ulcer should be swabbed to exclude infection. • Arterial sufficiency should be assessed with Doppler USS. • Venous sufficiency may be assessed with venography to highlight any surgically remediable venous disease. • Urinalysis to detect glycosuria ± a fasting glucose level should be taken to rule out diabetes.

LEG ULCERATION DUE TO VENOUS DISEASE

Clinical assessment

This is a common clinical problem in middle to old age. Clinical signs include:

• Varicose veins. • Haemosiderin deposition. • Oedema. • Lipodermatosclerosis: firm induration of the skin of the leg, with a shiny appearance, producing the 'inverted champagne bottle' sign. • Ulceration, typically on

17.5 CLINICAL FEATURES OF SOME IMMUNE-MEDIATED BLISTERING SKIN CONDITIONS

Disease	Age	Site of blisters	Nature of blisters	Involves mucous membranes	Treatment
Pemphigus vulgaris	40–60 yrs	Torso, head	Flaccid and fragile, many erosions	100%	Systemic steroids, cyclophosphamide
Bullous pemphigoid	60 yrs and over	Trunk (esp. flexures) and limbs	Tense (Fig. 17.1)	Occasionally	Systemic steroids, azathioprine
Dermatitis herpetiformis	Young, associated with coeliac disease	Elbows, lower back, buttocks	Excoriated and often not present	No	Dapsone, gluten-free diet
Pemphigoid gestationis	Young pregnant female	Peri-umbilical and limbs	Tense	Rare	
Epidermolysis bullosa acquisita	All ages	Widespread	Tense, scarring	Common (50%)	Cyclophosphamide, azathioprine, methotrexate
Bullous lupus erythematosus	Young, black female	Widespread	Tense	Rare	Dapsone

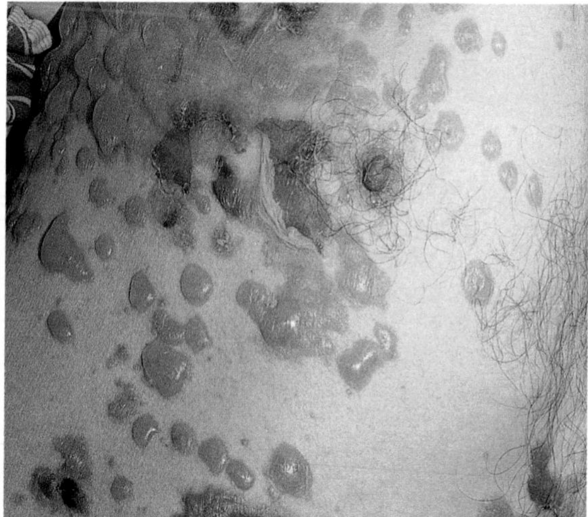

Fig. 17.1 Bullous pemphigoid. Large tense and unilocular blisters clustered in and around the axilla.

the medial malleolus. • Malignant transformation of a chronic ulcer into squamous cell carcinoma is termed 'Marjolin's ulcer'.

Management

• General management: dietary advice for the obese and encouragement to take gentle exercise. • Oedema: should be reduced with the use compression bandages (once arterial sufficiency is confirmed; ratio of ankle : brachial systolic pressure >0.8), elevation of the legs when sitting, and the judicious use of diuretics. • Antiseptic soaks, e.g. potassium permanganate. • Non-adhesive absorbent dressings (alginates, charcoals, hydrogels or hydrocolloids) for highly exudative ulcers. • Silver-containing dressings for infected wounds ± antibiotics, as guided by swabs. • Management of surrounding venous eczema with topical steroid. • Vein surgery: may help some younger patients with persistent venous ulcers.

LEG ULCERATION DUE TO ARTERIAL DISEASE

Deep, painful and punched-out ulcers on the lower leg, especially if they occur on the shin and foot and are preceded by a history of intermittent claudication, are likely to be due to arterial disease. Risk factors include smoking, hypertension, diabetes mellitus and hyperlipidaemia. The foot is cyanotic and cold, and the skin surrounding the ulcer is atrophic and hairless. The peripheral arterial pulses are absent or reduced. Doppler studies are required, and if arterial insufficiency is confirmed, compression bandaging should be prohibited and advice sought from a vascular surgeon.

17.6 MAIN CAUSES OF LEG ULCERATION	
Venous hypertension	
Arterial disease	Atherosclerosis, vasculitis, Buerger's disease
Small-vessel disease	Diabetes mellitus, vasculitis
Abnormalities of blood	Sickle-cell disease, cryoglobulinaemia, spherocytosis, immune complex disease
Neuropathy	Diabetes mellitus, leprosy, syphilis
Tumour	Squamous cell carcinoma, basal cell carcinoma, malignant melanoma, Kaposi's sarcoma
Trauma	Injury, artefact

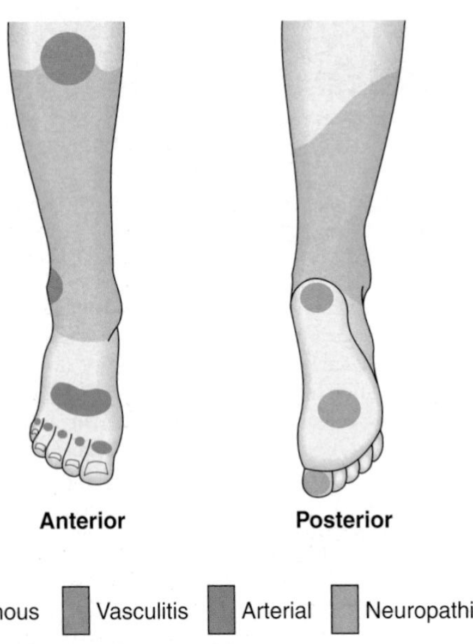

Fig. 17.2 Causes of lower leg ulceration.

LEG ULCERATION DUE TO VASCULITIS

These ulcers start as painful, palpable, purpuric lesions and turn into small, punched-out ulcers. The involvement of larger vessels is heralded by painful nodules which evolve into intractable, deep, sharply demarcated ulcers. Management includes treatment of the underlying disorder as well as immunosuppression with, for example, systemic corticosteroids or cyclophosphamide.

LEG ULCERATION DUE TO NEUROPATHY

The most common cause of a neuropathic ulcer is diabetes. The ulcers occur over weight-bearing areas such as the heel. Microangiopathy also contributes to ulceration in diabetes. This is discussed in detail on page 414.

TOO LITTLE OR TOO MUCH HAIR

ALOPECIA

The term means nothing more than loss of hair and is a sign rather than a diagnosis. There are many causes and patterns, but an important distinction is whether the alopecia is scarring or non-scarring. The causes of alopecia are summarised in Box 17.7; the most common are discussed here.

Tinea capitis: Fungal scalp infection is increasingly common in the UK. Any patient developing an area of hair loss and scaling in the scalp should have the area scraped and affected hairs plucked for mycological examination.

- Endothrix (within the hair shaft) infections, e.g. *Trichophyton tonsurans*, cause relatively uninflamed patchy baldness with breakage of the hairs at the skin surface ('black dot'). There is no fluorescence under Wood's light.
- Ectothrix (outside the hair shaft) species of fungi, such as *Microsporum audouinii,* show minimal inflammation, although *M. canis* infections (from dogs and cats) are more inflamed and can be identified by green fluorescence with Wood's light.

17.7 CLASSIFICATION OF ALOPECIA

Localised	Diffuse
Non-scarring	
Tinea capitis, alopecia areata, androgenetic alopecia, traumatic (trichotillomania, traction, cosmetic), syphilis	Androgenetic alopecia, telogen effluvium, metabolic, hypo- or hyperthyroidism, hypopituitarism, diabetes mellitus, HIV disease, nutritional deficiency, liver disease, post-partum, alopecia areata, syphilis
Scarring	
Developmental defects, discoid lupus erythematosus, herpes zoster, pseudopelade, tinea capitis/kerion, idiopathic	Discoid lupus erythematosus, radiotherapy, folliculitis decalvans, lichen planus pilaris

Kerions are boggy, highly inflamed areas of tinea capitis and are usually caused by zoophilic fungi (from animals, e.g. cattle ringworm, *T. verrucosum*). Treatment is systemic, with oral terbinafine, griseofulvin or itraconazole. Topical therapy with an antifungal shampoo is recommended as an adjunct and arachis oil is used to remove crusting.

Alopecia areata: This non-scarring condition appears as sharply defined, non-inflamed bald patches, usually on the scalp. During the active stage of hair loss pathognomonic 'exclamation mark' hairs are seen (broken-off hairs 3–4 mm long, which taper off towards the scalp). The condition may affect the eyebrows, eyelashes and beard. The hair usually regrows spontaneously in small bald patches, but the outlook is less good with larger patches and when the alopecia appears early in life or is associated with atopy. Alopecia totalis describes complete loss of scalp hair and alopecia universalis complete loss of all hair. There is an association of alopecia areata with autoimmune disorders, atopy and Down's syndrome.

Androgenetic alopecia: Male-pattern baldness is physiological in men >20 yrs old, although rarely it may be extensive and develop at an alarming pace in the late teens. It also occurs in females, most obviously after the menopause. The distribution is of bitemporal recession and then crown involvement.

Investigations

• Laboratory tests, including an FBC, ESR, U&Es, LFTs and TFTs, an autoantibody profile and, in cases where lupus or lichen planus is suspected, a biopsy should allow a diagnosis to be reached in most cases. • Mycological assessment is advisable in cases of localised hair loss with scaling.

Management

• Specific causes such as fungal infection should be treated. • Alopecia areata sometimes responds to topical or intralesional corticosteroids, such as 0.3 ml triamcinolone (10 mg/ml). • Some males with androgenetic alopecia may be helped by systemic finasteride or topical 2% minoxidil solution. • In females, anti-androgen therapy such as cyproterone acetate is sometimes useful. • A wig may be the most appropriate treatment for extensive alopecia.

HIRSUTISM

Hirsutism is the growth of terminal hair in a male pattern in a female. It should be distinguished from hypertrichosis, which describes the excessive growth of terminal hair in either sex in a non-androgenic distribution. The amount of terminal hair varies in people with different genetic ancestries and this should be remembered when reaching a clinical diagnosis of 'excessive'.

Investigations

Full endocrinological investigations are required if hirsutism:

• Occurs in childhood. • Is of sudden onset. • Is accompanied by signs of virilisation. • Is associated with menstrual irregularity or cessation.

In addition to the screening tests for hyperandrogenism, polycystic ovary syndrome (p. 354) and Cushing's syndrome (p. 362) need to be considered Usually no underlying hormonal abnormality is found.

Management

• Depilatory creams, waxing, electrolysis, bleaching and shaving are often used for physiological hirsutism. • In those with darkly pigmented hair, laser therapy may be useful. • Any remediable cause should be corrected by medical and surgical methods, sometimes with the help of the endocrinologist or gynaecologist. • Oral anti-androgen therapy may be helpful (e.g. Dianette, containing cyproterone acetate).

ABNORMAL SKIN COLOUR

DECREASED PIGMENTATION

Oculocutaneous albinism

Albinism results from genetic abnormalities of melanin biosynthesis in skin and eyes but the number of melanocytes is normal (in contrast to vitiligo). It is usually inherited as an autosomal recessive trait; several types can be distinguished by genetic analysis. Affected individuals have (from birth) an almost complete absence of pigment resulting in pale skin and white hair, and also failure of melanin production in the eye, in the iris and retina. Patients have photophobia, poor vision not correctable with refraction, rotatory nystagmus, and an alternating strabismus associated with abnormalities in the decussation of nerve fibres in the optic tract. Oculocutaneous albinos are at grossly increased risk of sunburn and skin cancer, and careful protection from sun damage is essential.

Vitiligo

Vitiligo is an acquired condition in which circumscribed depigmented patches develop; it affects 1% of the population world-wide.

Clinical assessment: Segmental vitiligo is restricted to one part of the body but not necessarily a dermatome. Generalised vitiligo is often symmetrical and frequently involves the hands, wrists, knees and neck, as well as the area around the body orifices. The hair of the scalp and beard may also depigment (Fig. 17.3). The patches of depigmentation are sharply defined. Some spotty perifollicular pigment may be seen within the depigmented patches and is sometimes the first sign of repigmentation. Sensation in the depigmented patches is normal (in contrast to tuberculoid leprosy). The course is unpredictable but most patches remain static or enlarge; a few repigment spontaneously.

Management: This is unsatisfactory. Patients should be warned that their patches of vitiligo will be more susceptible to sunburn, and should take appropriate precautions. Camouflage cosmetics are found useful by some patients. Phototherapy can produce some successful results, but must be used cautiously due to the susceptibility of the vitiliginous patches to burning. The patient should also be warned of the possibility of the vitiligo

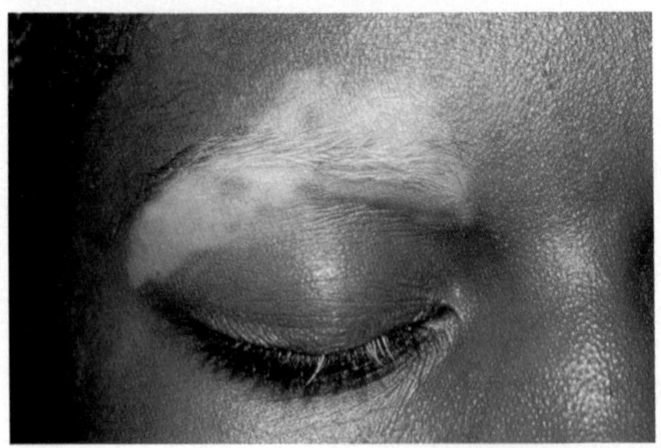

Fig. 17.3 Vitiligo. Localised patches of depigmented skin, including some white hairs.

becoming more prominent as surrounding skin darkens during the course of phototherapy. Repigmentation tends to occur perifollicularly.

Hypopituitarism

Hypopigmentation is due to decreased production of pituitary melanotrophic hormones (p. 375). The complexion has a pale, yellow tinge; there is skin atrophy and thinning or loss of the sexual hair.

INCREASED PIGMENTATION

This is mostly due to hypermelanosis but other pigments may occasionally be deposited in the skin, e.g. an orange tint in carotenaemia or a bronze hue in haemochromatosis.

Localised hypermelanosis

Freckles: These are sharply demarcated, light brown–ginger macules of up to 5 mm in diameter due to focal overproduction of melanin but with normal melanocyte number. They are most prominent on exposed sites, multiply and become darker with sun exposure, and are associated with a sun-sensitive phenotype.

Lentigines: These are dark brown macules 1 mm–1 cm across. They are associated with chronic sun exposure, a sun-sensitive phenotype and the Peutz–Jeghers syndrome (p. 470).

Diffuse hypermelanosis

Endocrine pigmentation: Chloasma describes discrete patches of facial pigmentation which occur in pregnancy and in some women taking oral contraceptives. A number of medical conditions may cause diffuse pigmentary change:

• Addison's disease. • Cushing's syndrome. • Nelson's syndrome. • Chronic renal failure.

Drugs: Drugs causing hyperpigmentation are shown in Box 17.8.

17.8 DRUG-INDUCED PIGMENTATION	
Drug	**Appearance**
Amiodarone	Slate-grey, exposed sites
Arsenic	Diffuse bronze pigmentation with superimposed raindrop depigmentation
Bleomycin	Often flexural, brown
Busulfan	Diffuse brown
Chloroquine	Blue-grey, exposed sites
Clofazimine	Brown-grey, exposed sites
Mepacrine	Yellow
Minocycline	Slate-grey, scars, temples, shins and sclera
Phenothiazines	Slate-grey, exposed sites
Psoralens	Brown, exposed sites

ABNORMAL NAILS

NAIL FOLD DISORDERS

Paronychia means inflamed and swollen nail folds. Chronic paronychia is seen frequently in those with a poor peripheral circulation, those involved in wet work, people with diabetes and those who are over-enthusiastic with manicure. Ragged cuticles and dilated or thrombosed capillaries in the proximal nail folds are important pointers to connective tissue disease (e.g. Fig. 17.4).

NAIL PLATE DISORDERS

Longitudinal ridging and beading of the nail plate is not abnormal and increases with age. Similarly, occasional white transverse flecks (striate leuconychia) are seen frequently in normal nails and are due to airspaces within the plate and not, contrary to popular belief, to insufficient calcium.

TRAUMA

Splinter haemorrhages: These are fine linear dark brown flecks running longitudinally in the plate. They are commonly due to trauma, particularly when distal, but may be seen in nail psoriasis. Less commonly, they are a sign of subacute bacterial endocarditis (p. 261).

Subungual haematomas: These may appear as a crimson, purple or grey-brown discoloration of the nail plate, most frequently that of the big toe. There is not always a history of trauma. They may be confused with melanoma, the difference being that a haematoma will 'grow out' gradually, leaving normal nail in its wake. Biopsy may be necessary to differentiate.

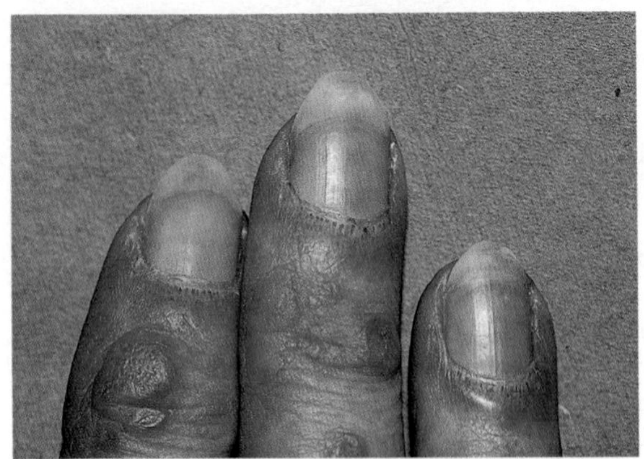

Fig. 17.4 Dermatomyositis. Erythema, dilated and tortuous capillaries in the proximal nail fold, and Gottron's papules on the digits are important diagnostic features (p. 607).

Habit-tic dystrophy: This is common, and is due to the habit of picking or fiddling with the proximal nail fold of the thumb. This produces a ladder pattern of transverse ridges and furrows up the centre of the nail.

THE NAIL IN SYSTEMIC DISEASE

Koilonychia: This concave or spoon-shaped deformity of the plate is a sign of iron deficiency.

Beau's lines: These are transverse grooves which appear at the same time on all nails, a few weeks after an acute illness, moving out to the free margins as the nails grow.

Digital clubbing: In its most gross form this is seen as a bulbous swelling of the tip of the finger or toe. The normal angle between the proximal part of the nail and the skin is lost. Causes may be:

• Respiratory: bronchogenic carcinoma, asbestosis, suppurative lung disease (empyema, bronchiectasis, cystic fibrosis), idiopathic pulmonary fibrosis. • Cardiac: cyanotic congenital heart disease, subacute bacterial endocarditis. • Other: inflammatory bowel disease, biliary cirrhosis, thyrotoxicosis, familial.

Whitening of the nails: This is a rare sign of hypoalbuminaemia. 'Half and half' nails (white proximally and red-brown distally) occur occasionally in patients with renal failure. Rarely, drugs (e.g. antimalarials) may discolour nails.

THE NAIL IN SOME COMMON SKIN DISEASES

Eczema: Shiny nails may signify frequent rubbing of eczematous skin elsewhere. When eczema involves the distal phalanges the nail may be deformed, with transverse ridging and thickening of the plate.

Lichen planus and severe alopecia areata: These may cause trachyonychia, a fine roughness and white discoloration of the nail plate.

ECZEMA

The terms 'eczema' and 'dermatitis' are synonymous. There are a number of clinical variants, which are all characterised by acute or chronic inflammation and spongiosis (oedema) of the dermis and epidermis on histology.

Atopic eczema: Atopy is a genetic predisposition to form excessive IgE, which leads to a generalised and prolonged hypersensitivity to common environmental antigens, including pollen and the house dust mite. Atopic individuals manifest one or more of a group of diseases that includes asthma, hay fever, urticaria, food and other allergies, and this distinctive form of eczema. The identification of null alleles in the filaggrin gene predisposing to atopic eczema (and asthma in association with atopic eczema) has dramatically increased our understanding of the pathogenesis of atopic eczema. Filaggrin is an important component of the skin barrier and it is the combination of this defect as well as exposure to environmental allergens that is likely to cause the clinical signs of atopic eczema.

In the acute phase, atopic eczema presents with severe itch, redness, swelling. Papules and vesicles may be evident, along with scaling and cracking of the skin, which is excessively dry. In patients with chronic eczema, lichenification may be found (dry leathery thickening of the skin with increased skin markings, secondary to constant rubbing/scratching). The distribution of atopic eczema varies according to the age of the patient: in infancy and adulthood, the eczema tends to affect the face and trunk, while in childhood, it affects the limb flexures, wrists and the ankles (Fig. 17.5).

Seborrhoeic eczema: This condition, which is characterised by a red scaly rash, classically affects the scalp (dandruff), central face, nasolabial folds, eyebrows and central chest. It is thought to be a reaction to *Pityrosporum ovale* infection of the skin. Management includes the use of ketoconazole or selenium-containing shampoo, in combination with a weak- to moderate-potency topical steroid.

Discoid eczema: This is a common form of eczema recognised from discrete coin-shaped lesions of eczema seen on the limbs of young men in association with alcohol excess, and of elderly men. It can occur in children with atopic eczema and tends to be more stubborn to treat.

Irritant eczema and allergic contact eczema: These terms refer to eczematous eruptions of the skin in response to exogenous agents. Allergic contact eczema is the more severe of the two, and represents a type IV hypersensitivity reaction to an exogenous agent. Detergents, alkalis, acids, solvents and abrasive dusts are common causes of irritant dermatitis. Nickel, parabens (a preservative in cosmetics and creams), colophony (found in sticking plasters) and balsam of Peru (found in per-

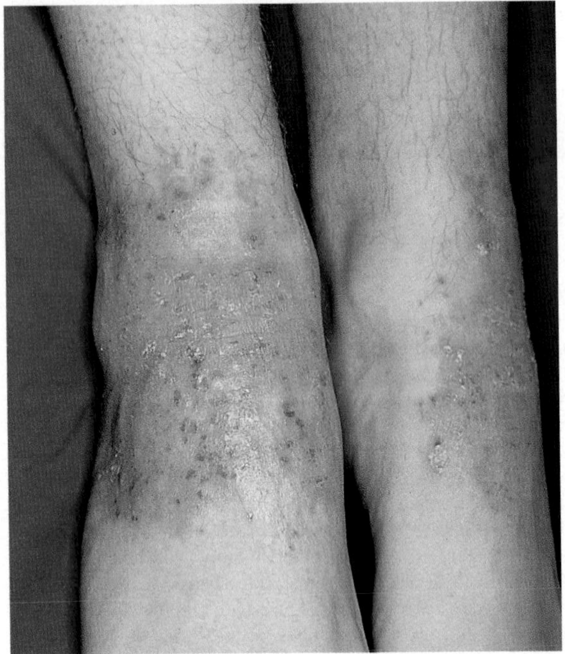

Fig. 17.5 Atopic subacute eczema on the fronts of the ankles of a teenager. These are sites of predilection, along with the cubital and popliteal fossae, in atopic eczema.

fumes) are common causes of allergic contact eczema. Both types account for a large amount of work loss. Patch testing may be helpful in diagnosis.

Asteatotic eczema: This occurs most often on the lower legs as a rippled or 'crazy paving' pattern of fine fissuring on an erythematous background. Low humidity caused by central heating, over-washing and diuretics are contributory factors.

Gravitational (stasis) eczema: This occurs on the lower legs and is often associated with signs of venous insufficiency (oedema, red or bluish discoloration, loss of hair, induration, haemosiderin pigmentation and ulceration).

Lichen simplex: This describes a plaque of lichenified eczema due to repeated rubbing or scratching, as a habit or in response to stress. Common sites include the nape of the neck, the lower legs and the anogenital area.

Pompholyx: Recurrent vesicles and bullae occur on the palms, palmar surface of the fingers and soles, and are excruciatingly itchy. This form of eczema can occur in atopic eczema and in irritant and contact allergic dermatitis. It can be provoked by heat, stress and nickel ingestion in a nickel-sensitive patient, but is often idiopathic.

General management of eczema

Bacterial and viral swabs should be taken where supra-infection is suspected. Swabbing for carriage of *Staphylococcus aureus* from the nose, axillae and inguinal areas is mandatory; if infection is found, eradication therapy should be prescribed (mupirocin or chlorhexidine/neomycin).

Important components of management of all types of eczema include:

• Use of a moisturising soap substitute such as Oilatum or Dermol 500. • Regular use of a greasy emollient. • Appropriate use of topical steroid of adequate potency.

Topical steroids: These are available in a range of potencies from highly potent (Dermovate) to potent (Betnovate), moderately potent (Eumovate) and weakly potent (hydrocortisone). Both cream (oil/water mix base) and ointment (oil base) preparations are available; the latter are preferable for their enhanced capacity to moisturise, and the fact that they contain fewer preservatives which might provoke an irritant or allergic reaction. Higher-potency topical steroids should be used for the shortest time possible, as side-effects of chronic use include:

• Thinning, striae, fragility and purpura. • Increased susceptibility to infection. • Rarely, systemic absorption causing suppression of the hypothalamic–pituitary–adrenal axis.

PSORIASIS AND OTHER ERYTHEMATOUS SCALY ERUPTIONS

Psoriasis and lichen planus will be described here in detail; other scaly conditions were covered on page 699.

PSORIASIS

Psoriasis is a non-infectious, chronic inflammatory disease of the skin, characterised by well-defined erythematous plaques with silvery scale, which have a predilection for the extensor surfaces and scalp, and by its chronic fluctuating course. The prevalence is 2% in European populations, but less in African and Asian populations. Pathology reveals keratinocyte proliferation and an inflammatory infiltrate. The cause is unknown, but there is a large familial component. Precipitating factors include:

• Trauma. • Intercurrent infection. • Certain drugs (β-blockers, antimalarials, lithium). • Stress/anxiety.

There are five main clinical presentations:

Stable plaque psoriasis: This the most common type, consisting of the well-recognised salmon-pink plaques with silvery scale arising on the elbows, knees and back (Fig. 17.6). The scalp is involved in ~60% of patients. Nail disease is common, with pitting of the nail plate, onycholysis or subungual hyperkeratosis (Fig. 17.7). Psoriasis of the flexures (e.g. natal cleft, axillae, submammary folds) looks red, shiny and symmetrical, but not scaly.

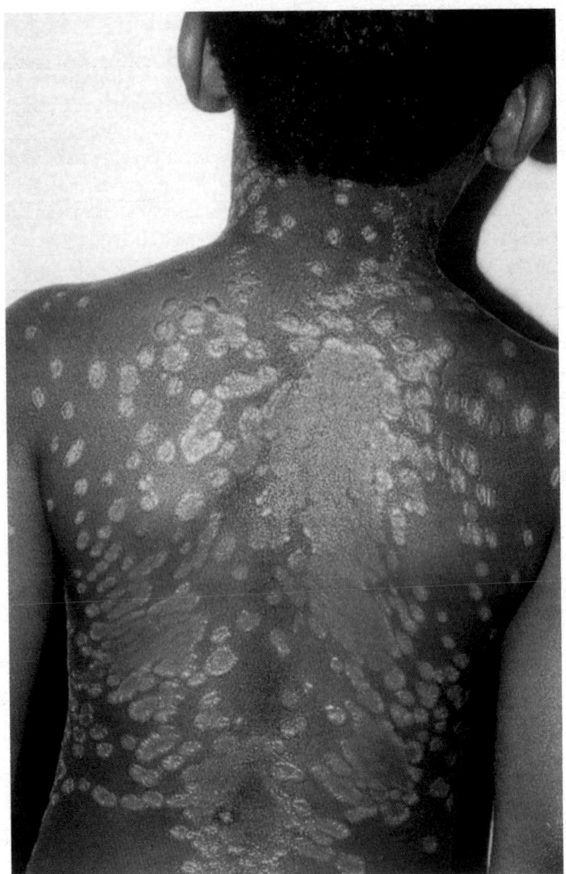

Fig. 17.6 Psoriasis: plaques of varying size in a child.

Guttate psoriasis: This occurs more frequently in children and adolescents, and often follows a streptococcal sore throat. The onset is rapid, and the lesions consist of small raindrop-sized scaly plaques. Guttate psoriasis responds well to phototherapy. The majority of these patients later develop plaque psoriasis.

Erythrodermic psoriasis: This is one of the dermatological emergencies. Over 90% of the body surface becomes erythematous and scaly. It is often accompanied by systemic upset due to the high losses of heat and fluid from the inflamed skin.

Pustular psoriasis: This may be generalised or localised. The rare generalised form is a dermatological emergency, presenting with large numbers

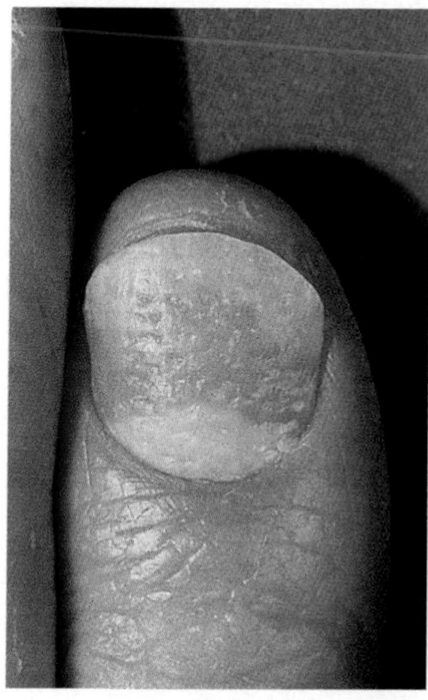

Fig. 17.7 Coarse pitting of the nail and separation of the nail from the nail bed (onycholysis). These are both classic features of psoriasis.

of sterile pustules on an erythematous base. The patient is unwell with swinging pyrexia, and requires hospital admission. The localised form is less serious, though extremely uncomfortable, and generally affects the palms and the soles (palmoplantar pustulosis). This condition particularly affects middle-aged female smokers.

Psoriatic arthropathy: See page 591.

Diagnosis and management

The diagnosis is clinical.

Management depends on the patient, his or her expectations, the subtype of psoriasis and the extent of the disease. Limited chronic plaque psoriasis should be manageable with topical agents only, whereas more extensive disease may require phototherapy or systemic agents. Inpatient treatment with a combination of dithranol and UVB (Ingram's regimen) is an excellent and safe option, which can clear psoriasis.

Topical agents: Dithranol, tar, and vitamin D analogues (calcitriol, calcipotriol) all reduce plaques. Corticosteroids should be used sparingly, mainly for flexures.

Phototherapy: UVB or psoralen (photosensitiser) plus UVA (PUVA) are effective in moderate to severe psoriasis, but carry a long-term risk of skin cancer.

Systemic agents: Acitretin (a retinoid), methotrexate and ciclosporin are effective but may cause significant side-effects.

Newer biological agents: Infliximab, etanercept and efalizumab may be considered when other treatments have failed.

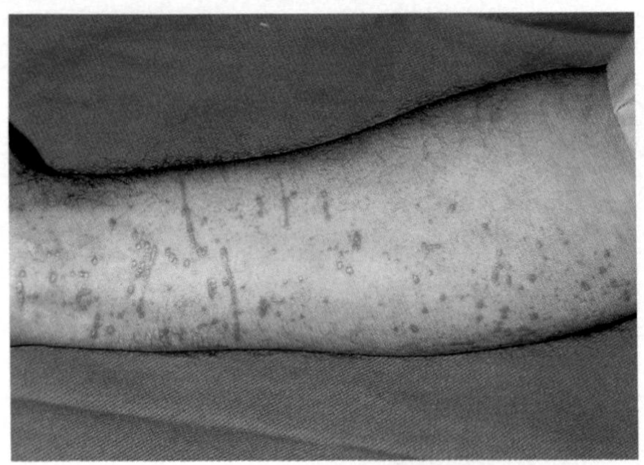

Fig. 17.8 Lichen planus. Glistening discrete papules involving the volar aspects of the forearm and wrist. Note the lesions along scratch marks (Köbner phenomenon).

LICHEN PLANUS

Lichen planus is a rash characterised by intensely itchy polygonal papules with a violaceous hue, most commonly involving the volar aspects of the wrists, and the lower back (Fig. 17.8). About two-thirds of patients have oral mucosal involvement: an asymptomatic fine white lacy network of papules known as Wickham's striae (p. 696).

The diagnosis is clinical but biopsy for histopathology may be required in atypical cases. Potent topical steroids may ease the itch; ciclosporin, retinoids and phototherapy have all been tried for more recalcitrant cases. Resolution usually occurs after ~1 yr, leaving post-inflammatory staining of the skin.

SOME COMMON SKIN INFECTIONS AND INFESTATIONS

BACTERIAL INFECTIONS

IMPETIGO

Impetigo is a common superficial purulent skin infection.

Non-bullous impetigo (Fig. 17.9): This can be caused by either *Staphylococcus aureus* or *Streptococcus*. It can affect all age groups but particularly involves young children, and is highly contagious. Other skin diseases, such as eczema and infestations, predispose to it.

The initial lesion is a thin-walled vesicle, which ruptures rapidly with the formation of a golden crust on an erythematous base. The sites usually affected are the face and the limbs. It is imperative to take a swab for

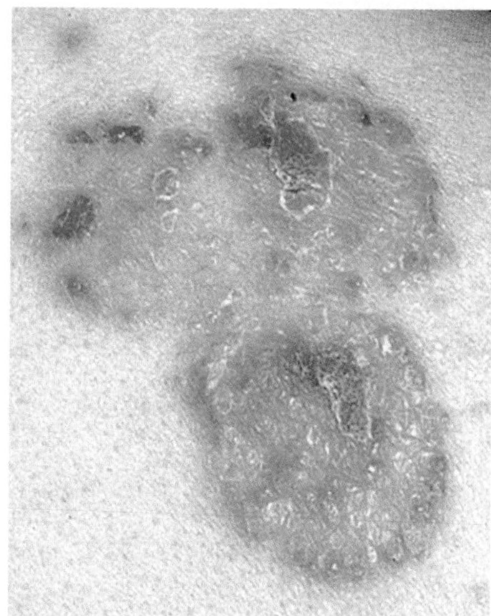

Fig. 17.9 Non-bullous impetigo.

microbiological assessment prior to starting treatment in order to determine the culprit organism. Treatment is usually with a topical preparation such as mupirocin, which is active against both organisms, or fusidic acid, in combination with an antiseptic wash. Severe cases may require oral antibiotics. Glomerulonephritis can follow infection with a nephritogenic *Streptococcus.*

Bullous impetigo: This primarily affects children and is caused by *Staphylococcus.*

Bullae (often quite large) develop and last for 2–3 days; they are initially clear but then become cloudy. Once the blisters have burst, crusts develop. Management is the same as for the non-bullous form of the disease.

ERYTHRASMA

Erythrasma is a mild localised infection of the skin caused by *Corynebacterium minutissimum*, which often is part of the normal skin flora.

C. minutissimum can provoke an asymptomatic or mildly itchy eruption between the toes and in the flexures. Lesions are well defined and reddish-brown, with some scale. The bacterium is identified by coral pink fluorescence with Wood's light. Treatments include a topical azole cream such as miconazole or a topical antibiotic.

FOLLICULITIS, FURUNCLES AND CARBUNCLES

Folliculitis can be superficial, involving just the ostium of the hair follicle (folliculitis), or deep (furuncles and carbuncles).

Superficial folliculitis: This is an extremely common condition that can be subacute or chronic. It is often infective, caused by *Staph. aureus*, but can also be due to physical (e.g. traumatic epilation) or chemical (e.g. mineral oils) injury. In these cases the folliculitis is usually sterile. Staphylococcal folliculitis is most common in children and often occurs on the scalp or limbs. The pustules usually heal in 7–10 days but can become more chronic, and in older children and adults can progress to a deeper form of folliculitis.

Deep folliculitis (furuncles and carbuncles): A furuncle (or boil) is an inflammatory nodule, follicularly based, which becomes pustular and fluctuant and is often exquisitely tender. The lesions eventually rupture to discharge pus and, because they are deep, leave a scar. They can progress to form a carbuncle, which is an exquisitely tender nodule, often on the neck, shoulders or hips and associated with severe constitutional symptoms. It implies the involvement of several contiguous hair follicles. Treatment, as for furuncles, is with an appropriate antistaphylococcal antibiotic.

STAPHYLOCOCCAL SCALDED SKIN SYNDROME (SSSS)

This is a serious exfoliating cutaneous disease predominantly affecting children, particularly neonates. Exfoliative toxins are released from a focus of *Staph. aureus* infection, which cause a split in the superficial epidermis, leading to peeling of the skin.

The child very rapidly develops fever, irritability, skin tenderness and erythema, often starting in the groin, in the axilla and around the mouth. Blisters and superficial erosions are seen within 24–28 hrs. As the toxins are spread via the blood stream, *Staph. aureus* will be isolated not on a skin swab from the sites of peeling, but from the primary site of infection. A bacterial swab should be taken from the nose and throat, as many cases arise from previously asymptomatic nasal staphylococcal carriage. Diagnosis is made on the clinical appearance and histological examination of a skin snip taken from the edge of one of the peeling areas, to determine the plane of cleavage and thus exclude the differential diagnosis of toxic epidermal necrolysis, which involves the full thickness of the epidermis. Management consists of immediate systemic antibiotics (e.g. flucloxacillin) and supportive measures in an HDU.

CELLULITIS AND ERYSIPELAS

Cellulitis and erysipelas may be difficult to distinguish clinically, the difference being the depth of involvement of the tissues. Erysipelas is the more superficial of the two conditions, with infective inflammation involving the epidermis and upper dermis. Cellulitis implies deeper involvement of subcutaneous tissues. The most common organism causing both conditions is group A streptococcus.

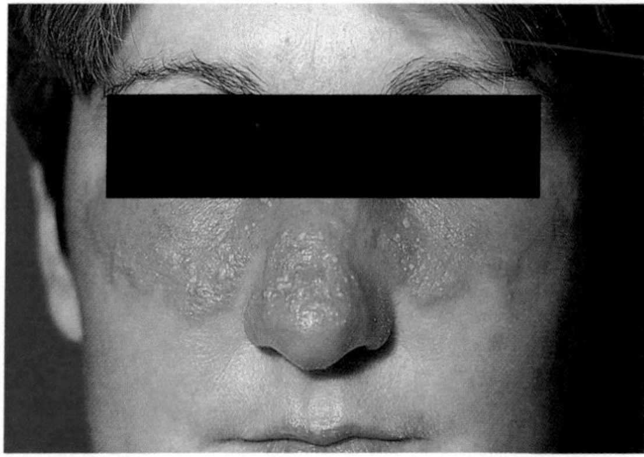

Fig. 17.10 Erysipelas. Note the blistering and crusted rash with raised erythematous edge.

Erysipelas has a characteristic raised erythematous edge (Fig. 17.10), indicating involvement of the dermis. It usually affects the face or the legs. Cellulitis most commonly involves the legs. Blistering may occur in both conditions. Diagnosis is based on clinical findings of erythema, heat, swelling, pain and sometimes fever, with a leucocytosis, raised inflammatory markers and a swab isolating a causative organism. There is often a predisposing cause, such as a portal of entry for infection, e.g. tinea pedis, or an underlying predisposition to infection such as varicose leg ulcer or diabetes. Treatment is with an appropriate antistreptococcal agent such as phenoxymethylpenicillin, or in cases of penicillin sensitivity, erythromycin or ciprofloxacin. In severe cases i.v. antibiotics are indicated.

VIRAL INFECTIONS

HERPES VIRUS INFECTIONS

These are described on pages 71–73.

PAPILLOMAVIRUSES AND VIRAL WARTS

Viral warts are caused by the DNA human papillomavirus (HPV) and are extremely common, being transmitted by direct contact with the virus in either living skin or shed skin fragments. Most people suffer from one or more warts at some point during their life. There are >90 different subtypes. HPV subtypes 16 and 18 are spread by sexual contact and are strongly associated with subsequent development of cervical carcinoma. A vaccine against these serotypes of HPV has been developed, raising the prospect that vaccination may reduce the incidence of cervical cancer. Immunosuppressed patients are at greater risk of infection with HPV.

Clinical features

Common warts appear initially as smooth, skin-coloured papules. As they enlarge, their surface becomes irregular and hyperkeratotic, producing the typical warty appearance. One method of classifying warts is based on their clinical appearance:

Plantar warts (verrucae): Found on the sole of the foot, these are characterised by a horny collar surrounding a roughened surface. Upon paring, pinpoint areas of bleeding corresponding to capillary loops can be discerned.

Mosaic warts: Plaques of tightly packed individual warts are seen.

Plane warts: These smooth, flat-topped papules are found on the face and the dorsum of the hands.

Filiform warts: These are often found on the face.

Genital warts: These are papillomatous and protuberant.

Management

Most viral warts resolve spontaneously, but often very slowly. Therapeutic options to speed resolution include:

- Cryotherapy.
- Topical salicylic acid.
- Topical formaldehyde solution.
- Imiquimod or podophyllin for genital warts.
- Intralesional bleomycin (for recalcitrant warts).

MOLLUSCUM CONTAGIOSUM

Molluscum contagiosum is a common cutaneous infection with a poxvirus. It can affect any age group but usually targets children over the age of 1 and the immunosuppressed. The classic lesion is a dome-shaped, 'umbilicated', skin-coloured papule with a central punctum. Lesions tend to be multiple and are often in sites of apposition such as the side of the chest and the inner arm. No treatment is required, as these lesions resolve spontaneously but can take several months to do so. If active resolution is sought, curettage or cryotherapy may be tried, or topical agents such as salicylic acid, podophyllin or imiquimod.

ORF

Orf is an occupational hazard for those who work with sheep and goats. It is a cutaneous infection with a parapoxvirus carried by these animals. Inoculation of the virus, usually into the skin of a finger, causes significant inflammation and necrosis, which resolve in 2–6 wks. No specific treatment is available unless there is evidence of secondary infection. Erythema multiforme can be triggered by orf virus infection.

FUNGAL INFECTIONS

Dermatophytes are fungi capable of causing superficial skin infections known as ringworm or dermatophytosis. The causative fungi belong to three genera (*Microsporum, Trichophyton, Epidermophyton*); they can originate from the soil (geophilic) or animals (zoophilic), or be confined to human skin (anthropophilic).

Clinical forms of cutaneous infection include:

• Tinea corporis (involvement of the body). • Tinea capitis (scalp involvement, see p. 707). • Tinea cruris (groin involvement). • Tinea pedis (involvement of the feet). • Onychomycosis (fungal infection of the nail).

Tinea corporis: This condition should be considered in the differential diagnosis of the red scaly rash (see p. 699). Lesions are erythematous, annular and scaly, with a well-defined edge and central clearing. They may be single or multiple and are usually asymmetrical. *Microsporum canis* and *Trichophyton verrucosum* are common culprits and are zoophilic (from dogs and cattle respectively). Inadvertent topical corticosteroid application leads to disguising and worsening of the signs (tinea incognito).

Tinea cruris: This is common world-wide and is usually caused by *T. rubrum.* Itchy erythematous plaques extend from the groin flexures on to the thighs.

Tinea pedis (athlete's foot): This is the most common fungal skin infection in the UK and USA, and is usually caused by anthropophilic fungi such as *T. rubrum, T. mentagrophytes* and *Epidermophyton floccosum.* Clinical features include an itchy rash between the toes, with peeling, fissuring and maceration.

Onychomycosis: This causes yellow-brown discoloration and crumbling of the plate, which usually starts distally and spreads proximally.

Diagnosis and management

In all cases of suspected dermatophyte infection, the diagnosis should be confirmed by skin scraping or nail clippings. Treatment can be topical (terbinafine or miconazole cream) or systemic (terbinafine, griseofulvin or itraconazole).

SCABIES

Scabies is caused by the Acarus mite, *Sarcoptes scabiei.* The infestation causes intense itch and can lead to secondary infection and complications such as post-streptococcal glomerulonephritis. Scabies spreads in households and environments where there is a high frequency of intimate personal contact.

Diagnosis is made by identifying the scabietic burrow, usually found on the edges of the fingers, toes or sides of the hands and feet. The clinical features include secondary eczematisation elsewhere on the body; the face and scalp are never involved except in the case of infants. Even after successful treatment the itch can continue and occasionally nodular lesions persist. Treatment involves two applications, 1 wk apart, of an aqueous solution of either permethrin or malathion to the whole body, excluding the head. Household contacts should also be treated. In some clinical situations such as poor compliance, immunocompromised individuals and heavy infestations (Norwegian scabies), systemic treatment with ivermectin as a single dose is appropriate.

LICE

Infestation with head louse, *Pediculus humanus capitis*, is common and highly contagious. Head lice are spread by direct head-to-head contact.

Itching of the scalp is the main symptom; scratching leads to secondary infection and cervical lymphadenopathy. The diagnosis is confirmed by identifying the living louse or nymph on the scalp or on a black sheet of paper after careful fine-toothed combing of wet hair that has had conditioner applied. The pale empty egg cases ('nits') are easily seen adhering strongly to the hair shaft. Treatment with malathion, permethrin, and carbaryl in lotion or aqueous form is recommended for the infected individual and any infected household/school contacts. Treatment is applied on two separate occasions at 7–10 days' interval. Body lice and pubic (crab) lice are similar, the latter being predominantly sexually transmitted. They also respond to malathion.

ACNE AND ROSACEA

ACNE VULGARIS

Acne is an inflammatory eruption almost ubiquitous in the teenage years, characterised clinically by open comedones (blackheads), closed comedones (white heads) and seborrhoea. More severe manifestations include inflammatory papules, pustules, nodules and cysts. The latter may cause significant scarring. The distribution is predominantly on the face, shoulders, upper chest and back. There are three pathogenetic factors:

• Elevated sebum excretion. • Occlusion or blockage of the pilosebaceous unit. • Colonisation with *Propionibacterium acnes*.

Management

• Mild disease may be treated with topical antibiotics such as erythromycin, dessicants such as benzoyl peroxide, or topical retinoids. • Oral antibiotics, particularly of the tetracycline group, are used as prolonged courses for more stubborn disease. • The anti-androgenic oral contraceptive Dianette (cyproterone acetate with ethinylestradiol) is also an option in female patients. • For the most severe cases, oral retinoid therapy with isotretinoin has revolutionised the management of acne. The side-effect profile includes drying of the skin and mucous membranes but this is generally manageable. Isotretinoin may elevate serum triglycerides and derange liver function; both should be checked prior to commencing the drug. Isotretinoin is highly teratogenic, and female patients must be counselled about this prior to commencing treatment.

ROSACEA

Rosacea is a persistent facial eruption of unknown cause, largely occurring in middle age (Fig. 17.11). It is characterised by erythema, telangiectasia,

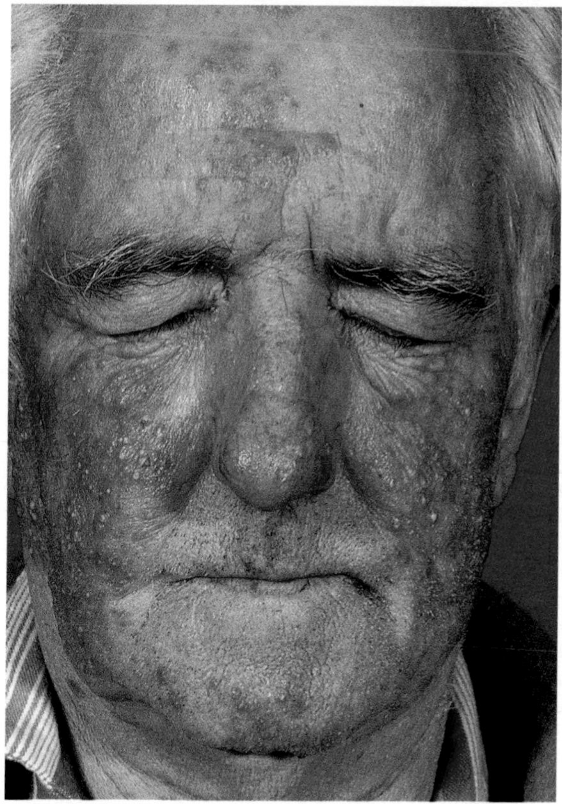

Fig. 17.11 Rosacea. The colour is distinctive and the typical papulo-pustular rash involves the cheeks, centre of forehead and chin.

papules and pustules. A bulbous appearance to the nose, known as rhinophyma, may be seen as part of the disease complex and is caused by sebaceous gland hypertrophy. The papulo-pustular element of disease usually responds well to tetracyclines, but the erythema and telangiectasia do not; these may require laser therapy.

SKIN TUMOURS

Only the most common benign tumours and a few malignant ones are described in this section.

BENIGN TUMOURS

MELANOCYTIC NAEVI

Melanocytic naevi (moles) are localised benign proliferations of melanocytes which are probably clonal. Moles are a usual feature of most human beings and it is quite normal to have 20–50. Individuals with high sun exposure also show more moles, i.e. there is clear evidence for both genetic and environmental factors. With the exception of congenital melanocytic naevi (which are present at birth or appear shortly after), most melanocytic naevi appear in early childhood, at adolescence, and during pregnancy or oestrogen therapy. The appearance of a new mole is less common after the age of 25.

Clinical features

Acquired melanocytic naevi are classified according to the microscopic location of the clumps of melanocytes in the skin.

Junctional naevi are usually circular and macular; their colour ranges from mid- to dark brown and may vary within a single lesion. Compound and intradermal naevi are similar to one another in appearance; both are nodules of up to 1 cm in diameter, although intradermal naevi are usually less pigmented than compound naevi. Their surface may be smooth, cerebriform or even hyperkeratotic and papillomatous, and they are often hairy.

Management

Melanocytic naevi are normal and do not require excision, except when malignancy is suspected or when they repeatedly become inflamed or traumatised. Some individuals wish to have them removed for cosmetic reasons.

SEBORRHOEIC WARTS (BASAL CELL PAPILLOMA)

Seborrhoeic warts are common benign epidermal tumours, which occur almost exclusively over the age of 35. They vary in colour from yellow to very dark brown, and have a greasy, ‘stuck-on’ appearance. Although they may be a cosmetic problem, their principal significance lies in the differential diagnosis of melanoma or other skin tumours. If treatment is required, seborrhoeic keratoses respond well to cryotherapy or alternatively to curettage.

KERATOACANTHOMA

This is a striking benign keratinocyte tumour characterised by a period of rapid growth of a lesion that may be 4 or 5 cm across or even larger, with a central keratin plug in a dome-shaped nodule. Spontaneous resolution occurs but may take months. Excision of these lesions is usually undertaken, as they can clinically resemble squamous cell carcinomas.

PRE-MALIGNANT TUMOURS

ACTINIC KERATOSIS

Actinic keratoses are small, scaly, red areas on sun-exposed sites that show focal areas of dysplasia on histological examination (Fig. 17.12). They are extremely common and frequently multiple. They are treated easily and effectively with liquid nitrogen. If there is a large number of lesions, then the topical cytotoxic 5-fluorouracil may be required; alternatively, the topical immunostimulant, imiquimod, or photodynamic therapy may be used. Lesions which do not respond to treatment may require curettage or excision and reconsideration of their nature.

INTRA-EPIDERMAL CARCINOMA (IEC; BOWEN'S DISEASE)

This usually presents as a slow-growing, red, scaly area (resembling a psoriatic plaque), in which histology demonstrates full-thickness dysplasia. IEC is most commonly found on the lower legs of elderly female patients, may develop into squamous cell carcinomas, and should always be treated. A biopsy may be required to make the diagnosis and distinguish from actinic keratosis, and subsequent treatment should be destructive—either surgery, cryotherapy or photodynamic therapy.

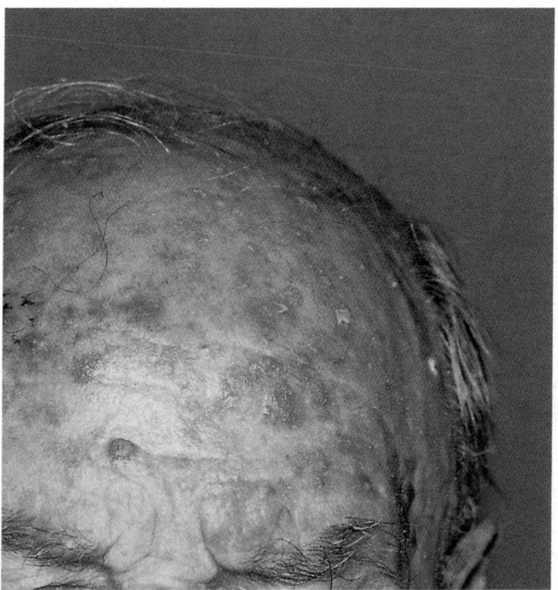

Fig. 17.12 Numerous actinic keratoses in a white patient who had lived for years in the tropics.

MALIGNANT TUMOURS

NON-MELANOMA SKIN CANCERS

This term incorporates both basal cell carcinomas and squamous cell carcinomas; these cutaneous cancers are rising in age-specific incidence. Risk factors include:

• UV exposure. • Pale skin type. • Previous radiotherapy. • Arsenic exposure. • Chronic inflammation (e.g. Marjolin's ulcer; see p. 705).

There is also an increased risk of non-melanoma skin cancers in those receiving long-term immunosuppressive medication such as transplant recipients, and in those who have received large amounts of PUVA therapy in the past.

Basal cell carcinoma (BCC; 'rodent ulcer')

This is the most common human cancer. It is a slow-growing tumour which rarely metastasises but which can invade locally. There are three morphological variants:

• Nodular BCC (Fig. 17.13): the most common type, this presents as a pearly-edged papule with central ulceration, and fine telangiectasia on its surface. It can reach several centimetres in diameter if not treated. A pigmented variant is recognised. • Morphoeic BCC: presents as a slowly enlarging, yellowy-grey, waxy-looking plaque with a shiny appearance and ill-defined edges. It may ulcerate. • Superficial BCC: seen most often on the trunk, this appears as a slowly enlarging, pink or brown scaly plaque with a fine 'whipcord' edge. It may resemble a patch of intra-epidermal carcinoma.

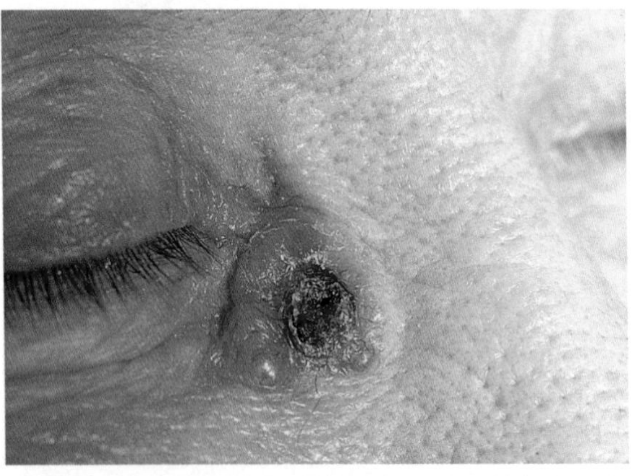

Fig. 17.13 Basal cell carcinoma. A slowly growing, pearly nodule just below the inner canthus. The central crust overlies an ulcerated area.

Management: The choice of treatment modality depends on local expertise and interest, and includes surgery, cryotherapy, radiotherapy, photodynamic therapy or the topical immunostimulant, imiquimod. All forms of treatment used optimally can produce excellent cure rates.

Squamous cell carcinoma (SCC)

SCC is a proliferative tumour that can present with a very heterogenous group of clinical pictures, including keratotic nodules, exophytic erythematous nodules, infiltrating firm tumours and ulcers with an indurated edge. Histological grade also varies from well-differentiated to anaplastic.

Management: As with BCC, a number of modalities may be used, including aggressive curettage and cautery, excision with a surrounding cuff of normal tissue, or radiotherapy. In general, excision with assessment of adequacy of margins is the preferred option because of the definite risk of metastasis. Surgical excision with a 3–4 mm margin has a cure rate of ≥90%.

MALIGNANT MELANOMA

Malignant melanoma is a tumour of the pigment cells (melanocytes) and has increased in incidence in the last two decades. Its importance lies in the significant mortality associated with thicker lesions, and the lack of effective therapies for metastatic disease. The main risk factors for melanoma are:

• Prolonged UVR exposure. • Pale skin. • Large numbers of naevi. • Positive family history.

Clinical features

There are five subtypes of melanoma, which can be discerned clinically:

Superficial spreading malignant melanoma (Fig. 17.14): Most common in Caucasians and is characterised by a superficial radial growth pattern, which over time may progress to vertical spread.

Lentigo maligna melanoma: Occurs most often on exposed skin of the elderly as a macular area of variable pigmentation. It is often preceded by an in situ phase known as lentigo maligna.

Nodular melanoma: Presents as a pigmented nodule without a preceding in situ phase.

Acral lentiginous melanoma: Occurs on the palms and soles and occasionally under nails.

Amelanotic malignant melanoma: Thought to be a non-pigment-producing variant of nodular melanoma, which can be confused with other benign skin lesions such as pyogenic granuloma.

Diagnosis

The ABCDE rule is a useful tool for detecting suspicious pigmented lesions:

• Asymmetry. • Border irregularity or bleeding. • Colour (moles developing pigment variegation). • Diameter (increase in size over time). • Evolving (any change noted by the patient in a pigmented lesion).

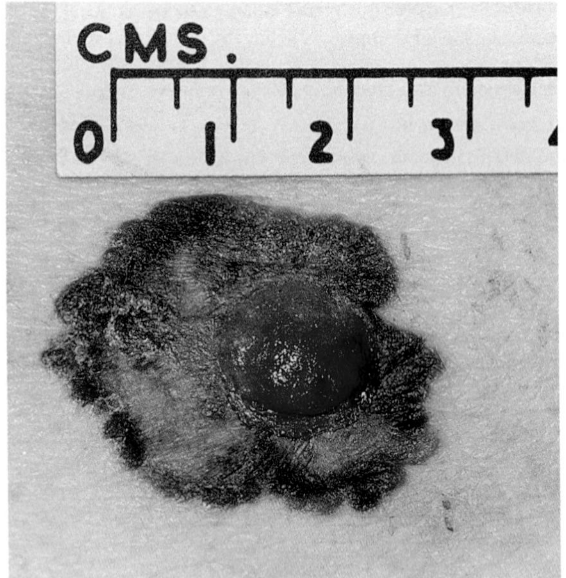

Fig. 17.14 Superficial spreading melanoma. The radial growth phase was present for ~3 yrs before the invasive amelanotic nodule developed within it. Note the irregular outline, asymmetrical shape and different hues, including depigmented areas signifying spontaneous regression.

Management

The lesion should be excised with a margin of clinically normal tissue around it. Histological classification using Clarke levels (based on the extent of invasion into the various anatomical levels of the skin) and Breslow thickness (based on the depth of invasion in millimetres) is used to determine prognosis and further treatment. This may involve wider local excision and sentinel lymph node mapping and biopsy.

CUTANEOUS T-CELL LYMPHOMA (MYCOSIS FUNGOIDES)

In contrast to B-cell lymphomas, which usually present as sudden focal skin tumours, cutaneous T-cell lymphoma often has an indolent course, developing slowly over many years from polymorphic patches and plaques through to nodules and then a systemic stage. Given that it can appear clinically similar to a number of other more common inflammatory skin conditions such as eczema and psoriasis, a high index of suspicion is required for diagnosis.

Staging with CT may be required. Treatment options include corticosteroids and phototherapy in early-stage disease. Chemotherapy and physical therapies such as radiotherapy and electron beam radiotherapy are reserved for more advanced disease.

THE SKIN IN SYSTEMIC DISEASE

NEUROFIBROMATOSIS

NF1 is one of the most common autosomal disorders and is caused by a mutation on chromosome 17. The characteristic cutaneous features are:

• Café au lait macules (also a feature of Albright's syndrome—polyostotic fibrous dysplasia). • Axillary freckling. • Lisch nodules (iris hamartomas). • Cutaneous neurofibromas.

Involvement of other organs, such as the eye (optic gliomas), the spine (scoliosis), the adrenal glands (phaeochromocytomas) and neurofibromas affecting any organ, demands a multidisciplinary approach to management of these patients.

NF2 presents with neurological disease and has few or no cutaneous features (p. 677).

TUBEROUS SCLEROSIS

This is an autosomal dominant condition with hamartomas affecting many systems. Diagnosis is made on the basis of the classical triad of mental retardation, epilepsy and the presence of characteristic skin lesions:

• Ash leaf macules (small white oval patches on the skin). • Adenoma sebaceum (pink-yellow papules on the face). • Peri-/subungual fibromas. • Shagreen patches (cobblestone-like plaques at the base of the spine).

Other features may include hyperplastic gums, retinal phakomas (fibrous overgrowth), renal, lung and heart tumours, cerebral gliomas and calcification of the basal ganglia.

XANTHOMAS

These deposits of fatty material in the skin, subcutaneous fat and tendons may be the first clue to primary or secondary hyperlipidaemia. Several patterns are recognised:

• Eruptive yellow papules on the buttocks (eruptive xanthomas). • Yellowish macules or plaques (plane xanthomas). • Small yellow-grey plaques around the eyes (xanthelasma palpebrarum). • Nodules over the elbows and knees (tuberous xanthomas). • Subcutaneous nodules attached to tendons, especially those on the dorsal aspect of the fingers and the Achilles tendons (tendinous xanthomas).

When xanthomas are detected, the fasting blood lipids and the electrophoretic pattern of plasma lipoproteins should be measured.

AMYLOIDOSIS (see also p. 159)

Cutaneous amyloidosis is a much more common feature of primary systemic amyloidosis and the amyloidosis associated with myeloma than of secondary amyloidosis. Deposits appear as waxy plaques around the eyes or as peri-orbital purpura. 'Pinch purpura', appearing where the skin is traumatised, is due to amyloid infiltration of blood vessels and may also be a striking feature.

PORPHYRIA

The porphyrias are a group of rare systemic diseases characterised by defects in the haem biosynthesis pathway (p. 161). Some of these diseases have cutaneous manifestations.

Porphyria cutanea tarda: This is the most common porphyria. It usually starts in adulthood and can be inherited or acquired due to alcohol, iron overload, oestrogens, hepatitis C and HIV disease. The cutaneous features are increased skin fragility, blistering, erosions and milia occurring on light-exposed areas. The skin manifestations of variegate porphyria are similar.

Erythropoietic protoporphyria: This is a rare porphyria that starts in childhood, with burning and pain on light-exposed areas due to ferrochelatase deficiency. Scars occur, particularly on the nose. Examination of the red cells, plasma and stool for protoporphyrins is confirmatory.

Pseudoporphyrias: Sun-bed usage, NSAIDs (particularly naproxen) and renal failure can give rise to skin lesions that mimic the photosensitive porphyrias, particularly porphyria cutanea tarda.

SARCOIDOSIS

Cutaneous manifestations of sarcoid are seen in about one-third of patients with systemic disease. The clinical features include:

• Erythema nodosum. • Dusky infiltrated plaques on the nose and fingers (lupus pernio). • Scattered brownish-red, violaceous or hypopigmented papules or nodules which vary in number, size and distribution.

ERYTHEMA MULTIFORME

This term describes a reactive eruption in which lesions may be urticaria-like and often have an obvious 'bull's-eye' or 'target' appearance. Blisters may be seen in the centre or around the edges of the lesions (Fig. 17.15). In some cases blisters dominate the picture; the Stevens–Johnson syndrome is severe bullous erythema multiforme with the emphasis on mucosal involvement including the mouth, eyes and genitals, with constitutional disturbance. This condition may be provoked by a variety of infective agents, including viruses (e.g. herpes simplex, orf), *Mycoplasma*, drugs (especially sulphonamides, penicillins, barbiturates) and, more rarely, internal malignancy.

Management is supportive, although the severest manifestation of the disease, Stevens–Johnson syndrome, can be treated with a short course of i.v. immunoglobulin. There is no evidence that systemic corticosteroids shorten the course of illness or diminish severity.

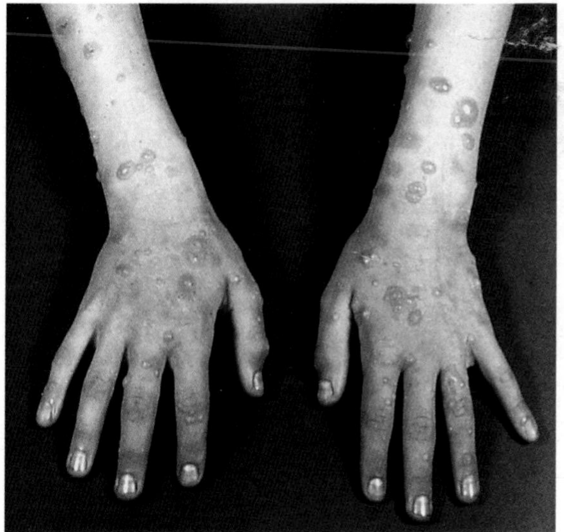

Fig. 17.15 Erythema multiforme with blistering lesions in a young woman.

ERYTHEMA NODOSUM

This characteristic reaction pattern is due to a vasculitis in the deep dermis and inflammation of subcutaneous fat (panniculitis).

Causes include:

- Infections including bacteria (streptococcus, *M. tuberculosis*, *Brucella*, *M. leprae*), viruses, rickettsiae, *Chlamydia*, *Mycoplasma* and fungi. • Drugs including sulphonamides and the oral contraceptive pill. • Systemic diseases especially sarcoidosis, ulcerative colitis and Crohn's disease.

Clinical features

Painful, palpable, dusky blue-red nodules are most commonly seen on the lower legs. Malaise, fever and joint pains are common. The lesions resolve slowly over a month, leaving bruise-like marks.

Management

• The underlying cause should be determined and treated. • Bed rest and oral NSAIDs may hasten resolution. • Tapering systemic corticosteroid courses may be required in stubborn cases.

PYODERMA GANGRENOSUM (PG)

PG predominantly occurs in adults between the ages of 25 and 54 yrs. The eruption starts as an inflamed nodule or pustule, which breaks down centrally and rapidly progresses to an ulcer with an indurated or undermined

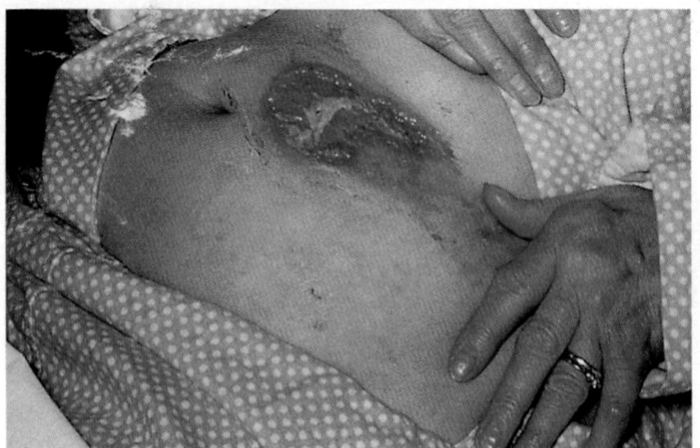

Fig. 17.16 Pyoderma gangrenosum. A large indolent ulcer in a patient with rheumatoid arthritis. Note healing in one part.

purplish or pustular edge, often demonstrating a cribriform (basket-weave) pattern (Fig. 17.16). Subtypes include ulcerative, pustular, bullous and vegetative. Although PG may arise in the absence of any underlying disease, it is often associated with a systemic disease, such as inflammatory bowel disease, arthritis (both rheumatoid arthritis and seronegative arthropathies), immunodeficiency and immunosuppression including HIV disease, monoclonal gammopathies and leukaemia.

• Local therapy includes pain relief, highly potent topical steroid, prevention of secondary bacterial infection and dressings. • Systemic therapy includes oral corticosteroids in a tapering dose, dapsone, minocycline, sulfasalazine and ciclosporin.

ACANTHOSIS NIGRICANS

This is a velvety thickening and pigmentation of the major flexures, particularly the axillae. Causes include obesity, insulin resistance syndromes and malignancy, particularly gastric cancer. Pruritus is a feature of malignancy-associated acanthosis and regression occurs after the tumour is excised.

NECROBIOSIS LIPOIDICA

This condition is important to recognise because of its association with diabetes mellitus. Fewer than 1% of people with diabetes have necrobiosis, but more than 85% of patients with necrobiosis will have or will develop diabetes.

Typically, the lesions appear as shiny, atrophic and slightly yellow plaques on the shins (Fig. 17.17). Underlying telangiectasia is easily seen. Minor knocks may precipitate slow-healing ulcers. No treatment is very effective. Topical and intralesional corticosteroids are used, as is long-term PUVA.

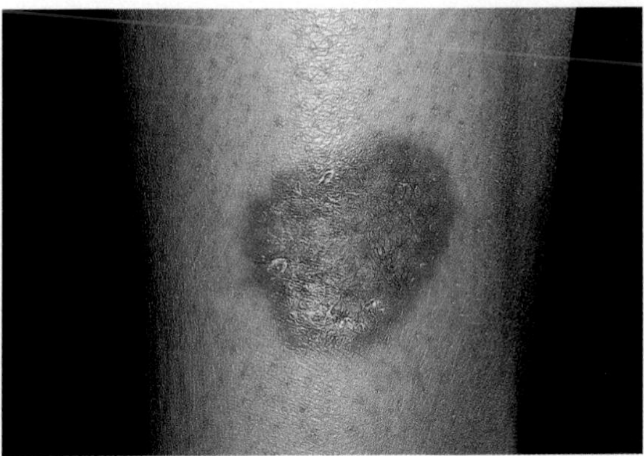

Fig. 17.17 Necrobiosis lipoidica. An atrophic yellowish plaque on the skin of a person with diabetes.

GRANULOMA ANNULARE

This is a common cutaneous condition of uncertain aetiology; any association with diabetes is now thought to be spurious. Dermal nodules occur singly or in an annular configuration. They are asymptomatic and commonly occur on highly visible sites such as the hands and feet. Intralesional corticosteroids can be helpful but most nodules spontaneously resolve over years.

DRUG ERUPTIONS

Cutaneous drug reactions are common and almost any drug can cause them. Drug reactions may reasonably be included in the differential diagnosis of most skin diseases. Presentations are summarised in Box 17.9. However, common to most drug eruption is symmetry, and a temporal relationship in onset to the commencement of the drug in question. There are no specific investigations which help.

Management

• Withdrawal of the offending drug. • Oral antihistamines for itch. • Short course of oral prednisolone or potent topical steroid for symptomatic relief. • Copious emollient.

DERMATOLOGICAL PROCEDURES

Many dermatological procedures can be carried out under local anaesthetic. Options include:

Biopsy: Incisional (where the aim is diagnostic) or excisional (where the aim is to remove the lesion in its entirety). Used in a wide variety of conditions, from rashes for the purposes of diagnosis to the definitive treatment

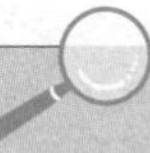

17.9 DRUG ERUPTIONS AND SOME DRUGS WHICH MAY CAUSE THEM		
Reaction pattern	**Clinical features**	**Examples of drugs commonly responsible**
Toxic erythema	Erythematous plaques, morbilliform rash	Antibiotics, sde, thiazides, pbz, PAS
Urticaria	Itchy weals, sometimes with angioedema	Salicylates, codeine, antibiotics, dextran, ACEI
Erythema and scaling	Scaly, pink/red papules, varying sizes	Antibiotics, anticonvulsants, ACEI, gold, penicillamine
Allergic vasculitis	Painful palpable purpura with ulcers	Sde, pbz, indometacin, phenytoin, o.c.
Erythema multiforme	Target-like lesions and bullae on limbs	Sde, pbz, barbiturates
Purpura	Exclude thrombocytopenia, coagulation defect	Thiazides, sde, pbz, sulphonylureas, barbiturates, quinine
Bullous eruptions	Sometimes with erythema and purpura	Barbiturates, penicillamine, nalidixic acid
Exfoliative dermatitis	Universal redness and scaling, shivering	Pbz, PAS, isoniazid, gold
Fixed drug eruptions	Erythematous, occasionally bullous plaques	Tetracyclines, quinine, sde, barbiturates
Acneiform eruptions	Rash resembles acne	Lithium, o.c., steroids, anti-TB drugs, anticonvulsants
Toxic epidermal necrolysis	Rash resembles scalded skin	Barbiturates, phenytoin, pbz, penicillin
Hair loss	Diffuse	Cytotoxics, acitretin, anticoagulants, antithyroid drugs, o.c.
Hypertrichosis		Diazoxide, minoxidil, ciclosporin
Photosensitivity	Rash limited to exposed skin	Thiazides, tetracyclines, phenothiazines, sde, psoralens

ACEI = ACE inhibitors; sde = sulphonamides; o.c. = oral contraceptives; pbz = phenylbutazone; PAS = para-aminosalicylic acid.

of skin cancers. Biopsy has the advantage of providing tissue for histological diagnosis to be made.

Cryotherapy: Application of liquid nitrogen to a lesion. Used to treat viral warts, seborrhoeic keratoses, actinic keratoses and IEC (Bowen's disease). Treatment can be uncomfortable and does not provide tissue for histological evaluation, but has the advantage of not requiring an anaesthetic.

Curettage: A method of removing lesions by scraping, with healing left to occur by secondary intention. Used to treat actinic keratoses, seborrhoeic warts, IEC and occasionally superficial BCC. Provides tissue for histological confirmation of diagnosis.

Laser therapy: Useful for treating vascular lesions and benign areas of pigmentation such as melasma, tattoos or drug-induced pigmentation following minocycline therapy.

18

Therapeutics and prescriptions

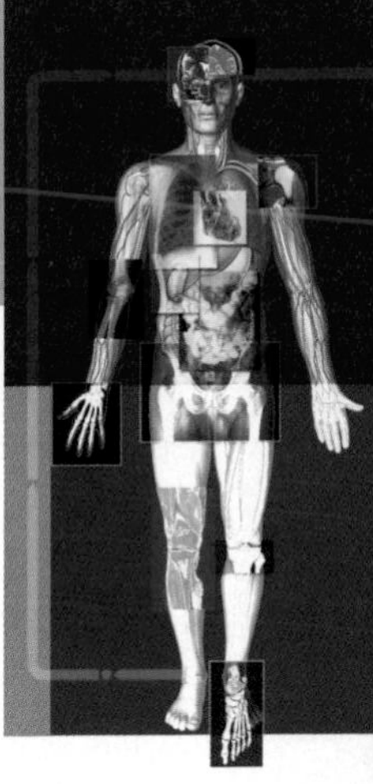

The purpose of drug therapy is to cure or ameliorate disease, or to alleviate symptoms. However, all drugs also have adverse effects and drug therapy is not always necessary. The good prescriber: The good prescriber prescribes only when the balance of benefit to harm is favourable. The choice of drug should be based on an understanding of the relevant pathophysiology and pharmacology, and the dose regimen must take into account the particular circumstances of each patient. The response to treatment should be monitored and the prescription reviewed if adverse effects emerge.

The knowledge and experience required to become a good prescriber may take many years to accrue and, for the newcomer to medicine, merely gaining some familiarity with the wide range of available treatments may seem daunting. This chapter provides concise summaries of some important and common drugs, including the mode of action, major side-effects, contraindications and interactions, and a guide to their use in everyday practice. Also included is some basic advice on writing prescriptions and on prescribing in renal impairment, hepatic impairment and the elderly. Neither the list of drugs nor the information on their side-effects and interactions is exhaustive, and we would advise readers to refer to the *British National Formulary* or other national equivalent for more detailed and regularly updated guidance.

WRITING A DRUG PRESCRIPTION

A prescription should be a precise, accurate, clear, readable set of instructions, sufficient for a nurse to administer a drug accurately in hospital, or for a pharmacist to provide a patient with both the correct drug and the instructions on how to take it. The information that should be written on a prescription is given in Box 18.1. Some abbreviations used in prescribing are listed in Box 18.2. Other abbreviations should be avoided and instructions should, whenever possible, be written in plain English. Because of the problems of drug addiction and misuse of drugs, drugs likely to be abused are, in the UK, the subject of the *Misuse of Drugs Act* (1971), the *Misuse of Drugs (Notification of and Supply to Addicts) Regulations* (1973) and the *Misuse of Drugs Regulations* (1985). The requirements for the prescription of controlled drugs are listed in Box 18.3. Doctors in other countries should make themselves familiar with local regulations.

18.1 INFORMATION TO BE GIVEN ON A UK PRESCRIPTION OUTSIDE HOSPITAL

- The date
- The patient's name, initials and address
- The age of a child under 12
- The name of the drug, preferably in capitals (use generic names when possible)
- The formulation to be prescribed
- The strength of the formulation
- The dose
- The frequency of administration
- The route of administration
- The doctor's name, address and signature

ALTERING DOSAGES IN RENAL INSUFFICIENCY

If a drug is more than 50% eliminated unchanged by the kidneys or has active metabolites that are eliminated by the kidneys (Box 18.4), the maintenance dosage must be altered in renal insufficiency, although it is not usually necessary to alter a one-off dose. Creatinine clearance can be used as a guide to reducing maintenance dosages.

Some drugs should be avoided entirely in renal insufficiency, for either pharmacokinetic or pharmacodynamic reasons (Box 18.5).

Diuretics are relatively ineffective in severe renal insufficiency, partly because they cannot gain access to their site of action, the luminal epithelium. High dosages of loop diuretics may be required for efficacy. Potassium-sparing diuretics should not be used, because of the increased risk of hyperkalaemia.

18.2 ACCEPTABLE ABBREVIATIONS IN PRESCRIPTIONS

Abbreviation	Latin meaning	English translation
b.d. or b.i.d.	Bis in die	Twice a day
gutt.	Guttae	Drops
i.m.	—	Intramuscular(ly)
i.v.	—	Intravenous(ly)
o.d.	Omni die	(Once) every day
o.m.	Omni mane[1]	(Once) every morning
o.n.	Omni nocte[1]	(Once) every night
p.o.	Per os	By mouth
PR	Per rectum	By the anal route
p.r.n.	Pro re nata	Whenever required
PV	Per vaginam	By the vaginal route
q.d.s.	Quater die sumendum[2]	Four times a day
s.c.	—	Subcutaneous(ly)
stat.	Statim	Immediately
t.d.s.	Ter die sumendum[2]	Three times a day

[1] Sometimes written simply as 'mane' or 'nocte'.
[2] The abbreviations t.i.d. and q.i.d. (ter/quater in die) are sometimes used instead; do not use q.d. to mean once a day.

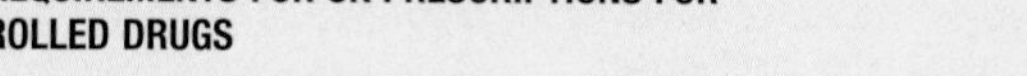

18.3 REQUIREMENTS FOR UK PRESCRIPTIONS FOR CONTROLLED DRUGS

Prescriptions for controlled drugs must:

- be completely written in the prescriber's handwriting in ink
- be signed and dated by the prescriber
- specify the prescriber's address
- specify the name and address of the patient
- state the form and strength (if appropriate) of the drug
- state the total quantity of the drug or the number of dose units to be dispensed in both words and figures
- state the exact size of each dose in both words and figures

ALTERING DOSAGES IN HEPATIC FAILURE

The liver has a large functional capacity, and chronic hepatic insufficiency usually has to be considerable before it affects drug dosages. In chronic liver disease, jaundice, ascites, a prolonged PT, hypoalbuminaemia, malnutrition and encephalopathy all make clinically important impairment of drug metabolism more likely.

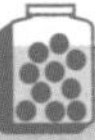

18.4 DRUGS WHOSE DOSAGES ARE AFFECTED BY RENAL INSUFFICIENCY[1]	
Mild renal insufficiency (creatinine clearance 20–50 ml/min)	
• ACE inhibitors • Aminoglycosides • Chlorpropamide • Digoxin	• Fibrates • Lithium • Zidovudine
Moderate renal insufficiency (creatinine clearance 10–20 ml/min)	
• Some β-blockers (e.g. atenolol, sotalol)	• Opioid analgesics
Severe renal insufficiency (creatinine clearance <10 ml/min)[2]	
• Azathioprine • Cephalosporins • Cimetidine	• Isoniazid • Penicillins • Sulphonylureas (gliclazide)

[1] These guidelines mirror those recommended in the *British National Formulary*.
[2] Many of these patients receive renal replacement therapy, which can affect drug pharmacokinetics.

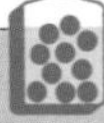

18.5 DRUGS TO AVOID IN RENAL INSUFFICIENCY	
Any degree of renal insufficiency	
• Mesalazine • Metformin	• NSAIDs • Tetracyclines (except doxycycline and minocycline)
Moderate to severe renal insufficiency	
• Lithium	• Methotrexate
Severe renal insufficiency	
• Chloramphenicol • Chloroquine	• Fibrates • Sulphonylurea hypoglycaemic drugs (chlorpropamide, glibenclamide)

In contrast to renal insufficiency, there is no easy way of calculating changes in dosage in patients with impaired hepatic function. Dosages of drugs that are metabolised by the liver should therefore be altered according to the therapeutic response, and with careful clinical monitoring for signs of adverse effects.

18.6 SOME DRUGS WITH HIGH HEPATIC CLEARANCE RATES	
• Clomethiazole	• Morphine
• Glyceryl trinitrate	• Pethidine
• Labetalol	• Propranolol
• Lidocaine	• Simvastatin

18.7 SOME DRUGS WHOSE ACTIONS ARE INCREASED IN LIVER DISEASE

Drug	Adverse effect
Oral anticoagulants	Increased anticoagulation (reduced clotting factor synthesis)
Metformin	Lactic acidosis
Chloramphenicol	Bone marrow suppression
NSAIDs	GI bleeding
Sulphonylureas	Hypoglycaemia

If a drug has a high rate of hepatic clearance (Box 18.6), it will be mostly cleared during its first passage through the liver (so-called 'first-pass' metabolism). In such cases hepatic impairment increases the amount of drug that escapes metabolism in the liver after oral administration, reducing oral dosage requirements but not altering i.v. dosage requirements. The pharmacological effects of some drugs are altered in liver disease, with increased risks of adverse effects (Box 18.7).

ALTERING DOSAGES IN OLDER PEOPLE

Both drug handling and responses to drugs change as people age, and there is much more variability in drug response in elderly people than in younger people. Adverse drug reactions are particularly likely in frail older people, partly because they tend to have poorer renal function and smaller livers, and partly because they are less able to maintain their homeostatic control mechanisms than younger people or fit older people.

Inappropriate polypharmacy is common in older people and the scope for drug interactions is large; in patients >60 yrs of age the error rate in taking drugs is ~60%, and this increases markedly if more than three drugs are prescribed.

Many older people find it difficult to swallow tablets, and the more frail they are, the more difficult this becomes. Tablets or capsules can adhere to the oesophageal mucosa, and tablets should be swilled down with at least 60 ml of water to avoid hold-up.

Drug distribution is sometimes altered in older people and dosages should be adjusted for body weight, particularly for drugs with a low therapeutic index. Older people have an increased proportion of body fat, and lipid-soluble drugs tend to accumulate to a greater extent than in younger patients.

The metabolism of some drugs (e.g. clomethiazole, nifedipine, propranolol, theophylline) is reduced in older people and dosages of these drugs should be reduced.

Renal function falls with age, and drugs with predominantly renal excretion may require dosage reductions (see above). Serum creatinine may be deceptively reassuring because of reduced muscle mass in old age; creatinine clearance should therefore be calculated using an equation such as Cockcroft–Gault.

In general, when prescribing for older people, try to use as few drugs as possible, start with low dosages, and increase the dosages carefully only if required. Choose easily swallowed formulations, and keep therapy as simple as possible (for example, with once-daily drugs and formulations).

DRUGS COMMONLY USED FOR INFECTIOUS DISEASES

The optimal selection of antimicrobial therapy requires knowledge of:
• The infecting organism (or most likely pathogen, given the clinical and geographical context). • Local patterns of antimicrobial resistance. • The relevant pharmacokinetics. • The clinical status of the patient.

ANTIBACTERIAL AGENTS

BETA-LACTAM ANTIBIOTICS (PENICILLINS, CEPHALOSPORINS, CARBAPENEMS)

Mode of action: Exert a bactericidal effect by disrupting bacterial cell wall synthesis.

Penicillins

Indications:

• *Natural penicillins (phenoxymethylpenicillin and benzylpenicillin)*: streptococcal infections including throat infections, otitis media, erysipelas, cellulitis, endocarditis; meningococcal infections; anthrax, diphtheria, syphilis, gas gangrene, leptospirosis.

• *Flucloxacillin:* staphylococcal infections including impetigo, cellulitis, osteomyelitis, septic arthritis, wound infections, endocarditis, pneumonia.
• *Aminopenicillins (ampicillin and amoxicillin):* exacerbations of chronic bronchitis, pneumonia, treatment and prophylaxis of endocarditis, urinary tract infection (UTI), otitis media, sinusitis, dental abscess, listerial meningitis.

Clinical use: Very cheap, well tolerated, safe and easy to use, but resistance is increasing. Natural penicillins are primarily effective against Gram-positive organisms (except staphylococci) and anaerobic organisms (Fig. 18.1).

• *Phenoxymethylpenicillin* (oral 250–500 mg 6-hourly): widely used for simple skin, ear and oral infections, but should not be given in serious infections due to unreliable oral absorption.

• *Benzylpenicillin* (i.v. 1.2–2.4 g 6-hourly): first-line treatment for streptococcal endocarditis (with gentamicin) and cellulitis (with flucloxacillin). It is also highly effective in meningococcal meningitis/sepsis, but less effective in pneumococcal meningitis; for this reason, a broad-spectrum cephalosporin is often preferred as empirical therapy for meningitis (p. 667).

• *Flucloxacillin* (oral/i.v. 500 mg–1 g 6-hourly): the mainstay of treatment for most staphylococcal infections (Fig. 18.2), but meticillin-resistant *Staph. aureus* (MRSA) is an increasing problem. If MRSA is suspected (low threshold in serious or hospital-acquired infections), vancomycin should be used in preference.

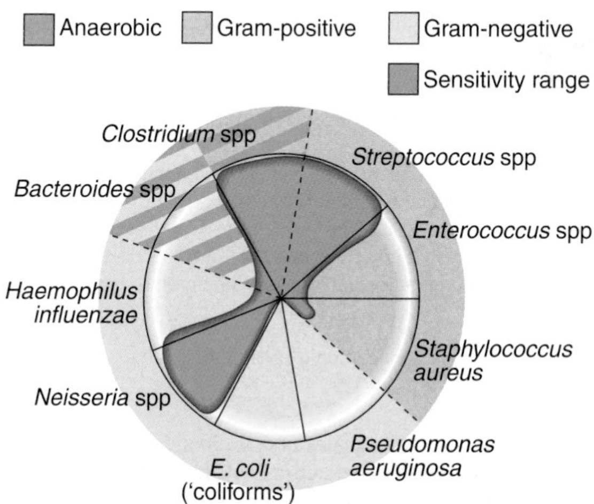

Fig. 18.1 Antibacterial spectrum of Natural Penicillin.

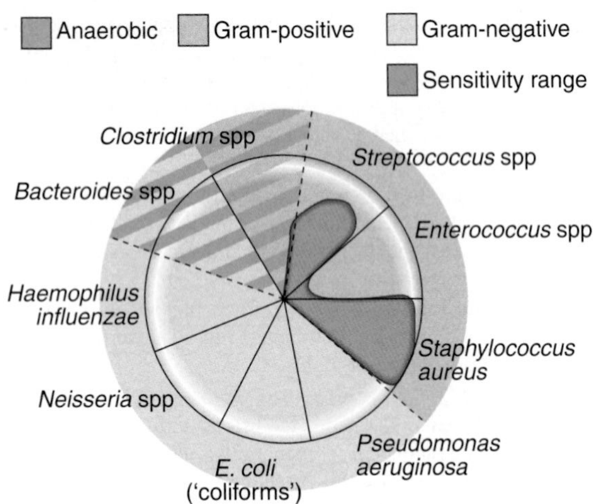

Fig. 18.2 Antibacterial spectrum of flucloxacillin.

Aminopenicillins have similar activity to natural penicillins with additional Gram-negative cover against Enterobacteriaceae and haemophilus (Fig. 18.3). Addition of the β lactamase inhibitor, clavulanic acid (producing 'co-amoxiclav'), prevents resistance due to bacterial β-lactamase production and extends the spectrum of activity.

• *Amoxicillin* (oral/i.v. 500 mg–1 g 8-hourly) and *co-amoxiclav* (oral 375–625 mg 8-hourly; i.v. 1.2 g 8-hourly) are widely used in the treatment of uncomplicated community-acquired pneumonia, exacerbations of chronic bronchitis and UTI.

• *Ampicillin* (i.v. 2 g 4-hourly) should be added to empirical therapy for bacterial meningitis where listerial infection is suspected (e.g. in patients >50 yrs).

Side-effects: Hypersensitivity reactions (generalised allergy to penicillin occurs in 0.7–10% of cases and anaphylaxis in <0.2%); diarrhoea (including antibiotic-associated colitis). Over 90% of patients with infectious mononucleosis develop a rash if given aminopenicillins; this does not imply lasting allergy. Cholestatic jaundice may occur with co-amoxiclav.

Cephalosporins

Indications: Include sepsis, pneumonia, meningitis, biliary infections, UTIs, peritonitis.

Clinical use:

• *First-generation compounds* (e.g. cefalexin: oral 250 mg 6-hourly): excellent activity against Gram-positive organisms but limited Gram-negative cover. They may be helpful in some urinary, skin and soft tissue infections but are rarely first-line treatment.

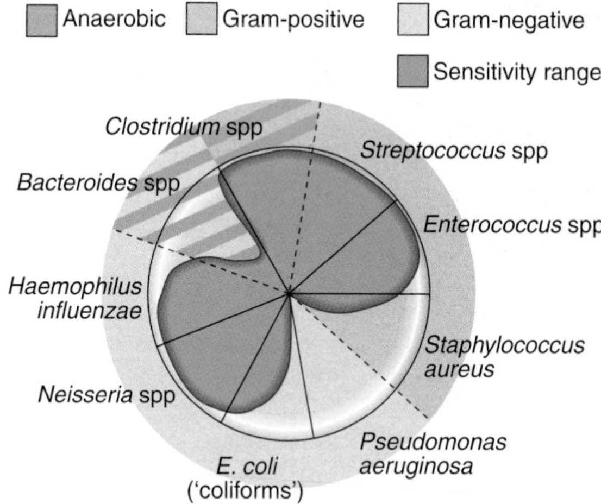

Fig. 18.3 Antibacterial spectrum of amoxicillin.

- *Second-generation cephalosporins* (e.g. cefuroxime): retain Gram-positive activity but have extended Gram-negative activity and some activity against anaerobes (Fig. 18.4). Oral cefuroxime (250–500 mg 12-hourly) has good activity against common respiratory pathogens but is poorly absorbed. I.V. cefuroxime (750 mg–1.5 g 8-hourly) is widely used with metronidazole in the treatment of colorectal and biliary tract infection and for prophylaxis in colorectal and hepatobiliary surgery.
- *Third-generation cephalosporins:* further improve anti-Gram-negative cover but are very expensive and only available i.v. Ceftriaxone (i.v. 1–2 g daily) and cefotaxime (i.v. 1–2 g 6–12-hourly) retain good activity against *Strep. pyogenes*, haemolytic streptococci and many staphylococci; they are widely used in serious infections including sepsis, meningitis, severe community-acquired pneumonia and acute pyelonephritis. Ceftazidime (e.g. i.v. 1 g 8-hourly) has particularly good antipseudomonal activity but less Gram-positive effectiveness; it has an important role in the treatment of hospital-acquired pneumonia and sepsis.

Side-effects: Many of the first-generation drugs are potentially nephrotoxic. Second- and third-generation cephalosporins have a low incidence of allergy and a very low rate of anaphylaxis, even in patients with established penicillin allergy; however, their broad spectrum of activity predisposes to antibiotic-associated colitis.

Carbapenems

Carbapenems (e.g. meropenem i.v. 500 mg 8-hourly) are very broad-spectrum antibiotics and include activity against anaerobes (Fig. 18.5). They

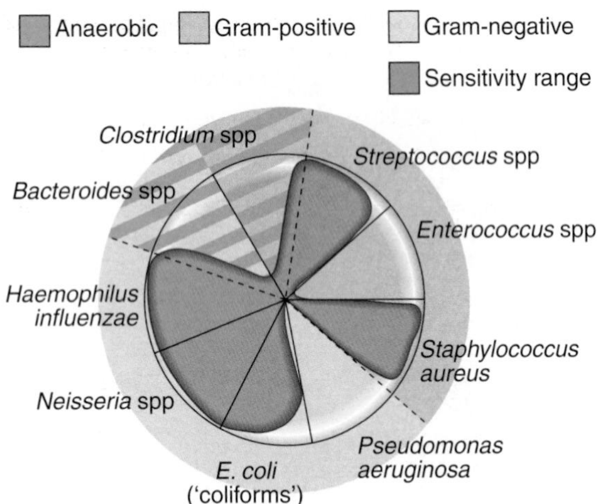

Fig. 18.4 Antibacterial spectrum of cefuroxime.

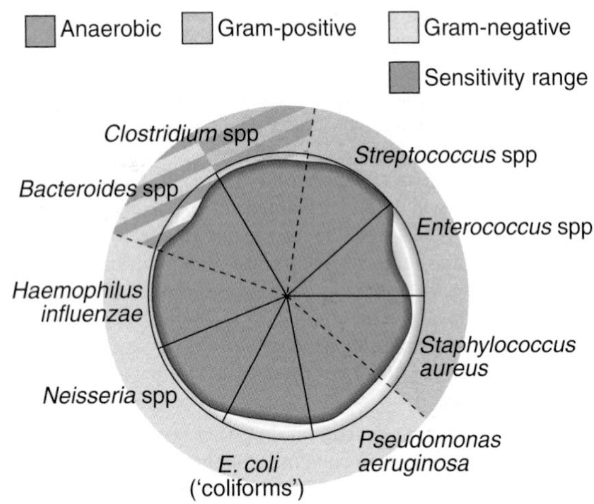

Fig. 18.5 Antibacterial spectrum of meropenem.

are very expensive, are only available in i.v. formulation, and are reserved for severe infections with organisms resistant to other antibiotics.

MACROLIDES (erythromycin, clarithromycin, arithromycin)

Mode of action: Bind to bacterial ribosomes, preventing protein synthesis.

Indications: Respiratory infections, *Campylobacter* enteritis, susceptible Gram-positive infections in patients with penicillin allergy.

Clinical use: Macrolides (e.g. erythromycin oral/i.v. 250–500 mg 6-hourly; clarithromycin oral/i.v. 250–500 mg 12-hourly) have a similar spectrum of activity to penicillin and are a useful alternative in patients with penicillin allergy. They are also active against *Legionella*, *Mycoplasma*, *Chlamydia* and *Rickettsia* infections, and are therefore used for the treatment of atypical pneumonia.

Azithromycin: has a long half-life and is particularly useful for single-dose or short-course treatment of genitourinary infection.

Side-effects: GI upset is common with erythromycin, but clarithromycin is better tolerated. Macrolides inhibit the cytochrome P450 system and may increase plasma concentrations of some drugs (e.g. carbamazepine, phenytoin, digoxin); they also cause prolongation of the QT interval (avoid concomitant use of other drugs that prolong the QT interval).

AMINOGLYCOSIDES (gentamicin, tobramycin)

Mode of action: Bind to ribosomes and interfere with bacterial protein synthesis.

Indications: Sepsis, endocarditis, biliary tract infection, acute pyelonephritis, prostatitis, adjunct in hospital-acquired pneumonia.

Clinical use: Very effective against Gram-negative organisms (Fig. 18.6), including *Pseudomonas aeruginosa*, and useful in Gram-negative sepsis or serious infections arising from the urinary or biliary tract. They also have some Gram-positive activity and show impressive synergy with penicillins; the combination of gentamicin and penicillin is frequently used in the treatment of endocarditis. They must be administered by injection (e.g. gentamicin i.v./i.m. 3–5 mg/kg 8-hourly), as absorption from the GI tract is negligible. Careful monitoring of renal function and drug levels can help to minimise oto- and nephrotoxicity.

Side-effects: Renal toxicity (usually reversible), worse with concomitant vancomycin; permanent cochlear damage; neuromuscular blockade after rapid i.v. infusion (contraindicated in myasthenia gravis).

QUINOLONES (ciprofloxacin, levofloxacin)

Mode of action: Inhibit bacterial DNA-gyrase, an essential enzyme for DNA replication and repair.

Indications: Infections of the respiratory, urinary and GI tracts; gonorrhoea, anthrax.

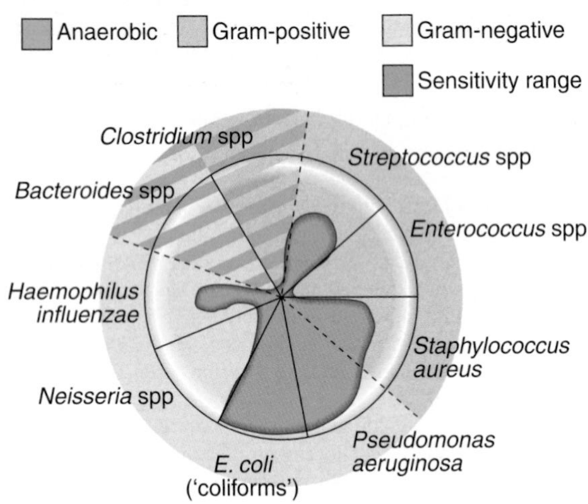

Fig. 18.6 Antibacterial spectrum of gentamicin.

Clinical use: Quinolones have very high bio-availability when given by mouth and should only be administered i.v. when the oral route is unavailable.

Ciprofloxacin (oral 250–750 mg 12-hourly; i.v. 200–400 mg 12-hourly) has excellent anti-Gram-negative activity and is also effective against atypical or intracellular organisms, e.g. *Mycoplasma* and *Chlamydia* and some Gram-positive organisms (Fig. 18.7). It is used for severe GI infections (e.g. shigellosis, invasive salmonellosis, *Campylobacter* enteritis) and urinary infections (e.g. acute pyelonephritis, prostatitis, persistent lower UTI).

Ciprofloxacin has relatively poor activity against *Strep. pneumoniae*, and should not be used routinely in the treatment of community-acquired pneumonia. However, newer 'extended-spectrum' quinolones (e.g. levofloxacin oral 500 mg 12-hourly) have greater activity against pneumococci and are useful alternatives to amoxicillin and clarithromycin in this condition.

Side-effects: Quinolones are usually well tolerated. GI upset in 1–5%; tremor, dizziness, confusion, occasional seizures (especially in the elderly). Bone and joint disease in animal studies limits use in children.

GLYCOPEPTIDES (vancomycin, teicoplanin)

Mode of action: Inhibit bacterial cell wall synthesis.

Indications: Endocarditis and other serious infections with Gram-positive cocci, including MRSA; antibiotic-associated colitis.

Clinical use: Glycopeptides (e.g. vancomycin i.v. 0.5–1 g 12-hourly; teicoplanin i.v./i.m. 200–400 mg daily) are effective against Gram-positive organisms and are particularly useful in infections with MRSA and resistant

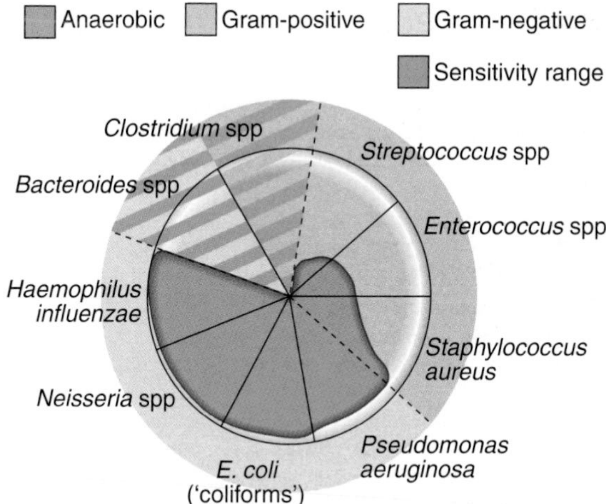

Fig. 18.7 Antibacterial spectrum of ciprofloxacin.

enterococci, though strains of coagulase-negative staphylococci, enterococci and MRSA resistant to glycopeptides are emerging. Glycopeptides are not active against Gram-negative organisms. Neither drug achieves any useful oral absorption, but oral vancomycin (125 mg 6-hourly for 7–10 days) is effective in diarrhoea due to *Cl. difficile* infection. The inappropriate use of vancomycin, particularly in the management of *Cl. difficile* infections (metronidazole is first-line treatment), should be limited to prevent further development of resistance.

Side-effects: Oto- and nephrotoxicity with vancomycin (teicoplanin is less toxic), particularly when used in combination with an aminoglycoside; monitoring of plasma concentration is required. Rapid i.v. infusion of vancomycin may cause an anaphylactoid reaction due to widespread histamine release ('red man' syndrome).

FOLATE ANTAGONISTS (trimethoprim)

Mode of action: Interfere with the bacterial synthesis of folate, an essential precursor for DNA nucleotide synthesis; this inhibits cell replication. Sulphonamides and trimethoprim interfere with two consecutive steps in the same metabolic pathway and are commonly used in combination.

Indications: UTI, *Pneumocystis jirovecii* pneumonia.

Clinical use: Resistance to these antibiotics and the risk of adverse effects (see below) have limited their clinical usefulness over the years.

• Short courses of *trimethoprim* (oral 200 mg 12-hourly for 3 days) are still used for uncomplicated UTI in the community. • *Co-trimoxazole*, a mixture of trimethoprim and sulfamethoxazole in a 1 : 5 ratio, is the first-line drug for the treatment (e.g. i.v. 120 mg/kg daily in divided doses) and prophylaxis (e.g. oral 960 mg every 1–3 days) of *Pneumocystis jirovecii* infection in HIV disease.

Side-effects: Most are dose- and time-dependent; they include fatal marrow dysplasia and haemolysis in glucose-6-phosphate dehydrogenase deficiency, and skin and mucocutaneous reactions, including Stevens–Johnson syndrome.

TETRACYCLINES (oxytetracycline, doxycycline and minocycline)

Mode of action: Prevent bacterial protein synthesis by binding to ribosomes; have a mainly bacteriostatic effect.

Indications: Acne vulgaris, rosacea, leptospirosis, periodontitis, anthrax, brucellosis, Lyme disease, infections due to *Chlamydia*, *Rickettsia*, *Mycoplasma.*

Clinical use: This has narrowed, as most streptococci, *Haemophilus*, *Moraxella*, *E. coli* and *Proteus* spp are now resistant. Important contemporary uses include the treatment of genital *Chlamydia* infection (e.g. doxycycline oral 100 mg 12-hourly for 7 days) and systemic infections with spirochaetes, brucellae or rickettsiae; tetracyclines are also effective in pneumonia due to *Mycoplasma pneumoniae* and *Chlamydia pneumoniae* or psittacosis (though macrolides are first-line empirical treatment for suspected atypical pneumonia).

- *Oxytetracycline* (oral 500 mg 12-hourly): valuable in rosacea (may require repeated intermittent treatments) and moderate to severe acne.
- *Doxycycline and minocycline:* show better absorption and distribution than older tetracyclines, but all should be taken in the fasting state to maximise absorption.

Side-effects: GI upset (due to alterations in gut flora), discoloration of teeth, and occasionally dental hypoplasia (avoid in children <12 yrs, pregnancy and breastfeeding) and photosensitive skin reactions. Tetracyclines also cause hypernatraemia (they are sometimes used to treat hyponatraemia). Older tetracyclines are contraindicated in renal failure, as they may exacerbate renal dysfunction, but doxycycline or minocycline may be used with caution.

NITROIMIDAZOLES (metronidazole)

Mode of action: Reduced by metabolic pathways particular to anaerobic bacteria, yielding intermediates that have toxic effects on DNA.

Indications: Antibiotic-associated colitis, peritonitis, anaerobic sepsis, bacterial vaginosis, pelvic inflammatory disease, acute oral infections and other anaerobic infections; giardiasis, amoebiasis.

Clinical use: Highly active against strictly anaerobic bacteria, especially *Bacteroides fragilis*, *Cl. difficile* and other *Clostridia* species.

Oral metronidazole (e.g. 400 mg 8-hourly) is first-line therapy for *Cl. difficile* infection, bacterial vaginosis, pelvic inflammatory disease (with ofloxacin) and some severe gum and dental infections. I.V. metronidazole

(500 mg 8-hourly) is used in patients with sepsis where anaerobic infection is suspected (e.g. post-colonic or pelvic surgery) and, with a broad-spectrum cephalosporin, in peritonitis.

Side-effects: May cause a metallic taste. Like disulfiram (Antabuse), nitroimidazoles cause a severe vomiting reaction if taken with alcohol.

ANTIFUNGAL AGENTS

AZOLE ANTIFUNGALS (clotrimazole, ketoconazole, itraconazole)

Mode of action: Inhibit fungal enzymes necessary for the construction of cell membranes.

Indications and clinical use:

- *Clotrimazole* (e.g. 1% cream topical application 2–3 times daily; pessary 500 mg nocte as single dose) and *miconazole:* only used for cutaneous and mucosal infections such as ringworm and vaginal candidiasis.
- *Fluconazole* (oral 50–400 mg daily or 150 mg as single dose for vaginal candidiasis): well absorbed orally, has an excellent safety profile and achieves very good CSF penetration; it lacks activity against *Aspergillus*, but has wide efficacy in *Candida* syndromes (including invasive candidiasis) and is useful in fungal meningitis.
- *Ketoconazole* and *itraconazole:* have reasonable activity against both *Candida* and *Aspergillus*; the latter requires a low gastric pH for effective oral absorption.
- *Voriconazole* is a new agent with an extended spectrum of activity and excellent efficacy via oral administration.

Side-effects: GI upset (e.g. nausea, vomiting, abdominal discomfort); rashes, pruritus. Ketoconazole (and rarely itraconazole) may cause potentially fatal hepatotoxicity. All are potent inhibitors of cytochrome P450 enzymes and interact with a wide range of drugs (see national formulary).

DRUGS COMMONLY USED FOR GASTROINTESTINAL DISEASES

ANTACIDS AND ANTISECRETORY DRUGS

Simple antacids, such as aluminium hydroxide and magnesium trisilicate, relieve symptoms of gastro-oesophageal reflux disease (GORD), acute gastritis and peptic ulceration. Alginate-containing antacid preparations aid symptomatic relief by forming a protective mucosal raft on the surface of the stomach contents. Aluminium salts inhibit absorption of some drugs (e.g. digoxin) and are constipating, while magnesium salts can cause diarrhoea; some preparations have high sodium content and can exacerbate cardiac failure.

H_2-RECEPTOR ANTAGONISTS (ranitidine)

Mode of action: Competitively inhibit H_2-receptors on the parietal and enterochromaffin-like cells, thereby reducing secretion of hydrogen ions.

Indications: Benign gastric or duodenal ulceration, GORD, prophylaxis of acid aspiration in obstetrics and surgery; prophylaxis of stress ulceration in critically ill patients.

Clinical use: H_2 antagonists (e.g. ranitidine oral 150 mg 12-hourly) have a good safety profile and are effective in the symptomatic relief of GORD and healing of peptic ulceration. However, they provide less potent acid suppression than proton pump inhibitors (see below) and, as a consequence, their use has declined.

Side-effects: Diarrhoea and other GI upset, altered LFTs, headache, dizziness. Cimetidine may interfere with the metabolism of warfarin, phenytoin and other drugs via the cytochrome P450 system.

PROTON PUMP INHIBITORS (PPIs) (omeprazole, lansoprazole)

Mode of action: Irreversibly inhibit H^+/K^+ATPase (the 'proton pump') on the surface of parietal cells, thereby reducing hydrogen ion secretion.

Indications: GORD, benign gastric and duodenal ulceration, eradication of *Helicobacter pylori*, prophylaxis of NSAID-associated ulcer, prophylaxis of acid aspiration due to general anaesthesia, Zollinger–Ellison syndrome, acid-related dyspepsia.

Clinical use: PPIs (e.g. omeprazole oral 10–40 mg daily; lansoprazole oral 15–30 mg daily) cause potent acid suppression and rapid ulcer healing, and have become the treatment of choice for many of the above conditions. They form a key component of *H. pylori* eradication therapy (p. 440) and are effective in both the prevention and treatment of NSAID-associated ulcer. They are superior to H_2 antagonists for healing ulcers and oesophagitis. I.V. PPI treatment reduces rates of rebleeding and need for surgery in post-endoscopic therapy for major peptic ulcer haemorrhage, but has not been shown to influence mortality.

Side-effects: Include GI upset (e.g. nausea, diarrhoea, flatulence), headache and dizziness, but PPIs are usually well tolerated. Reduced gastric acidity may increase the risk of GI infections.

ANTIEMETICS

A careful assessment of the cause of nausea and vomiting is required to make a rational choice of antiemetic. Reversible causes (e.g. hypercalcaemia, constipation, medication) should be sought and treated appropriately. Parenteral administration is often required initially.

ANTIHISTAMINES (cyclizine, promethazine)

Mode of action: Antagonise the actions of histamine at the H_1 receptor; these receptors are present in the vomiting centre within the medulla, and receive stimulation from the vestibular system and gut vagal afferents.

Indications: Nausea, vomiting, motion sickness, vertigo, labyrinthine disorders; also used for the treatment of allergies and urticaria and as an adjunct in anaphylaxis.

Clinical use: Antihistamines (e.g. cyclizine oral/i.v./i.m. 50 mg 8-hourly) are effective antiemetics in a wide variety of conditions, but are particularly useful in vomiting due to vestibular disorders (including motion sickness) and intracranial causes. Promethazine (25–100 mg oral nocte) is used for severe vomiting in pregnancy.

Side-effects: Most older antihistamines (particularly promethazine) cause sedation but this is less of a problem with cyclizine and chlorphenamine. They may also cause antimuscarinic effects, such as urinary retention, dry mouth and blurred vision, and must be used with caution in prostatic hypertrophy and glaucoma.

PROKINETIC ANTIEMETICS (metoclopramide, domperidone)

Mode of action: Block dopamine receptors in the chemoreceptor trigger zone (CTZ) and have a direct prokinetic effect on the GI tract.

Indications: Nausea and vomiting, defective gastric emptying.

Clinical use: Metoclopramide (oral/i.m./i.v. 10 mg 8-hourly) and domperidone (oral 10–20 mg 6-hourly) are useful in nausea and vomiting associated with gut stasis or treatment with cytotoxics or radiotherapy, but have limited efficacy in post-operative nausea and vomiting and are ineffective in motion sickness.

The use of metoclopramide is restricted, particularly in patients <20 yrs, due to extrapyramidal side-effects (see below). As domperidone does not cross the blood–brain barrier, it is less likely to cause CNS side-effects (note: the CTZ lies *outside* the blood–brain barrier); for the same reason it is also used to prevent vomiting associated with dopaminergic drugs in Parkinson's disease.

Side-effects: Extrapyramidal effects such as acute dystonic reactions may occur with metoclopramide, especially in young females; hyperprolactinaemia and galactorrhoea can occur with prolonged administration. Domperidone is usually well tolerated but GI disturbances may occur. Avoid both drugs in GI obstruction.

5HT3 ANTAGONISTS (ondansetron)

Mode of action: Block 5HT3 receptors in the GI tract and CTZ, thereby inhibiting activation of the vomiting centre by both gut (vagal) afferents and the CTZ.

Indications: Nausea and vomiting induced by cytotoxic chemotherapy and radiotherapy; prevention and treatment of post-operative nausea and vomiting.

Clinical use: These agents (e.g. ondansetron oral/i.v. 8 mg before treatment, then 8 mg 12-hourly for up to 5 days) are very effective in the prevention of nausea and vomiting associated with chemotherapy (addition of dexamethasone may provide further benefit).

Side-effects: Include constipation, headache, flushing.

LAXATIVES

BULK-FORMING LAXATIVES (bran, ispaghula, methylcellulose)

Mode of action: Stimulate peristalsis by increasing faecal mass.

Indications: Constipation (especially with small hard stools); colostomy, ileostomy, irritable bowel syndrome.

Clinical use: Wheat bran is very effective but may be unpalatable to some patients. Ispaghula husk (e.g. Fybogel 1 sachet 12-hourly) and methylcellulose are alternatives. Adequate fluid intake is essential for effect and to avoid risk of intestinal obstruction, especially in the elderly.

Side-effects: Flatulence, abdominal distention, intestinal obstruction.

STIMULANT LAXATIVES (senna, bisacodyl)

Mode of action: Stimulate intestinal motility.

Indications: Short-term treatment of constipation.

Clinical use: Senna (e.g. 15 mg nocte) and bisacodyl (5–10 mg nocte) take up to 12 hrs to act and are therefore usually administered at night. Co-danthramer is a combination laxative (stimulant/softener) usually reserved for use in patients with terminal disease due to concern over potential carcinogenicity in animal studies.

Side-effects: Abdominal cramps, hypokalaemia; with prolonged use, may lead to an atonic, poorly functioning colon (degeneration of the myenteric plexus).

OSMOTIC LAXATIVES (macroglycols, lactulose)

Mode of action: Draw water into the colon, thereby softening the stool.

Indications: Constipation; bowel preparation for investigation; hepatic encephalopathy (lactulose).

Clinical use:

• Macroglycols (e.g. Movicol oral 1–2 sachets daily) are effective laxatives, provided fluid intake is sufficient.

• Lactulose (oral 10–20 ml 12-hourly) is safe and can be used long-term for chronic constipation (may take 24–48 hrs to act); in higher doses (15–30 ml 8-hourly) it is used in hepatic encephalopathy, where it reduces the pH of colonic contents, thereby inhibiting ammonia-producing bacteria.

• Phosphate enemas are used in severe constipation (may require faecal softener, e.g. arachis oil enema, first if stool is very hard) and for bowel evacuation prior to endoscopic and surgical procedures.

Side-effects: Flatulence, cramps, abdominal distention; avoid lactulose in lactose intolerance.

DRUGS COMMONLY USED FOR CARDIOVASCULAR DISEASES

ANTI-ANGINAL DRUGS

These drugs help to restore the imbalance between myocardial O_2 supply and demand. Negatively chronotropic agents lower O_2 demand by reducing cardiac work and improve supply by prolonging diastole (coronary perfusion occurs during diastole). Vasodilating drugs reduce demand by lowering cardiac preload and afterload, and increase supply by dilating the coronary arteries.

NITRATES (glyceryl trinitrate, isosorbide mononitrate and dinitrate)

Mode of action: Act directly on vascular smooth muscle to produce venous and arteriolar dilatation.

Indications: Prophylaxis and treatment of angina; left ventricular failure.

Clinical use: Sublingual glyceryl trinitrate (GTN) in aerosol (400 μg per spray) or tablet (300 or 500 μg) form usually relieves an attack of angina in 2–3 mins and can be used prophylactically before exercise. Slow-release buccal tablets or GTN patches provide a more prolonged therapeutic effect, but long-acting oral nitrates (e.g. isosorbide mononitrate 20–60 mg once or twice daily; isosorbide dinitrate 10–20 mg 12-hourly) are usually preferred. Oral nitrates (in combination with hydralazine) are an effective treatment in patients with chronic heart failure intolerant of ACE inhibitors and angiotensin II receptor antagonists.

Continuous nitrate therapy causes pharmacological tolerance, necessitating a nitrate-free period of 6–8 hrs every day (usually overnight unless there are prominent nocturnal symptoms). I.V. GTN (10–200 μg/min gradually titrated to achieve symptomatic relief) is effective in the initial treatment of acute left ventricular failure and for the relief of persistent anginal pain in acute coronary syndromes.

Side-effects: Throbbing headache (may diminish over time), postural hypotension. Contraindicated in aortic stenosis and hypertrophic obstructive cardiomyopathy.

β-BLOCKERS (propranolol, atenolol, bisoprolol, labetalol)

Mode of action: Block cardiac β_1-adrenoceptors, thereby reducing heart rate and myocardial contractility. Individual β-blockers vary in their relative selectivity for β_1 and β_2 receptors; some cause bronchoconstriction by blocking β_2 receptors.

Indications: Prophylaxis of angina; unstable angina; hypertension; treatment and prevention of supraventricular tachycardia (SVT) and AF; stable heart failure; prophylaxis after MI; symptomatic relief in anxiety and thyrotoxicosis.

Clinical use:

• Propranolol (oral 40–120 mg 12-hourly) is not cardioselective and may aggravate obstructive airways disease, coronary vasospasm or peripheral vascular disease; it is now used mainly to relieve symptoms of palpitation and tremor in anxiety and thyrotoxicosis. • Cardioselective agents (oral atenolol 25–100 mg daily, bisoprolol 2.5–10 mg daily) are first-line therapy for stable angina and, unless contraindicated, should also be given to patients with unstable angina. In acute MI, i.v. β-blockers (e.g. atenolol 5–10 mg; metoprolol 5–15 mg) relieve pain, reduce arrhythmias and improve short-term mortality (avoid in heart failure, AV block or bradycardia); thereafter chronic oral therapy reduces long-term mortality by ~25%.

• β-blockers are effective antihypertensives, particularly in younger patients, but are no longer first-line treatment (p. 248) unless there is another specific indication (e.g. angina). In phaeochromocytoma, they must be combined with phenoxybenzamine (an α-blocker) to avoid a hypertensive crisis from unopposed α-receptor stimulation in blood vessels.

• Labetalol has combined β- and α-blocking properties; it is particularly useful for lowering BP in aortic dissection (e.g. 20 mg i.v. over 2 mins, repeated as necessary; max. 200 mg) and can be given as an infusion in malignant phase hypertension.

• In chronic heart failure, judicious use of β-blockers can improve symptoms and reduce mortality. Suitable agents include bisoprolol (oral 1.25 mg daily, increased gradually over 12 wks to a target dose of 10 mg daily). They may precipitate decompensation and must be initiated under careful supervision.

• For the use of β-blockers in arrhythmias see page 760.

Side-effects:

• Fatigue, reduced exercise capacity, cold peripheries and sexual dysfunction are common. Sleep disturbance and nightmares occur more frequently with lipid-soluble (e.g. propranolol) than water-soluble (e.g. atenolol) agents.

• Bradycardia and conduction disorders may occur (contraindicated in sick sinus syndrome; second- or third-degree AV block).

• Myocardial depression can precipitate or aggravate heart failure (contraindicated in uncontrolled heart failure).

• Even cardioselective β-blockers may provoke bronchospasm; they should be avoided in patients with asthma but may be tolerated in mild COPD.

• Other effects include exacerbation of psoriasis, decreased insulin sensitivity (increased incidence of diabetes), reduced awareness of hypoglycaemia and worsening of intermittent claudication and Raynaud's phenomenon.

• Abrupt withdrawal of a β-blocker may precipitate dangerous arrhythmias, worsening angina or MI.

CALCIUM CHANNEL BLOCKERS (CCBs) (nifedipine, amlodipine, verapamil, diltiazem)

Mode of action: Inhibit the slow inward calcium current in cardiac and arteriolar muscle cells, reducing contractility, sinus node activity, AV node conduction and vascular tone. Dihydropyridine CCBs (e.g. nifedipine, amlodipine) bind more selectively to vascular cells and principally cause arteriolar vasodilatation. Non-dihydropyridine CCBs (verapamil, diltiazem) bind equally to cardiac and vascular cells and possess powerful negative inotropic and chronotropic properties.

Indications: Prophylaxis and treatment of angina; hypertension, supraventricular arrhythmias.

Clinical use: Dihydropyridine CCBs (e.g. amlodipine oral 5–10 mg daily; nifedipine oral 30–90 mg daily) cause arteriolar and coronary vasodilatation and are used in the treatment of hypertension and angina. They have no anti-arrhythmic activity and often cause a reflex tachycardia, which may be counterproductive in angina (consider combining with a β-blocker). They are particularly helpful in disorders caused by vasospasm (e.g. Raynaud's phenomenon).

Verapamil (oral 40–120 mg 8-hourly) and diltiazem (oral 60–120 mg 8-hourly) slow heart rate and inhibit conduction through the AV node They are used in the treatment of supraventricular arrhythmias (p. 218) and are often employed for their rate-limiting properties (e.g. in angina, permanent AF) in patients unable to take β-blockers.

Side-effects: Peripheral oedema is common with dihydropyridine CCBs; other unwanted effects include flushing, headache and postural lightheadedness. The most common side-effect of verapamil is constipation. It is also highly negatively inotropic (more so than diltiazem) and chronotropic, and may cause profound bradycardia ± hypotension (especially when combined with β-blockers or when given i.v.). Use with caution in the elderly. CCBs are contraindicated in heart failure, significantly impaired LV function, sick sinus syndrome, second- or third-degree AV block.

NICORANDIL

Mode of action: Activates potassium channels in vascular smooth muscle, causing venous and arteriolar dilatation.

Indications: Prophylaxis and treatment of angina.

Clinical use: Nicorandil (oral 10–30 mg 12-hourly) is effective in the treatment of stable angina; it produces comparable effects to long-acting nitrate preparations but does not exhibit tolerance.

Side-effects: Throbbing headache (may diminish if patients persevere with treatment), flushing postural hypotension.

ANTI-ARRHYTHMIC DRUGS

Many arrhythmias are benign and do not require treatment. Optimum management often involves correction of precipitating factors (e.g. alcohol excess, hyperthyroidism, electrolyte disorders, myocardial ischaemia) or non-pharmacological measures (e.g. electrical cardioversion, radiofrequency ablation, implantable defibrillator) in addition to or instead of drug treatment.

CLASS I DRUGS (disopyramide, lidocaine, flecainide)

Mode of action: Stabilise membranes in atrial or ventricular muscle by blocking sodium channels, suppressing excitability and slowing conduction.

Indications: Prevention and treatment of atrial and ventricular tachyarrhythmias.

Clinical use:

- Disopyramide (i.v. 2 mg/kg at 30 mg/min, then 0.4 mg/kg/hr; oral 300–800 mg in divided doses), or flecainide (i.v. 2 mg/kg over 10 mins, then 1.5 mg/kg over 1 hr, then 0.1 mg/kg/hr; oral 50–100 mg 12-hourly) may be given to patients with atrial or ventricular arrhythmias to restore or maintain sinus rhythm, usually under specialist supervision.
- Lidocaine (i.v. 50–100 mg, then 4 mg/min for 30 mins; 2 mg/min for 2 hrs; 1 mg/min for 24 hrs) is mainly used for the urgent treatment of ventricular tachycardia (VT).

Side-effects:

- Myocardial depression, especially with flecainide and disopyramide (contraindicated in patients with impaired LV function).
- Pro-arrhythmic properties, including ventricular arrhythmias (flecainide is particularly hazardous in patients with prior MI).
- AV block.
- Disopyramide may cause dry mouth, blurred vision, urinary retention.
- Lidocaine may cause CNS depression or convulsions.

CLASS II DRUGS (β-blockers—see above)

Clinical use in arrhythmia: Cardioselective β-blockers (e.g. metoprolol oral 50–200 mg 12-hourly; bisoprolol oral 2.5–10 mg daily) are used to limit the ventricular rate in atrial fibrillation or flutter (usually more effective than digoxin) and as prophylactic therapy in paroxysmal AF and SVT. In the acute setting, the ultra short-acting i.v. agent esmolol (50–200 μg/kg/min) may be helpful if there is concern about potential adverse effects.

CLASS III DRUGS (amiodarone)

Mode of action: Prolongs the plateau phase of the action potential, thus lengthening the refractory period.

Indications: Serious or resistant atrial and ventricular tachyarrhythmias.

Clinical use: Used in cardiopulmonary resuscitation (i.v. 300 mg bolus) for refractory ventricular fibrillation (VF) or pulseless VT. I.V. amiodarone (5 mg/kg *in 5% dextrose* over 20–120 mins, then up to 15 mg/kg/24 hrs) may be used to attempt chemical cardioversion in VT without haemodynamic compromise, or in new-onset AF.

Given orally (usually 200 mg 8-hourly for 1 wk, then 200 mg 12-hourly for 1 wk, then 200 mg daily), it is used for controlling paroxysmal AF and arrhythmias associated with Wolff–Parkinson–White (WPW) syndrome; also for preventing recurrent VT, particularly in patients with poor LV function. Amiodarone has the added benefit of not causing significant myocardial depression.

However, extensive side-effects limit its use to the prevention of life-threatening arrhythmias or where other drugs have proved ineffective. Because it has a very long tissue half-life (25–110 days), the onset of action is delayed and it may take several months to reach steady state.

Side-effects: The most important are: photosensitisation, corneal deposits, GI upset, thyroid dysfunction, liver disease, pneumonitis leading to pulmonary fibrosis, peripheral neuropathy and torsades de pointes (caution is needed with other drugs that prolong the QT interval). May last for weeks or months after treatment has been stopped. Drug interactions are also common (e.g. amiodarone potentiates the effects of digoxin and warfarin)—see national formulary for full details.

CLASS IV DRUGS (calcium channel blockers: verapamil, diltiazem (see above))

Clinical use in arrhythmia: I.V. verapamil (5–10 mg over 2 mins) may be used to restore sinus rhythm in AV nodal re-entry tachycardia (AVNRT) or to achieve rapid rate control in atrial tachyarrhythmias. Oral verapamil is used as prophylactic therapy in recurrent AVNRT or for rate control in permanent AF. Note that verapamil does not help to maintain sinus rhythm in paroxysmal AF and should be avoided in WPW syndrome (shortens the refractory period of the accessory pathway) and ventricular arrhythmias.

ATROPINE SULPHATE

Mode of action: Competitive antagonist at muscarinic acetylcholine receptors.

Indications: Asystole, symptomatic bradycardia; drying of bronchial secretions; symptomatic relief of GI disorders characterised by smooth muscle spasm.

Clinical use: I.V. atropine (0.6 mg, repeated if necessary to a maximum of 3 mg) increases the sinus rate and sinoatrial and AV conduction, and is the treatment of choice for severe bradycardia due to vagal overactivity. It is also used in symptomatic bradyarrhythmias complicating the early stages of inferior MI and in asystolic cardiac arrest.

Side-effects: Dry mouth, blurred vision, urinary retention, tachycardia.

ADENOSINE

Mode of action: Transiently blocks conduction through the AV node by causing hyperpolarisation via the adenosine A1 receptor.

Indications: Treatment of AVRT and AVNRT; diagnostic aid in broad- or narrow-complex tachycardia.

Clinical use: Used to terminate SVTs when the AV node is part of the re-entry circuit or to assist with diagnosis by transiently slowing AV node conduction (e.g. atrial flutter with 2:1 AV block or broad-complex tachycardia). It is given as an i.v. bolus in escalating doses (3 mg over 2 secs, followed if necessary by 6 mg then 12 mg at intervals of 1–2 mins).

Side-effects: Short-lived flushing, breathlessness and chest pain (warn patients in advance). Can cause bronchospasm (avoid in asthmatics). Effects are potentiated by dipyridamole, and inhibited by theophylline.

DIGOXIN

Mode of action: Inhibits the Na^+/K^+ATPase pump on cardiac myocytes; leading indirectly to an increase in intracellular calcium, resulting in a small positive inotropic effect. Also increases vagal activity via a central effect, thereby slowing conduction through the AV node.

Indications: Heart failure, supraventricular arrhythmias.

Clinical use:

• Digoxin (oral 62.5–250 μg daily) is mainly used to limit the ventricular response rate in AF and is usually initiated with a loading dose (e.g. oral 500 μg 6-hourly for 2 doses; i.v. 500 μg over 30 mins then a further 250–500 μg over 4–8 hrs).

• In the acute setting it has the disadvantage of a slow onset of action (often several hours, even with i.v. loading) but avoids problems with myocardial depression associated with alternative drugs (e.g. β-blockers, CCBs).

• When used as maintenance therapy it may provide inadequate control of heart rate during exercise and is often combined with a β-blocker. It can be used to interrupt re-entry tachycardias involving the AV node but is not usually first choice.

• In chronic heart failure, it is helpful in patients with coexistent AF but of uncertain benefit in those who remain in sinus rhythm (no effect on overall survival but may reduce the need for hospitalisation).

• Digoxin is largely excreted by the kidneys, and the maintenance dose should be reduced in the elderly and those with renal impairment.

Side-effects: Anorexia, nausea, vomiting, altered colour vision, drowsiness and confusion are common; cardiac manifestations include bradycardia, increased ectopy and atrial and ventricular tachyarrhythmias. All are more common in the presence of hypokalaemia or renal impairment. Measurement of plasma digoxin concentration (at least 6 hrs post-dose) helps to confirm toxicity; treatment entails discontinuation of the drug, correction of hypokalaemia and, in severe cases, administration of digoxin-specific antibody fragments.

Contraindicated in SVT associated with WPW (increases conduction through accessory pathway), second- or third-degree AV block and hypertrophic obstructive cardiomyopathy.

ANTIHYPERTENSIVE DRUGS

DIURETICS

Mode of action: Thiazides (e.g. bendroflumethiazide) and loop diuretics (e.g. furosemide) inhibit sodium resorption in the renal tubule at the expense of increased potassium excretion. Potassium-sparing diuretics (e.g. amiloride) and aldosterone receptor antagonists (e.g. spironolactone) inhibit sodium resorption in the distal convoluted tubule but retain potassium.

Indications: Hypertension, oedema.

Clinical use:

• *Low-dose thiazides* (e.g. bendroflumethiazide oral 2.5 mg daily) are used to treat hypertension; higher doses cause greater side-effects without any additional BP-lowering effects. They are less effective than loop diuretics in relieving oedema, but the combination of a loop diuretic and thiazide (e.g. bendroflumethiazide 5–10 mg daily) or thiazide-like diuretic (e.g. metolazone 5–10 mg daily) may produce an intense diuresis and can be helpful in resistant oedema.

• *Loop diuretics* (e.g. furosemide oral 40 mg daily or bumetanide oral 1 mg daily) have few advantages over thiazides in hypertension unless there is substantial renal impairment. They are given in acute left ventricular failure (e.g. furosemide i.v. 50–100 mg) to relieve pulmonary oedema, where they also cause a small but significant degree of arterial and venous dilatation. They are usually first-line treatment in chronic heart failure and other serious oedematous disorders. In patients with oliguric renal failure or severe chronic heart failure very high oral doses (e.g. furosemide 250 mg daily), or an i.v. infusion (e.g. furosemide 10 mg/hr) can sometimes initiate a diuresis in resistant oedema.

• *Aldosterone receptor antagonists* (e.g. spironolactone oral 100–200 mg daily) potentiate the diuretic effects of loop and thiazide diuretics and prevent hypokalaemia. They are used in the treatment of ascites and oedema in hepatic cirrhosis. Lower doses (e.g. spironolactone 25 mg daily) are beneficial in selected patients with chronic heart failure.

• *Other potassium-sparing agents* (e.g. amiloride oral 10 mg daily) are weak diuretics but may be useful in combination with loop or thiazide diuretics to prevent hypokalaemia.

Side-effects:

• Excessive diuresis: hypovolaemia and hypotension.

• Electrolyte disturbances: hyponatraemia, hypokalaemia, hypomagnesaemia and metabolic alkalosis, as well as hypocalcaemia (loop) and hypercalcaemia (thiazide).

• Thiazides (and to a lesser extent loop diuretics) have a number of unwanted metabolic effects, including hyperglycaemia, hyperlipidaemia and hyperuricaemia.

• High-dose loop diuretics: ototoxicity.

• Potassium-sparing agents: hyperkalaemia, particularly in patients with renal impairment or taking an ACE inhibitor/angiotensin II receptor antagonist.

• Spironolactone: gynaecomastia (eplerenone is a suitable alternative).

ANGIOTENSIN-CONVERTING ENZYME (ACE) INHIBITORS

(enalapril, ramipril, lisinopril)

Mode of action: Inhibit the conversion of angiotensin I to angiotensin II; also inhibit the breakdown of the vasodilating hormone, bradykinin. The major haemodynamic effect is a reduction in peripheral vascular resistance.

Indications: Hypertension, heart failure, asymptomatic left ventricular systolic dysfunction, diabetic nephropathy, secondary prevention in coronary artery and cerebrovascular disease.

Clinical use:

- *Hypertension:* ACE inhibitors (e.g. enalapril 20 mg daily, ramipril 2.5–5 mg daily or lisinopril 10–40 mg daily) are first-line antihypertensive therapy for younger patients (<55 yrs) but are less effective in black patients. Their BP-lowering effect is potentiated by diuretics. They are particularly indicated in hypertensive patients with chronic renal impairment (with careful monitoring).
- *Diabetic nephropathy:* they retard the progression of renal failure and reduce proteinuria independently of BP reduction.
- *Heart failure* (p. 253): they relieve symptoms, improve exercise capacity and reduce hospital admissions and mortality. In addition, they reduce cardiovascular events and can delay the development of overt heart failure in patients with asymptomatic LV systolic dysfunction.
- *Secondary prevention* in all patients with established CHD or cerebrovascular disease, irrespective of the presence of hypertension or LV dysfunction.

Electrolytes and creatinine should be checked before and 1–2 wks after commencing therapy in all patients (discontinue if >15% rise in creatinine), with more frequent monitoring required in certain groups (e.g. patients with renal impairment; elderly patients).

Side-effects: Hypotension (including severe first-dose hypotension), dry cough (due to increased bradykinin), rash, angioedema, hyperkalaemia, renal dysfunction. Particular care is required in patients taking concomitant thiazide or loop diuretics (risk of severe hypotension), potassium-sparing diuretics (risk of hyperkalaemia) or NSAIDs (increased risk of nephrotoxicity) and those with impaired renal function (reduction in glomerular filtration pressure may exacerbate renal failure).

Contraindicated in pregnancy, bilateral renal artery stenosis and critical aortic stenosis.

ANGIOTENSIN RECEPTOR BLOCKERS (losartan, valsartan)

Mode of action: Block the angiotensin II type I receptor. The major haemodynamic effect is a reduction in peripheral vascular resistance.

Indications: Hypertension, heart failure, diabetic nephropathy in patients intolerant of ACE inhibitors.

Clinical use: These drugs (e.g. losartan oral 50–100 mg daily, valsartan oral 40–160 mg daily) have similar effects to ACE inhibitors and are better tolerated. They are generally used as an alternative for patients intolerant of ACE inhibitors, usually due to cough. The addition of an angiotensin II receptor antagonist to ACE inhibitor therapy in selected patients with CHF may produce a further reduction in the risk of cardiovascular events.

Side-effects: Better tolerated than ACE inhibitors and in particular do not cause dry cough; however, they share all the more serious adverse effects, including renal dysfunction and hyperkalaemia.

β-BLOCKERS, CALCIUM CHANNEL BLOCKERS

See above.

ALPHA-BLOCKERS (doxazosin)

Mode of action: Relax smooth muscle cells in blood vessels and the prostate/bladder neck through blockade of α_1-adrenoceptors, thereby causing vasodilatation and also relieving prostatic obstruction.

Indications: Hypertension, benign prostatic hyperplasia.

Clinical use: In hypertension, these drugs (e.g. doxazosin oral 1–16 mg daily) are generally used as add-on therapy when satisfactory control is not achieved with the agents above. In symptomatic benign prostatic hyperplasia, they produce rapid improvement in urinary flow in 60–70% of patients.

Side-effects: Include first-dose and postural hypotension, headache, tachycardia.

LIPID-LOWERING DRUGS

Lipid-lowering therapies have a key role in the primary and secondary prevention of cardiovascular disease. Assessment of absolute risk, treatment of all modifiable risk factors and optimisation of lifestyle factors are central to management in all cases.

STATINS

Mode of action: Inhibit HMG CoA reductase, the rate-limiting enzyme in cholesterol synthesis; the reduction in cholesterol synthesis upregulates hepatic LDL receptor activity, increasing clearance of LDL from the circulation.

Indications: Prevention of cardiovascular events in patients with atherosclerotic vascular disease or diabetes mellitus; hypercholesterolaemia (particularly with an estimated 10-yr risk of cardiovascular disease >20%).

Clinical use: Statins (e.g. simvastatin oral 10–80 mg daily, atorvastatin oral 10–80 mg daily) reduce LDL cholesterol by up to 60%, reduce triglycerides by up to 40%, and increase HDL cholesterol by up to 10%. They are most effective when given at night. In patients with established coronary disease, ischaemic stroke or diabetes mellitus, statins offers clear protection against adverse cardiovascular outcomes and should be prescribed irrespective of plasma cholesterol concentration. Statin treatment also lowers cardiovascular events in patients with high cholesterol without evidence of vascular disease; however, as benefit is related to the absolute risk of such events, decisions on treatment should be informed by individual assessments of the 10-yr risk of cardiovascular disease.

Side-effects: Serious side-effects are rare (<2%). Statins may alter liver function tests; monitor LFTs and stop the drugs if there is a persistent increase in transaminases >3× the upper limit of normal. Myalgia, myositis and, very rarely, rhabdomyolysis may occur (more likely with higher doses or concurrent treatment with fibrates or ciclosporin); stop if creatine kinase >5× the upper limit of normal. Contraindicated in pregnancy, breastfeeding and active liver disease.

FIBRATES

Mode of action: Stimulate peroxisome proliferator-activated receptor-α (PPARα), which controls the expression of gene products that mediate the metabolism of triglycerides and HDL.

Indications: Dyslipidaemia with predominant hypertriglyceridaemia.

Clinical use: Fibrates (e.g. bezafibrate oral 200 mg 8-hourly) reduce triglycerides by up to 50% and increase HDL cholesterol by up to 20%, with a variable effect on LDL cholesterol. They are usually considered first-line therapy in patients with predominant hypertriglyceridaemia. Reduced rates of cardiovascular disease have been reported in studies amongst patients with low HDL cholesterol levels but statins are usually preferred.

Side-effects: These drugs are generally well tolerated but they exhibit a similar profile and frequency of side-effects as statins, including myalgia, myopathy (especially with impaired renal function or concurrent statin treatment) and abnormal LFTs. They may also increase the risk of cholelithiasis and prolong the action of anticoagulants.

OTHER LIPID-LOWERING DRUGS

Anion exchange resins (colestyramine)

These deplete hepatic cholesterol by preventing the reabsorption of bile acids and thereby increasing de novo bile acid synthesis from hepatic cholesterol. They are safe and can achieve substantial reductions in LDL cholesterol, but are poorly tolerated because of their GI effects and may interfere with bio-availability of other drugs (which should be taken at least 1 hr before or 4–6 hrs after colestyramine).

ANTI-PLATELET DRUGS

ASPIRIN

Mode of action: Irreversibly inactivates the cyclo-oxygenase (COX) enzyme in platelets, thereby blocking production of thromboxane A2, a potent mediator of platelet aggregation. Inactivation of COX also inhibits production of pro-inflammatory prostaglandins, producing an equivalent effect to NSAIDs (see below).

Indications: Coronary heart disease (CHD), cerebrovascular disease, peripheral arterial disease; primary prevention of vascular disease in patients with a 10-yr CHD risk >15%; atrial fibrillation (AF; selected patients); mild to moderate pain and inflammation; pyrexia.

Clinical use: A cheap, effective and relatively safe treatment for the prevention of arterial thrombotic events. Acute treatment with oral aspirin (e.g. 300 mg followed by 75 mg daily) reduces the incidence of death, reinfarction and stroke in patients with acute MI; death and MI in unstable angina; and death and dependency in acute ischaemic stroke (can be administered PR if necessary). In patients with established atherosclerotic vascular disease, low-dose maintenance treatment (e.g. oral 75 mg daily) reduces the risk of MI, stroke and cardiovascular death; it may also provide a small net benefit in patients with high vascular risk, provided BP is well controlled.

Aspirin is less effective than warfarin for reducing the risk of ischaemic stroke in patients with AF and is generally reserved for those at lower risk or with a contraindication to anticoagulation.

In regular high dosage (e.g. 600 mg 4-hourly) aspirin has similar analgesic, anti-inflammatory and antipyretic properties to NSAIDs; the latter are now usually preferred but aspirin is still recommended for arthritis in rheumatic fever.

Side-effects: GI haemorrhage (may occur even with low doses and is common with anti-inflammatory doses), other haemorrhage (e.g. subconjuctival), bronchospasm (caution in patients with asthma) and, at anti-inflammatory doses, dizziness and tinnitus (reduce dose).

Contraindicated in patients with a bleeding disorder or active peptic ulceration (co-prescribe a PPI in antiplatelet doses if there is a past history of ulcer) and in children <16 yrs (risk of Reye's syndrome).

CLOPIDOGREL

Mode of action: Blocks ADP receptors on the platelet membrane, preventing ADP-dependent platelet activation.

Indications: Alternative antiplatelet agent in patients intolerant of aspirin; also given with aspirin in acute coronary syndromes and following coronary stent insertion.

Clinical use: Clopidogrel (oral 75 mg daily) is an equally effective alternative to aspirin in patients with established atherosclerotic vascular disease who are unable to tolerate aspirin. In acute coronary syndromes, the addition of clopidogrel (oral 300 mg followed by 75 mg daily for 4 wks in STEMI (ST segment elevation MI) or 3–9 mths in NSTEMI) to aspirin produces further improvement in outcomes. Combination therapy also reduces cardiac events and vascular complications after coronary stenting.

Side-effects: Dyspepsia, GI bleeding, diarrhoea; rarely, thrombotic thrombocytopenic purpura. Contraindicated in active bleeding.

DIPYRIDAMOLE

Mode of action: Inhibits breakdown of cyclic AMP by phosphodiesterases; the mechanism of antiplatelet action in vivo is uncertain.

Indications: Secondary prevention of ischaemic stroke and TIA.

Clinical use: The addition of modified-release dipyridamole (oral 200 mg 12-hourly) to aspirin in patients who have experienced a stroke or TIA whilst on aspirin therapy reduces the risk of further vascular events.

Side-effects: GI effects, dizziness, flushing, tachycardia.

ANTICOAGULANTS AND FIBRINOLYTICS

HEPARIN

Mode of action:

• Standard (unfractionated) heparin potentiates the activity of antithrombin, which inhibits clotting factors IIa, VIIa, IXa, Xa and XIa (see Fig. 14.1, p. 531). This results in prolongation of the activated partial thromboplastin time (APTT). • Low molecular weight heparins (LMWHs) augment antithrombin activity preferentially against factor Xa; they do not prolong the APTT.

Indications: Treatment and prevention of DVT and PE; treatment of acute coronary syndromes and acute peripheral arterial occlusion; post-thrombolysis for MI.

Clinical use: Standard heparin is initiated with a loading dose of 5000 U i.v. followed by a continuous infusion, adjusted to maintain the APTT at 1.5–2.5 times the control time. LMWHs are given by s.c. injection once or twice daily in a weight-related dose with no need for monitoring (e.g. enoxaparin: 20–40 mg daily for DVT prophylaxis; 1.5 mg/kg daily for treatment of DVT/PE; 1 mg/kg 12-hourly for acute coronary syndromes). Because of their convenience and the predictability of their anticoagulant effect, LMWHs are now the usual treatment of choice. However, standard heparin may be preferable in patients at high risk of bleeding complications (e.g. peptic ulcer, severe renal impairment), as it has a short half-life (1 hr) and, unlike LMWH, can be rapidly neutralised by protamine.

Side-effects: Bleeding is the main side-effect. A small number of patients develop heparin-induced thrombocytopenia (HIT)—a decline in the platelet count after 5–7 days due to the development of an antibody directed against a factor on the platelet surface. Heparin should be discontinued immediately and the direct thrombin inhibitor, hirudin, given instead.

WARFARIN

Mode of action: Vitamin K-dependent carboxylation of clotting factors II, VII, IX and X is essential for their biological activity. Following this reaction, vitamin K must be regenerated by a reductase enzyme. By inhibiting this enzyme, warfarin prevents activation of these clotting factors, thereby prolonging the prothrombin time (PT).

Indications: Prophylaxis and treatment of DVT and PE (target INR 2.5), thromboembolic prophylaxis in patients with AF, mural thrombus post-MI, extensive anterior MI (target INR 2.5) and mechanical prosthetic cardiac valves (target INR 3.5).

Clinical use: Treatment is initiated with a loading dose (e.g. oral 10 mg), and subsequent daily doses depend on the INR—the ratio of the patient's

PT to a normal control. The full anticoagulant effect of warfarin takes several days to develop, so where rapid anticoagulation is required (e.g. venous thromboembolism), heparin should be administered until the INR is >2.0 for 2 consecutive days. Warfarin is usually given for 3–6 mths after a single episode of venous thromboembolism but may be continued indefinitely following a second.

Side-effects: Bleeding is the main side-effect. If the INR is above the desired therapeutic level, the warfarin dose should be reduced or withheld. The anticoagulant effect of warfarin may be reversed by administering vitamin K, but this takes about 6 hrs. Where necessary, rapid reversal can be achieved by giving coagulation factor concentrate or fresh frozen plasma. Contraindicated in haemorrhagic states (e.g. haemophilia, severe liver disease, thrombocytopenia), uncontrolled hypertension, recent surgery (especially to the eye or CNS) or cerebral haemorrhage, active peptic ulcer, frequent falls or cognitive impairment in the elderly.

Interactions: Numerous drugs interact with warfarin—check the national formulary for a full list. The frequency of INR monitoring should be increased whenever one of these drugs is initiated or discontinued.

- *Drugs that enhance the anticoagulant effect of warfarin* include alcohol, amiodarone, some antibiotics (e.g. ciprofloxacin, macrolides), fluconazole, tamoxifen, statins, fibrates, thyroxine and antiplatelet agents.
- *Drugs that reduce its anticoagulant effect* include rifampicin, carbamazepine, barbiturates, oestrogen, raloxifene, St John's wort.
- *Drugs that may enhance or reduce its effect* include colestyramine, phenytoin and corticosteroids.

FIBRINOLYTIC AGENTS

Mode of action: Cleave plasminogen to plasmin, a proteolytic enzyme that degrades cross-links between fibrin strands, and thereby dissolve thrombus.

Indications: Acute MI, PE, acute ischaemic stroke.

Clinical use: Fibrinolytic agents such as streptokinase (i.v. 1.5 million units over 60 mins) and alteplase (tPA; i.v. 15 mg bolus, followed by 50 mg over 30 mins, and then 35 mg over 60 mins) have been shown to reduce mortality in patients with acute MI who are eligible for reperfusion therapy (p. 237).

These agents are also used in massive PE associated with hypotension. In acute ischaemic stroke tPA increases the risk of fatal intracranial haemorrhage but, given within 3 hrs of onset, improves longer-term outcome amongst survivors.

- *Streptokinase:* antigenic; circulating neutralising antibodies formed following treatment can render subsequent infusions of the drug ineffective; therefore use a different agent if the patient requires further thrombolysis in the future. Streptokinase may also cause hypotension, which can often be managed by stopping the infusion and restarting at a slower rate.
- *Alteplase:* a genetically engineered drug that is not antigenic and seldom causes hypotension.

• *Newer-generation analogues of tPA* (e.g. tenecteplase): some have been generated that have a longer plasma half-life and can be given as an i.v. bolus.

Side-effects: Bleeding, including intracranial haemorrhage, is the major side-effect. Streptokinase may cause allergic reactions, hypotension and back pain. Contraindications to thrombolysis are shown in Box 8.10 (p. 237).

DRUGS COMMONLY USED FOR RESPIRATORY DISEASES

BRONCHODILATORS

SELECTIVE β_2-AGONISTS

Mode of action: Stimulate β_2-adrenoceptors, thereby relaxing airway smooth muscle; may exert additional anti-inflammatory effects by reducing mediator release from mast cells.

Indications: Asthma, COPD.

Short-acting β_2-agonists (salbutamol, terbutaline)

Clinical use: Salbutamol (100–200 μg) and terbutaline (250–500 μg) are best administered by inhalation using metered-dose aerosol or dry powder inhalers. In asthma and COPD they are used 'as required' for relief of wheeze. In acute severe asthma, salbutamol is given by nebuliser (2.5–5 mg) in repeated doses until bronchospasm is relieved; there is no evidence that i.v. administration is more effective. In COPD, nebulised administration may help if adequate doses by inhaler fail to relieve symptoms. Always check inhaler technique.

Long-acting β_2-agonists (LABA) (salmeterol, formoterol)

Clinical use: Salmeterol (50 μg 12-hourly) and formoterol (9–18 μg 12-hourly), given by inhaler, improve asthma control in patients who remain symptomatic despite inhaled corticosteroids and short acting β-agonists. In severe COPD there is some evidence that regular LABA given with inhaled corticosteroids reduce exacerbation frequency and improve quality of life.

Side-effects: Muscle tremor (especially hands) is the main dose-limiting side-effect; also tachycardia, palpitation, arrhythmia, headache, sleep disturbance. Hypokalaemia may occur at high doses.

ANTICHOLINERGIC BRONCHODILATORS (ipratropium, tiotropium)

Mode of action: Block M_3 muscarinic receptors, inhibiting parasympathetic bronchoconstrictor tone.

Indications: Asthma, COPD.

Clinical use: Ipratropium (250–500 μg by nebuliser) is used in addition to nebulised salbutamol in acute severe asthma. Tiotropium (18 μg daily) and ipratropium (20–40 μg 4-hourly) from appropriate inhalers may improve exercise capacity and relieve hyperinflation in COPD.

Side-effects: Dry mouth, urinary retention and angle-closure glaucoma (due to conjunctival absorption of nebulised aerosol).

LEUKOTRIENE RECEPTOR ANTAGONISTS (montelukast, zafirlukast)

Mode of action: Block the bronchoconstrictor and pro-inflammatory effects of cysteinyl leukotrienes in the airway.

Indications: Asthma.

Clinical use: Montelukast (oral 10 mg daily) or zafirlukast (oral 20 mg 12-hourly) can be used as 'add-on' therapy for persistent asthma (step 3/4) to improve symptom control; they are *not* a replacement for inhaled corticosteroid. They are particularly useful in patients with concomitant rhinitis, also in the prevention of exercise-induced asthma.

Side-effects: These drugs are usually well tolerated, but can cause abdominal pain, thirst or headache. Rare cases of Churg–Strauss syndrome have been reported, although it is difficult to establish direct causation.

THEOPHYLLINE

Mode of action: Non-selective phosphodiesterase inhibitor that causes weak bronchodilatation (additive effect with inhaled β_2-agonists) by increasing intracellular cyclic AMP concentration. It may also have some respiratory stimulant and anti-inflammatory effects.

Indications: Asthma, COPD.

Clinical use: Can be considered as an 'add-on' therapy in asthma (step 4), if asthma symptoms remain uncontrolled. It is occasionally used in stable severe COPD with persistent symptoms, where it may enhance the effects of inhaled corticosteroids. Because toxic plasma levels are close to the therapeutic range (narrow therapeutic index), plasma levels should be monitored and the dose adjusted to maintain plasma levels in the range 10–20 mg/l (see national formulary for preparations). Use has declined following the introduction of safer alternative long-acting bronchodilators.

Side-effects: Nausea, tachycardia, palpitations, arrhythmias, convulsions. Theophylline levels are increased in hepatic impairment and heart failure, or by drugs that inhibit its metabolism (e.g. macrolide antibiotics). Levels are decreased by smoking, alcohol excess and drugs that accelerate hepatic metabolism.

MAGNESIUM SULPHATE

Mode of action: Direct relaxation of airway smooth muscle.

Indications: Acute severe asthma unresponsive to first-line treatment.

Clinical use: Given as an i.v. infusion (1.2–2 g over 20 mins) in acute severe asthma, where there has been a limited response to nebulised bronchodilators. There is no evidence that its use reduces mortality but it was shown to reduce admissions to hospital in a subset of patients with severe exacerbations.

Side-effects: Very few but may cause hypotension.

CORTICOSTEROIDS

Mode of action: Reduce airway inflammation, thereby decreasing mucous secretion and reducing bronchial reactivity.

Indications: Asthma, COPD.

Inhaled corticosteroids (ICS) (beclometasone, budesonide, fluticasone, mometasone)

Clinical use: In asthma, recommended as prophylactic treatment (beclometasone 200–400 μg 12-hourly or equivalent) if using a β_2-agonist more than twice a week, nocturnal symptoms occur more once a week or there has been an exacerbation within the last year (step 2—see p. 282). Beclometasone and budesonide are approximately equivalent, whilst fluticasone and mometasone provide equal clinical activity at half the dosage. Regular use is needed for maximum benefit. Treatment compliance and inhaler technique should be checked before treatment is intensified. In moderate/severe COPD, inhaled steroids may reduce the frequency of exacerbations and are indicated if there are more than two infective exacerbations/yr and FEV_1 is <50% predicted. Inhaled steroid/LABA combination inhalers (Seretide, Symbicort) are commonly used when both drugs are indicated, e.g. COPD, asthma (step 3/4).

Side-effects: The common side-effects of oral candidiasis and dysphonia can be reduced by rinsing the mouth with water or using a spacer device; systemic effects are considerably fewer than with oral corticosteroids, although there is still some systemic effect due to absorption from the lung and/or the GI tract. Long-term use of high-dose ICS may inhibit growth in children and reduce bone mineral density; therefore the lowest dose of ICS that maintains control of asthma symptoms should be used.

Oral prednisolone

Clinical use: In exacerbations of asthma, oral prednisolone (40 mg daily for 5–7 days) is used to reduce airway inflammation. The dose should be gradually reduced if there is a history of poor asthma control, or if the course of treatment lasts >2 wks. In exacerbations of COPD, prednisolone 30 mg daily for 5–7 days is used.

Side-effects: See below.

DRUGS COMMONLY USED FOR ENDOCRINE DISEASES

THYROID HORMONES (levothyroxine and levo-tri-iodothyronine)

Mode of action: Synthetic hormones, acting on intracellular receptors. Levo-tri-iodothyronine is the active form, which has a more rapid effect.

Indications: Hypothyroidism, Hashimoto's thyroiditis, thyroid carcinoma, myxoedema coma.

Clinical use:

• Oral L-thyroxine (starting dose 50 μg daily, increased by 50 μg every 3 wks to 100–150 μg daily) is used as maintenance therapy in hypothyroidism. It can also be used to shrink goitres associated with Hashimoto's, and to suppress TSH production following thyroidectomy for TSH-dependent carcinoma.

• I.V. L-tri-iodothyronine (5–20 μg 8-hourly), in combination with i.v. fluids and hydrocortisone, is used in myxoedema coma, where rapid thyroid replacement is required.

• L-tri-iodothyronine 20 μg is equivalent to L-thyroxine 100 μg.

Side-effects: Symptoms of hyperthyroidism; exacerbation of angina. Caution in suspected hypoadrenalism: replace corticosteroids prior to administering thyroid hormone.

ANTI-THYROID DRUGS (carbimazole, propylthiouracil)

Mode of action: Inhibit the iodination of tyrosine, thereby reducing synthesis of new thyroid hormones.

Indications: Hyperthyroidism, thyrotoxic crisis, induction of euthyroid state pre-thyroidectomy.

Clinical use: In hyperthyroidism, high-dose oral carbimazole (40–60 mg daily) or propylthiouracil (200–400 mg daily) is given until the patient is clinically and biochemically euthyroid (typically 3–4 wks). Thereafter, maintenance treatment at a lower dose (determined by measurement of T_4 and TSH) is usually continued for 12–18 mths.

Side-effects: Rash is common. Agranulocytosis is rare but important; patients should be told to discontinue treatment if a sore throat or fever develops, and to attend their doctor for an FBC to exclude neutropenia. Carbimazole is contraindicated during breastfeeding but propylthiouracil may be used instead.

CORTICOSTEROIDS (hydrocortisone, fludrocortisone, prednisolone, dexamethasone)

Mode of action: Regulate the transcription of genes in various cells and tissues.

• *Mineralocorticoids* (e.g. fludrocortisone) promote sodium retention at the expense of potassium.

• *Glucocorticoids* regulate metabolism and cardiovascular homeostasis and limit inflammatory responses.

• Some glucocorticoids (e.g. hydrocortisone) also exert significant mineralocorticoid effects, while others (e.g. dexamethasone) have negligible mineralocorticoid activity.

Indications: Glucocorticoid and/or mineralocorticoid deficiency (e.g. Addison's disease); suppression of inflammatory and immune-mediated conditions (e.g. rheumatic disease, asthma, COPD, inflammatory bowel disease, glomerulonephritis, vasculitis, prevention of transplant rejection); cerebral oedema; postural hypotension in autonomic neuropathy (mineralocorticoids).

Clinical use:

• *Replacement therapy:* oral hydrocortisone (e.g. 15–20 mg on waking and 5–10 mg at 18:00 hrs) is the usual maintenance treatment for adrenal insufficiency and, in primary adrenal failure, is supplemented with oral fludrocortisone (50–300 μg daily). The dose should be doubled during an acute illness. I.V. hydrocortisone succinate (100 mg 6-hourly) is used in hypoadrenal crisis.

• *Other indications:* oral prednisolone (20–60 mg for acute illness; 2.5–15 mg for maintenance therapy) has minimal mineralocorticoid activity and is the corticosteroid used most commonly for anti-inflammatory purposes. The lowest effective dose should be used to minimise side-effects; maintenance doses >7.5 mg are associated with a higher incidence of side-effects. I.V. methylprednisolone (10–500 mg) provides powerful suppression of inflammatory, autoimmune and allergic disorders, with higher doses reserved for treatment of transplanted graft rejection. Dexamethasone (0.5–10 mg daily by mouth; 4 mg 6-hourly i.v.) is used to relieve cerebral oedema, as its lack of mineralocorticoid activity avoids counterproductive fluid retention.

Side-effects:

Glucocorticoid effects include dyspepsia, peptic ulceration (signs of perforation may be masked), osteoporosis (bone protection required with long-term treatment), skin atrophy, bruising, proximal myopathy, diabetes mellitus, increased susceptibility to infections and psychosis. Patients taking glucocorticoids for >2 wks are at risk of adrenal suppression and should not discontinue treatment abruptly (such patients should carry a steroid treatment card).

Mineralocorticoid effects include hypertension, sodium and water retention, and hypokalaemia.

DRUGS COMMONLY USED FOR DIABETES MELLITUS

METFORMIN

Mode of action: Increases insulin sensitivity and peripheral glucose uptake, and may also impair glucose absorption from the gut; requires some endogenous insulin secretion for effects.

Indications: Type 2 diabetes mellitus inadequately controlled with dietary measures.

Clinical use: Oral metformin (starting dose 500 mg 12-hourly increased to maximum of 1 g 8-hourly with meals) is the hypoglycaemic drug of choice in obese patients (does not cause weight gain) and may also be used in non-obese patients. Its glucose-lowering effect is synergistic with that of sulphonylureas, so the two drugs may be usefully combined. It may also be used in combination with thiazolidinediones, acarbose or insulin.

Side-effects: GI side-effects (e.g. nausea, diarrhoea) are common and troublesome, but may lessen with time. There is a risk of severe lactic acidosis, particularly when renal function is impaired. Metformin is contraindicated in renal impairment (even mild), pregnancy and breastfeeding; it should be withheld in patients receiving iodine-containing contrast agents or general anaesthesia and those with shock or conditions associated with tissue hypoxia (replace with insulin if necessary). It does not cause hypoglycaemia.

SULPHONYLUREAS (tolbutamide, gliclazide, glibenclamide)

Mode of action: Stimulate release of insulin from pancreatic β-cells; only effective with some residual pancreatic function.

Indications: Type 2 diabetes mellitus inadequately controlled with dietary measures.

Clinical use: Oral sulphonylureas (e.g. tolbutamide 500 mg 12-hourly or 8-hourly; gliclazide 40–160 mg 12-hourly; glibenclamide 5–15 mg daily) can promote weight gain so are most beneficial in non-obese patients. They are also used in obese patients who are unable to take metformin (contraindication or side-effects) or have poor glycaemic control despite metformin treatment. Shorter-acting agents (e.g. tolbutamide, gliclazide) are preferred in the elderly (hypoglycaemia less likely) and both can be used in mild to moderate renal impairment.

Side-effects: Sulphonylureas are generally well tolerated; weight gain and hypoglycaemia (particularly with long-acting agents, e.g. glibenclamide) may occur. They are contraindicated in severe hepatic or renal impairment, breastfeeding and pregnancy.

INSULINS

Mode of action: Replacement polypeptide hormone that acts on endogenous insulin receptors. Unmodified insulin is short-acting. Longer-acting preparations can be derived by adding protamine and zinc at neutral pH (isophane) or excess zinc ions (lente).

Indications: Type 1 diabetes mellitus; type 2 diabetes mellitus in which satisfactory glucose control cannot be achieved with oral hypoglycaemics and diet, during intercurrent illness or pregnancy, or perioperatively.

Clinical use: Human insulin, produced by recombinant DNA technology, is now the most widely used form.

• Soluble insulin is usually given s.c. 15–30 mins before a meal but is also given as an infusion in hospital during emergency treatment and perioperatively. It has a very short half-life when administered i.v.

• Insulin analogues (insulin aspart and lispro) have a faster action and shorter duration of action than soluble insulin, and are therefore administered immediately before or shortly after meals; they carry a lower incidence of hypoglycaemia.
• Intermediate and long-acting insulins have an onset of action 1–2 hrs following injection, and a duration of action of 16–35 hrs.

Insulin regimens are described on page 406.

Side-effects: Hypoglycaemia is common, and more likely with tight blood sugar control; frequent hypoglycaemic episodes or β-blockers may cause loss of hypoglycaemic warning symptoms. At the injection site, local reaction and fat hypertrophy can occur, which may delay onset of effect.

DRUGS COMMONLY USED FOR MUSCULOSKELETAL DISEASES

DRUGS USED FOR PAIN RELIEF

PARACETAMOL

Mode of action: Inhibits CNS production of prostaglandins; little effect on peripheral prostaglandin production.

Indications: Mild to moderate pain; pyrexia.

Clinical use: Paracetamol (1 g 4-hourly oral/i.v.) is an effective first-line analgesic for mild to moderate pain. It is safe, inexpensive and widely available, and has few contraindications and drug interactions.

Side-effects: Rare. Serious risk of liver damage in overdose; see page 37.

NON-STEROIDAL ANTI-INFLAMMATORY DRUGS (NSAIDs)

Mode of action: NSAIDs reduce prostaglandin levels by inhibiting cyclo-oxygenases (COX; see Fig. 15.1). COX-1 is constitutively expressed and affects gut mucosal integrity, renal blood flow and platelet aggregation. COX-2 is induced at sites of inflammation both locally, where it produces prostaglandins involved in inflammation and pain, and in the CNS, where it mediates pain and fever.

Indications: Mild to moderate pain; inflammation in musculoskeletal disorders.

Clinical use: Oral NSAIDs relieve mild to moderate pain and, in regular full dosage, reduce inflammation. They are particularly useful in inflammatory musculoskeletal disorders such as rheumatoid arthritis and gout.

• *Ibuprofen:* at standard doses (1.2–1.8 g daily in 3–4 divided doses), provides effective pain relief and causes fewer side-effects than other NSAIDs, but has weaker anti-inflammatory effects. • *Naproxen* (0.5–1 g daily in 1–2 divided doses) and *diclofenac* (75–150 mg daily in 2–3 divided doses): combine good anti-inflammatory properties with a low incidence of side-effects (but more than ibuprofen), and are more suitable than ibuprofen for conditions with a prominent inflammatory component such as acute gout.

• *COX-2 inhibitors* (e.g. celecoxib): selectively inhibit COX-2; they have similar efficacy to traditional NSAIDs with less GI toxicity (see below), but may be associated with an increased risk of MI and stroke.

Side-effects: By depleting mucosal prostaglandins (COX-1 inhibition), NSAIDs impair gastroduodenal defences; they may cause erosions and ulceration, and increase the risk of bleeding and perforation from existing ulcers. Start with a safer NSAID (e.g. ibuprofen) and always use the lowest effective dose. Co-prescription of a gastroprotective drug (e.g. omeprazole 20 mg daily) should be considered in patients with risk factors for ulceration, particularly age >60 yrs, past history of peptic ulcer, and concomitant steroid or antiplatelet use.

NSAIDs also impair autoregulation of renal blood flow and may precipitate renal failure, especially patients with pre-existing renal impairment. Other side-effects include bronchospasm and worsening of asthma, fluid retention, non-ulcer dyspepsia and interstitial nephritis (rare).

Contraindications include active peptic ulcer, current anticoagulant use and a history of hypersensitivity reactions to aspirin or any NSAID.

OPIOIDS (codeine, dihydrocodeine, morphine, fentanyl, diamorphine)

Mode of action: Agonists at central opioid receptors.

Indications: Moderate to severe pain.

Clinical use:

• Weak opioids (e.g. codeine oral 30–60 mg 4-hourly; dihydrocodeine oral 30–60 mg 4-hourly) are mild analgesics that provide effective relief for moderate pain, especially in combination with paracetamol.

• Strong opioids (e.g. morphine s.c./i.m. 10 mg 2–4-hourly) are used to relieve severe acute pain and post-operative pain. They are also used for chronic pain, particularly in the setting of palliative care, where dependence and tolerance resulting from prolonged administration are not limiting factors.

• In severe, continuous cancer pain, oral immediate-release (IR) morphine (5–20 mg) should be given 4-hourly with the same dose available on an as-required basis for breakthrough pain. The regular dose should be adjusted daily, taking account of breakthrough requirements and side-effects. Once the correct dose has been established, IR morphine can be replaced by a controlled-release preparation (usually 12-hourly).

• Oxycodone or transdermal fentanyl is an alternative to morphine that may produce a better balance of benefit against side-effects and is useful in renal failure (no renal excretion of active metabolites).

• Pethidine is used in acute pain management but should not be used to manage chronic pain because of its short half-life and ceiling dose.

• Diamorphine is a highly soluble strong opioid used for s.c. infusions, particularly in the last few days of life.

Side-effects: Nausea and vomiting occur initially but usually settle after a few days (co-prescribe an antiemetic). Constipation is common and often requires regular laxative administration. Confusion and drowsiness are dose-related and reversible. Respiratory depression can occur.

DRUGS USED IN THE MANAGEMENT OF GOUT

NSAIDs

See above.

COLCHICINE

Mode of action: Potent inhibitor of neutrophil microtubular assembly.

Indications: Treatment of acute attacks of gout.

Clinical use: Oral colchicine (1 mg loading dose, then 0.5 mg 4-hourly until symptoms abate; max. 6 mg per course) provides effective symptomatic relief in acute gout and is a useful alternative in patients unable to take NSAIDs.

Side-effects: Nausea, vomiting, abdominal pain and diarrhoea are common.

ALLOPURINOL

Mode of action: Lowers serum uric acid levels by inhibiting xanthine oxidase and thereby reducing conversion of hypoxanthine and xanthine to uric acid.

Indications: Long-term management of gout in patients with recurrent attacks of acute gout, tophi, bone or joint damage, or renal disease.

Clinical use: Drug of choice for the long-term prophylaxis of gout (100–300 mg daily). The sharp reduction in tissue uric acid levels following initiation of treatment can partially dissolve monosodium urate monohydrate crystals and trigger acute attacks. Allopurinol should therefore be commenced *after* the acute attack has settled, and can be co-prescribed with an NSAID or colchicine.

Side-effects: Rashes and GI upset can occur but are uncommon. Allopurinol greatly increases the risk of azathioprine toxicity (reduce the azathioprine dose).

DRUGS USED IN THE MANAGEMENT OF BONE DISEASES

BISPHOSPHONATES (alendronate, risedronate, pamidronate)

Mode of action: Synthetic analogues of pyrophosphate that adsorb on to bone surfaces and become incorporated within the bone matrix. When osteoclasts resorb bone containing bisphosphonate, the drug inhibits intracellular pathways, decreasing bone resorption.

Indications: Treatment of postmenopausal osteoporosis and osteoporosis in men; prevention and treatment of corticosteroid-induced osteoporosis; hypercalcaemia of malignancy; bone pain secondary to metastases; Paget's disease of bone.

Clinical use:
• Oral *alendronate* (10 mg daily or 70 mg weekly) and *risedronate* (5 mg daily or 35 mg weekly) prevent postmenopausal bone loss, reduce the risk of vertebral and non-vertebral fractures in patients with established osteoporosis, and are effective in the prevention and treatment of corticosteroid-induced osteoporosis. Risedronate is also used for pain control in patients with Paget's disease of bone (PDB). Due to poor absorption, they should be taken on an empty stomach, 45–60 mins before food with plain water only.
• I.V. *pamidronate* is used in the management of hypercalcaemia of malignancy (15–60 mg in single infusion), bone pain secondary to metastases (90 mg every 4 wks) and PDB (30 mg/wk for 6 wks).

Side-effects: Principally GI upset, e.g. nausea, dyspepsia, oesophageal reactions (including erosions and ulceration), abdominal pain and altered bowel habit. Pamidronate can also causes flu-like symptoms. Use with caution in patients with GORD; avoid in patients with oesophageal stricture.

DRUGS COMMONLY USED FOR PSYCHIATRIC DISEASES

ANTIDEPRESSANTS

Both cognitive behavioural and interpersonal therapy are as effective as antidepressants for mild to moderate depression but antidepressant drugs are preferred for severe depression. The agents below are equally effective in moderate to severe depression; about three-quarters of patients respond to treatment but, typically, no improvement is seen until 2–4 wks after initiation of treatment (though side-effects may occur immediately).

TRICYCLIC ANTIDEPRESSANTS (TCAs) (amitriptyline, imipramine)

Mode of action: Inhibit the re-uptake of noradrenaline (norepinephrine) and 5-hydroxytryptamine (5-HT; serotonin) at synaptic clefts in the CNS.

Indications: Depressive illness, neuropathic pain.

Clinical use: These agents (e.g. amitriptyline 75–150 mg daily; imipramine 75–150 mg daily) are effective, but their use is limited by side-effects and dangerous toxicity in overdose. Tricyclic-related drugs (e.g. trazodone 150–300 mg daily in 1–2 divided doses) are particularly useful where sedation is required and have fewer antimuscarinic and cardiac effects. In lower doses, TCAs (e.g. amitriptyline 10–25 mg) are effective against neuropathic pain.

Side-effects: Sedation (less with imipramine); antimuscarinic effects (dry mouth, blurred vision, urinary retention, constipation); confusion (especially in elderly patients); tachycardia, arrhythmias (cardiotoxic in overdose). Caution with angle-closure glaucoma, history of urinary retention; contraindicated in recent MI and arrhythmias.

SELECTIVE SEROTONIN RE-UPTAKE INHIBITORS (SSRIs)

(fluoxetine, citalopram)

Mode of action: Selectively inhibit the re-uptake of 5-HT.

Indications: Depressive illness, anxiety disorders, obsessive-compulsive disorder.

Clinical use: These widely used agents (e.g. fluoxetine 20 mg daily; citalopram 20–40 mg daily) have similar efficacy to TCAs but are less toxic in overdose, and cause less sedation and fewer antimuscarinic side-effects. They are most useful in patients who cannot tolerate a TCA or who are at significant risk of overdose.

Side-effects: Headache, nausea, anorexia and sexual dysfunction; may cause hyponatraemia (syndrome of inappropriate ADH secretion).

ANTIPSYCHOTICS

- Phenothiazines (e.g. chlorpromazine).
- Butyrophenones (e.g. haloperidol).
- Thioxanthines (e.g. flupentixol).
- Atypical antipsychotics (e.g. clozapine, olanzapine).

Mode of action: Exert an antipsychotic effect by blocking D_2 dopamine receptors in the CNS; may also have anticholinergic, anti-adrenergic, anti-serotonergic and antihistaminergic effects.

Indications: Schizophrenia and other psychoses; short-term treatment of psychomotor agitation and other disturbed behaviour (especially violent or dangerous); nausea and vomiting.

Clinical use:

These drugs (e.g. haloperidol oral/i.m. 1–5 mg) are used widely to sedate patients with acutely disturbed and aggressive behaviour. Lower doses (e.g. haloperidol oral 0.5–1.5 mg once or twice daily, chlorpromazine oral 10–25 mg once or twice daily) may be helpful in agitated elderly patients, but are not a substitute for good community support for patients and carers or attentive nursing care.

Both traditional (e.g. haloperidol, flupentixol) and newer ‘atypical’ antipsychotics (e.g. olanzapine, risperidone) are effective against the positive symptoms of schizophrenia in the majority of cases. They take 2–3 wks to be maximally effective, but have some immediate beneficial effects. For long-term use, antipsychotic agents are often given in slow-release (depot) injected form to improve adherence. Atypical antipsychotics are less likely to cause extrapyramidal side-effects and are now often used as first-line treatment; they may also be effective (especially clozapine) in patients who are unresponsive to traditional drugs.

Side-effects:

- Extrapyramidal symptoms, including parkinsonism (more common in the elderly), dystonic reactions (more common in children or young adults), akathisia (restlessness) and tardive dyskinesia (involuntary facial movements which may be irreversible on withdrawing therapy), are most common with butyrophenones (e.g. haloperidol) and some phenothiazines (e.g. prochloperazine) and less common with atypical drugs.

• Drowsiness, apathy, confusion, insomnia, convulsions; antimuscarinic symptoms (e.g. blurred vision, dry mouth, urinary retention); menstrual disturbances, galactorrhoea, gynaecomastia; and cholestatic jaundice also occur.

• Neuroleptic malignant syndrome is uncommon but life-threatening; it is characterised by fever, tremor and rigidity, confusion and elevated creatine kinase (stop antipsychotic medication immediately and treat with dantrolene sodium and intensive supportive therapy).

• Prolongation of the QT interval may predispose to torsades de pointes (avoid other drugs which prolong the QT interval).

• The atypical agents (especially olanzapine) tend to cause greater metabolic side-effects such as hyperglycaemia, insulin resistance and weight gain. Clozapine can cause agranulocytosis and requires regular monitoring of the WBC, initially on a weekly basis.

DRUGS COMMONLY USED FOR NEUROLOGICAL DISEASES

ANTICONVULSANTS (carbamazepine, valproate, phenytoin)

The aim of therapy should be to control seizures with a simple regimen; this is likely to promote compliance and minimise adverse effects or interactions. Monotherapy is sufficient for most but not all patients. Interactions between antiepileptics and with other drugs are usually caused by hepatic enzyme induction or inhibition. The risk of toxicity is increased when using combinations of anticonvulsants.

Pregnancy and breastfeeding

Many antiepileptic drugs carry a risk of teratogenicity; women should be informed of these risks and offered specialist advice prior to pregnancy. Folate supplemention taken before and during pregnancy reduces the risk of neural tube defects. Breastfeeding is acceptable with most anticonvulsants, excepting the barbiturates and some of the newer agents.

CARBAMAZEPINE

Mode of action: Only partially elucidated—stabilises hyperexcited nerve membranes; prevents repetitive firing of sodium-dependent action potentials in depolarised neurons.

Indications: Primary and secondary generalised tonic-clonic seizures, absences, partial seizures.

Clinical use: Initially 100–200 mg orally once or twice daily, followed by a slow increase until best response is obtained, often 800–1200 mg daily. A modified-release preparation is available for once-daily use. Steady-state levels occur within 1–2 wks (therapeutic range 20–50 μmol/l).

Side-effects:

• *Dose-related:* paraesthesia, anorexia, headache, nausea, diarrhoea, visual changes. • *Idiosyncratic:* rashes, agranulocytosis, thrombocytopenia, photosensitivity, liver damage.

Contraindicated in AV conduction disorders, bone marrow depression and porphyria. Use with caution in hepatic, renal and cardiac disease and in pregnancy.

Interactions: Carbamazepine is catalysed by cytochrome P450 3A4. Inhibitors or inducers of this enzyme will interact by altering plasma carbamazepine—see national formulary.

SODIUM VALPROATE

Mode of action: Potentiation of the inhibitory action of gamma aminobutyric acid (GABA).

Indications: Primary and secondary generalised tonic-clonic seizures, absences, myoclonus.

Clinical use: Initially 600 mg daily in 2 divided doses, increasing by 200 mg every 3 days until control is achieved (usually between 1000 and 2000 mg/day). Modified-release preparations are available. Sodium valproate can also be administered by i.v. injection (400–800 mg over 3–5 mins) or infusion; for continuation of treatment the dose is the same as the current oral dose. There is no clear relationship between drug levels and clinical efficacy.

Side-effects:

• *Dose-related:* drowsiness, nausea, ataxia, nystagmus, diplopia, tremor. • *Idiosyncratic:* alopecia, rashes, blood dyscrasias, liver damage, pancreatitis. • *Long-term:* weight gain.

Contraindicated in active liver disease; use with caution in renal insufficiency and in pregnancy. Liver function should be measured at baseline and during the first 6 mths of therapy. Valproate has no enzyme-inducing effect and does not reduce efficacy of the oral contraceptive pill.

PHENYTOIN

Mode of action: Not fully elucidated. Effects include inhibition of sodium and calcium channels in neuronal cell membranes and increased GABA-mediated inhibition of excitatory synaptic transmission.

Indications: Partial and secondary generalised tonic-clonic seizures.

Clinical use: Initially 3–4 mg/kg/day or 150–300 mg daily is appropriate. This is increased slowly to the lowest dose achieving seizure control; for most adults this will be 200–500 mg daily in single or divided doses. Serum measurement (therapeutic range 40–80 μmol/l) can help to confirm the correct dose and also aid compliance with treatment. Phenytoin has a narrow therapeutic index and small changes in dose can produce large effects on serum concentrations over days. Dose changes should be gradual.

Side-effects:
• *Dose-related:* drowsiness, ataxia, nystagmus, diplopia, tremor, dystonia, asterixis. • *Idiosyncratic:* rashes, blood dyscrasias, liver damage, SLE. • *Long-term:* gum hypertrophy, facial dysmorphism, hirsutism, folate deficiency, osteomalacia, neuropathy.

Phenytoin should be avoided in porphyria, hepatic impairment, pregnancy and breastfeeding. Abrupt withdrawal should be avoided.

Interactions: Common; see national formulary.

DRUGS USED IN PARKINSON'S DISEASE

Treatment is usually not started until the disease has caused significant disability. Patients should be advised about limitations of treatment and potential side-effects. Antiparkinsonian medication should not be stopped abruptly, as there is a small risk of neuroleptic malignant syndrome. Side-effects are more common in the elderly (particularly confusion and hallucinations), so treatment should be initiated gradually.

LEVODOPA

Mode of action: Levodopa is the amino-acid precursor of dopamine and acts by replenishing depleted striatal dopamine.

Indications: Parkinson's disease.

Clinical use:

Levodopa is given together with a peripheral dopa-decarboxylase inhibitor, which reduces the peripheral conversion to dopamine and limits side-effects. Peripheral dopa-decarboxylase inhibitors include benserazide (in co-beneldopa) and carbidopa (in co-careldopa). There are several such combined preparations available, including modified-release agents and the national formulary should be consulted for details.

An initial low dose is increased in small steps, keeping the final dose as low as possible. The usual maintenance dose of levodopa is 400–800 mg daily in divided doses.

Motor complications include response fluctuations and dyskinesias. 'End-of-dose deterioration' may be improved by using smaller, more frequent doses or a slow-release preparation. More complex fluctuations present as periods of severe parkinsonism alternating with dyskinesia and agitation (the 'on-off' phenomenon).

Side-effects: Common: nausea, vomiting, taste disturbances, dry mouth, arrhythmias, postural hypotension, drowsiness, dementia, psychoses, confusion, euphoria, abnormal dreams, insomnia, depression, dystonia, dyskinesia and chorea. Levodopa should be used with caution in severe cardiovascular or pulmonary disease, psychiatric illness, endocrine disorders, convulsions, malignant melanoma, open-angle glaucoma, and in hepatic or renal impairment.

Interactions: Levodopa can interact with a variety of medications; non-selective monoamine oxidase inhibitors are contraindicated, as there is a risk of hypertensive crisis, and must be stopped at least 2 wks prior to levodopa therapy.

19

Interpreting key investigations

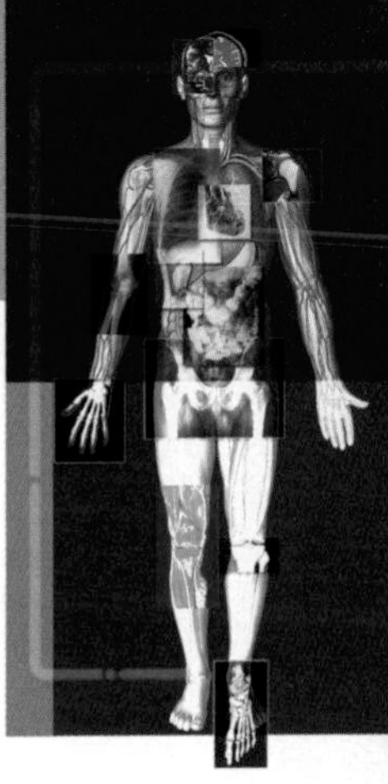

Although the history and examination remain the key to most clinical problems, investigations are usually required to confirm the diagnosis or to narrow the differential diagnosis. Such investigations are frequently performed in emergency situations, so familiarity with the key tests is vital to practising physicians in all specialties.

The biochemical and haematological abnormalities specific to particular conditions are covered in the relevant chapter. This chapter deals with basic aspects of the ECG, chest X-ray and respiratory function tests, together with the common problem of interpreting raised markers of inflammation, which can occur in the presence of a wide range of disorders.

ELECTROCARDIOGRAPHY (ECG)

ECG is used to detect the cardiac rhythm, conducting tissue disease, ventricular hypertrophy, myocardial ischaemia and infarction, and the effects of some drugs on the heart. ECGs can appear difficult to interpret at first, but a systematic approach will ensure that important findings are not missed.

SYSTEMATIC APPROACH TO ECG INTERPRETATION

PATIENT DETAILS AND ECG CALIBRATION

Always record and check the patient's name and date of birth, as well as the date and time, on an ECG. Also check the calibration; ECGs are usually recorded at a paper speed of 25 mm/s and calibrated so that a signal of 1 mV = 10 mm.

THE NORMAL ECG

Figure 19.1 shows a normal 12-lead ECG, and the terminology and limits of normality for the key waves and intervals are shown in Figure 19.2.

P WAVE

The P wave is caused by atrial depolarisation, and is normally <0.2 mV (2 small squares) in amplitude and <0.12 s (3 small squares) in duration. • Broad bifid P waves >0.12 s (P mitrale) can be due to left atrial abnormality or enlargement. • Tall P waves >2.5 mm (P pulmonale) indicate right atrial enlargement and often accompany pulmonary hypertension.

PR INTERVAL

The PR interval is from the onset of the P wave to the onset of the QRS complex, and is normally 0.12–0.2 s in duration (3–5 small squares). • A long PR interval indicates AV block. • A short PR interval suggests pre-excitation, e.g. Wolff–Parkinson–White syndrome (see p. 219).

QRS COMPLEX

The QRS complex is caused by ventricular depolarisation.
• A Q wave is defined as any negative deflection preceding an R wave. • An R wave is any positive deflection. • An S wave is any negative deflection after an R wave.

Non-pathological small Q waves are often seen in leads I, aVL, III, V_5 and V_6.

QRS duration: Normally <0.1 s (2.5 small squares). A broad QRS complex (>0.12 s) can occur with delayed ventricular depolarisation (e.g. bundle branch block) or if the impulse is generated from a focus outside the bundle branches (e.g. ventricular ectopic or ventricular tachycardia).

QRS amplitude: Affected by LV mass, axis and patient build. Large-amplitude complexes can be normal in thin patients, while small complexes can be seen in patients with thick chest walls, emphysema, pericardial effusions or hypothermia.

• Left ventricular hypertrophy (LVH) can cause large-voltage QRS complexes; voltage criteria for LVH are present if the S wave in V_1 plus the tallest R wave in V_5 or V_6 is >35 mm. Other ECG criteria for LVH exist, but all scoring systems suffer from relatively low sensitivity. If non-voltage criteria for LVH, such as ST/T wave abnormalities in I, aVL, V_{5-6} ('abnormal repolarisation' or 'strain'), are also present, the likelihood of LVH is higher. • Right ventricular hypertrophy (RVH) may cause a dominant R wave in V_1, T wave inversion in V_{1-3}, deep S waves in V_6 and right axis deviation.

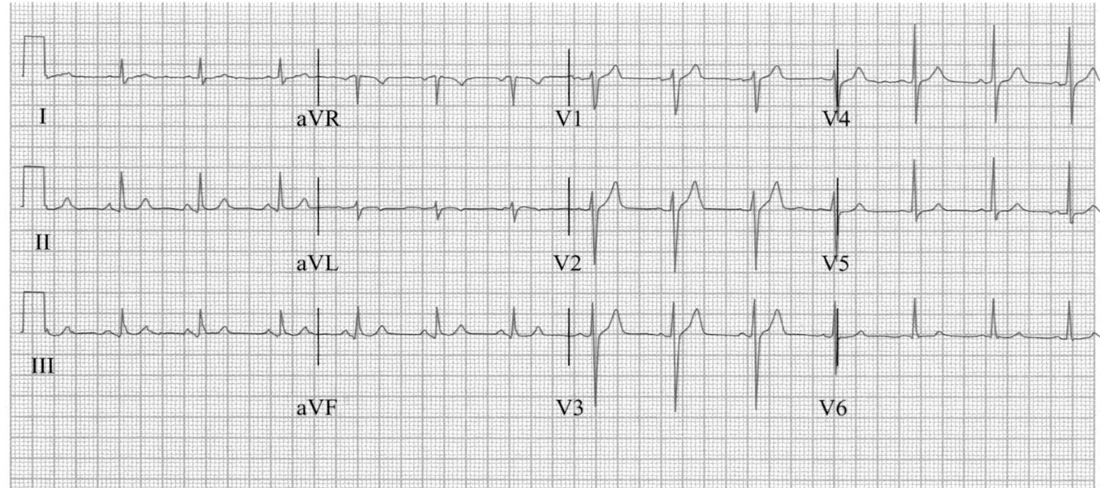

Fig. 19.1 A normal 12-lead ECG. Note how the R wave becomes gradually move positive from V_1 to V_6.

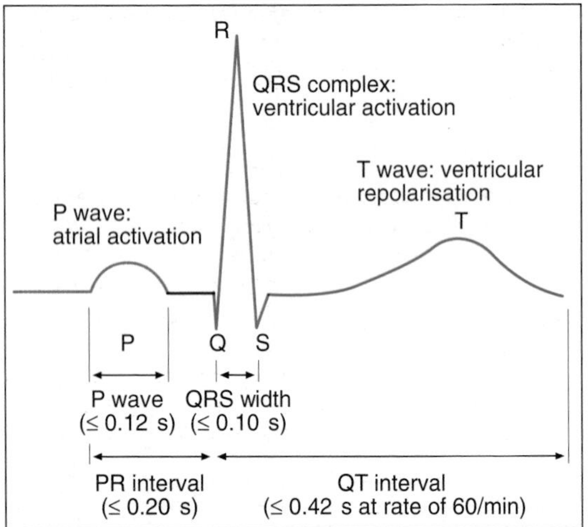

Fig. 19.2 The components of the ECG correspond to the depolarisation and repolarisation. The upper limit of the normal range for each interval is given in brackets.

ST SEGMENT

The ST segment is usually isoelectric.

• ST segment elevation can occur in acute myocardial infarction, pericarditis or LV aneurysm. It can be normal ('early repolarisation' or 'high take-off') in some individuals. • ST segment depression usually occurs in myocardial ischaemia, abnormal repolarisation with LVH, with digoxin therapy, and with other drugs and metabolic disorders.

T WAVE

T waves are caused by ventricular repolarisation. They can be inverted in lead III, V_1 or V_2 in normal individuals. T wave abnormalities are common and non-specific.

• T wave inversion may be due to myocardial ischaemia/infarction, drugs, stroke, hyperventilation, exercise or anxiety. • Tall T waves can be normal but may also be seen with myocardial ischaemia/infarction, hyperkalaemia, LVH and pericarditis.

QT INTERVAL

The QT interval is from the beginning of the QRS complex to the end of the T wave. It varies with heart rate and should be corrected for this:

$$QT_C \text{ (corrected QT)} = QT \text{ (s)}/\sqrt{R - R \text{ interval (s)}}$$

The QT_C is normally 0.38–0.46 s. Prolonged QT can predispose to VT and may be caused by:

• Electrolyte abnormalities (hypokalaemia, hypocalcaemia). • Drugs. • Hypothermia. • Long QT syndrome.

U WAVE

U waves follow the T wave and are not always present. Prominent U waves can be seen with bradycardia, hypokalaemia and some drugs.

RATE

Heart rate is calculated from the R–R interval. At a standard paper speed of 25 mm/s, the number of large squares between each R wave divided into 300 indicates the heart rate in beats per minute (bpm). For example, 2 large squares between R waves = 150 bpm, 3 large squares = 100 bpm, and so on. If the heart rate is irregular, take an average over 5 R–R intervals.

RHYTHM

This is best assessed in lead II where the P waves are usually clearly seen. Firstly, note if the rhythm (R–R interval) is regular or irregular. Then look for P waves and establish their relationship to the QRS complexes. In sinus rhythm:

• R–R intervals are regular. • There are normal P waves (upright in leads I and II) before each QRS complex. • The rate is between 60 and 100 bpm.

CARDIAC AXIS

This is the mean direction of ventricular depolarisation in the coronal plane. It is most accurately estimated from the limb leads using the hexaxial system (Fig. 19.3). Firstly, identify the equiphasic lead (where the positive and negative deflections of the QRS complex are roughly equal). Then find the lead at 90° to this on the hexaxial diagram.

• If the QRS complex in this lead is predominantly positive, then this indicates the axis. • If it is negative, then the axis is directly opposite (at 180° to) this lead.

Normal axis: From –30° to +90°.
Left axis deviation: From –30° to –90°.
Right axis deviation: From +90° to +180°.

Quick method

As lead I is oriented horizontally across the chest, it reveals whether the axis is to the left or right.

• A predominantly negative QRS in lead I indicates right axis deviation. • As the normal axis extends above the horizontal to –30°, left axis deviation is revealed by a mainly negative QRS in lead II (which lies at right angles to –30°). • If the QRS complexes in leads I and II are mainly positive, the axis is normal.

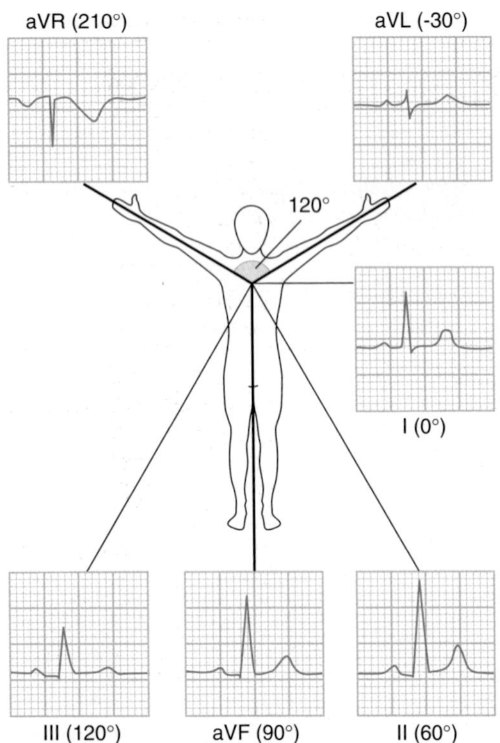

Fig. 19.3 The normal appearance of the ECG from different leads in the coronal plane.

CHEST X-RAY (CXR)

The chest radiograph remains the most common X-ray examination. It contains a large amount of information and a systematic approach is imperative to correct interpretation.

THE NORMAL CHEST X-RAY

An example of a normal chest X-ray with key features highlighted, is given in Figure 19.4.

SYSTEMATIC APPROACH TO CXR INTERPRETATION

PATIENT DETAILS AND DATE

Note the patient's name and date of birth, as well as the date and time the CXR was performed, to ensure you are looking at the correct film.

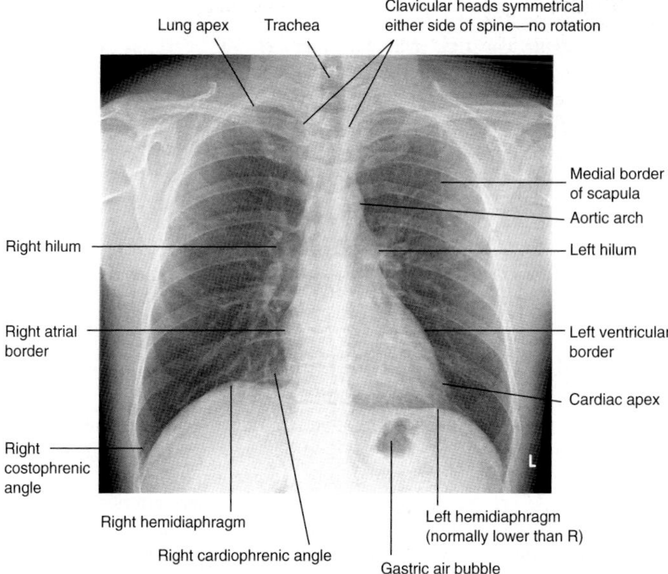

Fig. 19.4 The normal chest X-ray. Note: Lung markings consist of branching and tapering lines radiating out from the hila; where airways and vessels turn towards the film they can appear as open or filled circles (see upper pole of R. hilum). The scapula may overlie the lung fields—trace the edge of bony structures to avoid mistaking them for pleural or pulmonary shadows. To check for hyperinflation, count the ribs. If you can see more than ten ribs posteriorly above the diaphragm then the lungs are hyperinflated.

TECHNICAL QUALITY

Several technical factors affecting the quality of the X-ray should be assessed before proceeding further:

Orientation: Most CXRs are taken using a postero-anterior (PA) view: the patient stands with their chest towards the plate and the X-ray source behind them. If patients are too unwell to stand, then an antero-posterior (AP) X-ray will be done with the X-ray source in front of them and the plate behind them. With an AP film the heart appears magnified relative to a PA film.

Posture: If the patient is supine, the distribution of air and fluid is changed and it is impossible to exclude a pneumothorax, pleural effusion or subdiaphragmatic air.

Rotation: If the patient is not rotated, the spinous processes of the thoracic vertebrae will be projected midway between the medial borders of the clavicles.

Penetration: The thoracic vertebral bodies should be just visible behind the heart. If they cannot be seen at all, the film is under-exposed and will appear too white. If they can be seen in detail, then the film is over-exposed and will be too dark.

Inspiration: The right hemidiaphragm should be at the level of the anterior end of the 6th rib or the posterior end of the 9th–10th ribs. If more ribs are seen, hyperinflation is present.

Field of view: All of the lungs should be visible; make sure that lung apices and especially costophrenic angles have not been missed.

TRACHEA

The trachea should be central. It may be deviated towards an area of loss of volume (e.g. lobar collapse) or away from an area of increased pressure (e.g. tension pneumothorax).

HEART AND MEDIASTINAL CONTOURS

Superior mediastinum: This should be central.

Widening may represent a normal variant (the aorta dilates and becomes more tortuous with increasing age), aortic aneurysm or soft tissue mass (primary tumour, retrosternal thyroid or lymphadenopathy).

Hila: These are the shadows cast by the pulmonary arteries and veins. The largest hilar structure is the lower lobe pulmonary artery, which tapers downwards and outwards in health. The left hilum is usually higher than the right.

Rounded shadows which fail to taper and branch may indicate lymph nodes or tumours.

Heart: Note the following:

A cardiac shadow of >50% of the total thoracic width on a PA film is abnormal and occurs with ventricular dilatation or pericardial effusion. The left heart border consists of the left ventricle and left atrium, while the right heart border is made up of the right atrium. Consolidation in the immediately adjacent lung blurs the heart borders.

LUNG FIELDS AND PLEURA

Lungs: For the purposes of description, assess and compare the upper, middle and lower zones of both lungs (these do not correspond with the lobes which overlie each other in the frontal view). Common lung abnormalities are listed in Box 19.1.

Pleura: Not normally visible on a CXR. Pleural thickening appears on the chest X-ray as a dense line on the inner surface of the lateral chest wall, separating the inner cortex of the ribs from the underlying aerated lung. At the lung apices, pleural thickening forms a 'cap' which opacifies the first intercostal space on the X-ray.

• Thickened pleura occur after empyema, pleurodesis or industrial exposure to asbestos. • Well-defined dense calcified pleural plaques are typical of asbestos exposure. • With a pleural effusion, the lung 'floats' in a dependent pool of radiodense fluid, which is displaced peripherally up the sides of the

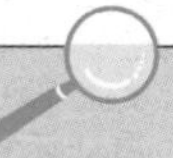

19.1 COMMON CHEST X-RAY APPEARANCES AND UNDERLYING CAUSES
Increased opacity
• Consolidation: infection, infarction, inflammation, rarely bronchoalveolar cell carcinoma • Lobar collapse: mucus plugging, tumour, compression by lymph nodes • Solitary nodule: bronchial carcinoma, abscess, single metastasis, pneumonia, tuberculoma • Multiple nodules: miliary TB, dust inhalation, malignancy, varicella pneumonia, rheumatoid • Ring shadows, tramlines and tubular shadows: bronchiectasis • Cavitating shadows: tumour, abscess, infarct, pneumonia, Wegener's granulomatosis • Reticular (intersecting lines), nodular and reticulonodular shadows: diffuse parenchymal lung disease, infection • Pleural abnormalities: fluid, tumours, calcified plaques due to asbestos
Increased translucency
• Bullae, severe emphysema • Pneumothorax • Oligaemia (congenital or pulmonary embolism)
Hilar abnormalities
• Unilateral hilar enlargement: TB, bronchial carcinoma, lymphoma • Bilateral hilar enlargement: sarcoid, lymphoma, TB, silicosis
Other abnormalities
• Hiatus hernia • Surgical emphysema

lung. • Complete pneumothorax causes the lung to shrink to the size of a fist. • In partial pneumothorax a subtle lung edge is separated from the chest wall by a radiolucent region devoid of lung markings.

DIAPHRAGM

The hemidiaphragms should have well-defined edges, and the costophrenic and cardiophrenic angles should be sharp. The right hemidiaphragm is usually higher due to the liver below. Pneumonia consolidating the lower lobes where they abut the pleura leads to blurring or loss of the diaphragmatic shadow.

SOFT TISSUES AND BONES

Assess the soft tissues, including breast shadows. Look for surgical emphysema and free air under the diaphragm. Examine each rib, looking for

19.2 PATTERNS OF RESPIRATORY FUNCTION ABNORMALITIES IN DISEASE

	Asthma	Chronic bronchitis	Emphysema	Pulmonary fibrosis
FEV_1	↓↓	↓↓	↓↓	↓
VC	↓	↓	↓	↓↓
FEV_1/VC	↓	↓	↓	→/↑
TL_{CO}	→	→	↓↓	↓↓
K_{CO}	→	→	↓	→/↓
TLC	→/↑	↑	↑↑	↓
RV	→/↑	↑	↑↑	↓

FEV_1 = forced expiratory volume in 1 sec; VC = vital capacity (relaxed); TL_{co} = gas transfer factor for carbon monoxide; K_{co} = gas transfer per unit lung volume; TLC = total lung capacity; RV = residual volume.

fractures or metastatic lesions, then check the clavicles and scapulae. Although the thoracic vertebrae and shoulder joints are not optimally seen on CXR, they should be assessed for collapse and fractures, respectively.

REVIEW AREAS

Finally, recheck areas in which abnormalities are commonly missed:

• Lung apices. • Subdiaphragmatic air. • Behind the cardiac shadow. • Behind hemidiaphragms. Possible opacitices behind the heart or diaphragm may be confirmed using a lateral chest X-ray.

RESPIRATORY FUNCTION TESTS

Respiratory function tests are used to aid diagnosis, assess functional impairment and monitor treatment or progression of disease. Airway narrowing, lung volume and gas exchange capacity are quantified and compared with normal values adjusted for age, gender, height and ethnicity. Common respiratory function abnormalities are summarised in Box 19.2.

PEAK EXPIRATORY FLOW

Airway narrowing is assessed by forced expiration into a peak flow meter or a spirometer. Peak flow meters are cheap and convenient for home monitoring (e.g. in asthma), but values are efford dependent.

SPIROMETRY

The forced expiratory volume in 1 sec (FEV_1) and vital capacity (VC) are obtained from maximal forced and relaxed expirations into a spirometer.

Airflow obstruction (asthma, COPD): FEV_1 is disproportionately reduced, resulting in FEV_1/VC ratios <70%. Spirometry should be repeated following inhaled short-acting β_2-adrenoceptor agonists (e.g. salbutamol); an increase in FEV_1 or VC of at least 200 ml and 12% of baseline is significant; reversibility of FEV_1 by >400 ml is suggestive of asthma.

Restriction: FEV_1 and VC are reduced in proportion, resulting in FEV_1/VC ratios of ≥70%. Causes of a restrictive defect include lung fibrosis, respiratory muscle weakness, thoracic cage deformity and obesity.

FLOW-VOLUME LOOPS

In addition to obstructive and restrictive patterns, flow-volume loops recorded during maximum expiratory and inspiratory efforts can distinguish large airway narrowing (e.g. tracheal stenosis or compression) from small airway narrowing, as each produces specific patterns of flow limitation.

LUNG VOLUMES

These can be measured by dilution of an inhaled inert gas (usually helium) or by determining the pressure/volume relationship of the thorax by body plethysmography. Obstructive lung disease is usually accompanied by hyperinflation, while fibrosis reduces lung volume.

TRANSFER FACTOR

To measure the capacity of the lungs to exchange gas, patients inhale 0.3% carbon monoxide, which is taken up by haemoglobin in pulmonary capillaries. The rate of CO disappearance into the circulation is calculated from a sample of expirate, and expressed as the TL_{CO} or carbon monoxide transfer factor. Transfer factor expressed per unit lung volume is termed K_{CO} and is typically reduced in emphysema.

INFLAMMATORY MARKERS

The changes associated with inflammation are reflected in many laboratory investigations (e.g. leucocytosis, increased platelets, normocytic normochromic anaemia). The C-reactive protein is the most widely used measure of acute inflammation, but fibrinogen, ferritin and complement may also be increased as part of the acute phase response, while albumin levels are reduced.

C-REACTIVE PROTEIN (CRP)

CRP is an acute phase reactant which opsonises invading pathogens. Levels of CRP increase within 6 hrs of an inflammatory stimulus. The short plasma half-life of CRP (19 hrs) means it can be used to monitor disease activity. Some diseases (e.g. SLE, systemic sclerosis, ulcerative colitis and leukaemia) cause only minor elevations of CRP despite the presence of inflam-

19.3 COMMON CONDITIONS ASSOCIATED WITH ABNORMAL CRP AND/OR ESR

Condition	Consequence	Effect on CRP (mg/l)[1]	Effect on ESR[2]
Acute infection	Stimulation of acute phase response	↑ (50–150; if severe, >300)	↑
Necrotising bacterial infection	Profound acute inflammation	↑↑↑ (may be >300)	↑
Chronic bacterial/fungal infection, e.g. abscess, endocarditis, TB	Stimulation of acute and chronic inflammatory response	↑ (range 50–150)	↑↑↑
Acute inflammatory diseases, e.g. Crohn's, vasculitides, polymyalgia rheumatica	Stimulation of acute phase response	↑ (range 50–150)	↑
SLE, Sjögren's syndrome	Chronic inflammatory response	Normal (paradoxically)	↑
Myeloma	Increase in Ig without inflammation	Normal	↑
Pregnancy, old age, renal failure	Increased fibrinogen	Normal	Moderately ↑
Macrocytic anaemia	Increased red cell viscosity	Normal	Moderately ↑

[1] Normal range <10 mg/l.
[2] Normal range: adult males <10 mm/hr, adult females <20 mm/hr.

mation. Intercurrent infection, however, does provoke a significant CRP response in these conditions.

ERYTHROCYTE SEDIMENTATION RATE (ESR)

The rate of fall of erythrocytes through plasma (ESR) is an indirect measure of the acute phase response. Normal erythrocytes repel each other because of their negative charge. Plasma proteins are positively charged, and raised levels overcome the repulsion between erythrocytes, causing them to stack up in rouleaux and increasing sedimentation rate.

• The most common cause of an increased ESR (and CRP) is an increase in acute phase proteins. Increased monoclonal or polyclonal immunoglobulin levels also increase the ESR. • Changes in erythrocyte size, morphology and density influence sedimentation; therefore an abnormally low ESR occurs in spherocytosis, sickle cell anaemia, microcytic anaemia and with low plasma protein levels.

CRP versus ESR

CRP is a simpler and more sensitive early indicator of the acute phase response and is used increasingly in preference to the ESR. If both are used, any discrepancy should be resolved by assessing the individual determinants of the ESR (full blood count/film, serum immunoglobulins and protein electrophoresis). Common conditions associated with raised CRP or ESR are shown in Box 19.3.

Unexplained raised ESR

Although the ESR should not be used to screen asymptomatic patients, an unexplained raised ESR is a common problem. Comprehensive history and examination are crucial. Extreme elevations in the ESR (>100 mm/hr) rarely occur in the absence of significant disease.

Investigations: The following are useful:

• CRP, immunoglobulins and urine electrophoresis will help determine whether the increased ESR is due to an acute inflammatory process. • FBC may show a normocytic, normochromic anaemia which occurs in many chronic diseases. • Neutrophilia suggests infection or acute inflammation. • Atypical lymphocytes may occur in some chronic infections (e.g. CMV, EBV). • Abnormal LFTs suggest either a local infective process (hepatitis, hepatic abscess or biliary sepsis) or systemic disease including malignancy. • Blood and urine cultures should be taken.

Imaging: Must be guided by clinical assessment:

• CXR and abdominal CT (occult infection, malignancy). • Abdominal/pelvic USS (hepatic lesions, intra-abdominal abscesses). • MRI (soft tissue or bone/joint infections). • Echocardiography (suspected bacterial endocarditis). • White cell scan (occasionally useful in identification of site of infection). • Isotope scan (malignancy or focal bone infection).

20 Objective structured clinical examination (OSCE)

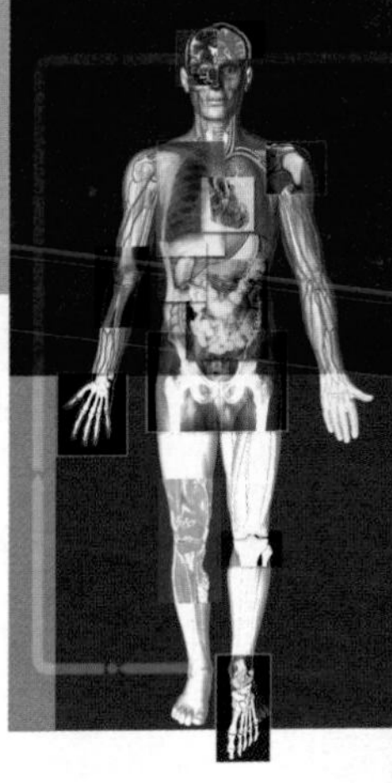

This mode of assessment is frequently used in exams to test clinical skills, including history-taking, examination, explanation and advice, and prescribing. It usually involves a 5–10 min 'station' with a single examiner. The aim is to create a standardised test that is the same for all candidates. For each OSCE station, marks are allocated to each component of the assessment that is considered important. Although this may lead to a 'tick-box' mentality, the key to performing well is to have a clear and systematic approach to each case. Chronic conditions with clear physical signs dominate this environment, as examiners need to be certain of what students should find. Some typical examples are provided to illustrate the process, although clearly a wide range of additional topics may appear. The mark schemes will vary depending on the level of the exam, with greater emphasis on correct diagnosis in addition to competent technique in more senior assessments.

A. CARDIOVASCULAR EXAMINATION

CASE 1: AORTIC STENOSIS

Instruction: This 65-yr-old woman has been admitted, complaining of chest tightness and faintness on exertion. Examine her cardiovascular system.

Key positive findings

- *Pulse:* sinus rhythm, slow rising major pulse (carotid), narrow pulse pressure on BP measurement.

- *JVP:* not elevated until late stage of disease when heart failure develops.
- *Apex beat:* not displaced (dilatation, not concentric hypertrophy, displaces apex) but has sustained quality.
- *Heart sounds:* S1 normal; S2 normal or quiet, and often a single sound; S4 may occur.
- *Murmur:* harsh ejection systolic murmur separated from both S1 and S2, loudest over aortic area and left sternal edge. Usually radiates to both carotid arteries.

Example mark scheme (10 marks)

1.	Introduces self to patient, explains what he/she is about to do	1 mark
2.	Assesses pulse and BP	1/2 mark
3.	Comments on narrow pulse pressure/slow rising pulse	1 mark
4.	Assesses JVP	1 mark
5.	Determines position of apex beat	1/2 mark
6.	Accurately comments on character of apex beat	1/2 mark
7.	Auscultates in relevant areas of precordium and neck	1 mark
8.	Comments on S1 and S2; notes soft S2	1 mark
9.	Identifies ejection systolic murmur, where it is loudest and its radiation	1 mark
10.	Sits patient forward to listen for aortic regurgitation	1/2 mark
11.	Gives most likely diagnosis as aortic stenosis	1 mark
12.	Suggests echocardiogram and ECG to assess	1 mark

Additional questions which could be included

1. What are markers of severity in aortic stenosis?
   a. *Clinical symptoms:* angina and syncope. Breathlessness may occur but cardiac failure is a late and poor prognostic sign.
   b. *Examination:* slow rising pulse, abnormal apex beat and absence of second heart sound. Loudness of murmur misleading—murmur often quiet in severe stenosis.
   c. *Investigations:* ECG showing evidence of left ventricular hypertrophy (LVH). Echocardiogram showing concentric LVH. Gradient estimated by Doppler from aortic jet velocity; gradient >40 mmHg considered severe.
2. How would you explain to the patient that he/she has aortic stenosis?
3. How would you explain to the patient what further investigations are required?

CASE 2: MITRAL REGURGITATION

This is a common murmur that is often secondary to other cardiovascular disease: in particular, rheumatic heart disease, ischaemic heart disease and dilated cardiomyopathy. Other causes include infective endocarditis and connective tissue diseases.

Instruction: The GP has noted that this 72-yr-old man has a murmur. Can you examine his cardiovascular system and determine the nature of the murmur?

Key positive findings

- *Pulse:* often irregular due to atrial fibrillation, pulse pressure usually normal.
- *JVP:* may be elevated.
- *Apex beat:* displaced with a thrusting quality.
- *Heart sounds:* S1 soft; S2 overlapped by murmur; S3 may be present.
- *Murmur:* commences immediately after a soft S1, lasts throughout systole and may obscure S2. Murmur is loudest at apex and radiates into axilla.
- *Other signs of cardiac failure:* may be present and include bi-basal inspiratory crackles and peripheral oedema.
- *Mitral valve prolapse:* has mid-systolic click followed by murmur. Associated with connective tissue diseases, including Marfan's and Ehlers–Danlos syndrome.

Example mark scheme (10 marks)

1. Introduces self to patient, explains what he/she is about to do — 1 mark
2. Determines presence of irregular pulse/atrial fibrillation — 1 mark
3. Assesses that JVP is elevated — 1 mark
4. Determines position and character of apex beat — 1 mark
5. Comments on S1 and S2; notes soft/absent S1 — 1 mark
6. Identifies systolic murmur, where it is loudest and its radiation — 1 mark
7. Gives most likely diagnosis as mitral regurgitation — 2 marks
8. Able to give two possible causes (e.g. LV dilatation in ischaemic heart disease, rheumatic valvular disease) — 1 mark
9. Suggests echo/Doppler as most valuable investigation — 1 mark

N.B.: Compared to case 1, this mark scheme gives more points for correctly identifying abnormalities rather than correct procedure.

B. RESPIRATORY EXAMINATION

CASE 1: IDIOPATHIC PULMONARY FIBROSIS

Instruction: This 56-yr-old man has presented with a 3-mth history of worsening breathlessness on exertion and a non-productive cough. Examine his respiratory system to identify a possible cause. At the end of your examination, please tell me your diagnosis and what further tests you would like to carry out.

Key positive findings

- *Finger clubbing.*
- *Central cyanosis.*
- *Elevated respiratory rate*: at rest.
- *Signs of pulmonary hypertension:* may be present, with elevated JVP and v-wave of tricuspid regurgitation.
- *Chest expansion:* may be reduced but symmetrical.
- *Vesicular breath sounds:* with fine inspiratory crackles.

Example mark scheme (12 marks)

1.	Appropriate introduction and explanation	1 mark
2.	Examines for presence of flapping tremor	½ mark
3.	Identifies finger clubbing	1 mark
4.	Identifies central cyanosis	½ mark
5.	Examines trachea to check for deviation and cricosternal distance	1 mark
6.	Assesses for cervical lymphadenopathy	½ mark
7.	Inspects for respiratory rate and chest wall movement	½ mark
8.	Assesses chest expansion	½ mark
9.	Percusses chest wall	1 mark
10.	Auscultates all areas of chest wall	½ mark
11.	Identifies vesicular breath sounds with fine inspiratory crackles	1 mark
12.	Gives most likely diagnosis as idiopathic pulmonary fibrosis	2 marks
13.	Additional investigations and likely results a. ABGs—type 1 respiratory failure b. CXR—small lungs, bi-basal reticular interstitial shadowing c. Pulmonary function tests—restrictive defect d. High-resolution CT—honeycomb basal fibrosis	2 marks

N.B.: Complete respiratory examination within 10 mins is challenging. Often examiners will direct candidates to the front or back of the chest. Follow a strict routine (inspection/palpation/percussion/auscultation) to avoid missing signs.

CASE 2: PLEURAL EFFUSION

This is a common clinical problem with a wide range of causes. The main distinction is between a transudate (e.g. cardiac failure, nephrotic syndrome, liver disease) and an exudate (e.g. infection, malignancy, pulmonary embolus and autoimmune disease). Distinguishing these conditions may not be obvious clinically.

Instruction: This 65-yr-old man presented with a 1-mth history of cough, breathlessness and left-sided chest pain. Can you examine his chest and tell me your findings?

Key positive findings

- *Peripheral clues:* may be provided by presence of finger clubbing (malignancy), elevated JVP (states of fluid overload) or lymphadenopathy (malignancy).
- *Trachea:* usually central (rarely, deviated away from side of effusion if this is very large).
- *Expansion:* reduced on side of effusion (can be subtle).
- *Percussion note:* stony dull on side of effusion (usually obvious).
- *Breath sounds:* reduced or absent over effusion. Often there is area of bronchial breathing ± crackles at upper edge of effusion.

Example mark scheme (10 marks)

1. Appropriate introduction and explanation	1 mark
2. Checks for finger clubbing	$^1/_2$ mark
3. Inspects respiratory rate and chest wall movement	1 mark
4. Checks trachea central	$^1/_2$ mark
5. Assesses chest expansion	$^1/_2$ mark
6. Identifies reduced expansion of left lung	$^1/_2$ mark
7. Correctly percusses chest wall	$^1/_2$ mark
8. Identifies dull percussion note at left base	1 mark
9. Auscultates all areas of chest wall	$^1/_2$ mark
10. Identifies reduced breath sounds at left base	1 mark
11. Correctly diagnoses left pleural effusion	2 marks
12. Differential diagnosis	1 mark

   a. Transudate: fluid overload
   b. Exudate:
      i. Infection
      ii. Malignancy
      iii. Pulmonary embolus

Additional questions which could be included

1. What further investigations would you carry out?
   a. CXR
   b. CT of chest
   c. Diagnostic pleural tap, with measurement of protein, LDH and cellular content
2. How can you distinguish a transudate from an exudate?
   a. *Clinical context:* in a patient with obvious fluid overload pleural effusions are likely to be transudates. It is usual to treat fluid overload and observe progress.
   b. *Appearance:* presence of pus suggests infection whilst blood suggests malignancy or pulmonary embolus/infarction.
   c. *Pleural fluid protein:* transudate protein is <30 g/l, whilst exudate is >30 g/l. This distinction is not absolute.
   d. *Light's criteria:* the presence of one of the following diagnoses an exudate:

   i. Pleural fluid/serum protein ratio >0.5
   ii. Pleural fluid/serum LDH ratio >0.6
   iii. Pleural fluid LDH >$^2/_3$ the upper laboratory limit for serum LDH

C. GASTROINTESTINAL EXAMINATION

CASE 1: CHRONIC LIVER DISEASE

Instruction: This 40-yr-old man describes increasing swelling of his abdomen over the last few months. Please examine his GI system and formulate a differential diagnosis. Please tell me what tests you would like to perform.

Key positive findings

- *Stigmata of chronic liver disease in the hands:* clubbing, leuconychia, palmar erythema, asterixis, Dupuytren's contracture.
- *Other signs of chronic liver disease:* spider naevi, bruising, jaundice, gynaecomastia, lymphadenopathy, scratch marks, signs of anaemia, hair loss.
- *Hepatomegaly:* non-tender and firm (cirrhosis; in later stages liver may shrink); firm, smooth and tender (cardiac failure); nodular and hard (malignancy).
- *Splenomegaly, ascites, peripheral oedema.*

Example mark scheme (12 marks)

1. Appropriate introduction and asks if abdomen is tender — 1 mark
2. Examines hands, including checking for flapping tremor — 1 mark
3. Looks at sclerae for jaundice — $^1/_2$ mark
4. Palpates for lymph nodes (at least supraclavicular) — 1 mark
5. Examines for spider naevi — $^1/_2$ mark
6. Examines for gynaecomastia — $^1/_2$ mark
7. Elicits hepatomegaly and liver span — 1 mark
8. Elicits splenomegaly — 1 mark
9. Examines kidneys using correct bi-manual technique — 1 mark
10. Checks for shifting dullness — 1 mark
11. Auscultates abdomen for bruits and bowel sounds — $^1/_2$ mark
12. Differential diagnosis — 1 mark
    a. Alcohol excess
    b. Hepatitis B
    c. Malignancy
13. Investigations — 2 marks
    a. FBC (checking Hb and platelets)
    b. LFTs
    c. Liver USS
    d. Ascitic fluid analysis

CASE 2: POLYCYSTIC KIDNEY DISEASE

Autosomal dominant polycystic kidney disease (ADPKD) occurs in around 1 in 800 live births but has a variable presentation ranging from minor abnormalities on urinalysis (microscopic haematuria) to end-stage renal failure.

Instruction: This 44-yr-old woman has been referred by her GP with hypertension and an eGFR of 50 ml/min (normal >60 ml/min). Examine her abdomen to determine a possible cause. What additional investigations would you like to perform?

Key positive findings

- *Limited peripheral stigmata:* but check for presence of arteriovenous fistula if patient is already established on dialysis.
- *Distension:* may be present in loin.
- *Bilateral palpable flank/para-umbilical masses:* can be ballotted. Masses are usually resonant to percussion (unlike liver and spleen); hand can get between mass and costal margin. The correct technique is essential to feel the kidneys accurately.

Example mark scheme (12 marks)

1.	Appropriate introduction and asks if abdomen is tender	1 mark
2.	Checks patient's BP	$^1/_2$ mark
3.	Examines eyes for signs of anaemia	$^1/_2$ mark
4.	Inspects abdomen and comments on flank distension	1 mark
5.	Palpates abdomen lightly whilst observing patient's face	1 mark
6.	Appropriately examines for liver and spleen	1 mark
7.	Correct technique to feel for kidneys, including balloting	1 mark
8.	Checks for ascites	1 mark
9.	Listens for abdominal bruits	1 mark
10.	Comments on bilateral kidney enlargement	2 marks
11.	Gives most likely diagnosis as PKD	1 mark
12.	Additional investigations: USS of abdomen	1 mark

Additional questions which could be included

1. Family history:
   a. How would you explain to the patient the risk of passing this disease to her children, aged 10 and 8 yrs?
   Autosomal dominant condition, thus 50% risk of being passed on to children. There is no preceding family history in ~25% of cases.
   b. What screening can be offered?
   USS will diagnose condition. There is no point screening people under age of 18 yrs. Presence of two cysts under age of 30 is diagnostic. Screening can be undertaken after appropriate counselling. Genetic testing not routinely available.
2. What are the complications of this disease?
   a. Hypertension
   b. Haematuria

c. Episodes of loin pain from bleeding into cyst
d. Chronic kidney disease (CKD)
e. Kidney stones; patients are at increased risk, compared to other forms of CKD
f. Subarachnoid haemorrhage; cerebral aneurysms are recognised associations.

D. RHEUMATOID HANDS (see Fig. 15.5)

This is a common OSCE station at all levels of examination. Place the patient's hands palms down on a pillow, with the patient sitting in a chair or upright in bed. The basic outline of the examination is 'look, feel, move', followed by an assessment of function. It is important to examine both palmar and dorsal aspects of the hands, taking care to avoid causing discomfort. Ensure that you look for symmetry/asymmetry of pathological changes.

Instruction: Please examine this lady's hands.

Key positive findings

- *Skin changes:* palmar erythema, wasting of small muscles of hand, surgical scars (e.g. tendon release), atrophic skin due to previous steroid use.
- *Rheumatoid nodules:* briefly scan for these on dorsal surface of elbow.
- *Psoriatic skin and nail changes:* nail changes include pitting, onycholysis, ridging and hyperkeratosis. Psoriatic arthropathy is the major differential.
- *Deformities:* subluxation and ulnar deviation at MCP joints, swan-necking (hyperextension of PIP joints, fixed flexion of DIP joints), Boutonnière deformity (hyperextension of DIP joints, fixed flexion of PIP joints), Z deformity of thumb (hyperextension of IP joint, fixed flexion and subluxation of MCP joint), dorsal subluxation of ulna at carpal joint, ulnar deviation of wrist.

Example mark scheme (12 marks)

1. Appropriate introduction and asks if hands are sore	1 mark
2. Notes presence of swan-necking and Boutonnière changes	1 mark
3. Looks for nail and skin changes	2 marks
4. Comments on activity of disease (warmth, redness, tenderness)	1 mark
5. Palpates individual sets of joints and compares two sides	1 mark
6. Looks for evidence of rheumatoid nodules	1 mark
7. Assesses wrist extension (prayer sign) and flexion (inverted prayer sign)	1 mark
8. Assesses hand function appropriately (e.g. doing up/undoing buttons, combing hair, writing)	2 marks

9. Comments on other systems to examine (lungs for fibrosis, heart for murmurs) — 1 mark
10. Gives appropriate differential diagnosis — 1 mark

Additional questions which could be included

1. Which joints are commonly affected in rheumatoid arthritis?
   a. Wrists
   b. PIP and MCP joints of hands
   c. Metatarsophalangeal joints
   d. Knees
2. What is the significance of the presence of rheumatoid nodules?
   These suggest positivity for rheumatoid factor and more aggressive arthritis.
3. What are the poor prognostic factors in rheumatoid arthritis?
   a. Systemic features (weight loss, extra-articular manifestations)
   b. Insidious onset
   c. Rheumatoid nodules
   d. Presence of the rheumatoid factor
   e. Persistent disease activity >12 mths
   f. Early bone erosions

E. NEUROLOGICAL EXAMINATION

Neurological short cases are often the most feared. The key is to spend as much time practising for these as for other stations and to have a polished and confident examination routine (as for all OSCE stations), which then gives you time to consider your findings. Outlined below are standard examination techniques followed by some common cases.

EXAMINATION OF THE EYES

Instruction: Examine this man's eyes.

Example mark scheme (10 marks)

1. Appropriate introduction and explanation — ½ mark
2. Observes eyes from front/side/above — 1 mark
3. Tests visual acuity in both eyes (if patient wears glasses. these should be worn) — 1 mark
4. Assesses eye movements (asks patient to report any double vision) — 1 mark
5. Observes for nystagmus — 1 mark
6. Checks for visual inattention — ½ mark
7. Tests visual fields in both eyes — 1 mark
8. Examines pupils: reactions to light and accommodation — 1 mark
9. Checks for red reflex — 1 mark
10. Examines fundi appropriately — 2 marks

CASE 1: HORNER'S SYNDROME

This results from damage to the sympathetic nerves supplying the eyes and face, and gives rise to ipsilateral signs. Malignant lymph nodes at the root of the neck are a common cause.

Instruction: Examine this man's eyes and face.

Key positive findings

- *Ptosis and meiosis (small constricted pupil):* should be apparent.
- *Associated features of ipsilateral enophthalmos and loss of forehead sweating:* may be present
- *Reactions to light and accommodation:* should be present and normal.
- *Iris:* in congenital cases, remains blue/grey.

Additional examination

1. Inspect the neck for scars of cervical sympathectomy or thyroidectomy.
2. Palpate for cervical ribs and cervical lymphadenopathy.
3. Examine for weakness of the small muscles of the hand (T1) and for loss of sensation over the T1 dermatome (T1 involvement commonly due to Pancoast's syndrome).
4. Test for loss of pain and temperature sensation in the arm/face, loss of arm reflexes, bulbar palsy and nystagmus (syringomyelia/syringobulbia).
5. Percuss the supraclavicular area, looking for the dullness of Pancoast's tumour.

Additional questions which could be included

1. How do you differentiate a ptosis that is due to Horner's syndrome from one due to a 3rd nerve palsy?
   a. The pupil is constricted in Horner's syndrome but dilated in a 3rd nerve palsy.
   b. Movement of the eye by the extra ocular muscles is affected in a 3rd nerve palsy but not in Horner's syndrome.
   c. The light reflex is intact in Horner's syndrome.
   d. Horner's syndrome causes partial ptosis; 3rd nerve palsy causes complete ptosis.

CASE 2: VISUAL FIELD DEFECTS (see Fig. 16.6)

Instruction: Examine this man's eyes.

- A number of visual field defects may appear in short cases. These include homonymous hemianopia (e.g. due to stroke), bitemporal hemianopia (e.g. chiasmal compression due to a pituitary tumour), central scotoma (e.g. retrobulbar neuritis) and concentric constriction (e.g. retinitis pigmentosa).
- Homonymous hemianopia is the most common of these and implies a lesion posterior to the optic chiasm (in the optic tract, radiation or occipital cortex).

- A lesion in the occipital cortex (e.g. due to a posterior cerebral artery occlusion) causes a hemianopia which may spare the macula.
- Lesions in the optic tract may lead to an incongruous hemianopia.
- Lesions of the optic radiation may produce an upper quadrantic hemianopia with a temporal lobe lesion, or a lower quadrantic hemianopia with a parietal lobe lesion.

EXAMINATION OF SPEECH

CASE 3: EXPRESSIVE/RECEPTIVE DYSPHASIA

Expressive and/or receptive dysphasias most commonly occur as a result of a stroke. Simple bedside testing enables these to be identified and distinguished from dysarthria. Dysphasia is usually due to a lesion in the left fronto-parietal area, and may be associated with right upper motor neuron facial palsy and weakness of the right arm.

Instructions: This 70-yr-old male patient has been admitted with sudden onset of difficulty with speaking. Could you assess his speech?

Key positive findings

- *Expressive dysphasia:* patients have difficulty naming objects. The key is gradually to increase level of difficulty in your testing. Start with asking patients to identify watch, then to name hands, strap and buckle. Similar approach can be taken with pen, shirt or glasses.
- *Receptive dysphasia:* patients have difficulty following instructions. Best identified by asking patients to follow increasingly complex set of instructions. Start by asking them to lift right arm; then to lift right arm and turn it palm up; finally, to lift right arm, turn palm up and touch right ear.
- *Dysarthria:* patients have slurred speech. Ask them to repeat complex phrases, such as 'British constitution', 'Manchester constabulary' or 'West Register Street'. Dysarthria may occur with cerebellar, brain-stem or upper motor neuron lesions.

Example mark scheme (10 marks)

1. Introduces self to patient, explains what he/she is about to do	1 mark
2. Asks patient simple introductory questions (could include name, date of birth, address, what problems have provoked visit, or how speech has been affected)	2 marks
3. Assesses expressive dysphasia by naming objects (or similar)	2 marks
4. Assesses receptive dysphasia by asking patient to follow instructions (or similar)	2 marks
5. Assesses dysarthria	1 mark
6. Correctly diagnoses nature of speech defect	2 marks

CASE 4: PERIPHERAL NEUROPATHY

The key is to identify whether this is predominantly sensory, motor or mixed. There is a long list of causes, diabetes mellitus being the most common.

Instruction: This 48-yr-old man has noticed a painful burning sensation in both feet. Examine the nervous system of his lower limbs.

Key positive findings

- *Inspection:* signs of chronic peripheral neuropathy, such as pes cavus, high-arched feet and claw toes. Signs of muscle-wasting, giving classic 'inverted champagne bottle' appearance to legs. Look for signs of injury, including ulcers and infection. Long-standing disease may lead to Charcot joints at ankle.
- *Tone:* normal.
- *Power:* will predominantly affect distal muscles (dorsiflexion, plantar flexion) if motor neuropathy present with preserved proximal muscles.
- *Sensation:* exams will vary in what they leave at your disposal but test all modalities available. Should include a minimum of light touch (cotton wool), pin-prick, joint position sense and vibration sense (tuning fork). For light touch and pin-prick, assess each dermatome, as well as determining if stocking pattern of numbness present.
- *Reflexes:* ankle jerk often absent; knee jerk absent in severe cases.
- *Gait:* patient may have obvious foot drop. Romberg's sign may be positive.
- *Clues to cause:* evidence of diabetes mellitus (insulin injection sites, blood glucose testing on fingers), chronic liver disease or chronic renal failure (arteriovenous fistula).

Example mark scheme (12 marks)

1. Introduces self to patient, explains what he/she is about to do — 1 mark
2. Inspection: identifies claw toes and ulcer — 1 mark
3. Checks tone and clonus — 1 mark
4. Assesses all motor groups in lower limb — 1 mark
5. Checks for weakness of dorsiflexion in both feet — 1 mark
6. Assesses all modalities of sensation in appropriate areas — 1 mark
7. Identifies loss of sensation in both feet — 1 mark
8. Delineates extent of numbness in both feet — 1 mark
9. Identifies loss of ankle jerk reflexes in both feet — 1 mark
10. Assesses abnormal gait and Romberg's test — 1 mark
11. Concludes that patient has sensorimotor peripheral neuropathy — 2 marks

Additional questions which could be included

1. What are the most likely causes?
   a. Diabetes
   b. Alcohol

c. Chronic renal failure
d. Paraneoplastic
e. Vasculitis (usually mononeuritis multiplex)
f. Critical illness: may occur post-ICU
g. Multiple myeloma (usually motor neuropathy)
h. Charcot–Marie–Tooth disease (predominantly motor neuropathy)
i. B_{12} deficiency

Additional tests can be determined from this list.

2. How would you treat his painful peripheral neuropathy?
   a. Gabapentin (first-line)
   b. Amitriptyline
   c. Carbamazepine
   d. Ensure suitable podiatry care

Index